Baillière's
DICTIONARY

T0200384

Baillière's
DICTIONARY
for Nurses and Health Care Workers

27th Edition

Edited by

Jayne Taylor PhD MBA BSc(Hons)
DipN(Lond) RN HV RNT
Head of Organisational Development, West
Hertfordshire Hospitals NHS Trust Watford,
UK

ELSEVIER

Edinburgh   London   New York   Oxford
Philadelphia   St Louis   Sydney   2019

Elsevier

© 2019, Elsevier Limited. All rights reserved.

First published in 1912
© Elsevier Ltd, 2002
25th edition 2009 (main and international)
26th edition 2014 (main and international)
27th edition 2019 (main and international)

ISBN: 9780702072796
ISBN: 9780702072789

Printed in Poland

Last digit is the print number: 9 8 7 6 5 4 3

Content Strategist: Alison Taylor
Senior Content Development Specialist: Helen Leng
Content Coordinator: Deanna Sorenson
Project Manager: Andrew Riley
Design: Bridget Hoette
Illustration Manager: Paula Catalano
Marketing Manager: Samantha Page

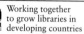

Working together
to grow libraries in
developing countries

www.elsevier.com • www.bookaid.org

Contents

Preface

I am incredibly honoured and privileged that Barbara Weller, who has updated the dictionary through several editions over a number of years, has entrusted the updating of the 27th edition of the dictionary to me. It is not a vast tome in terms of its size but it is packed with information – the extent of which I had not fully appreciated. A dictionary is something that you delve into rather than read from cover to cover. When I took on the task I had very little idea about the amount of work it would involve but as the months have gone by and letter by letter the work has been completed I have come to fully appreciate the vast scope of what we, as nurses, do in our everyday work. We work with people who have mild or serious, common or rare conditions; we work with people of every age; we work in many different settings and fields of nursing; we work with people who have lived and come from all over of the world; and we work with other health professionals, with colleagues from local authorities, the voluntary sector and most of all we work with patients, service users, carers and their families to deliver the very best care for every patient every day.

While talking with our patients/service users/carers/families and others for whom we are providing care and support, and with colleagues, we use words. These words must be appropriate to the context of the person with whom we are communicating, without the use of jargon, and as far as possible avoiding the use of medical terminology. This will help to ensure that they not only receive the message, but that they also understand the content and the context. This we do by sharing the right words with compassion and sensitivity. I hope this little dictionary will help you to better achieve great communication.

I am grateful to Barbara for giving me this opportunity – Barbara was the person who got me started in writing back in the late 1980s and it has been something that I have done continuously with great enjoyment ever since. As ever, behind this new edition of the dictionary has been a team of talented contributors. I am most grateful to them for their professional expertise and contributions. I would also like to thank Anna Wood, Renton L'Heureux and Victoria Taylor-Simpson for their help on particularly tricky entries. The support and enthusiasm of the Elsevier publishing team and particularly Helen Leng and Alison Taylor has made my job run smoothly and has helped me to meet the deadline set for publication. Finally, I should like to acknowledge the support of my partner Dudley Walton who has a definite love/hate relationship with 'the dictionary' but is, I know, proud of me now that it is finished.

Jayne Taylor

List of Contributors

The editor(s) would like to acknowledge and offer grateful thanks for the input of all previous editions' contributors, without whom this new edition would not have been possible.

Nicola Bramley BSc(Hons) DipDiet RD
Diabetes Specialist Dietician, Imperial College Healthcare NHS Trust, London, UK

Susan Clements BSc TechIOSH VMSM
Safety Practitioner and Trainer, Clements Training, Cambridge, UK

Sandra Ellis PhD RD
Cardiovascular Prevention and Rehabilitation Dietician, Imperial College Healthcare NHS Trust, London, UK

Jonathan Green LLB(Hons)
Solicitor and Head of In-house Fitness to Practise, General Dental Council, London, UK

Caroline King BSc SRD
Specialist Neonatal and Paediatric Dietician, Imperial College Healthcare NHS Trust, London, UK

Lucy Oughton DipHE(Health and Social Care) RN
Resuscitation Officer, Cambridge University Hospitals NHS Trust, Cambridge, UK

Gerii Reilly
Critical Care Dietician, Imperial College Healthcare NHS Trust, London, UK

Jayne Taylor PhD MBA BSc(Hons) DipN(Lond) RN HV RNT
Head of Organisational Development, West Hertfordshire Hospitals NHS Trust, Watford, UK

Tejal Vaghela BPharm PgDIP
Pharmacy Team Leader – Antimicrobials and AAU, West Hertfordshire Hospitals NHS Trust, Watford, UK,

Barbara F. Weller BA MSc RGN RSCN RNT

Independent Nurse Consultant; formerly Editor, Infant (Journal for Neonatal and Paediatric Healthcare Professionals) and Nursing Officer, Department of Health and Chief Nursing Adviser, British Red Cross Society, London, UK

Elizabeth Whittaker RGN ALS EPLS GIC

Instructor, Resuscitation Officer, Resuscitation Services, Cambridge University Hospitals NHS Trust, Cambridge, UK

Acknowledgements

The figures and tables below have been reproduced or adapted with permission from the following Elsevier publications:

Australian Nurses' Dictionary 6e 978-0-7295-4229-6
Jennie King, Rhonda Hawley

Mosby's Dictionary of Medicine, Nursing and Health Professions UK Edition 1E
978-0-7234-3504-4
Edited by Chris Brooker BSc MSc RGN SCM RNT

Dorland's Gray's Pocket Atlas of Anatomy 1E 978-0-443-06761-7
Richard L. Drake, A. Wayne Vogl, Adam W. M. Mitchell

Churchill Livingstone Medical Dictionary 16E 978-0-443-10412-1
Edited by Chris Brooker BSc MSc RGN SCM RNT

All other illustrations reused with permission from Ballière's Nurses' Dictionary for Nurses and Health Care Workers 1E (South Asia) 978-81-312-4456-2
Annu Kaushik

Style Guide

Subentries

The term being sought may be a main entry or a subentry under the main entry. In subentries, the main entry is represented by its initial letter if it is singular, and by the addition of an apostrophe and *s* if it is plural. Subentries are listed alphabetically under the main entry. For example:

> **abdomen**...
>> *Acute a*....
>> *Pendulous a*....
>> *Scaphoid (navicular) a*....

Cross-referencing

Throughout the dictionary, cross-references are given within the text as SMALL CAPITALS. For example:

> **fibrin** an insoluble protein that is essential to CLOTTING of blood, formed from fibrinogen by action of thrombin.

There are also situations where it is simply more convenient to define the word in a different location, to which the reader is then referred.

Translations

Where a translation of a foreign term occurs, it is indicated in *italic type* immediately after the abbreviation for the language (which is in square brackets). For example:

> **acus** [L.] *a needle*

Abbreviations Used in this Dictionary

b. born		L. Latin	
Fr. French		*pl.* plural	
Ger. German		*sing.* singular	

Drug Names

Where possible, only generic names are used; however, some proprietary drug names and names for preparations are included, with information (and sometimes cross-references) about the generic drug(s) involved. Inclusion of a drug in the dictionary does not imply endorsement.

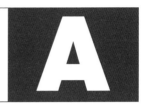

@ at.

A accommodation; anode (anodal); anterior; axial; symbol for *ampere* and *mass number.*

AAA ABDOMINAL AORTIC ANEURYSM.

abatement a decrease in the severity of a pain or a symptom.

abdomen the cavity between the diaphragm and the pelvis, lined by a serous membrane, the peritoneum, and containing the stomach, intestines, liver, gallbladder, spleen, pancreas, kidneys, suprarenal glands, ureters and bladder. For descriptive purposes, its area can be divided into nine regions (*see* Figure). *Acute a.* any abdominal condition urgently requiring treatment, usually surgical. *Pendulous a.* a condition in which the anterior part of the abdominal wall hangs down over the pubis. *Scaphoid (navicular) a.* a hollowing of the anterior wall so that it presents a concave rather than convex contour.

abdominal pertaining to the abdomen. *A. aorta* that part of the aorta below the diaphragm. *A. aortic aneurysm* a dilatation of the abdominal aorta. Men are most at risk and all men are invited for an AAA screening test at 65 years involving a simple ultrasound. Also known as TRIPLE A screening. *A. breathing* deep breathing; hyperpnoea. *A. examination* a systematic examination of the abdomen by inspection, palpation and auscultation carried out by midwives during pregnancy and after

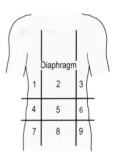

1. Right hypochondriac region
2. Epigastric region
3. Left hypochondriac region
4. Right lumbar region
5. Umbilical region
6. Left lumbar region
7. Right iliac fossa
8. Hypogastric region
9. Left iliac fossa

REGIONS OF THE ABDOMEN

delivery. The purpose is to determine the equality of uterine size with the calculated period of gestation and later in the pregnancy to determine the position of the fetus. Postnatally the examination is used to ascertain that the uterus is regaining its former non-pregnant size and position. *A. reflex* reflex contraction of abdominal wall muscles observed when skin is lightly stroked. *A. section* incision through the abdominal wall. *A. thrust* (formerly called the Heimlich manoeuvre) *see* Appendix 2.

abdominoperineal pertaining to the abdomen and the perineum. *A. excision* an operation performed through the abdomen and the perineum for the excision of the rectum or bladder. Often done as a synchronized operation by two surgeons, one working at each approach.

abdominoplasty also known as a tummy tuck, is a cosmetic surgery procedure to remove fat and excess loose skin to improve the shape of the abdominal area.

abduce to abduct or to draw away.

abducent leading away from the midline. *A. muscle* the external rectus muscle of the eye, which rotates it outward. *A. nerve* the cranial nerve that supplies this muscle.

abductor a muscle that draws a limb away from the midline of the body. The opposite of adductor.

aberrant taking an unusual course. Used of blood vessels and nerves.

aberration deviation from the normal. In optics, failure to focus rays of light. *Mental a.* mental disorder with a deviation from linear or normal thinking.

ability the power to perform an act, either mental or physical, with or without training. *A. test* a test that measures a person's level of performance or estimates future performance. Sometimes also known as an intelligence test, achievement test or aptitude test. *Innate a.* the ability with which a person is born.

ablation removal or destruction, by surgical or radiological means, of neoplasms or other body tissue.

abnormal varying from what is regular or usual.

ABO system *see* BLOOD GROUPS.

abort 1. to terminate a process or disease before it has run its normal course. 2. to remove or expel from the womb an embryo or fetus before it is capable of independent existence.

abortifacient an agent or drug that may induce abortion.

abortion 1. premature cessation of a normal process. 2. emptying of the pregnant uterus before the end of the 24th week or a miscarriage (the preferred term). 3. the product of such an abortion. *Complete a.* one in which the contents of the uterus are expelled intact. *Criminal a.* the termination of a pregnancy for reasons other than those permitted by law (i.e., danger to mental or physical health of mother or child or family) and without medical approval. *Incomplete a.* one in which some part of the fetus or placenta is retained in the uterus. *Induced a.* the intentional emptying of the uterus. *Inevitable a.* abortion where bleeding is profuse and accompanied by pains, the cervix is dilated and the contents of the uterus can be felt. *Missed a.* one where all signs of pregnancy disappear and later the uterus discharges a blood clot surrounding a shrivelled fetus, i.e., a carneous mole. *Septic a.* abortion associated with infection. *Therapeutic (legal) a.* one induced on medical advice because the continuance of the pregnancy would involve risk to the life of the pregnant woman, or injury to the physical or mental health of the pregnant woman or any existing children of her family, greater than if the pregnancy were terminated; or because there is a substantial risk that if the child were born it would suffer from such physical or mental abnormalities as to be seriously handicapped (1967 Abortion Act, as amended by the Human Fertilization and Embryology Act Amendments 1990 and 2008). *Threatened a.* the appearance of signs of premature expulsion of the fetus; bleeding is slight, the cervix is closed. *Tubal a.* the termination of a tubal pregnancy caused by rupture of the uterine tube.

abrasion a superficial injury, where the skin or mucous membrane is rubbed or torn, sometimes called a graze. *Corneal a.* this can occur when the surface of the cornea has been removed, e.g., by a scratch or other injury.

abreaction the reliving of a painful experience, with the release of repressed emotion.

abruptio placentae premature detachment of the placenta, causing maternal shock.

abscess a collection of pus in a cavity. Caused by the disintegration and replacement of tissue damaged by mechanical, chemical or bacterial injury. *Alveolar a.* an abscess in a tooth socket. *Brodie's a.* a bone abscess, usually on the head of the tibia. *Cold a.* the result of chronic tubercular infection and so called because there are few, if any, signs of inflammation. *Psoas a.* a cold abscess that has tracked down the psoas muscle from caries of the lumbar vertebrae. *Subphrenic a.* one situated under the diaphragm.

absorbent 1. able to take in, or suck up and incorporate. 2. a tissue structure involved in absorption. 3. a substance that absorbs or promotes absorption.

absorption 1. in physiology, the taking up by suction of fluids or other substances by the tissues of the body. 2. in psychology, great mental concentration on a single object or activity. 3. in radiology, uptake of radiation by body tissues.

abstinence a refraining from the use of or indulgence in food, stimulants or coitus. *A. syndrome* withdrawal symptoms.

abstract a brief, comprehensive summary of a research study or other academic report.

abuse misuse, maltreatment, or excessive use—may be physical, sexual, psychological or neglect. Can apply to any group of people, e.g., the vulnerable, children, women, people with learning disabilities or the elderly. May also apply to the misuse of power,

authority, drugs and other substances, e.g., solvents and equipment.

abusive head injury commonly called shaken baby syndrome resulting in traumatic brain injury in infants and young children.

acanthosis nigricans darkened, thickened patches of skin that develop around the groin, neck and axilla. Patches can sometimes be itchy and may indicate underlying disease.

Acarus a genus of small mites. *A. scabiei* (former term for *SARCOPTES SCABIEI*) the cause of scabies.

acataphasia loss of the ability to express connected thought, resulting from a cerebral lesion.

acceleration 1. An increase in the speed or velocity of an object or reaction. 2. An increase in the fetal heartbeat of at least 15 beats per minute over the baseline rate for at least 15 seconds.

access to health care records there are three pieces of legislation which govern access to patient health care records. Patients (or in the case of deceased patients, their representative) can apply for access to health care records, unless it is considered that serious physical or mental harm to the patient may result or where information would be disclosed relating to a third party who has not consented.

accessory supplementary. *A. nerve* the 11th cranial nerve. It is made up of two portions: the cranial and the spinal.

accident and emergency sometimes referred to as casualty, the emergency department or trauma medicine. A setting for dealing with problems which require immediate attention and where patients can be directed or referred by a general practitioner or the emergency services.

acclimatization the ability of the body to adapt physiologically to changes in the environment. Taking exercise in a hotter climate than the body is used to will lead to increased sweating with lower sodium levels in an attempt to cool the body but which may lead to dehydration. Climbing, for example, at a high altitude can produce altitude sickness with low oxygen levels in the blood, associated with increased cardiac output and respiratory effort. Athletes participating in sport events at international venues held in hot climates or at high altitudes will require training to adapt to the physiological adjustments that will affect the athletic performance.

accommodation adjustment. In ophthalmology, the term refers specifically to adjustment of the ciliary muscle, which controls the shape of the lens. *Negative a.* the ciliary muscle relaxes and the lens becomes less convex, giving long-distance vision. *Positive a.* the ciliary muscle contracts and the lens becomes more convex, giving near vision.

accountable liable to be held responsible for a course of action. A qualified nurse has a duty of care according to law; in nursing, being accountable refers to the responsibility the qualified nurse takes for prescribing and initiating nursing care. Nurses are accountable to their patients, their peers and their employing authority, according to the Code for Nurses and Midwives. Registered practitioners are accountable at all times for their actions, on or off duty and whether engaged in current practice or not. Accountability is also identified as one of the three foundations of public service. Everything done by those who work in the NHS must be able to stand the test of parliamentary scrutiny, public judgements on propriety and professional codes of conduct.

accreditation 1. to officially recognize someone as having particular status or being qualified to perform particular activity. 2. An acknowledgement of a person's responsibility or achievement of something . 3. The granting of approval to an institution that meet a satisfactory level of organizational achievement. *A. for Prior Experiential Learning (APEL)* credit gained for non-academic work (clinical or work experience) that can be used to give credit to academic course work and programmes of study in colleges and universities. *A. for Prior Learning* abbreviated APL or APCL (accreditation for prior certificated learning). A system used by academic institutions and other establishments to grant credit for previous academic achievements. Usually used to gain credit transfer between institutions leading to academic qualifications.

accretion growth. The accumulation of deposits, e.g., of salts to form a calculus in the bladder. In dentistry, the growth of tartar on the teeth.

acculturation the process by which a person absorbs the beliefs, values and customs of another culture, usually through direct contact, e.g., migrants resident in another country.

ACE inhibitors a group of drugs used in the treatment of hypertension. Their name, angiotensin converting enzyme inhibitors, explains part of their mode of action, although it is thought that some of their other actions may also be important in reducing blood pressure.

acet- combining form denoting acid. From the Latin *acetum*, vinegar.

acetabuloplasty an operation performed to improve the depth and shape of the hip socket in correcting congenital dislocation of the hip or in treating osteoarthritis of the hip.

acetabulum the cup-like socket in the innominate bone, in which the head of the femur moves.

acetate a salt of acetic acid.

acetoacetic acid diacetic acid. A product of fat metabolism. It occurs in excessive amounts in diabetes and starvation, giving rise to acetone bodies in the urine.

acetonaemia the presence of acetone bodies in the blood.

acetone a colourless inflammable liquid with a characteristic odour. Traces are found in the blood and in normal urine. *A. bodies* ketones found in the blood and urine of uncontrolled diabetic patients and also in acute starvation as a result of the incomplete breakdown of fatty and amino acids.

acetonuria the presence of an excess quantity of acetone bodies in the urine, giving it a peculiar sweet smell.

acetyl coenzyme A active form of acetic acid, to which carbohydrates, fats and amino acids not needed for protein synthesis are converted.

acetylcholine a chemical transmitter that is released by some nerve endings at the synapse between one neurone and the next or between a nerve ending and the effector organ it supplies. These nerves are said to be cholinergic, e.g., the parasympathetic nerves and the lower motor neurones to skeletal muscles. Acetylcholine is rapidly destroyed in the body by cholinesterase.

achalasia failure of relaxation of a muscle sphincter causing dilatation of the part above, e.g., of the oesophagus above the cardiac sphincter.

ache a dull continuous pain.

Achilles Greek mythological hero who could be wounded only in the heel. *A. tendon* tendo calcaneus, connecting the soleus and gastrocnemius muscles of the calf to the heel bone (os calcis). Tapping the Achilles tendon normally produces the Achilles reflex or ankle jerk.

achlorhydria the absence of free hydrochloric acid in the stomach. May be found in pernicious anaemia, pellagra and gastric cancer.

acholia lack of secretion of bile.

acholuria deficiency or lack of bile in the urine.

acholuric pertaining to acholuria. *A. jaundice* jaundice without bile in the urine.

achondroplasia an inherited condition in which there is early union of the epiphysis and diaphysis of long bones. Growth is arrested resulting in short stature.

achromasia 1. lack of colour in the skin. 2. absence of normal reaction to staining in a tissue or cell.

achromatopsia complete colour-blindness caused by disease or trauma. It may be congenital.

achylia absence of hydrochloric acid and enzymes in the gastric secretions. *A. gastrica* a condition in which gastric secretion is reduced or absent.

acid 1. sour or sharp in taste. 2. a substance which, when combined with an alkali, will form a salt. Any acid substance will turn blue litmus paper red. Individual acids are given under their specific names. *A. alcohol-fast* descriptive of stained bacteria that are resistant to decolourization by both acid and alcohol. *A.–base balance* the normal ratio between the acid ions and the basic or alkaline ions required to maintain the pH of the blood and body fluids. Most of the body's metabolic processes produce acids as their end products, but a somewhat alkaline body fluid is required as a medium for vital cellular activities. Therefore chemical exchanges of hydrogen ions must take place continuously in order to maintain a state of equilibrium. An optimal pH (hydrogen ion concentration) between 7.35 and 7.45 must be maintained; otherwise, the enzyme systems and other biochemical and metabolic activities will not function normally.

acidaemia abnormal acidity of the blood, which contains an excess of hydrogen ions in which the pH of the blood falls below 7.35.

acidity 1. sourness or sharpness of taste. 2. the state of being acid.

acidosis a pathological condition resulting from accumulation of acid or depletion of the alkaline reserve (bicarbonate content) in the blood and body tissues, and characterized by increase in hydrogen ion concentration (decrease in pH to below 7.30). *Metabolic a.*

acidosis resulting from accumulation in the blood of ketoacids (derived from fat metabolism) at the expense of bicarbonate, thus diminishing the body's ability to neutralize acids. Occurs in diabetic ketoacidosis, lactic acidosis and failure of renal tubules to reabsorb bicarbonate. *Respiratory a.* acidosis resulting from ventilatory impairment and subsequent retention of carbon dioxide. Carbon dioxide accumulates in the blood and unites with water to form carbonic acid. Occurs with severe birth asphyxia and other respiratory conditions affecting the newborn and in adults with depression of the respiratory centre of the brain due to cerebral disease or drugs.

acidotic 1. pertaining to acidosis. 2. a person suffering from acidosis.

acinus a minute saccule or alveolus of a compound gland, lined by secreting cells. The secreting portion of the mammary gland consists of acini.

acme 1. the highest point. 2. the crisis of a fever when the symptoms are fully developed.

acne an inflammatory condition of the sebaceous glands in which blackheads (comedones) are usually present together with papules and pustules. *A. keratitis* inflammation of the cornea associated with acne rosacea. *A. rosacea* a redness of the forehead, nose and cheeks due to chronic dilatation of the subcutaneous capillaries, which may become permanent with the formation of pustules in the affected areas. *A. vulgaris* form that occurs commonly in adolescents and young adults, affecting the face, chest and back.

acneiform resembling acne.

acousma the hearing of imaginary sounds.

acoustic relating to sound or the sense of hearing. *A. neuroma* a benign tumour of the brain. The tumour grows on the acoustic nerve and can affect hearing and balance. Whilst the tumours are generally slow growing they can become large if not treated. Also known as vestibular schwannoma.

acquired pertaining to disease, habits or immunity developed after birth; not inherited.

acquired immune deficiency syndrome (AIDS) *see* AIDS.

acrocephalia a malformation of the head, in which the top is pointed.

acromegaly a chronic condition producing gradual enlargement of the hands, feet, and bones of the head and chest. Associated with overactivity of the anterior lobe of the pituitary gland in adults.

acromioclavicular pertaining to the joint between the acromion process of the scapula and the lateral aspect of the clavicle.

acromion the outward projection of the spine of the scapula, forming the point of the shoulder.

acroparaesthesia condition in which pressure on the nerves of the brachial plexus causes numbness, pain and tingling of the hand and forearm.

acrophobia extreme or irrational fear of height.

acrosclerosis a combination of RAYNAUD'S DISEASE and scleroderma that affects the hands, feet, face or chest.

acrosome part of the head of a spermatozoon containing enzymes that break down the cell membrane of the ovum and allow penetration.

ACTH adrenocorticotrophic hormone; corticotrophin.

actin the protein of myofibrils responsible for contraction and relaxation of muscles.

actinic keratoses also known as SOLAR KERATOSES rough patches of skin caused by sun exposure over a prolonged period of time.

actinodermatitis inflammation of the skin due to the action of ultraviolet or X-rays.

Actinomyces a genus of the actinobacteria class of bacteria which may give rise to actinomycosis.

actinomycosis a rare chronic infective disease chiefly affecting the lung and jaw, and more rarely the intestine and pelvis.

action the accomplishment of an effect, whether mechanical or chemical, or the effect so produced. *A. research* a method of undertaking social research that incorporates the researcher's involvement as a direct and deliberate part of the research, i.e., the researcher acts as a change agent. *Cumulative a.* the sudden and markedly increased action of a drug after administration of several doses. *Reflex a.* an involuntary response to a stimulus conveyed to the nervous system and reflected to the periphery, passing below the level of consciousness (*see also* REFLEX).

activator a substance, hormone or enzyme that stimulates a chemical change, although it may not take part in the change. In chemistry, a catalyst. For example, yeast is the activator in the process by which sugar is converted into alcohol; the digestive secretions are activated by hormones to carry out normal digestion.

active causing change; energetic. *A. immunity* an immunity in which individuals have been stimulated to produce their own antibodies. *A. labour* the normal progress of the birth process, including uterine contractions, dilation of the cervix to at least 3–4 cm and the descent of the fetus into the birth canal. *A. listening* the act of alert, intentional hearing and demonstration of an interest in what a person has to say through verbal signs, non-verbal gestures and body language. *A. movements* movements made by the patient, as distinct from passive movements. *A. principle* the ingredient in a drug that is primarily responsible for its therapeutic action. *A. transport* the movement of ions or molecules across the cell membranes and epithelial layers, usually against a concentration gradient, resulting directly from the expenditure of metabolic energy. Under

normal circumstances more potassium ions are present within the cell and more sodium ions extracellularly. The process of maintaining these normal differences in electrolytic composition between the intracellular fluids is active transport. The process differs from simple diffusion or osmosis in that it requires the expenditure of metabolic energy.

activities of daily living (ADL) those activities usually performed in the course of a person's normal daily routine, such as eating, cleaning teeth, washing and dressing: forms part of a health assessment.

activities of living (ALs) those activities which meet the physical, psychological and social needs of the individual, e.g., eating, elimination, communication, breathing, expressing sexuality, working, play, etc.

activity theory describes a psychosocial process whereby ageing people disengage from some activities of their earlier life and replace these with other hobbies and pastimes, according to their changing physical abilities and economic situation.

activity tolerance the amount of physical activity tolerated by a patient. It may be assessed in patients with cardiac or chronic respiratory disease. Graded exercise, including walking, cycling and going up and down stairs, may be used to rebuild confidence during the convalescent phase after any serious illness or injury as an important part of any rehabilitation programme.

actomyosin muscle protein complex; the myosin component acts as an enzyme which causes the release of energy.

acuity sharpness. *A. of hearing* an acute perception of sound. *A. of vision* clear focusing ability.

acupressure a system of complementary medicine in which pressure is applied to various points on the body to stimulate the innate self-healing capacity of the individual. *See* ACUPUNCTURE, SHIATSU.

acupuncture a Chinese medical system which aims to diagnose illness and promote health by stimulating the body's self-healing powers. The insertion of special needles into specific points along the 'meridians' of the body is used for the production of anaesthesia, the relief of pain and the treatment of certain conditions.

acute a term applied to a disease in which the attack is sudden, severe and of short duration. *A. respiratory distress syndrome (ARDS)* a severe form of acute lung function failure which occurs after an event such as trauma, inhalation of a toxic substance or septic shock. There is severe breathlessness and a dangerous reduction in the supply of oxygen to the blood. *A. stress disorder* an anxiety disorder that is usually transient which occurs within 4 weeks following exposure or involvement to a traumatic event. The staff of the emergency services may be affected, e.g., following a major road traffic incident.

acyclic occurring independently of a natural cycle of events (such as the menstrual cycle).

Adam's apple the laryngeal prominence, a protrusion of the front of the neck formed by the thyroid cartilage.

adamantine pertaining to the enamel of the teeth.

adaptation 1. the process of modification that a living organism undergoes when adjusting itself to new surroundings or circumstances. 2. a function of the stimulus to which the individual is exposed and of the individual's accommodation to the situation. The adaptation response may relate to physiological needs, role, 'self' concept and interdependence. 3. the process of overcoming difficulties and adjusting to changing circumstances. 4. used in ophthalmology to mean the adjustment of visual function according to the ambient illumination. *Colour a.* 1.

changes in visual perception of colour with prolonged stimulation. 2. adjustment of vision to degree of brightness or colour tone of illumination. *Dark a.* adaptation of the eye to vision in reduced illumination. *Light a.* adaptation of the eye to vision in bright illumination (photopia), with reduction in the concentration of the photosensitive pigments of the eye.

addict a person exhibiting addiction.

addiction 1. the taking of drugs or alcohol leading to physiological and psychological dependence with a tendency to increase use. 2. the state of being devoted to a particular activity or interest, e.g., gambling, exercise or computer games to the exclusion of the normal activities of daily living. *See* DEPENDENCE and DRUG ADDICTION.

Addison's disease *T. Addison, British physician, 1793–1860.* Deficiency disease of the suprarenal cortex. There is wasting, brown pigmentation of the skin and extreme debility. Also known as primary adrenal insufficiency or hypo-adrenalism.

additives substances added to improve, enhance or preserve something. *Food a.* used in the food industry to preserve and make the food look more attractive; these are given serial numbers, e.g., E102 (tartrazine) E200 (sorbic acid). Some additives may produce an allergic reaction in some people and a few are thought to be implicated in behavioural problems in children.

adducent leading towards the midline. *A. muscle* the medial rectus muscle of the eye, which turns it inwards.

adductor a muscle that draws a limb towards the midline of the body. The opposite of abductor.

adenine one of the purine bases found in DNA.

adenitis inflammation of a gland, also referred to as LYMPHADENITIS.

adenoid small lumps of tissue at the back of the nose, above the roof of the mouth. Part of the immune system.

Only present in children and by the age of 7–8 years the adenoids start to shrink. They disappear by adulthood.

adenoidectomy the surgical removal of adenoid tissue from the nasopharynx.

adenoma a benign growth involving glandular tissue including the adrenal glands, the thyroid, prostate and pituitary glands. Whilst usually benign they can become cancerous.

adenomyosis a condition in which the endometrium of the uterus breaks through the muscle wall of the uterus usually resulting in painful and profuse periods.

adenopathy enlargement of any gland, especially those of the lymphatic system.

adenosine a nucleoside consisting of adenine and D-ribose (a pentose sugar). *A. triphosphate (ATP)* a compound containing three phosphoric acids. It is present in all cells and serves as a store for energy.

adenovirus a virus of the Adenoviridae family. Many types have been isolated, some of which cause respiratory tract infections, while others are associated with conjunctivitis, epidemic keratoconjunctivitis or gastrointestinal infection.

ADH antidiuretic hormone. Vasopressin.

adhesion union between two surfaces normally separated. Usually the result of inflammation when fibrous tissue forms, e.g., peritonitis may cause adhesions between organs. A possible cause of intestinal obstruction.

adhesive capsulitis *see* FROZEN SHOULDER.

adipose of the nature of fat. Fatty.

adiposity the state of being too fat. Obesity.

adiposogenital dystrophy a condition occurring in adolescent boys with increased body fat accompanied by underdevelopment of the genitalia and altered secondary sexual characteristics caused by damage to the HYPOTHALAMUS usually as a result of a tumour or infection. Also known as FROHLICH'S SYNDROME.

aditus an opening or passageway; often applied to that between the middle ear and the mastoid antrum.

adjustment in psychology, the ability of a person to adapt to changing circumstances or environment.

adjuvant 1. any treatment used in conjunction with another to enhance its efficacy. 2. a substance administered with a drug to enhance its effect.

ADL activities of daily living.

Adler's theory *A. Adler, Austrian psychiatrist, 1870–1937.* The theory that neuroses develop as a compensation for feelings of inferiority, either social or physical.

adolescence the period between puberty and maturity. In the male, 14–25 years. In the female, 12–21 years.

adopt 1. to take a person, especially another's child, into a legal relationship as one's own. 2. to choose to follow a course of action.

adoption the legal procedure by which a child is transferred from its natural parents to adopting parents. Regulated by law, the child's welfare is paramount. Local authorities offer advice and social work support and may act as an adoption agency, and there are also private and charitable agencies registered with the local authority.

adrenal 1. near the kidneys. 2. a triangular endocrine gland situated above each kidney.

adrenalectomy surgical excision of an adrenal gland.

adrenaline a hormone secreted by the medulla of the adrenal gland. Has an action similar to normal stimulation of the sympathetic nervous system: (a) causing dilatation of the bronchioles; (b) raising the blood pressure by constriction of surface vessels and stimulation of the cardiac output; (c) releasing glycogen from the liver. It is therefore used to treat such conditions as asthma, collapse and hypoglycaemia. It acts as a haemostat in local anaesthetics.

adrenergic pertaining to nerves that release the chemical transmitter noradrenaline in order to stimulate the muscles and glands they supply.

adrenocorticotrophin adrenocorticotrophic hormone (ACTH); secreted by the anterior lobe of the pituitary body. Stimulates the adrenal cortex to produce cortisol. *See* CORTICOTROPHIN.

adrenogenital relating to both the adrenal glands and the gonads. *A. syndrome* a condition of masculinization caused by overactivity of the adrenal cortex resulting in precocious puberty in the male infant and masculinization in the female. Both sexes are liable to Addisonian crises.

adrenolytic a drug that inhibits the stimulation of the sympathetic nerves and the activity of adrenaline.

adsorbent a substance that has the power of attracting gas or fluid to itself, e.g., charcoal.

adsorption the power of certain substances to attach gases or other substances in solution to their surface and so concentrate them there. This is made use of in chromatography.

adult mature. A mature person.

adulteration addition of an impure, cheap or unnecessary ingredient to cheat with, cheapen or falsify a preparation.

advance care planning discussions about the wishes and preferences for end of life care which are documented and shared with permission with relevant agencies and individuals.

advance decision sometimes also referred to as advanced decision to refuse treatment, advance directive or a living will is a written declaration made by a mentally competent person, which sets out their wishes with regard to life-prolonging medical interventions if they are incapacitated by an irreversible disease or are terminally ill which prevents them making their wishes known to health professionals at the time. *See* LIVING WILL.

advanced life support (ALS) resuscitation techniques used during a cardiac arrest that follows on from basic life support. They include defibrillation and the administration of appropriate drugs. Paediatric advanced life support (PALS) is a structured and algorithm method of life support for children with severe medical emergencies. *See* Appendix 2.

advanced trauma life support (ALS) a set of protocols recommended for use by doctors and paramedics when dealing with seriously injured people at the scene of an accident. The immediate treatment of shock from reduced blood volume by the infusion of fluids is an integral component of the life support regime.

advancement in surgery, an operation to detach a tendon or muscle and reattach it further forward. Used in the treatment of strabismus and plastic surgery.

adventitia the outer coat of an artery or vein.

advocacy the process whereby a nurse or health care professional provides a patient and/or the family with information to enable them to make informed decisions relating to the care situation. The nurse is then able to support the patient's decision vis-à-vis other professionals and also to incorporate the informed decisions into care planning.

A-EQUIP a model of clinical supervision for midwives. Abbreviation for advocating for education and quality improvement.

aeration supplying with air. Used to describe the oxygenation of blood which takes place in the lungs.

aerobe an organism that can live and thrive only in the presence of oxygen.

aerobic exercise physical exercises for which the degree of effort is such that it can be maintained for long periods without undue breathlessness. The aim of this form of exercising is to increase the effectiveness of the heart and lungs and the supply of oxygen to the tissues of the body.

aeropathy commonly called 'the bends' (decompression sickness).

aerophagy the excessive swallowing of air.

aerosol finely divided particles or droplets. *A. sprays* used in medicine to humidify air or oxygen, or for the administration of drugs by inhalation.

aetiology the science of the causes of disease.

afebrile without fever.

affect in psychiatry, the feeling experienced in connection with an emotion or mood.

affection 1. a morbid condition or disease state. 2. a warm feeling for someone or something.

affective pertaining to the emotions or moods. *A. psychoses* major mental disorders in which there is grave disturbance of the emotions.

afferent conveying towards the centre. *A. nerves* the sensory nerve fibres that convey impulses from the periphery towards the brain. *A. paths* or *tracts* the course of the sensory nerves up the spinal cord and through the brain. *A. vessels* arterioles entering the glomerulus of the kidney, or lymphatics entering a lymph gland. *See* EFFERENT.

affiliation the judicial decision about the paternity of a child with a view to the issue of a maintenance order.

affinity in chemistry, the attraction of two substances to each other, e.g., haemoglobin and oxygen.

afibrinogenaemia absence of fibrinogen in the blood. The clotting mechanism of the blood is impaired as a result.

African tick fever disease caused by a spirochaete, *Borrelia duttonii*. Transmitted by ticks. *See* RELAPSING FEVER.

afterbirth a lay expression used to describe the placenta, cord and membranes expelled after childbirth.

afterimage a visual impression that remains briefly after the cessation of sensory stimulation.

afterpains the pains due to uterine contraction after childbirth.

agammaglobulinaemia a condition in which there is a lack of gamma-globulin in the blood. The patients are therefore susceptible to infections because of an inability to form antibodies.

aganglionosis *see* HIRSCHSPRUNG'S DISEASE.

agar a gelatinous substance prepared from seaweed. Used as a culture medium for bacteria and as a laxative because it absorbs liquid from the digestive tract and swells, so stimulating peristalsis.

age 1. the duration, or the measure of time, of the existence of a person or object. 2. to undergo change as a result of the passage of time. *Chronological a.* the actual measure of time elapsed since a person's birth. *Gestational a.* an expression of age of a developing fetus, usually given in weeks. It is measured from the date of the mother's last menstrual period, and so is approximately 2 weeks longer than time from conception. *Mental a.* the age level of intellectual ability of a person as gauged by intelligence tests. *Age-related macular degeneration. See* MACULA.

age-associated memory impairment with age short-term memory declines; most elderly people learn to overcome and compensate for this deficit. However, for some it may be a considerable problem in daily living. Memory loss associated with dementia is often due to Alzheimer's disease or cerebral vascular disease. *See* DEMENTIA and ALZHEIMER'S DISEASE.

age spots with increasing age skin blemishes appear; most commonly they are seborrhoeic keratoses, which are brown or yellow and can occur anywhere on the body. Also common with increasing age are freckles, red pinpoint blemishes on the trunk and solar keratoses due to overexposure to the sun. Treatment is usually unnecessary except occasionally for solar keratoses which may eventually progress to skin cancer.

ageing the structural changes that take place with time and are not caused by accident or disease. Heredity is an important determinant of life expectancy, but factors such as smoking, an excessive intake of alcohol, obesity, poor diet and insufficient exercise can all contribute to physical and mental deterioration. *A. population* as the number of older people increase, the demand for health care increases. Expectations for health care delivery and provision too are changing as patients become increasingly knowledgeable about their health.

ageism the systematic discrimination against people on the grounds of age, based on stereotyping of the elderly as helpless, infirm, confused, requiring health care and supportive social services.

Agenda for Change the grading and pay system for NHS staff with the exception of doctors, dentists and some very senior managers.

agenesis failure of a structure to develop properly.

agent any substance or force capable of producing a physical, chemical or biological effect. *Alkylating a.* a cytotoxic preparation. *Chelating a.* a chemical compound that binds metal ions. *Wetting a.* a substance that lowers the surface tension of water and promotes wetting.

agglutination collecting into clumps, particularly of cells suspended in a fluid and of bacteria affected by specific immune serum. *A. test* a means of aiding diagnosis and identification of bacteria. If serum containing known agglutinins comes into contact with the specific bacteria, clumping will take place (*see* WIDAL REACTION). *Cross a.* a simple test to decide the group to which blood belongs (*see* BLOOD GROUPS).

agglutinin any substance causing agglutination (clumping together) of

cells, particularly a specific antibody formed in the blood in response to the presence of an invading agent. Agglutinins are proteins (IMMUNOGLOBULIN) and function as part of the immune mechanism of the body. When the invading agents that bring about the production of agglutinins are bacteria, the agglutinins produced bring about agglutination of the bacterial cells.

agglutinogen any substance that, when present in the bloodstream, can cause the production of specific antibodies or agglutinins.

aggregation the massing together of materials, as in clumping. *Familial a.* the increased incidence of cases of a disease in a family compared with that in control families. *Platelet a.* the clumping together of platelets, which may be induced by a number of agents, such as thrombin and collagen.

aggression animosity or hostility shown towards another person or object as a response to opposition or frustration.

agitation 1. shaking. 2. mental distress causing extreme restlessness.

aglutition difficulty in the act of swallowing. Dysphagia.

agnosia an inability to recognize objects because the sensory stimulus cannot be interpreted, in spite of the presence of a normal sense organ.

agonist the prime mover. A muscle opposed in action by another (the antagonist).

agony extreme suffering, either mental or physical.

agoraphobia a fear of being in situations where escape might be difficult or help would not be available if things go wrong.

agranulocyte a white blood cell without granules in its cytoplasm. The term includes monocytes and lymphocytes.

agranulocytosis a condition in which there is a marked decrease or complete absence of granular leukocytes in the blood, leaving the body defenceless against bacterial invasion. May result from: (a) the use of toxic drugs; (b) irradiation. Characterized by a sore throat, ulceration of the mouth and pyrexia. It may result in severe prostration and death.

agraphia absence of the power of expressing thought in writing. It arises from a lack of muscular coordination or as a result of motor dysfunction.

ague malaria.

AHP allied health professional.

AID artificial insemination of a woman with donor semen.

AIDS acquired immunodeficiency syndrome. The late symptomatic stage of chronic disease caused by human immunodeficiency virus (HIV) infection which progressively impairs the body's cell-mediated immune responses to infections and cancers. This results in serious 'opportunistic infections' caused by microorganisms that do not usually cause illness in people with a healthy immune system, e.g., *Pneumocystis jirovecii* pneumonia (PCP), or cancers such as Kaposi's sarcoma (KS) and lymphoma. Additionally, this late stage of HIV disease is characterized by a high and rising level (viral load) of HIV and a progressively decreasing number (less than 200 cells/mm^3) of CD4$^+$ T lymphocytes in the plasma. Prior to AIDS, many HIV-infected people experience a variety of recurrent signs and symptoms, including lymphadenopathy, night sweats, diarrhoea, weight loss, malaise, oropharyngeal or vaginal candidiasis (thrush), and herpes zoster (shingles). Formerly known as the AIDS-related complex, this stage is now generally referred to as early symptomatic HIV disease (as opposed to AIDS which is also known as late symptomatic HIV disease).

AIH artificial insemination of a woman with her partner's semen.

ailment any minor disorder of the body.

air a mixture of gases that make up the earth's atmosphere. It consists of non-active nitrogen 79%; oxygen 21%, which supports life and combustion; traces of neon, argon, hydrogen, etc.; and carbon dioxide 0.03%, except in expired air, when 6% is exhaled as a result of diffusion that has taken place in the lungs. Air has weight and exerts pressure, which aids in syphonage from body cavities. *A.-bed* a rubber mattress inflated with air. *A. embolism* an embolism caused by air entering the circulatory system. *A. hunger* a form of dyspnoea in which there are deep sighing respirations, characteristic of severe haemorrhage or acidosis. *Residual a.* air remaining in the lungs after deep expiration. *Stationary a.* that retained in the lungs after normal expiration. *Supplemental a.* the extra air forced out of the lungs with expiratory effort. *Tidal a.* that which passes in and out of the lungs in normal respiratory action.

airway 1. the passage by which the air enters and leaves the lungs. 2. a mechanical device (tube) used for securing unobstructed respiration during general anaesthesia or on other occasions when the patient is not ventilating or exchanging gases properly. It may be passed through the mouth or nose. The tube prevents a flaccid tongue from resting against the posterior pharyngeal wall and causing obstruction of the airway (*see* Figure).

akinesia loss of muscle power. This may be the result of a brain or spinal cord lesion or, temporarily, of anaesthesia.

akinetic relating to states or conditions where there is lack of movement.

alalia loss or impairment of the power of speech due to muscle paralysis or a cerebral lesion.

alacrima a deficiency or absence of the secretion of tears.

alanine an amino acid formed by the ingestion of dietary protein. *A. transaminase (ALT)* a transaminase found in plasma and the liver which catalyses the two parts of the alanine cycle.

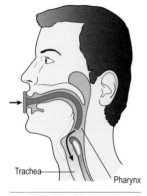

Trachea

Pharynx

OROPHARYNGEAL AIRWAY

albinism a condition in which there is congenital absence of pigment in the skin, hair and eyes. It may be partial or complete.

albino a person affected with albinism.

albumin 1. any protein that is soluble in water and moderately concentrated salt solutions and is coagulable by heat, e.g., egg white. 2. serum albumin; a plasma protein, formed principally in the liver and constituting about four-sevenths of the 6%–8% protein concentration in the plasma. Albumin is a very important factor in regulating the exchange of water between the plasma and the interstitial compartment (space between the cells). A drop in the amount of albumin in the plasma results in an increase in tissue fluid, which, if severe, becomes apparent as oedema. Albumin serves also as a transport protein.

albuminuria the presence of albumin in the urine, occurring e.g., in renal disease, in most feverish conditions and sometimes in pregnancy. *Orthostatic* or *postural a.* a non-pathological form that affects some individuals after prolonged standing but disappears after bedrest for a few hours.

alcohol a volatile liquid distilled from fermented saccharine liquids and forming the basis of wines and spirits. The official (British Pharmacopoeia) preparation of ethyl alcohol (ethanol) contains 95% alcohol and 5% water. Used: (a) as an antiseptic; (b) in the preparation of tinctures; (c) as a perspective for anatomical specimens. Taken internally, it acts as a temporary heart stimulant, and in large quantities as a depressant poison. It has some value as a food, 30 ml brandy producing about 400 J. *Absolute a.* that which contains not more than 1% by weight of water. *A.-fast* pertaining to bacteria that, once having been stained, are resistant to decolorization by alcohol. *A. related disorders* A variety of physical and mental disorders associated with prolonged and excessive consumption of alcohol including hepatitis, cirrhosis, some cancers, e.g., of the oesophagus, larynx and throat. Heavy alcohol consumption in pregnancy increases the risk of miscarriage and fetal alcohol syndrome. Alcoholics are more likely to suffer from personality changes, depression and to develop dementia. Many alcoholics suffer from a poor diet and are prone to nutritional deficiency. *See* WERNICKE—KORSAKOFF SYNDROME. *A. withdrawal syndrome* a group of symptoms that develop in a person suffering from alcoholism within 6–24 hours of taking the last drink of alcohol. The symptoms include restlessness, tremors, loss of appetite, nausea, vomiting, insomnia, disorientation, seizures and delirium tremens. Treatment involves sedation, improving nutrition, counselling and social support.

alcoholic 1. pertaining to alcohol. 2. a person addicted to excessive, uncontrolled alcohol consumption. This results in loss of appetite and vitamin B deficiency, leading to peripheral neuritis with eye changes and cirrhosis of the liver and to progressive deterioration in the personality.

alcoholism the state of poisoning resulting from alcoholic addiction.

aldosterone a compound, isolated from the adrenal cortex, that aids the retention of sodium and the excretion of potassium in the body, and by so doing aids the maintenance of electrolyte balance. *A. antagonists* a group of drugs which block the action of aldosterone.

aldosteronism an excess secretion of aldosterone caused by an adrenal neoplasm. The serum potassium is low and the patient has hypertension and severe muscular weakness.

aleukaemia an acute condition in which there is an absence or deficiency of white cells in the blood.

Alexander technique *F.M. Alexander, Australian actor and physiotherapist, 1869–1955.* A process of psychophysical postural re-education. Body posture is believed to affect physical and psychological wellbeing and the postural re-education process aims to assist individuals in monitoring how they consciously use their bodies to promote good health.

alexia a form of aphasia in which there is an inability to recognize written or printed words. Word blindness.

algorithm a process or set of rules used in calculations, e.g., of medications, or for other problem solving. Computer programs are the most familiar examples of algorithms in everyday use.

alienation a feeling of estrangement or separation from others or from self. A symptom of schizophrenia. Sufferers often believe that they are under the control of someone else. *See* DEPERSONALIZATION.

alignment the state of being arranged in a line, i.e., in the correct anatomical position.

aliment food or nourishment.

alimentary relating to the system of nutrition. *A. canal* alimentary tract. The passage through which the food passes, from mouth to anus. *A. system* the alimentary tract together with the liver and other organs concerned in digestion and absorption. *A. tract* alimentary canal.

alimentation the giving or receiving of nourishment. The process of supplying the patient's need for nutrition.

alkalaemia an increase in the alkali content of the blood. *See* ALKALOSIS.

alkali a substance capable of uniting with acids to form salts, and with fats and fatty acids to form soaps. Alkaline solutions turn red litmus paper blue. *A. reserve* the ability of the combined buffer systems of the blood to neutralize acid. The pH of the blood is normally slightly on the alkaline side, between 7.35 and 7.45. The principal buffer in the blood is bicarbonate; the alkali reserve is essentially represented by the plasma bicarbonate concentration.

alkaline having the reactions of an alkali. *A. phosphatase* an enzyme localized on cell membranes that hydrolyses phosphate esters, liberating inorganic phosphate, and has an optimal pH of about 10.0. Serum alkaline phosphatase activity is elevated in obstructive jaundice and bone disease.

alkalinity 1. the quality of being alkaline. 2. the combining power of a base, expressed as the maximum number of equivalents of acid with which it reacts to form a salt.

alkaloid one of a group of active nitrogenous compounds that are alkaline in solution. They usually have a bitter taste and are characterized by powerful physiological activity. Examples are morphine, cocaine, atropine, quinine, nicotine and caffeine. The term is also applied to synthetic substances that have structures similar to plant alkaloids, such as procaine.

alkalosis an increase in the alkali reserve in the blood. It may be confirmed by estimation of the blood carbon dioxide content and treated by giving normal saline or ammonium chloride intravenously to encourage the excretion of bicarbonate by the kidneys.

alkylating agent a drug that damages the deoxyribonucleic acid (DNA) molecule of the nucleus of the cell. Many are nitrogen mustard preparations; they are used in cancer chemotherapy.

all-or-none law principle that states that in individual cardiac and skeletal muscle fibres there are only two possible reactions to a stimulus: either there is no reaction at all or there is a full reaction, with no gradation of response according to the strength of the stimulus. Whole muscles can grade their response by increasing or decreasing the *number* of fibres involved.

allantois a membranous sac projecting from the ventral surface of the fetus in its early stages. It eventually helps to form the placenta.

allele allelomorph. One of a pair of genes that occupy the same relative positions on homologous chromosomes and produce different effects on the same process of development.

allelomorph allele.

Allen Test is used to test the blood supply to the hand, specifically the patency of the radial and ulnar arteries. It is performed prior to radial arterial sampling or cannulation.

allergen a substance that can produce an allergy or manifestation of an immune response.

allergic rhinitis a common condition where there is inflammation of the inside of the nose caused by an allergen such as pollen, dust, mould or animal skin.

allergy a hypersensitivity to some foreign substances that are normally harmless but which produce a violent reaction in the patient. Asthma, hay fever, angioneurotic oedema, migraine and some types of urticaria and eczema are allergic states. *See* ANAPHYLAXIS.

allograft an organ or tissue transplanted from one person to another of a dissimilar genotype but of the same species. *Non-viable a.* skin, taken from a cadaver, which cannot regenerate. *Viable a.* living tissue transplanted. *See* HOMOGRAFT.

alloimmunization the immune response to donated blood, bone marrow or transplanted organ; rhesus-negative pregnant women with a rhesus-positive fetus can become alloimmunized following a sensitizing event, e.g., antepartum haemorrhage or miscarriage, through the development of antibodies that target the foreign material, causing haemolytic disease of the newborn.

allopathy the practice of conventional medicine, i.e., with drugs having opposite effects to the symptoms.

alopecia baldness. Loss of hair. The cause of simple baldness is not yet fully understood, although it is known that the tendency to become bald is limited almost entirely to males, runs in certain families and is more common in certain racial groups than in others. Baldness is often associated with ageing. *A. areata* hair loss in sharply defined areas, usually the scalp or beard. *Cicatricial a., a. cicatrisata* irreversible loss of hair associated with scarring, usually on the scalp. Also known as scarring alopecia. *Male-pattern a.* loss of scalp hair, genetically determined and androgen-dependent, beginning with frontal recession and progressing symmetrically to leave ultimately only a sparse peripheral rim of hair.

alpha the first letter of the Greek alphabet, a. *A. cells* cells found in the islet of Langerhans in the pancreas. They produce the hormone glucagon. *A. fetoprotein (AFP)* a plasma protein originating in the fetal liver and gastrointestinal tract. The serum AFP level is used to monitor the effectiveness of cancer treatment; the amniotic fluid AFP level is used in the prenatal diagnosis of neural tube defects. *A.*

receptors tissue receptors associated with the stimulation (contraction) of smooth muscle.

alternative medicine a form of medicine differing from conventional health care. Consists of a range of treatments essentially based upon a holistic approach to health and wellbeing, including homeopathy, aromatherapy, hypnosis, acupuncture and others. These therapies fall into three categories: touch and movement, medicinal and psychological. Commonly called complementary therapies (*see* COMPLEMENTARY).

altitude sickness condition caused by hypoxia that occurs as a result of lower oxygen pressure at high altitudes before acclimatization to the increased altitude. *See* ACCLIMATIZATION.

altruism a sense of unconditional concern for the welfare of others.

aluminium *symbol* Al. A silver-white metal with a low specific gravity, compounds of which are astringent and antiseptic. *A. hydroxide* compound used as an antacid in the treatment of gastric conditions.

alveolar concerning an alveolus, or air sac of the lung. *A. air* air found in the alveoli.

alveolitis inflammation of the alveoli. *Extrinsic allergic a.* inflammation of the alveoli caused by inhalation of an antigen, such as pollen.

Alzheimer's cells *A. Alzheimer, German neurologist, 1864–1915.* 1. giant astrocytes with large prominent nuclei found in the brain in hepatolenticular degeneration and hepatic comas. 2. degenerated astrocytes.

Alzheimer's disease a progressive form of neuronal degeneration in the brain and the most common cause of dementia in people of all ages. It is more common in older than younger people and is not just a form of presenile dementia, as was originally thought. The degeneration of neurones is accompanied by changes in the brain's biochemistry. At the moment, there is no cure for Alzheimer's disease but medication is available to help relieve some of the symptoms. Other aspects of treatment are the provision of appropriate health and social care, together with ongoing support for their families.

amalgam a compound of mercury and other metals. *Dental a.* now rarely used for filling teeth.

amaurosis loss of vision, resulting from a systemic cause without damage to the eye. The visual loss may be partial or complete, and is usually temporary.

ambidextrous equally skilful with either hand.

ambivalence the existence of contradictory emotional feelings towards an object, commonly of love and hate for another person. If these feelings occur to a marked degree they lead to psychological disturbance.

amblyopia dimness of vision without any apparent lesion of the eye. Uncorrectable by optical means.

ambulant able to walk.

ambulatory having the capacity to walk. *A. treatment* or *care* health services provided on an outpatient or day care basis.

amelioration improvement of symptoms; a lessening of the severity of a disease.

amenorrhoea absence of menstruation. *Primary a.* the non-occurrence of the menses. *Secondary a.* the cessation of the menses, after they have been established, owing to disease or pregnancy.

ametropia defective vision. A general word applied to incorrect refraction.

Ames Test a biological assay to assess the mutagenic potential of chemical compounds. A positive test indicates that the chemical is mutagenic and therefore may act as a carcinogen, since cancer is often linked to mutation.

amino acid a chemical compound containing both NH_2 and $COOH$ groups. The end product of protein digestion.

	Essential amino acids
1	Threonine
2	Lysine
3	Methionine
4	Valine
5	Phenylalanine
6	Leucine
7	Tryptophan
8	Isoleucine
9	Histidine

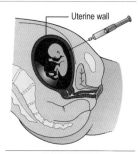

AMNIOCENTESIS

Essential a. one required for replacement and growth but which cannot be synthesized in the body in sufficient amounts and must be obtained in the diet (*see* Table). Histidine is also essential in childhood. *Non-essential a. a.* one necessary for proper growth but that can be synthesized in the body and is not specifically required in the diet.

aminoglycoside any of a group of bacterial antibiotics, derived from various species of *Streptomyces*, that interfere with the function of bacterial ribosomes. The aminoglycosides include gentamicin, tobramycin, streptomycin, tobramycin, amikacin, kanamycin and neomycin. They are used to treat infections caused by gram-negative organisms and are classified as bactericidal agents because of their interference with bacterial replication. All the aminoglycoside antibiotics are highly toxic, requiring monitoring of blood serum levels and careful observation of the patient for early signs of toxicity, particularly ototoxicity and nephrotoxicity.

amitosis multiplication of cells by simple division or fission.

ammonia NH_3. A naturally occurring compound of nitrogen and hydrogen formed by the decomposition of proteins and amino acids. Converted into urea by the liver.

amnesia partial or complete loss of memory. *Anterograde a.* loss of memory of events that have taken place since an injury or illness. *Retrograde a.* loss of memory for events prior to an injury. It often applies to the time immediately preceding an accident.

amniocentesis the withdrawal of fluid from the uterus through the abdominal wall by means of a syringe and needle (*see* Figure) with guided ultrasound. It is primarily used in the diagnosis of chromosome disorders in the fetus and in cases of hydramnios. Mothers who are rhesus-negative should be given a reduced dose of anti-D immunoglobulin after the procedure to prevent them making antibodies.

amniography radiography of the gravid uterus.

amnion the innermost membrane enveloping the fetus and enclosing the liquor amnii, or amniotic fluid.

amniotic pertaining to the amnion. *A. fluid* the albuminous fluid contained in the amniotic sac. Liquor amnii.

amoeba a minute unicellular protozoon. It is able to move by pushing out parts of itself (called pseudopodia). Capable of reproduction by amitotic fission. Infection of the intestines by *Entamoeba histolytica* causes 'amoebic dysentery'.

amoebiasis infection with amoeba, particularly *Entamoeba histolytica*.

amoebic pertaining to, caused by, or of the nature of an amoeba. *A. abscess* an abscess cavity of the liver resulting from liquefaction necrosis due to entrance of *Entamoeba histolytica* into the portal circulation in amoebiasis; amoebic abscesses may affect the lung, brain and spleen. *A. dysentery* a form of dysentery caused by *Entamoeba histolytica* and spread by contaminated food, water and flies; called also amoebiasis. Amoebic dysentery is mainly a tropical disease but many cases occur in temperate countries. Symptoms are diarrhoea, fatigue and intestinal bleeding. Complications include involvement of the liver, liver abscess and pulmonary abscess.

amoeboid resembling an amoeba in structure or movement.

amorphous without definite shape. The term may be applied to fine powdery particles, as opposed to crystals.

amphiarthrosis a form of joint in which the bones are joined together by fibrocartilage, e.g., the junctions of the vertebrae.

amphoric pertaining to a bottle. Used to describe the sound sometimes heard on auscultation over cavities in the lungs, which resembles that produced by blowing across the mouth of a bottle.

ampoule a small glass or plastic phial in which sterile drugs of specified dose for injection are sealed.

ampulla the flask-like dilatation of a canal, e.g., of a uterine tube.

amputation surgical removal of a limb or other part of the body, e.g., the breast.

amputee a person who has had one or more limbs amputated.

amylase an enzyme that reduces starch to maltose. Found in saliva (ptyalin) and pancreatic juice (amylopsin).

amyloid 1. pertaining to starch. 2. a waxy starch-like material that is a complex protein forming in tissues and organs leading to disturbance of function, called amyloidosis.

amylopsin an enzyme found in the pancreas. Amylase.

amylum [L.] *starch.*

amyotonia atonic condition of the muscles.

anabolic relating to anabolism. *A. compound* a substance that aids in the repair of body tissue, particularly protein. Androgens may be used in this way.

anabolism the building up or synthesis of cell structure from digested food materials. *See* METABOLISM.

anacidity decrease in normal acidity.

anaclitic denoting the dependence of the infant on the mother or mother substitute for its sense of wellbeing. *A. choice* a psychoanalytical term for the adult selection of a loved one who closely resembles one's mother (or another adult on whom one depended as a child). *A. depression* severe and progressive depression found in children who have lost their mothers and have not found a suitable substitute.

anacrotism an abnormal pulse wave tracing embodying a secondary expansion.

anaemia deficiency in either quality or quantity of red corpuscles in the blood that reduces the oxygen carrying capacity of the blood, giving rise especially to symptoms of anoxaemia. There is pallor, breathlessness on exertion, with palpitations, lassitude, headache, giddiness and often a history of poor resistance to infection. Anaemia may be due to many different causes. Increasingly, with the advent of electronic cell counters, anaemia is now classified according to the morphological characteristics of the erythrocytes. *Aplastic a.* the bone marrow is unable to produce red blood corpuscles. A rare condition. *Deficiency a.* any type that is due to the lack of the necessary factors for red cell formation, e.g., hormones or vitamins. *Haemolytic a.* a variety in which there is excessive destruction of red blood corpuscles caused by antibody formation in the blood (*see* RHESUS FACTOR), by drugs or by severe toxaemia, as in extensive burns. *Iron-deficiency a.* the most common type of anaemia, due to a lack of absorbable iron in the diet. It may also be due to excessive or chronic blood loss, or to poor absorption of dietary iron. *Macrocytic a.* a type in which the cells are larger than normal; present in pernicious anaemia. *Microcytic a.* a variety in which the cells are smaller than normal, as in iron deficiency. *Pernicious a.* a variety caused by the inability of the stomach to secrete the intrinsic factor necessary for the absorption of vitamin B_{12} from the diet. *Sickle-cell a.* a hereditary haemolytic anaemia seen most commonly in people living in or originating from the Caribbean islands, Africa, Asia, the Middle East and the Mediterranean. The red blood cells are sickle-shaped. *Splenic a.* a congenital, familial disease in which the red blood cells are fragile and easily broken down.

anaerobe a microorganism that can live and thrive in the absence of free oxygen. These organisms are found in body cavities or wounds where the oxygen tension is very low. Examples are the bacilli of tetanus and gas gangrene.

anaesthesia loss of feeling or sensation in a part or in the whole of the body, usually induced by drugs. *Basal a.* basal narcosis. Loss of consciousness, although supplemental drugs have to be given to ensure complete anaesthesia. *Epidural a.* injection into the extradural space between the vertebral spines and beneath the ligamentum flavum. *General a.* unconsciousness produced by inhalation or injection of a drug. *Inhalation a.* drugs or gas are administered by a face mask or endotracheal tube to cause general anaesthesia. *Intravenous a.* unconsciousness is produced by the introduction of a drug into a vein. *Local a.* local analgesia. Nerve conduction is blocked by injection of a local anaesthetic, or by

freezing with ethyl chloride or by topical application. *Spinal a.* injection of anaesthetic agent into the spinal subarachnoid space.

anaesthetic a drug causing anaesthesia.

anaesthetist a person who is medically qualified to administer an anaesthetic and in the techniques of life support for the critically ill or injured.

anal pertaining to the anus. *A. eroticism* sexual pleasure derived from anal functions. *A. fissure see* FISSURE. *A. fistula see* FISTULA. *A. stage* the second stage of a child's psychosexual development, characterized by the child's sensual interest in the anal area and the passing or retention of faeces.

analeptic a drug that stimulates the central nervous system.

analgesia insensibility to pain, especially the relief of pain without causing unconsciousness. *Patient-controlled a.* a preset dose of analgesic, which the patient controls according to need. In-built safety measures prevent accidental overdose.

analgesic 1. relating to analgesia. 2. a remedy that relieves pain. *A. cocktail* an individualized mixture of drugs used to control pain.

analogue 1. an organ with a different structure and origin to but the same function as another one. 2. a compound with a similar structure to another but differing in respect of a particular element.

analysis 1. the act of determining the component parts of a substance. 2. in psychiatry, a method of trying to understand the complex mental processes, experiences and relationships with other individuals or groups of individuals to determine the reasons for an individual's behaviour. *A. of covariance (ANCOVA)* a statistic that measures differences among group means and uses a statistical technique to equate the groups under study in relation to another given variable. *A. of variance (ANOVA)* a statistic that tests whether groups differ from each other, rather than testing each pair of means separately. ANOVA considers the variation among all groups.

anaphase part of the process of mitosis or meiosis.

anaphylaxis anaphylactic shock. A severe reaction, often fatal, occurring in response to drugs, e.g., penicillin, but also to bee stings and food allergy, e.g., nuts, in sensitive individuals. The symptoms are severe dyspnoea, rapid pulse, profuse sweating and collapse.

anaplasia a change in the character of cells, seen in tumour tissue.

anarthria inability to articulate speech sounds owing to a brain lesion or damage to peripheral nerves innervating articulatory muscles.

anastomosis 1. in surgery, any artificial connection of two hollow structures, e.g., gastroenterostomy. 2. in anatomy, the joining of the branches of two blood vessels.

anatomy the science of the structure of the body.

Ancylostoma hookworm. A genus of nematode roundworms which may inhabit the duodenum and cause extreme anaemia and malnutrition. *A. duodenale* a hookworm very widespread in tropical and subtropical areas.

androgen one of a group of hormones secreted by the testes and adrenal cortex. They are steroids which can be synthesized and produce the secondary male characteristics and the building up of protein tissue. *A. insensitivity syndrome* (AIS) a rare genetic condition that affects the development of a child's genitals and reproductive organs.

android resembling a man. *A. pelvis* a female pelvis shaped like a male pelvis with a wedge-shaped entrance and narrow anterior segment.

anergy 1. specific immunological tolerance in which T cells fail to respond normally. The state can be reversed. 2. tiredness, lethargy, lack of energy.

aneurine thiamin. An essential vitamin involved in carbohydrate metabolism. The main sources are unrefined cereals and pork. Vitamin B_1.

aneurysm a local dilatation of a blood vessel, usually an artery. Atherosclerosis is responsible for most arterial aneurysms; any injury to the arterial wall can predispose to the formation of a sac. Smoking is the strongest risk factor in developing aortic aneurysm . The pressure of blood causes it to increase in size and rupture is likely. Surgery, either open or endovascular, can prevent rupture, *see* ABDOMINAL AORTIC ANEURYSM. *Dissecting a.* a condition in which a tear occurs in the aortic lining when the middle coat is necrosed and blood gets between the layers, stripping them apart. *Fusiform a.* a spindle-shaped arterial aneurysm. *Saccular a.* a dilatation of only a part of the circumference of an artery.

angina a tight strangling sensation or pain. *A. cruris* intermittent claudication. Severe pain in the leg after walking. *A. pectoris* cardiac pain that occurs on exertion owing to insufficient blood supply to the heart muscles. *Vincent's a.* infection and ulceration of the tonsils by a spirochaete, *Borrelia vincentii*, and a bacillus, *Bacillus fusiformis*.

angiocardiography radiological examination of the heart and large blood vessels by means of cardiac catheterization and an opaque contrast medium.

angiography radiological examination of the blood vessels using an opaque contrast medium.

angioma a benign tumour composed of dilated blood vessels.

angioedema a type of reaction; most commonly caused by an allergy, characterized by well-defined swellings or weals of sudden and rapid onset in the skin, throat, mouth, eyes and other areas. Fatal oedema of the glottis may occur resulting in a medical emergency. *See* OEDEMA.

angioplasty surgery of a narrowed artery to promote the normal flow of blood. *Balloon a.* technique in which a catheter with an elastic, flexible (balloon-like) tip that can be inflated to widen the narrowed blood vessel, e.g., in the heart. Usually a stent is inserted to keep the artery open. Stents have now been developed coated in slow-release drugs that reduce further risk of arterial narrowing. *See* STENT.

angiosarcoma a malignant vascular growth.

angiospasm a spasmodic contraction of an artery, causing cramping of the muscles.

angiotensin a substance that raises the blood pressure. It is a polypeptide produced by the action of renin on plasma globulins. Hypertensin.

anhidrosis marked deficiency in the secretion of sweat.

anhidrotic an agent that decreases perspiration. An adiaphoretic.

anhydraemia deficiency of water in the blood.

aniline a chemical compound derived from coal tar, used for making antiseptic dyes. It is an important cause of serious industrial poisoning and methaemoglobinaemia.

anima 1. the soul. 2. Jung's term for the unconscious, or inner being, of the individual, as opposed to the personality presented to the world (persona). In Jungian psychoanalysis, the more feminine soul or feminine component of a man's personality.

anion a negatively charged ion which travels towards the anode, e.g., chloride (Cl⁻), carbonate (CO_3^{2-}). *See* CATION.

aniridia lack of part or the whole of the iris.

anisocoria inequality of diameter of the pupils of the two eyes.

anisocytosis inequality in the size of the red blood cells.

anisometropia a marked difference in the refractive power of the two eyes.

ankle the joint between the leg and foot, formed by the tibia and fibula articulating with the talus.

ankle-brachial pressure index (ABPI) The measurement of the ratio of systolic blood pressure at the ankle

measured by a Doppler ultrasound probe to that measured at the brachial artery to quantify the degree of arterial occlusion in the leg. Forms an important part of a leg ulcer assessment regarding the patient's suitability for compression bandaging.

ankyloblepharon adhesions and scar tissue on the ciliary borders of the eyelids, giving the eye a distorted appearance.

ankylosing spondylitis a long-term condition in which there is inflammation of the spine and other areas of the body leading to back pain and stiffness, pain and swelling of other parts of the body and extreme tiredness. The cause is unknown but there may be a genetic link.

ankylosis consolidation, immobility and stiffness of a joint as a result of disease.

annular ring-shaped.

anoci-association the exclusion of pain, fear and shock in surgical operations, brought about by means of local anaesthesia and basal narcosis.

anodyne 1. pain-relieving or relaxing. 2. a drug or other treatment that relieves pain.

anomaly considerable variation from normal.

anomie a feeling of hopelessness and lack of purpose.

Anopheles a genus of mosquito. Many are carriers of the malarial parasite and infect humans by their bite. Other species transmit filariasis.

anophthalmia congenital absence of a seeing eye.

anorexia loss of appetite for food. *A. nervosa* a condition in which there is complete lack of appetite, with extreme emaciation. It is owing to psychological causes and most commonly occurs in young women with poor self esteem and fear of obesity associated with a distorted body image, leading them to perceive themselves as fat and to take extreme forms of dietary control in order to lose weight.

anosmia loss of the sense of smell.

anovular applied to the absence of ovulation. Usually refers to uterine bleeding when there has been no ovulation, the result of taking contraceptive pills.

anoxaemia complete lack of oxygen in the blood.

anoxia lack of oxygen to an organ or tissue.

antacid a substance neutralizing acidity, particularly of the gastric juices.

antagonist 1. a muscle that has an opposite action to another, e.g., the biceps to the triceps. 2. in pharmacology, a drug that inhibits the action of another drug or enzyme, e.g., methotrexate is a folic acid antagonist. 3. in dentistry, a tooth in one jaw opposing one in the other jaw.

anteflexion a bending forward, as of the body of the uterus. *See* RETROFLEXION.

antenatal before birth. *A. care* care provided by midwives, GPs and obstetricians during pregnancy to ensure that the fetal and maternal health are satisfactory. Deviations from normal can be detected and treated early. The mother can be prepared for labour and parenthood and health education offered.

antepartum shortly before birth, i.e., in the last 3 months of pregnancy. *A. haemorrhage* bleeding occurring before parturition. *See* PLACENTA PRAEVIA.

anterior situated at or facing towards the front. The opposite of posterior. *A. capsule* the anterior covering of the lens of the eye. *A. chamber of the eye* the space between the cornea in front and the iris and lens behind.

anterograde extending or moving forwards.

anteversion the forward tilting of an organ, e.g., the normal position of the uterus. *See* RETROVERSION.

anthelmintic (anthelminthic) 1. destructive to worms. 2. an agent destructive to worms.

anthracosis a disease of the lungs, caused by inhalation of coal dust. A form of pneumoconiosis. 'Miner's lung'.

anthrax an acute, notifiable, infectious disease due to *Bacillus anthracis*, acquired through contact with infected animals or their by-products. A worldwide zoonosis, anthrax is now very uncommon in the UK.

anthropoid resembling a human. *A. pelvis* female pelvis in which the anteroposterior diameter exceeds the transverse diameter.

anthropology the study of human beings that focuses on origins, historical and cultural development, and races. *Cultural a.* that branch of anthropology that is concerned with individuals and their relationship to others and to their environment. *Medical a.* biocultural discipline concerned with both the biological and sociocultural aspects of human behaviour, and the ways in which the two interact to influence health and disease. *Physical a.* that branch of anthropology that concerns the physical and evolutionary characteristics of human beings.

anthropometry the science that deals with the comparative measurement of parts of the human body, such as height, weight, body fat, etc.

anti-D immunoglobulin anti-rhesus antibody which is given by intramuscular injection to a rhesus-negative woman within 72 hours of delivery of her infant or following termination of her pregnancy, miscarriage or invasive investigations such as amniocentesis, to prevent haemolytic disease of the newborn in the next pregnancy. Anti-D is also available to all rhesus-negative women as antenatal prophylaxis. *See* RHESUS FACTOR.

anti-inflammatory a drug that reduces or acts against inflammation. May belong to one of several groups.

antibacterial a substance that destroys or suppresses the growth of bacteria.

antibiotic substances (e.g., penicillin), produced by certain bacteria and fungi, that prevent the growth of, or destroy, other bacteria. *A. resistance* the evolution and survival, as a result of worldwide antibiotic misuse, of bacteria undergoing the process of natural selection, despite the use of antibiotics to which they were once sensitive.

antibody also known as immunoglobulin, an antibody is one of a group of these glycoprotein molecules found either on the cell surface of B lymphocytes (membrane antibody) where they act as antigen receptors, or produced and secreted by B lymphocytes that have been stimulated and transformed by an antigen into plasma cells. Secreted antibodies are found in blood, serum and in other body fluids and tissues. Antibodies react and combine with specific antigens during humoral immune responses, forming immune complexes. Antibodies are an important component of acquired (learned) immunity. There are five different types, or classes of antibody, each named by the abbreviation for immunoglobulin (Ig) and a letter of the alphabet, i.e., IgM, IgG, IgA, IgD, IgE. IgG (also called gamma-globulin) is the most abundant of the five classes of antibody and is the major immunoglobulin in the secondary humoral immune response.

anticholinergic a drug that inhibits the action of acetylcholine.

anticholinesterase an enzyme that inhibits the action of the enzyme acetylcholinesterase, thereby potentiating the action of acetylcholine at postsynaptic receptors in the parasympathetic nervous system, thus allowing return of normal muscle contraction.

anticoagulant a substance that prevents or delays the blood from clotting, e.g., warfarin. New anticoagulants are available and are becoming increasingly more common, e.g., rivaroxaban, dabigatran which require less frequent blood monitoring.

anticonvulsant a substance that will arrest or prevent convulsions. Anticonvulsant drugs such as phenytoin are used in the treatment of epilepsy and other conditions in which convulsions occur.

antidepressant one of a group of drugs which elevate mood, often diminish anxiety and increase coping behaviour. Tricyclic antidepressants and selective serotonin uptake inhibitors are the most commonly used in treatment of depression. These drugs are usually successful in relieving the symptoms of depression, but may take 2–3 weeks before any improvement is noted. Antidepressant drugs are not addictive, but abrupt withdrawal may result in physical symptoms and should be avoided. Monoamine oxidase inhibitors (MAOIs) are used in the treatment of panic disorders and bipolar depression.

anti-discriminatory practice the professional policies, practice and provisions that actively seek to reduce institutional discrimination experienced by individuals and groups, particularly on the grounds of age, race, gender, disability, social class or sexual orientation. Anti-discriminatory practice can utilize particular the Equalities Act 2010 to challenge discrimination.

antidiuretic a substance that reduces the volume of urine excreted. *A. hormone (ADH)* a hormone which is secreted by the posterior pituitary gland. Vasopressin.

antidote an agent that counteracts the effect of a poison.

antiembolic against embolism. Anti-embolic hose/stockings are worn to prevent the formation or decrease the risk of deep vein thrombosis, especially in patients after surgery or those confined to bed.

antiemetic a drug that prevents or overcomes nausea and vomiting.

antifungal a preparation effective in treating fungal infections.

antigen any substance, bacterial or otherwise, which in suitable conditions can stimulate the production of an immune response.

antihaemophilic *see* COAGULATION FACTOR CONCENTRATE.

antihistamine any one of a group of drugs which block the tissue receptors for histamine. They are used to treat allergic conditions, e.g., drug rashes, hay fever and serum sickness, and include promethazine.

antihypertensive 1. effective against hypertension. 2. an agent that reduces high blood pressure.

antimalarial against malaria. Drugs that are used both in the treatment of an attack and for prophylaxis. All visitors to malarial countries should take preventative antimalarial drugs. Expert advice should be sought regarding the appropriate drug and dose. *See* MALARIA.

antimetabolite one of a group of chemical compounds which prevent the effective utilization of the corresponding metabolite, and interfere with normal growth or cell mitosis if the process requires that metabolite.

antineoplastic effective against the multiplication of malignant cells.

antiperistalsis contrary contractions which propel the contents of the intestines backwards and upwards.

antiperspirant a substance applied to the body as a lotion, cream or spray to reduce sweating. Use can sometimes result in irritation especially if the skin is broken.

antiphospholipid syndrome (APS) also known as Hughes syndrome. An immune disorder causing increased risk of blood clots.

antipruritic an external application or drug that relieves itching.

antipyretic an agent that reduces fever.

antisepsis the prevention of infection by destroying or arresting the growth of harmful microorganisms.

antiseptic 1. preventing sepsis. 2. any substance that inhibits the growth of bacteria, in contrast to a germicide, which kills bacteria outright.

antiserum animal or human blood serum which contains antibodies to infective organisms or to their toxins. The serum donor must have previously been infected with the identified organism.

antisocial against society. *A. behaviour* in psychiatry, the refusal of an individual to accept the normal obligations and restraints imposed by the community upon its members.

antispasmodic any measure used to prevent or relieve the occurrence of muscle spasm.

antitoxin a substance produced by the body cells as a reaction to invasion by bacteria, which neutralizes their toxins. *See* IMMUNITY.

antitussive 1. effective against cough. 2. an agent that suppresses coughing.

antivenin an antitoxic serum to neutralize the poison injected by the bite of a snake or insect.

antiviral 1. acting against viruses. 2. a drug that is effective against viruses causing disease, e.g., aciclovir.

antrum a cavity in bone. *Mastoid a.* the tympanic antrum, which is an air-conditioning cavity in the mastoid portion of the temporal bone. *Maxillary a.* antrum of Highmore. The air sinus in the upper jawbone.

anuria cessation of the secretion of urine.

anus the extremity of the alimentary canal, through which the faeces are discharged. *Imperforate a.* one where there is no opening because of a congenital defect.

anxiety a chronic state of tension, which affects both mind and body. *A. neurosis see* NEUROSIS.

anxiolytic a substance, such as diazepam or pentobarbital, used for relief of anxiety. Anxiolytics may quickly cause dependence and are not suitable for long-term administration.

aorta the large artery rising out of the left ventricle of the heart and supplying blood to all the body. *Abdominal a.* that part of the artery lying in the abdomen. *Arch of the a.* the curve of the artery over the heart. *Thoracic a.* that part which passes through the chest.

aortic pertaining to the aorta. *A. incompetence* owing to previous inflammation the aortic valve has become fibrosed and is unable to close completely, thus allowing backward flow of blood (*a. regurgitation*) into the left ventricle during diastole. *A. stenosis* a narrowing of the aortic valve. *A. valve* the valve between the left ventricle of the heart and the ascending aorta, which prevents the backward flow of blood through the artery.

aortography radiographic examination of the aorta. A radio-opaque contrast medium is injected into the blood to render visible lesions of the aorta or its main branches.

APACHE abbreviation for Acute Physiology And Chronic Health Evaluation. A classification system for indicating severity of illness in intensive care patients.

apathy an appearance of indifference, with no response to stimuli or display of emotion.

aperient a drug that produces an action of the bowels. A laxative.

aperistalsis lack of peristaltic movement of the intestines.

Apert's syndrome *E. Apert, French paediatrician, 1868–1940.* A congenital abnormality in which there is fusion at birth of all the cranial sutures, in addition to syndactyly (webbed fingers).

apex the top or pointed end of a cone-shaped structure. *A. beat* the beat of the heart against the chest wall which can be felt during systole. *A. of the heart* the end closing the left ventricle. *A. of the lung* the extreme upper part of the organ.

Apgar score *V. Apgar, American anaesthetist, 1909–1974.* A system used in the assessment of the newborn: reflex irritability and colour. The Apgar score is assessed 1 minute after birth and again at 5 minutes. Most healthy infants score 9 at birth. A score below 7 would indicate cause for concern (*see* Table).

APEL *see* ACCREDITATION.

APH antepartum haemorrhage.

aphagia loss of the power to swallow.

aphakia absence of the lens of the eye. Aphacia.

aphasia a communication disorder owing to brain damage; characterized by complete or partial disturbance of language comprehension, formulation or expression. Partial disturbance is also called dysphasia. *Broca's a.* disorder in which verbal output is impaired, often owing to STROKE, and in which verbal communication may be affected as well. Speech is slow and laboured and writing is often impaired. *Developmental a.* a childhood failure to acquire normal language when deafness, learning difficulties, motor disability or severe emotional disturbance are not causes.

aphonia inability to produce sound. The cause may be organic disease of the larynx or may be purely functional.

aphrodisiac a drug which excites sexual desire.

Apgar score			
Sign	**Score**		
	0	*1*	*2*
Appearance	Blue/pale	Body pink, extremities blue	Pink
Pulse rate	Absent	Below 100	Above 100
Grimace	None	Grimace (on stimulation)	Cries
Activity	Limp	Some (flexion of extremities)	Active
Respiration	Absent	Weak cry, hypoventilation	Strong cry

aphthae small ulcers surrounded by erythema on the inside of the mouth (aphthous ulcers).

apical pertaining to the apex of a structure.

apicectomy excision of the root of a tooth. Root resection.

APL see ACCREDITATION.

aplasia incomplete development of an organ or tissue or absence of growth.

aplastic without power of development. *A. anaemia see* ANAEMIA.

apnoea cessation of respiration. *A. mattress* a mattress designed to sound an alarm if the infant lying on it ceases breathing. *A. monitor* designed to give an audible signal when a certain period of apnoea has occurred. *A. of prematurity* apnoeic periods occurring in the respiration of newborn infants in whom the respiratory centre is immature or depressed. *Cardiac a.* the temporary cessation of breathing caused by a reduction of the carbon dioxide tension in the blood, as seen in Cheyne–Stokes respiration. *Sleep a.* transient attacks of failure of autonomic control of respiration, becoming more pronounced during sleep.

apocrine pertaining to modified sweat glands that develop in hair follicles, such as are mainly found in the axillary, pubic and perineal areas.

aponeurosis a sheet of tendon-like tissue which connects some muscles to the parts that they move.

apophysis a prominence or excrescence, usually of a bone.

apoplexy a sudden fit of insensibility, usually caused by rupture of a cerebral blood vessel or its occlusion by a blood clot producing coma and paralysis of one side of the body. Rarely used term for a stroke.

apparition a hallucinatory vision, usually the phantom appearance of a person. A spectre.

appendectomy appendicectomy.

appendicectomy removal of the vermiform appendix.

appendicitis inflammation of the vermiform appendix.

appendix a supplementary or dependent part. *A. epiploicae* small tag-like structures of peritoneum containing fat, which are scattered over the surface of the large intestine, especially the transverse colon. *Vermiform a.* a worm-like tube with a blind end, projecting from the caecum in the right iliac region. It may be from 2.5 to 15 cm long.

apperception conscious reception and recognition of a sensory stimulus.

appetite the desire for food. It is stimulated by the sight, smell or thought of food, and accompanied by the flow of saliva in the mouth and gastric juice in the stomach. The stomach wall also receives an extra blood supply in preparation for its digestive activity. Appetite is psychological, dependent on memory and associations, as compared with hunger, which is physiologically aroused by the body's need for food. Appetite can be discouraged by unattractive food, surroundings or company, and by emotional states such as anxiety, irritation, anger and fear.

apposition the bringing into contact of two structures, e.g., fragments of bone in setting a fracture.

appraisal a formal review, usually annually, of a health care professional's performance by a trained appraiser in order to provide feedback on past performance, identifying progress made and together agreeing future goals and objectives.

apprehension a feeling of dread or fear.

approved name the non-proprietary or generic name for a drug. The approved name should always be used in prescribing except where the bio-availability may vary between brands.

apraxia the inability to perform correct movements because of a brain lesion and not because of sensory impairment or loss of muscle power in the limbs. *Oral a.* inability to perform volitional movements of the tongue and lips in the absence of paralysis or paresis. Involuntary movements may, however, be observed, e.g., patients may purse their lips in order to blow out a match.

aptitude the natural ability or capacity to acquire mental and physical skills. *A. test* the evaluation of a person's ability for learning certain skills or carrying out specific tasks.

apyrexia the absence of fever.

aqua [L.] *water. A. destillata* distilled water.

aqueduct a canal for the passage of fluid. *A. of Sylvius* the canal connecting the third and fourth ventricles of the brain.

aqueous watery. *A. humour* the fluid filling the anterior and posterior chambers of the eye.

Arachis a genus of leguminous plants used in various preparations such as earwax softeners and skin medications.

arachnodactyly abnormally long and thin fingers and toes. A congenital condition.

arachnoid 1. resembling a spider's web. 2. a web-like membrane covering the central nervous system between the dura and pia mater.

arborization the branching terminations of many nerve fibres and processes.

arbovirus one of a large group of viruses transmitted by insect vectors (arthropod-borne), e.g., mosquitoes, sandflies or ticks. The diseases caused include many types of encephalitis, also yellow, dengue, sandfly and Rift Valley fevers.

arcus [L.] *bow, arch. A. senilis* an opaque circle appearing round the edge of the cornea in old age.

ARDS acute respiratory distress syndrome.

areola 1. a space in connective tissue. 2. a ring of pigmentation, e.g., that surrounding the nipple.

arginase an enzyme of the liver that splits arginine into urea and ornithine.

arginine an essential amino acid produced by the digestion of protein. It forms a link in the excretion of nitrogen, being hydrolysed by the enzyme arginase.

Argyll Robertson pupil *D. Argyll Robertson, British ophthalmologist, 1837–1909. See* PUPIL.

Arnold–Chiari malformation *J. Arnold, German pathologist, 1835–1915; H. Chiari, German pathologist, 1851–1916.* Herniation of the cerebellum and elongation of the medulla oblongata; occurs in hydrocephalus associated with spina bifida. Also known as CHIARI MALFORMATION.

aromatherapy the therapeutic use of specially prepared essential or aromatic oils obtained from the different parts of plants, including the flowers, leaves, seeds, wood, roots and bark. The oils may be diluted for use in massage, baths or infusions.

arousal a state of alertness and increased response to stimuli.

arrector pili a small muscle attached to the hair follicle of the skin. When contracted it causes the hair to become erect, producing the appearance known as gooseflesh.

arrest a cessation or stopping. *Cardiac a.* cessation of ventricular contractions. *Developmental a.* discontinuation of a child's mental or physical development at a certain stage. *Respiratory a.* cessation of breathing. *See* Appendix 2.

arrhenoblastoma a rare ovarian tumour that secretes male hormones and causes virilization.

arrhythmia variation from the normal rhythm, e.g., in the heart's action. *Sinus a.* an abnormal pulse rhythm due to disturbance of the sinoatrial node, causing quickening of the heart on inspiration and slowing on expiration.

art therapy the use of the creative arts as a medium to encourage patients to express their feelings when unable to do so verbally.

artefact something that is man-made or introduced artificially.

arterial blood gases (ABGs) normally present in arterial blood include oxygen, carbon dioxide and nitrogen. Measurements of the partial pressures of oxygen and carbon dioxide together with the blood's pH provide important information on the oxygen saturation of the haemoglobin and acid–base state of the blood indicating the adequacy of ventilation in critical care situations.

arteriectomy the removal of a portion of artery wall, usually followed by anastomosis or a replacement graft. *See* ARTERIOPLASTY.

arteriography radiography of arteries after the injection of a radio-opaque contrast medium.

arterioplasty the reconstruction of an artery by means of replacement or plastic surgery.

arteriosclerosis a gradual loss of elasticity in the walls of arteries due to thickening and calcification. It is accompanied by high blood pressure, and precedes the degeneration of internal organs associated with old age or chronic disease.

arteriotomy an incision or puncture into an artery.

arteriovenous both arterial and venous; pertaining to both artery and vein, e.g., an arteriovenous aneurysm, fistula or shunt for haemodialysis.

arteritis inflammation of an artery. *Giant cell a.* a variety of polyarteritis resulting in partial or complete occlusion of a number of arteries. The carotid arteries are often involved. *Temporal a.* occlusion of the extracranial arteries, particularly the carotid arteries.

artery a tube of muscle and elastic fibres, lined with endothelium, which distributes blood from the heart to the capillaries throughout the body.

arthralgia neuralgic pains in a joint.

arthrectomy excision of a joint.

arthritis inflammation of one or more joints. Movement in the joint is restricted, with pain and swelling. Arthritis and the rheumatic diseases in general constitute the major cause of chronic disability in the UK. *Acute rheumatic a.* rheumatic fever. *Osteoa.* (DJD) a degenerative condition attacking the articular cartilage and aggravated by an impaired blood supply, previous injury or overweight, mainly affecting weight-bearing joints and causing pain. *Rheumatoid a.* a chronic inflammation, usually of unknown origin. The disease is progressive and incapacitating, owing to the resulting ankylosis and deformity of the bones. Usually affects the elderly. A juvenile form is known as STILL'S DISEASE.

arthroclasia the breaking down of adhesions in a joint to produce freer movement.

arthrodesis the fixation of a movable joint by surgical operation.

arthrography the examination of a joint by means of X-rays. An opaque contrast medium may be used.

arthrogryposis 1. a congenital abnormality in which fibrous ankylosis of some or all of the joints in the limbs occurs. 2. a tetanus spasm.

arthroplasty plastic surgery for the reorganization of a joint. *Charnley's a. see* MCKEE FARRAR a. *Cup a.* reconstruction of the articular surface, which is then covered by a vitallium cup. *Excision a.* excision of the joint surfaces affected, so that the gap thus formed then fills with fibrous tissue or muscle. *Girdlestone a.* an excision arthroplasty of the hip. *McKee Farrar a.* replacement of both the head and the socket of the femur; *Charnley's a.* is similar. *Replacement a.* partial removal of the head of the femur and its replacement by a metal prosthesis.

arthroscope an endoscope for examining the interior of a joint.

arthroscopy keyhole surgery used to diagnose and treat joint problems.

articular pertaining to a joint.

articulation 1. a junction of two or more bones. 2. the enunciation of words.

artificial not natural. *A. feeding* 1. the giving of food other than by placing it directly in the mouth. It may be provided via the mouth, using an oesophageal tube; the food may be introduced into the stomach through a fine tube via the nostril (the nasal route); an opening through the abdominal wall into the stomach (i.e., a gastrostomy) may allow direct introduction; or food may be injected intravenously (*see* PARENTERAL). 2. in reference to the feeding of infants, giving food other than human milk. *A. insemination* the insertion of sperm into the uterus by means of syringe and cannula instead of coitus. The husband's, partner's or donor semen may be used. *A. kidney* a dialysis machine to remove unwanted waste materials from the patient with acute or chronic renal failure. *See* HAEMODIALYSIS. *A. respiration* a means of resuscitation from asphyxia. *A. tears* sterile solutions designed to maintain the moisture of the cornea when the latter is abnormally dry due to inadequate tear production. Methylcellulose is a common ingredient.

arytenoid resembling the mouth of a pitcher. *A. cartilages* two cartilages of the larynx; their function is to regulate the tension of the vocal cords attached to them.

asbestos a fibrous non-combustible silicate of magnesium and calcium that is a good non-conductor of heat. There are three types of asbestos fibre—white, brown and blue—that were widely used in the building industry. White fibre was the most commonly used and blue and brown fibres the most dangerous to health. In many countries there are now strict regulations controlling the use of asbestos (which has declined), including its removal from buildings. Contact with asbestos over a prolonged period may result in asbestosis, bronchial and laryngeal cancer and mesothelioma.

asbestosis a form of pneumoconiosis (chronic lung disease), due to the inhalation of asbestos fibres causing scarring of the lung tissue. It results in breathlessness and leads to respiratory failure. It may be latent for many years. *See* MESOTHELIOMA.

ascariasis the condition in which roundworms are found in the gastrointestinal tract. Treatment is with anthelmintic drugs to eliminate the infestation.

ascites free fluid in the peritoneal cavity. It may be the result of local inflammation or venous obstruction, or be part of a generalized oedema.

ascorbic acid vitamin C. This acid is found in many vegetables and fruits and is an essential dietary constituent for humans. Vitamin C is destroyed by heat and deteriorates during storage. It is necessary for connective tissue and collagen fibre synthesis and promotes the healing of wounds. Deficiency causes scurvy.

asepsis freedom from pathogenic microorganisms.

aseptic free from sepsis. *A. technique* a method of carrying out sterile procedures so that there is the minimum risk of introducing infection. Achieved by the sterility of equipment and a non-touch technique.

asexual without sex. *A. reproduction* the production of new individuals without sexual union, e.g., by cell division or budding.

asparaginase an enzyme that catalyses the deamination of asparagine; used as an antineoplastic agent against cancers, e.g., acute lymphocytic leukaemia, in which the malignant cells require exogenous asparagine for protein synthesis.

aspartame a synthetic compound of two amino acids (L-aspartyl-L-phenylalanine methyl ester) used as a low-calorie sweetener. It is 180 times as sweet as sucrose (table sugar); the amount equal in sweetness to a teaspoon of sugar contains 0.1 calorie (4.2 J). Aspartame does not promote the formation of dental caries. It should be avoided by patients with phenylketonuria.

aspartate transaminase (AST) an enzyme released when the liver or muscles are damaged. Levels of AST are measured as markers of liver health.

aspect that part of a surface facing in a particular direction. *Dorsal a.* that facing and seen from the back. *Ventral a.* that facing and seen from the front.

aspergillosis a bronchopulmonary disease in which the mucous membrane is attacked by the fungus *Aspergillus*.

Aspergillus a genus of fungi. *A. fumigatus* a common cause of aspergillosis, found in soil and manure.

aspermia absence of sperm.

asphyxia a deficiency of oxygen in the blood and an increase in carbon dioxide in the blood and tissues. Symptoms include irregular and disturbed respirations, or a complete absence of breathing, and pallor or cyanosis. Asphyxia may occur whenever there is an interruption in the normal exchange of oxygen and carbon dioxide between the lungs and the outside air. Common causes are drowning, electric shock, lodging of a foreign body in the air passages, inhalation of smoke and poisonous gases and trauma to or disease of the lungs or air passages. Treatment includes immediate remedy of the situation (*see* RESPIRATION (ARTIFICIAL) and Appendix 2) and removal of the underlying cause whenever possible.

aspiration 1. the act of inhaling. 2. the drawing off of fluid from a cavity by means of suction.

assault unlawful personal attack or trespass upon another person including threatening words.

assay a quantitative examination to determine the amount of a particular constituent of a mixture, or of the biological or pharmaceutical potency of a drug.

assent agreement to undergo medical care and treatment that is obtained from an adult or child who is legally incompetent to consent.

assertiveness a form of behaviour characterized by a confident declaration or affirmation of a statement without need of proof. To assert oneself is to compel recognition of one's rights or position without either aggressively transgressing the rights of another and assuming a position of dominance, or submissively permitting another to deny one's rights or rightful position. *A. training* instruction and practice in techniques for dealing with interpersonal conflicts and threatening situations in an assertive manner, avoiding the extremes of aggressive and submissive behaviour.

assessment 1. the critical analysis and valuation or judgement of the status or quality of a particular condition, situation or other subject of appraisal. In the nursing process, assessment involves the gathering of information about the health status of the patient/client, analysis and synthesis of the data, and the making of a clinical nursing judgement. The outcome of the nursing assessment is the establishment of a nursing DIAGNOSIS, the identification of the nursing problems and establishing a nursing care plan. 2. an examination set by an examining authority to test a candidate's skills and knowledge.

assimilation the process of transforming food so that it can be absorbed and utilized as nourishment by the tissues of the body.

association coordination of function of similar parts. *A. fibres* nerve fibres linking different areas of the brain. *A. of ideas* a mental impression in which a thought or any sensory impulse will call to mind another object or idea connected in some way with the former. *Free a.* a method employed in psychoanalysis in which the patient is encouraged to express freely whatever comes to mind. By this method material that is in the unconscious can be recalled.

associative play a form of play in which a group of children participate in similar activities without formal organization or direction.

asthenia lack of energy or strength. Debility. Loss of tone.

asthenic description of a type of body build: a pale, lean, narrowly built person with poor muscle development.

asthenopia eye strain likely to arise in long-sighted people when continual effort of accommodation is required for close work.

asthma paroxysmal dyspnoea characterized by wheezing and difficulty in expiration. The illness often commences in childhood but can commence at any age and in about half of the children affected it may be outgrown. *Bronchial a.* attacks of dyspnoea in which there is wheezing and difficulty in expiration due to muscular spasm of the bronchi. The attacks may be precipitated by hypersensitivity to foreign substances, air pollution, exertion or infection, or associated with emotional upsets. There is often a family history of asthma or other allergic condition. Management involves avoidance of known allergens and treatment is with bronchodilators with or without corticosteroids, usually via an aerosol. Other drug therapies used include sodium cromoglycate useful in preventing exercise-induced asthma and inhaled anticholinergic drugs may also be used to assist bronchodilation. An asthmatic person with an acute attack that does not respond to initial drug therapy should be referred to hospital for immediate assessment and treatment. *Cardiac a.* attacks of dyspnoea and palpitation, arising most often at night, associated with left-sided heart failure and pulmonary congestion. Treatment is with diuretic therapy.

astigmatism inequality of the refractive power of an eye, due to curvature of its corneal meridians. The curve across the front of the eye from side to side is not quite the same as the curve from above downwards. The focus on the retina is then not a point but a diffuse and indistinct area. May be congenital or acquired.

astringent an agent causing contraction of organic tissues, thereby checking secretions, e.g., silver nitrate.

astrocytoma a malignant tumour of the brain or spinal cord. It is slow-growing. A glioma.

asymmetry inequality in size or shape of two normally similar structures or of two halves of a structure normally the same.

asymptomatic without symptoms.

asynergy lack of coordination of structures which normally act in harmony.

asystole absence of heartbeat. Cardiac arrest.

at risk whereby an individual or population may be vulnerable to a particular disease, hazard or injury. At risk situations are those involving possible problems that may be preventable with appropriate intervention, or, if they should occur, treatment.

ataraxia a state of detached serenity with depression of mental faculties or impairment of consciousness.

ataxia, ataxy failure of muscle coordination resulting in irregular jerky movements, and unsteadiness in standing and walking from a disorder of the controlling mechanisms in the brain, or from inadequate input to the brain from joints and muscles. *Hereditary a.* Friedreich's ataxia.

atelectasis a collapsed or airless state of the lung, which may be acute or chronic and may involve all or part of the lung: (a) from imperfect expansion of pulmonary alveoli at birth (*congenital a.*); (b) as the result of disease or injury.

atheroma an abnormal mass of fatty or lipid material with a fibrous covering, existing as a discrete, raised plaque within the intima of an artery.

atherosclerosis a condition in which the fatty degenerative changes of atheroma are accompanied by arteriosclerosis, a narrowing and hardening of the vessels.

athetosis a recurring series of slow, writhing movements of the hands, usually affecting people with cerebral palsy.

Athlete's foot a fungal infection between the toes, easily transmitted to other people. *See* TINEA.

atlas the first cervical vertebra, articulating with the occipital bone of the skull.

atmosphere 1. the gases that surround the earth, extending to an altitude of 16 km. 2. the air or climate of a particular place, e.g., a smoking atmosphere. 3. mental or moral environment, tone or mood.

atomizer an instrument by which a liquid is divided to form a fine spray or vapour (nebulizer).

atony lack of tone, e.g., in the muscle detrusor of the bladder resulting in incontinence.

atopy a state of hypersensitivity to certain antigens. There is an inherited tendency that includes asthma, eczema and hay fever.

ATP adenosine triphosphate.

atresia absence of a natural opening or tubular structure, e.g., of the anus or vagina; usually a congenital malformation.

atrial relating to the atrium. *A. fibrillation* overstimulation of the atrial walls so that many areas of excitation arise and the atrioventricular node is bombarded with impulses, many of which it cannot transmit, resulting in a highly irregular pulse. *A. flutter* rapid regular action of the atria. The atrioventricular node transmits alternative impulses or one in three or four. The atrial rate is usually about 300 beats per minute. *A. septal defect* the non-closure of the foramen ovale at the time of birth, giving rise to a congenital heart defect.

atrioventricular pertaining to the atrium and ventricle. *A. bundle see* BUNDLE OF HIS. *A. node* a node of neurogenic tissue situated between the atrium and ventricle and transmitting

impulses. *A. valves* the bicuspid and tricuspid valve on the left and right sides of the heart, respectively.

atrium *pl.* atria. 1. a cavity, entrance or passage. 2. one of the two upper chambers of the heart. Formerly called auricle.

atrophy wasting of any part of the body, owing to degeneration of the cells, from disuse, or lack of nourishment or nerve supply. *Progressive muscular a.* a rare form of motor neurone disease with degeneration of the lower motor neurones with wasting of muscle tissue.

atropine an alkaloid which inhibits respiratory and gastric secretions, relaxes muscle spasm and dilates the pupil.

attack an episode or onset of illness. *A. rate* number of cases of a disease in a particular group, e.g., a school, over a given period, related to the population of that group. *Transient ischaemic a.* brief attack (a few hours or less) of cerebral dysfunction of vascular origin, with STROKE-like symptoms, without lasting neurological deficit.

attention deficit syndrome a disorder of childhood characterized by marked failure of attention, impulsiveness and increased motor activity. Affects more boys than girls. Treatment involves medication, behaviour therapy and social support. Also known as attention deficit hyperactivity disorder (ADHD).

attenuation a bacteriological process by which organisms are rendered less virulent by culture in artificial media through many generations, exposure to light, air, etc.; it is used for vaccine preparations.

attitude 1. a posture or position of the body; in obstetrics, the relation of the various parts of the fetal body to one another. 2. a pattern of mental views established by cumulative prior experience.

atypical irregular; not conforming to type.

audiogram a graph produced by an audiometer.

audiologist an allied health professional specializing in audiology, who provides services that include: (a) evaluation of hearing function to detect hearing impairment and, if there is a hearing disorder, to determine the anatomical site involved and the cause of the disorder; (b) selection of appropriate hearing aids; and (c) training in lip reading, hearing aid use and maintenance of normal speech.

audiology the science concerned with the sense of hearing, especially the evaluation and measurement of impaired hearing and the rehabilitation of those with impaired hearing.

audiometer an instrument for testing hearing, whereby the threshold of the patient's hearing can be measured.

audit systematic review and evaluation of records and other data to determine the quality of the services or products provided in a given situation. *A. trail* the process in which careful documentation of the research process makes it possible for students and other researchers to understand how any particular finding was reached. *Medical a.* the systematic critical analysis of the quality of medical treatment and care, including the procedures for diagnosis and treatment, the use of resources, outcomes and the resultant quality of life for the patient. *Nursing a.* an evaluation of structure, process and outcome as a measurement of the quality of nursing care. *Concurrent audits* are conducted at the time the care is being provided to clients/patients. They may be conducted by means of observation and interview of clients/patients, review of open charts, or conferences with groups of consumers and providers of nursing care. *Retrospective audits* are conducted after the patient's discharge. Methods include the study of closed patient's charts and nursing care plans, questionnaires,

interviews and surveys of patients and families.

auditory relating to the ear or to the sense of hearing.

aura the premonition, peculiar to an individual, which often precedes an epileptic fit.

aural referring to the ear.

auricle 1. the external portion of the ear. 2. obsolete term for the atrium.

auriscope an instrument for examining the drum of the ear. An otoscope.

auscultation examining the internal organs by listening to the sounds that they give out. In *direct* or *immediate a.* the ear is placed directly against the body. In *mediate a.* a stethoscope is used.

autism neurodevelopment disorder characterized by impaired social interactions, verbal and non-verbal communication and restricted and repetitive behaviour. *Infantile a.* failure of a child to relate to people and situations, leading to complete withdrawal into a world of private fantasies.

autistic pertaining to autism.

autistic spectrum disorder also known as autism spectrum disorder. A range of conditions which encompass the previous diagnosis of autism, Asperger's syndrome, pervasive developmental disorder and childhood disintegrative disorder.

autoagglutination 1. clumping or agglutination of cells by an individual's own serum, as in autohaemagglutination. Autoagglutination occurring at low temperatures is called cold agglutination. 2. agglutination of particulate antigens, e.g., bacteria, in the absence of specific antigens.

autoantibody an antibody formed in response to and reacting against the individual's own tissues.

autoantigen a tissue constituent that stimulates production of autoantibodies in the organism in which it occurs.

autoclave a steam-heated sterilizing apparatus in which the temperature is raised by reducing the air pressure inside; steam is injected under pressure, bringing about efficient sterilization of instruments and dishes treated in this way.

autodigestion dissolution of tissue by its own secretions. Autolysis.

autoeroticism sexual pleasure derived from self-stimulation of erogenous zones (the mouth, the anus, the genitals and the skin). *See* MASTURBATION.

autogenic therapy a complementary therapy combining self-hypnosis and relaxation.

autogenous generated within the body and not acquired from external sources.

autograft the transfer of skin or other tissue from one part of the body to another to repair some deficiency.

autoimmune disease condition in which the body develops antibodies to its own tissues, e.g., in autoimmune thyroiditis (Hashimoto's disease).

autoimmunization the formation of antibodies against the individual's own tissue.

autoinfection self-infection, transferred from one part of the body to another by fingers, towels, etc.

autoinoculation inoculation with a microorganism from the body itself.

autointoxication poisoning by toxins generated within the body itself.

autologous related to self; belonging to the same organism. *A. blood transfusion (ABT)* the patient donates blood before elective surgery for transfusion postoperatively. ABT may also be obtained as a blood salvage procedure during operation or postoperatively. Avoids cross-matching, compatibility and transfusion infection problems.

autolysis a breaking up of living tissues, e.g., as may occur if pancreatic ferments escape into surrounding tissues. It also occurs after death.

automated auditory brainstem response (AABR) one of two hearing tests in the Newborn Hearing Screening Programme that records brain activity in response to clicking sounds via sensors placed on the infant's head. Those infants who fail to respond to this test are referred for a full auditory diagnostic assessment.

automatic performed without the influence of the will.

automatism performance of non-reflex acts without apparent volition, and of which the patient may have no memory afterwards, as in somnambulism. *Post-epileptic a.* automatic acts following an epileptic fit.

autonomic self-governing. *A. nervous system* the sympathetic and parasympathetic nerves that control involuntary muscles and glandular secretion, over which there is no conscious control.

autonomy the right of personal freedom of action, which is regarded as one of the hallmarks of a profession.

autoplasty 1. replacement of missing tissue by grafting a healthy section from another part of the body. 2. in psychoanalysis, instinctive modification within the psychic systems in adaptation to reality.

autopsy postmortem examination of a body to determine the cause of death.

autosome any chromosome other than the sex chromosomes. In humans there are 22 pairs of autosomes and one pair of sex chromosomes.

autosuggestion suggestion arising in one's self. Uncritical acceptance of an idea arising in the individual's own mind.

autotransfusion reinfusion of a patient's own blood.

autotransplantation transfer of tissue from one part of the body to another part.

avascular not vascular. Bloodless. *A. necrosis* death of bone owing to deficient blood supply, usually following an injury.

average 1. the value or score that is typical of a group. The result is obtained by adding several amounts together and then dividing the total by the number of amounts. Sometimes also referred to as the mean. 2. A colloquial term used to mean 'usual' or 'ordinary'.

aversion intense dislike. *A. therapy* a method of treating addictions by associating the craving for what is addictive with painful or unpleasant stimuli. It is rarely used.

avian influenza commonly known as bird flu, a disease of poultry and other birds caused by strains of the influenza virus that can occasionally infect people who are in close contact with infected birds. The severity of the disease depends upon the strain of the virus involved; the strain caused by the H5N1 virus is particularly virulent. At the present time, normal influenza vaccines do not protect against the H5N1 virus. *See* ORTHOMYXOVIRUS and swine influenza.

aviation medicine the medical speciality concerned with the effects of air travel and with the causes and treatment of health problems that may occur in flight.

avitaminosis a condition resulting from an insufficiency of vitamins in the diet. A deficiency disease.

avoidance a conscious or unconscious defence mechanism whereby an individual seeks to escape or avoid certain situations, feelings or conflicts.

avulsion the tearing away of one part from another. *Phrenic a.* a tearing away of the phrenic nerve. It paralyses the diaphragm on the affected side.

axilla an armpit.

axiom a statement or proposition that can be accepted without evidence as it is obviously true.

axis 1. a line through the centre of a structure. 2. the second cervical vertebra. *See* PLANES.

axon the process of a nerve cell along which electrical impulses travel. The nerve fibre.

axonotmesis nerve injury characterized by disruption of the axon and myelin sheath but with preservation of the connective tissue fragments, resulting in degeneration of the axon distal to the injury site; regeneration of the axon is spontaneous.

azoospermia absence of spermatozoa in the semen.

azygos something that is unpaired.

azygous vein an unpaired vein that ascends the posterior mediastinum and enters the superior vena cava.

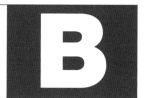

Ba symbol for *barium*.

Babinski's reflex or sign *J.F.F. Babinski, French neurologist, 1857–1932.* On stroking the sole of the foot, the great toe bends upwards instead of downwards (dorsal instead of plantar flexion). Present in disease or injury to the spinal cord or brain. Babies who have not walked react in the same way, but normal flexion develops later.

baby an infant or very young child. *B. blues* the transient feelings of unhappiness and tearfulness that affect many women after the birth of their baby. *B. Friendly Initiative (BFI)* part of a global campaign by the United Nations Children's Fund (UNICEF) to ensure that all mothers are facilitated in breast feeding to enable babies to benefit from the health and social advantages. *Battered b.* one suffering from the result of continued violence; extensive bruising, fractures of limbs, rib and skull, or an internal trauma may be found. *See* ABUSE. *Blue b.* one suffering from cyanosis at birth as a result of atelectasis or congenital heart malformation.

Bach flower remedies a system of complementary medicine, devised by Dr Edward Bach and based on homeopathic principles. Flower remedies can be used to treat emotional and psychological disorders. There are 38 flower remedies. *See also* HOMEOPATHY.

bacillaemia the presence of bacilli in the blood.

bacilluria the presence of bacilli in the urine.

Bacillus a genus of aerobic, spore-bearing gram-positive bacteria. *B. anthracis* the causative agent of ANTHRAX.

bacillus loosely, the cause of any bacterial infection by a rod-shaped microorganism, e.g., *Escherichia coli*, the colon bacillus.

back dorsum. Posterior trunk from neck to pelvis. *B. bone* the vertebral column. *B. slab* plaster or plastic splint in which a limb is supported. *Hunch b.* kyphosis.

backache any pain in the back, usually the lower part. The pain is often dull and continuous, but sometimes sharp and throbbing. Backache, or LUMBAGO, is one of the most common ailments and can be caused by a variety of disorders. In most cases, the pain is not caused by anything serious and will usually get better over time.

bacteraemia the presence of bacteria in the bloodstream.

bacteria a general name given to minute organisms which may live on organic matter. There are many species, only some of which are pathogenic to humans, animals and plants. Each bacterium consists of a single cell and, given favourable conditions, multiplies by subdivision. Bacteria are classified according to their shape (a) *bacilli*, rod-shaped and (b) *cocci*, spherical subdivided into (i) *streptococci*, in chains; (ii) *staphylococci*, in groups; (iii) diplococci, in pairs; (c) *spirilla, spiro-chaetes,* spiral. *Pathogenic b.* those whose growth in the body gives rise to disease, either by destruction of tissue or by formation of toxins, which circulate in the blood. Pathogenic bacteria thrive on organic matter in the presence of warmth and moisture.

bacterial pertaining to bacteria. *B. arthritis see* SEPTIC ARTHRITIS. *B. vaginosis* a condition in which the balance of bacteria in the vagina becomes disrupted resulting in an unusual vaginal discharge.

bactericidal capable of killing bacteria, e.g., disinfectants, great heat, intense cold or sunlight.

bacteriologist one who is qualified in the science of bacteriology.

bacteriology the scientific study of bacteria.

bacteriolysin an antibody produced in the blood to assist in the destruction of bacteria. The action is specific.

bacteriolysis the dissolution of bacteria by a bacteriolytic agent.

bacteriophage a virus that only infects bacteria. Many strains exist, some of which are used for identifying types of staphylococci and salmonellae.

bacteriostat an agent that inhibits the growth of bacteria.

bacteriostatic inhibiting the growth of bacteria.

bag a sac or pouch. *B. of waters* the membranes enclosing the AMNIOTIC (FLUID) and the developing fetus in utero. *Ambu b.* is a bag valve mask (BVM). It is a hand-held device used to provide positive pressure ventilation to a patient who is not breathing or who is breathing inadequately. Use of the Ambu bag to ventilate a patient is frequently called 'bagging'. *Colostomy b.* a receptacle worn over the stoma by the patient, to receive the faecal discharge. *Douglas b.* a receptacle for the collection of expired air, permitting measurement of respiratory gases. *Ileostomy b.* a receptacle worn over the stoma for the collection of faecal material after ILEOSTOMY. *Politizer b.* a soft bag of rubber for inflating the pharyngotympanic (Eustachian) tube. *Urine b.* a receptacle used for urine by patients with urinary incontinence.

Baker's cyst *see* POPLITEAL CYST.

balance the ability to remain upright and to move without falling over. In physiological terms the harmonious relationship between parts and organs of the body and their functions or between substances in the body. *See* ACID–BASE BALANCE. *B. of probabilities* the standard of proof required in civil proceedings.

balanced diet a varied diet that contains all the nutritional elements in the correct quantities required for growth and repair of body tissues.

balanced salt solution (BSS) a solution that is made to a physiological pH with appropriate concentrations of salts and electrolytes. Used during intraocular surgery to replace intraocular fluids.

balanitis inflammation of the glans penis and of the prepuce, usually associated with phimosis. Balanoposthitis.

baldness absence of hair, especially from the scalp. Alopecia.

ballottement [Fr.] manoeuvre used in physical examination to estimate the size of an organ not near the surface, particularly in the presence of ascites.

bandage 1. a strip or roll of gauze or other material for wrapping or binding any part of the body. 2. to cover by wrapping with such material. Bandages may be used to stop the flow of blood, to provide a safeguard against contamination, or to hold a dressing in place. They may also be used to hold a splint in position or otherwise immobilize an injured part of the body to prevent further injury and to facilitate healing.

banding placing a band round a vessel to restrict the flow from it.

bank an institution offering services, or a store of donated human tissues for use in the future by other individuals, e.g., *blood b., human milk b., sperm b. Nurse b.* a group of nurses who are known to the employing authority and available for employment on an on-call basis.

Bankhart's operation *A.S.B. Bankhart, British orthopaedic surgeon, 1879–1951.* An operation to repair a defect in the glenoid cavity that causes repeated dislocation of the shoulder joint.

barbiturates a group of sedative and hypnotic drugs derived from barbituric acid. Prolonged use may lead to addiction.

bariatrics a branch of medicine, surgery and dietetics that deals with obesity, its effects, treatment and control. *See* OBESITY.

barium *symbol Ba.* A soft silvery metallic element. *B. enema* a rarely used procedure where a form of liquid barium is passed into the bowel to enable abnormalities to be seen. *B. sulphate* a heavy mineral salt that is comparatively impermeable to X-rays and can therefore be used as a contrast medium, given as a meal or as an enema. Used to demonstrate abnormality in the stomach or intestines, and to show peristaltic movement. *B. sulphide* the chief constituent of depilatory preparations, i.e., those which remove hair.

baroreceptors the sensory branches of the glossopharyngeal and vagus nerves that influence the blood pressure. The receptors are situated in the walls of the carotid sinus and aortic arch.

barotrauma injury due to pressure, such as to structures of the ear, owing to differences between atmospheric and intratympanic pressures. May affect air travellers or scuba divers.

Barr body *M.L. Barr, Canadian anatomist, 1908–1995.* Small, dark-staining area underneath the nuclear membrane of female cells. Represents an inactive X chromosome.

Barré–Guillain syndrome *see* GUILLAIN–BARRÉ SYNDROME.

barrier an obstruction. *B. contraceptive* mechanical barrier preventing the sperm from entering the cervical canal, e.g., diaphragm, sheath. *B. cream* a cream used to protect the skin against irritant substances and water, e.g., hand cream. *B. nursing* a method of preventing the spread of infection from one patient to other patients and/or staff. This normally involves nursing the patient in a separate room or cubicle and the use of isolation techniques. *See* Appendix 11. *Blood–brain b.* the selective barrier which separates the circulating blood from the cerebrospinal fluid. *Placental b.* semipermeable membrane between maternal and fetal blood. *Protective b.* radiation-absorbing shield, e.g., lead, concrete, to protect the body against ionizing radiations. *Reverse b. nursing* an isolation technique used to prevent the transmission of infection to the patient who may be especially vulnerable, e.g., the immunosuppressed patient. *See* UNIVERSAL PRECAUTIONS.

Bartholin's glands *C.T. Bartholin, Danish anatomist, 1655–1738.* Two glands situated in the labia majora, with ducts opening inside the vulva. *B. cyst* a small fluid-filled sac which, if it becomes infected, will lead to pyrexia, pain and discomfort.

basal 1. fundamental. 2. referring to a base. *B. cell carcinoma* a common type of skin cancer. Generally occurs in later life, most usually on the face, scalp or neck and is caused by skin damage from the ultraviolet irradiation in sunlight over many years. Without treatment, the carcinoma invades and destroys the surrounding tissues but rarely invades other parts of the body. Treatment is usually with surgery. People who have had a basal cell carcinoma should be alert to any changes in their skin as they may develop new tumours. The risk of further tumours is also further reduced by avoiding overexposure to sunlight, wearing protective clothing and a sunscreen preparation on the skin. Also known as a rodent ulcer or BCC. *B. ganglia* the collections of nerve cells or grey matter in the base of the cerebrum. They consist of the caudate nucleus and putamen, forming the corpus striatum, and the globus pallidus. Such cells are concerned with modifying and coordinating voluntary muscle movements. *B. metabolic rate (BMR)* an indirect method of estimating the rate of metabolism in the body by measuring the oxygen intake and carbon dioxide output on breathing. The age, sex, weight and size of the patient have to be taken into account.

base 1. the lowest part or foundation. 2. the main constituent of a compound. 3. an alkali or other substance that can unite with an acid to form a salt.

basement membrane a thin layer of modified connective tissue supporting layers of cells, found at the base of the epidermis and underlying mucous membranes.

basic life support (BLS) a protocol of resuscitation of a collapsed patient which comprises initial assessment, airway maintenance, expired air ventilation and chest compression. BLS implies that no equipment is available to be used. Its purpose is to maintain adequate ventilation and circulation until further means are available to reverse the underlying condition. *See* Appendix 2 Resuscitation.

basilar situated at the base. *B. artery* midline artery at the base of the skull, formed by the junction of the vertebral arteries.

basilic prominent. *B. vein* a large vein on the inner side of the arm.

basophil adj. *basophilic.* 1. any structure, cell or histological element staining readily with basic dyes. 2. a granular leukocyte with an irregularly shaped, relatively pale-staining nucleus that is partially constricted into two lobes, and with cytoplasm

containing coarse bluish-black granules of variable size. 3. a beta cell of the adenohypophysis.

basophilia 1. an affinity of cells or tissues for basic dyes. 2. the reaction of relatively immature erythrocytes to basic dyes whereby the stained cells appear blue, grey or greyish-blue, or bluish granules appear. 3. abnormal increase of basophilic leukocytes in the blood. 4. basophilic leukocytosis.

bath 1. a medium, e.g., water, vapour, sand or mud, with which the body is washed or in which the body is wholly or partially immersed for therapeutic or cleansing purposes; application of such a medium to the body. 2. the equipment or apparatus in which a body or object may be immersed. *Bed b.* washing a patient in bed. *Emollient b.* a bath in a soothing and softening liquid, used in various skin disorders. It is prepared by adding soothing emollient substances to the bathwater, for the purpose of relieving skin irritation and pruritus. The skin should be dried by patting rather than rubbing after the bath. Care must be taken to avoid chilling. *Hot b.* one taken in water at 36–44°C. Care must be taken to avoid faintness. *Sponge b.* one in which the patient's body is not immersed but is wiped with a wet cloth or sponge. Sponge baths are most often employed for reduction of body temperature in the presence of a fever, in which case the water used is tepid. *Tepid b.* one taken in water at 30–33°C. *Warm b.* one taken in water at 32–40°C. *Whirlpool b.* (Jacuzzi) one in which the water is kept in constant motion by mechanical means. It has a gentle massaging action that promotes relaxation.

B cell *see* IMMUNITY.

BCG vaccine bacillus Calmette–Guérin vaccine, a tuberculosis vaccine prepared from artificially weakened stain of bovine tubercle bacillus (*Mycobacterium bovis*). BCG is given to those at risk of tuberculosis. This includes some health care workers, close contacts of people with tuberculosis, and immigrants and their families from countries with a high rate of tuberculosis. *See* Appendix 10.

'bearing down' 1. the expulsive pains in the second stage of labour. 2. a feeling of heaviness and downward strain in the pelvis, present with some uterine growths or displacements.

beat pulsation of the heart or an artery. *Apex b.* pulsation of the heart felt over its apex. The beat of the heart is felt against the chest wall. *Dropped b.* the occasional loss of a ventricular beat. *Ectopic b.* one that originates somewhere other than the sinoatrial node.

Beck inventory of depression (BDI) a scoring system used to determine the presence and severity of depression.

Beck scale for suicide ideation (BSS) an assessment tool used to identify the potential and risk of suicide in vulnerable patients.

Becquerel (Bq) the SI unit of radioactivity equal to the quantity of material undergoing one disintegration per second.

bed 1. a supporting structure or tissue. 2. a couch or support for the body during sleep. *B. cradle* a frame placed over the body of a bed patient. *See* CRADLE. *Capillary b.* the capillaries of a tissue, area or organ considered collectively, and their volume capacity. *Nail b.* the area of modified epidermis beneath the nail over which the nail plate slides as it grows.

bedboard a rigid board placed beneath the mattress of a bed to give firm support to the patient lying upon it.

bedbug a bug of the genus *Cimex*, a flattened, oval, reddish insect that inhabits houses, furniture and neglected beds, and feeds on humans, usually at night.

bedpan a shallow vessel used for defecation or urination by patients confined to bed.

bedrest limiting the patient to staying in bed for a prescribed period for therapeutic reasons.

bedsore an ulcer-like sore caused by prolonged pressure of the patient's body. Pressure ulcer is now the preferred term, as these sores are primarily due to pressure and can also occur in patients who are not confined to bed. *See* PRESSURE ULCER.

bed-wetting enuresis; involuntary voiding of urine. *See also* ENURESIS.

bee sting injury caused by the venom of a bee. Symptoms of a severe allergic reaction, such as collapse or swelling of the body, indicate anaphylaxis and require that medical help be sought.

behaviour the way in which an organism reacts to an internal or external stimulus. *B. disorders* may take many forms including anxiety, disruptive behaviour, dissociative, emotional and pervasive developmental disorders. *B. therapy* a therapeutic approach in which the focus is on positive behaviour change (*see also* COGNITIVE BEHAVIOUR THERAPY). *Incongruous b.* behaviour that is out of keeping with the person's normal reaction or has the opposite effect to that consciously desired.

behavioural sciences the application of scientific principles to the study of the behaviour of organisms, e.g., sociology, psychology and anthropology, etc.

behaviourism the purely objective study and observation of the behaviour of individuals.

Behçet's syndrome *H. Behçet, Turkish dermatologist, 1889–1948.* A rare chronic condition, which is a form of systemic vasculitis, resulting in painful, recurring mouth and genital ulcers, arthritis, skin lesions and inflammation of the eyes.

bejel a non-venereal but infectious form of syphilis caused by a treponema indistinguishable from that causing syphilis. Occurs mainly in children of Africa and the Middle East. The primary lesion is on the mouth, spreading to the trunk, arms and legs. Treated with penicillin.

belching the noisy expulsion of gas from the stomach through the mouth. Eructation.

beliefs thoughts, ideas and concepts developed by an individual over a period of time from cultural influences, education, religion, parents and family. *Health b.* those beliefs held by an individual regarding the maintenance of their physical and mental wellbeing, which may be at variance with those beliefs held by the health care practitioner, possibly leading to conflict and non-compliance with prescribed treatment.

belle indifference [Fr.] an indication of conversion hysteria, in which the patient describes symptoms, appearing not to be distressed by them.

Bell's palsy *Sir C. Bell, British physiologist, 1774–1842.* Facial paralysis due to oedema of the facial nerve.

bench marking comparing 'like with like' in order to identify best practice; or a process whereby organizations identify the best performers in order to improve their own performance. A scoring system is used which enables one hospital, department or other health care facility to compare their practices and services with another similar to their own. A quality-assurance technique.

bends a colloquial term for CAISSON DISEASE. Decompression sickness.

beneficence the duty to do good, to avoid harm to other people and to protect the weak and the vulnerable. In the health care setting this involves the staff acting in the best interests of their patients, and if necessary acting as advocate for them.

benign 1. the opposite to malignant. 2. describes a non-invasive condition or illness that is not usually serious even though treatment may be required for health or cosmetic reasons.

bereavement the experience of suffering loss, usually of a loved one by death or separation, but may also include the loss of previous good health,

position or wealth. Produces a psychological reaction that has recognized 'stages' that may overlap; these include anger, denial, disbelief and finally acceptance. Collectively recognized as mourning or grieving. There are specialist voluntary groups that provide help and support to those who have lost a family member or loved one e.g., CRUSE, Macmillan.

beriberi a deficiency disease due to insufficiency of vitamin B_1 in the diet. The disease is more common in areas where refined rice is the main staple in the diet. It is a form of neuritis, with pain, paralysis and oedema of the extremities.

berylliosis an industrial lung disease due to the inhaling of the metallic element beryllium. Interstitial fibrosis arises, impairing lung function.

beta the second letter in the Greek alphabet, β. *B. blockers* drugs used to block the action of adrenaline on beta-adrenergic receptors in cardiac muscle, thus decreasing the workload of the heart. *B. cells* insulin-producing cells found in the islets of Langerhans in the pancreas. *B. rays* electrons used therapeutically for treatment of lesions of the eye and bone. *B. receptors* associated with the inhibition (relaxation) of smooth muscle. They also bring an increase in the force of contraction and rate of the heart.

bezoar a mass formed usually in the stomach by ingested food which compacts and does not pass normally into the intestine.

bias in research, any tendency for results to differ from the true value in some consistent way. It is always associated with some systematic, non-random, usually undesirable phenomenon.

bicarbonate any salt containing the HCO_3 anion. *Blood b., plasma b.* the bicarbonate of the blood plasma, an important parameter of acid–base balance (*see* ACID) measured in blood gas analysis.

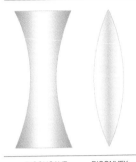

BICONCAVE   BICONVEX

bicellular composed of two cells.

biceps a muscle with two heads; a flexor of the arm; one of the hamstring muscles of the thigh.

biconcave pertaining to a lens or other structure with a hollow or depression on each surface (*see* Figure).

biconvex pertaining to a lens or other structure that protrudes on both surfaces (*see* Figure).

bicornuate having two horns. *B. uterus* a congenital malformation in which there is a partial or complete vertical division into two parts of the body of the uterus.

bicuspid having two cusps or projections. *B. teeth* the premolars. *B. valve* the mitral valve of the heart between the left atrium and ventricle.

bifid divided or cleft into two parts.

Bifidus factor present in human milk; promotes growth of gram-positive bacteria in gut flora, particularly *Lactobacillus bifidus*. This microorganism reduces the pH in the gut preventing the multiplication of pathogens.

bifocal having two foci, as with spectacles in which the lenses have two different foci.

bifurcate to divide into two branches; arteries bifurcate frequently, thereby getting smaller.

bifurcation the junction where a vessel divides into two branches, e.g., where the aorta divides into the right and left iliac vessels.

bigeminal double. *B. pulse* two pulse beats which occur together, regular in time and force. A regular irregularity.

biguanides oral hypoglycaemic agents for treating diabetes. They exert their effect by decreasing gluconeogenesis in muscle tissue. Only effective in those diabetics with functioning islet of Langerhans cells. Most commonly used in non-insulin-dependent diabetics, especially those who are overweight.

bilateral pertaining to both sides.

bile a secretion of the liver, greenish-yellow to brown in colour. It is concentrated in the gallbladder and passes into the small intestine, where it assists digestion by emulsifying fats and stimulating peristalsis. *B. ducts* the canals or passageways that conduct bile. The hepatic and cystic ducts join to form the common bile duct. *B. pigments* bilirubin and biliverdin, produced by haemolysis in the spleen. Normally these colour the faeces only, but in jaundice the skin and urine may also become coloured. *B. salts* sodium taurocholate and sodium glycocholate, which cause the emulsification of fats.

Bilharzia T.M. Bilharz, German physician, 1825–1862. A genus of blood fluke now known as *Schistosoma*.

bilharziasis schistosomiasis.

biliary pertaining to bile, the bile ducts and gallbladder. *B. colic* spasm of muscle walls of the bile duct causing often excruciating pain when gallstones are blocking the tube. Pain is usually in the right upper quadrant of the abdomen and referred to the shoulder. *B. fistula* an abnormal opening between the gallbladder and the surface of the body.

biliousness a symptom complex comprising nausea, abdominal discomfort, headache and constipation.

bilirubin an orange bile pigment produced by the breakdown of haem and reduction of biliverdin; it normally circulates in plasma and is taken up by liver cells and conjugated to form bilirubin diglucuronide, the water-soluble pigment excreted in the bile. Bilirubin may be classified as indirect ('free' or unconjugated) while en route to the liver from its site of formation by reticuloendothelial cells, and direct (diglucuronide) after its conjugation in the liver with glucuronic acid. Normally the body produces a total of about 260 mg of bilirubin per day. Almost 99% of this is excreted in the faeces; the remaining 1% is excreted in the urine as UROBILINOGEN. The typical yellowness of jaundice is caused by the accumulation of bilirubin in the blood and body tissues.

bilirubinaemia the presence of bilirubin in the blood.

Billings method a method of contraception. Ovulation time is estimated by observing changes in the cervical mucus and sensation at the vulva that occur during the menstrual cycle.

bimanual using both hands. *B. examination* examination with both hands. Used chiefly in gynaecology, when the internal genital organs are examined between one hand on the abdomen, and the other hand or a finger within the vagina.

binary made up of two parts. *B. fission* the multiplication of cells by division into two equal parts. *B. scale* one used in calculating, in which only two digits, 0 and 1, are used. Digital electronics use this scale.

binaural pertaining to both ears. *B. stethoscope. See* STETHOSCOPE.

Binet's test *A. Binet, French physiologist, 1857–1911.* A method of ascertaining the mental age of children or young persons by using a series of questions standardized on the capacity of normal children at various ages.

Bing test *A. Bing, German otologist, 1844–1922.* A vibrating tuning fork is held to the mastoid process and the auditory meatus is alternately occluded and left open; an increase and decrease in loudness (positive Bing) is perceived by the normal ear and in sensorineural hearing impairment, but in conductive hearing impairment no difference in loudness is perceived (negative Bing).

binge eating disorder (BED) an eating disorder characterized by frequent and recurring binge eating associated with negative psychological and social problems, without subsequent purging (vomiting). An alternative term for bulimia.

binocular relating to both eyes.

binovular derived from two ova. *B. twins* twins, who may or may not be of different sexes.

bioassay biological assay. The use of animals or an isolated organ preparation to determine the effect of the active power of a sample of a drug. Comparison is made with the effect of a standard preparation.

bioavailability the proportion of a drug that reaches the target organs of the body. Bioavailability is dependent upon metabolism, diet and administrative route. Intravenous administration results in 100% bioavailability. Orally administered drugs have a much lower bioavailability.

biochemical screening tests in pregnancy when the maternal serum is analysed for biochemical markers that identify babies with fetal Down's syndrome or inherited metabolic disorders. The newborn blood-spot screening test screens for nine conditions and also relies on biochemical markers to identify those infants with cystic fibrosis.

biochemistry the chemistry of living matter.

biofeedback visual or auditory evidence provided to an individual of the satisfactory performance of an autonomic body function, e.g., sounding a tone when blood pressure is at a satisfactory level, so that, through conditioning, the patient may assert control over that function.

biogenesis 1. the origin of life. 2. the theory that living organisms can originate only from those already living and cannot be artificially produced.

biohazard any hazard arising from inadvertent human biological processes, e.g., accidental inoculation, needlestick injury.

biology the science of living organisms, dealing with their structure, function and relations with one another.

biomechanical engineering the application of engineering knowledge and methods to the functions of the body. Used both as a means of explanation of bodily function and in the treatment of disorders of the body. Practical applications include the use of artificial joints, electronic hearing aids and pacemakers.

biometrics, biometry 1. anthropometry. 2. the use of statistics in biological science.

biomicroscopy a microscopic examination of living tissues, e.g., of the structures of the anterior of the eye during life. *See* SLIT LAMP.

biophysical profile a non-invasive test of fetal wellbeing using ultrasound to measure fetal heart rate, fetal tone, somatic movements, breathing movements and amniotic fluid volume. Each factor is scored to obtain a total biophysical score, which is an accurate predictor of fetal death in high-risk pregnancies. The score may be affected by gestation, maternal illness, therapeutic medication, substance abuse or fetal abnormality.

biopsy the removal of some tissue or organ from the living body, e.g., a lymph gland, for examination to establish a diagnosis. *Aspiration b.* biopsy in which the tissue is obtained by suction through a needle and syringe. *Cone b.* biopsy in which an inverted cone of tissue is excised, as from the uterine cervix. *Excisional b.* removal of an entire lesion and significant portion of normal-looking tissue for examination. *Needle b.* tissue obtained by the puncture of a lesion with a needle. Rotation of the needle removes tissue within the lumen of the needle.

biorhythm any cyclic biological event, e.g., sleep cycle and menstrual cycle, affecting daily life.

biosensors non-invasive instruments that measure the result of biological processes, e.g., body temperature.

biostatistics that branch of biometry that deals with the data and laws of human mortality, morbidity, natality and demography; called also vital statistics.

biosynthesis the creation of a compound within a living organism.

biotin formerly termed vitamin H, now part of the vitamin B complex and present in all normal diets.

biparietal pertaining to both parietal eminences or bones.

biparous giving birth to two infants at a time.

bipolar with two poles. *B. disorder* formerly known as manic-depressive illness, characterized by swings in mood between opposite extremes of severe depression and mania or overexcitability. Initially, the mood disturbance may consist of depression or excitability, but eventually it alternates between the two. Often accompanied by grandiose ideas or negative delusions. *B. nerve cells* cells having two nerve fibres, e.g., ganglionic cells.

birth the act of being born. *B. certificate* statement issued by the General Register Office (GRO) for births, marriages and deaths for the district in which the baby is born, which certifies details of parentage, name and sex of child, and date and place of birth. This certificate must be obtained by the parents or, failing them, anyone present at the delivery within 42 days of birth in England, Wales and Northern Ireland (21 days in Scotland). It gives legal status to the child and is necessary before Child Benefit can be paid. A birth certificate is issued to any baby born alive, irrespective of the period of gestation. *B. control* limiting the size of the family by abstention from sexual intercourse or the use of contraceptives. *B. mark* a naevus present from birth. *B. notification* a person present, or in attendance, at the birth or up to 6 hours afterwards must notify the Personal Demographic Service within 36 hours (Public Health Act 1936). This responsibility is accepted by the midwife when in attendance. *B. plan* a plan prepared by the expectant mother, usually in conjunction with her partner and midwife, which records her preferences for care during and after labour. *B. rate* the number of births during one year per 1000 total estimated mid-year population (crude birth rate), per 1000 estimated mid-year female population (refined birth rate), or per 1000 estimated mid-year female population of child-bearing age (true birth rate)—that is, between the ages of 15 and 45. *B. registration* either parent must register the birth within 42 days at the General Register Office in the district in which the birth took place in England and Wales or within 21 days in Scotland. Failure to do so incurs a fine. *Premature b.* one taking place before term.

birthing chair a specially designed chair for use in labour and delivery to promote greater mobility for the mother.

birthing pool a specially designed pool allowing mothers to give birth underwater.

bisexual 1. having gonads of both sexes. 2. hermaphrodite. 3. having both active and passive sexual interests or characteristics. 4. capable of the function of both sexes. 5. both heterosexual and homosexual. 6. an individual who is both heterosexual and homosexual. 7. of, relating to or involving both sexes, as in bisexual reproduction.

bite 1. to seize with the teeth. 2. a wound made by biting from either a human or animal. Treatment for both types of bite is through cleansing and, if necessary, a dressing. Consideration should be given to the immunization status of the patient as there is a risk of tetanus. For human bites there is also a risk of transmission of hepatitis B, hepatitis C, herpes simplex and HIV infection. With animal bites, preventive antibiotics may be prescribed together with anti-rabies vaccine and immunoglobulin, if the patient's history indicates that the animal is infected with the rabies virus. 3. an impression made by the teeth on a thin sheet of malleable material such as wax.

Bitot's spots *P.A. Bitot, French physician, 1822–1888.* Collections of dried epithelium, microorganisms, etc., forming shiny, greyish spots on the cornea. A sign of vitamin A deficiency.

bivalve 1. having two valves, as the shells of molluscs such as oysters. 2. to cut a plaster cast into an anterior and a posterior section. *B. speculum* a vaginal speculum with two blades that can be adjusted for easy insertion.

blackhead a comedo.

blackout momentary failure of vision and unconsciousness due to cerebral circulatory insufficiency.

blackwater fever a form of malignant malaria in which severe haemolysis causes a dark discoloration of the urine. *See* MALARIA.

bladder a membranous sac for holding fluid or gas (*see* Figure on p. 47). *Atonic b.* a condition in which there is lack of tone in the urinary bladder wall, which may be the result of incomplete emptying over a long period. *B. retraining* a process of education used by nurses to reduce urgency of micturition and episodes of urinary incontinence by increasing the time intervals between emptying the bladder. *B. worm* a cysticercus. *Irritable b.* a condition in which there is frequent desire to micturate. *Urinary b.* the reservoir for urine.

bland non-stimulating. *B. fluids* mild and non-irritating fluids such as barley water and milk.

blast 1. an immature cell. 2. a wave of high air pressure caused by an explosion.

BLADDER

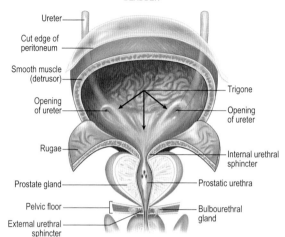

Ureter

Cut edge of peritoneum

Smooth muscle (detrusor)

Opening of ureter

Trigone

Opening of ureter

Rugae

Internal urethral sphincter

Prostate gland

Prostatic urethra

Pelvic floor

Bulbourethral gland

External urethral sphincter

blastocyst blastula.
blastoderm the germinal cells of the embryo consisting of three layers: the ectoderm, mesoderm and entoderm.
blastolysis the destruction of germ substance.
blastomycosis a fungal infection, which, after invasion of the skin, may cause granulomatous lesions in the mouth, pharynx and lungs.
blastula blastocyst. An early stage in the development of the fertilized ovum. This stage precedes the gastrula.
bleb a blister.
bleeder 1. a colloquial name for one who suffers from haemophilia. 2. a vessel that is difficult to seal at operation.
bleeding 1. escape of blood from an injured vessel. 2. venesection. *B. gums* See GINGIVITIS. *B. time* the time taken for oozing to cease from a sharp prick of the finger or ear lobe. The normal

value is 1–3 minutes. *Functional b.* bleeding from the uterus when no organic lesion is present.
blennorrhagia 1. an excessive discharge of mucus, e.g., leukorrhoea. 2. gonorrhoea.
blennorrhoea blennorrhagia.
blepharitis inflammation of the eyelids. *Allergic b.* that associated with response to drugs or cosmetics applied to the eye or eyelids. *Squamous b.* the edge of the eyelid is covered in small white or grey scales.
blepharon the eyelid.
blepharophimosis abnormal narrowing of the aperture between the eyelids. Usually congenital but may arise from chronic inflammation.
blepharospasm prolonged spasm of the orbicular muscles of the eyelids.
blind without sight. *B. spot* the point where the optic nerve leaves the retina, which is insensitive to light.

blind loop syndrome a condition of stasis in the small intestine, which aids bacterial multiplication, leading to diarrhoea and salt deficiencies. The cause may be intestinal obstruction or surgical anastomosis.

blindness lack or loss of ability to see; lack of perception of visual stimuli. Blindness is defined as less than 6/60 vision with glasses (vision of 6/60 is the ability to see only at 6 metres what the normal eye can see at 60 metres). A person with this level of vision may be registered as severely sight impaired (blind). A person may also be registered as sight impaired (partially sighted) if they are substantially and permanently disabled by defective vision caused by congenital defect, illness or injury.

blister a bleb or vesicle. A collection of serum between the epidermis and the skin. *Blood b.* a blister containing blood, usually caused by a pinch or bruise.

block a stoppage or obstruction. The term is used to describe: (a) various forms of regional anaesthesia, e.g., epidural block; (b) obstruction to the passage of a nervous impulse due to disease, e.g., heart block (*see* HEART); (c) an interruption of mental function.

blood the fluid that circulates through the heart and blood vessels, supplying nutritive material to all parts of the body and carrying away waste products. Blood is a red viscid fluid and consists of plasma in which are suspended erythrocytes (red blood cells), leukocytes (white blood cells) and lymphocytes, and platelets or thrombocytes. (a) The red corpuscles or ERYTHROCYTES contain haemoglobin, which combines with oxygen in passing through the lungs. This oxygen is released into the tissues from the capillaries and oxidation takes place. (b) The white corpuscles or LEUKOCYTES defend against invading microorganisms, which they have power to destroy. (c) Blood platelets or thrombocytes are concerned with the clotting of blood. Plasma also contains many other specialized substances that have important roles to play in immunity and clotting of blood.

blood bank 1. a place of storage for blood. 2. an organization that collects, processes, stores and transfuses blood.

blood-borne viruses viruses that are transmitted by blood and some other body fluids (e.g., semen, amniotic fluid), such as hepatitis B virus, hepatitis C virus and human immunodeficiency viruses (HIV-1, HIV-2).

blood–brain barrier (BBB) the membranous barrier separating the blood from the brain. It is permeable to water, oxygen, carbon dioxide, glucose, alcohol, general anaesthetics and some drugs.

blood casts casts of coagulated red blood cells formed in the renal tubules and found in the urine.

blood clotting coagulation. The formation of a jelly-like substance over the ends or within the walls of a blood vessel, with resultant stoppage of the blood flow. Clotting is one of the natural defence mechanisms of the body when injury occurs. A clot will usually form within 5 minutes of a blood vessel being damaged. The exact process of clotting or coagulation is triggered by exposure of coagulation factors in the blood plasma to tissue factor which is expressed beneath the surface of the blood vessel wall lining (called endothelium) when trauma occurs or pathology exists in the patient such as infection, inflammation or even cancer. This exposure of tissue factor activates one of the most important coagulation factors called factor VII (7) which then activates the rest of the extrinsic coagulation cascade. This results in the formation of thrombin factor XI (11) which converts fibrinogen to fibrin. Normal levels of functioning platelets are required for the coagulation factors to work as they are used as a lipid platform or scaffold. Fibrin, platelets and embedded red and white cells then form this mesh or clot. Factor XIII (13) then cross-links the fibrin to stabilize it further. Von Willebrand factor and platelets also help to repair traumatized vessels and prevent bleeding. Plasma coagulation factors are:

I	Fibrinogen
II	Prothrombin
	Tissue factor
IV	Calcium ions
VII	Factor VII (7)
VIII	Factor VIII (8)
IX	Christmas factor
X	Stuart factor (Prower factor)
XI	Factor XI (11)
XII	Hageman factor or contact factor
XIII	Fibrin stabilizing factor

blood count the number of blood cells in a given sample of blood, usually expressed as the number of cells per litre of blood (as the red blood cell, white blood cell or platelet count). A differential white cell count determines the number of various types of leukocyte in a sample of blood. For the range of normal values, *see* Appendix 9.

blood dyscrasia any abnormality of the blood cells or of the clotting elements.

blood gas analysis laboratory studies of arterial and venous blood for the purpose of measuring oxygen and carbon dioxide levels and pressure or tension, and hydrogen ion concentration (pH). Analyses of blood gases provide the following information: Pa_{O_2}, partial pressure (P) of oxygen (O_2) in the arterial blood (a); Sa_{O_2}, percentage of available haemoglobin that is saturated (Sa) with oxygen (O_2); Pa_{CO_2}, partial pressure (P) of carbon dioxide (CO_2) in arterial blood (a); pH, an expression of the extent to which the blood is alkaline or acidic; HCO_3, the level of plasma bicarbonate; an indicator of the metabolic acid–base status.

blood groups ABO system (*see* Table). In clinical practice, there are four main blood types: A, B, O and AB. In addition to this major grouping there is a rhesus (Rh) system that is important in the prevention of haemolytic disease of the newborn resulting from incompatibility of blood groups in mother and fetus. In determining blood group, a sample of blood is taken and mixed with specially prepared sera. One serum, anti-A agglutinin, causes blood of group A to agglutinate; another serum, anti-B agglutinin, causes blood of group B to agglutinate. Thus, if anti-A serum alone causes clumping, the blood is group A; if anti-B serum alone causes clumping, the blood group is B. If both cause clumping, the blood group is AB, and if it is not clumped by either, it is identified as group O. Transfusion with an incompatible ABO group will cause severe haemolytic reaction and death may occur.

blood pressure (BP) the pressure exerted on the artery walls by the blood as it flows through them. It can be measured in milligrams of mercury using a manual or semi-automated sphygmomanometer. Two readings are made.

ABO system		
Group	Antigen present in red cell	Antibody present in plasma
AB	A and B	—
A	A	Anti-B
B	B	Anti-A
O	—	Anti-A and Anti-B

Arterial pressure fluctuates with each heart beat and one measure records the pressure while the heart is in systole (when the heart is ejecting blood into the arteries) and is the higher, or systolic, pressure. The other records while the heart is in diastole (when the aortic and pulmonary valves are closed and the heart is relaxed) and is the lower, or diastolic, pressure. The range of normal blood pressure recording varies according to age and body size, but in the normal young adult is approximately 100–120/70–80 mmHg.

blood sugar the amount of glucose present in the blood. The normal range is 4.0-6.0 mmol/litre. When the amount exceeds 10 mmol/litre, glucose is excreted in the urine, as in diabetes mellitus.

blood transfusion introduction of blood from the vein of one person (donor) or from a blood bank into the vein of another (recipient) in cases of severe loss of blood, trauma, septicaemia, etc. It is used to supplement the volume of blood and also to introduce constituents, such as clotting factors or antibodies, that are deficient in the patient. *Autologous b.t.* the use of a person's own blood donated earlier for transfusion. The patient's blood may also be salvaged during surgery, filtered and returned to the circulation, thus reducing the need for donated blood transfusion.

blood and transplant NHS Blood and Transplant (NHSBT) special health authority for England and Wales set up for the purpose of providing a reliable and efficient supply of blood, tissues, stem cells and organs for transplantation throughout the NHS.

blood urea excretory product of protein present in the blood. The normal range is 2.5–7.8 mmol/litre; this increases in renal failure when the kidneys cease to function normally.

'blue baby' *see* BABY and FALLOT'S TETRALOGY.

blush growing redness of the face, usually a reaction to emotion or heat.

BMI body mass index.

BMR basal metabolic rate.

Bobath technique also known as neurodevelopmental treatment (NDT). An approach to the treatment of neurological conditions developed by Dr K. (1906–1991) and Mrs B. Bobath (1907–1991). It aims to facilitate movement by inhibiting abnormal tone, abnormal patterns of movement and abnormal balance reactions. It has largely been superseded by other treatments.

body 1. the trunk, or animal frame, with its organs. 2. the largest and most important part of any organ. 3. any mass or collection of material.

body dysmorphic disorder an anxiety disorder that causes a person to have a distorted view of how they look and to worry excessively about their appearance.

body image the total concept of the body, including conscious and unconscious feelings, thoughts and perceptions that a person has of it as an object in space, which is dependent and apart from other objects.

body language the expression of thoughts or emotions by means of posture or gestures. Body language may include unintended 'signs' as well as intended communication. Detailed studies of the importance of human non-verbal communication have been documented by several observers.

body mass index (BMI) the weight (kg) divided by the square of the height (m). A BMI of 18.5–24.9 indicates an ideal weight (below 23 for people of black, Asian or other ethnic groups who have slightly different thresholds defined due to increased risks of type 2 diabetes and cardiovascular disease); below 18.4 is underweight; a BMI of 25–29.9 is overweight; a BMI of 30–39.9 is classified as obese and over 40 very obese. These figures apply to adults under the age of 60 years only and are not applicable to children, people over 60 years, those with chronic health problems, athletes or to pregnant or breast-feeding women.

Body Substance Isolation (BSI) an INFECTION CONTROL system, developed in 1987, that further elaborated UNIVERSAL PRECAUTIONS and focused on the isolation of all moist and potentially infectious body substances (blood, faeces, urine, sputum, saliva, wound drainage and other body fluids) from all patients, regardless of their presumed infection status, primarily through the use of gloves. This concept has now been further developed and is known by the term STANDARD PRECAUTIONS. *See* TRANSMISSION-BASED PRECAUTIONS. *See also* Appendix 11.

boil an acute staphylococcal inflammation of the skin and subcutaneous tissues round a hair follicle. It causes a painful swelling with a central core of dead tissue (SLOUGH), which is eventually discharged. A furuncle.

bolus 1. a large pill. 2. a rounded mass of masticated food immediately before being swallowed or one passing through the intestines. 3. a quantity of a drug injected directly to raise its concentration in the blood to a therapeutic level.

bonding the attachment process that occurs between an infant and its parents, especially the mother, during the first hours and days following birth. Bonding is a reciprocal process and is considered a biological need for the future development, both physical and emotional, of the infant. *Dental b.* the use of bonding agents to repair, restore or improve the appearance of damaged or defective teeth.

bone the dense connective tissue forming the skeleton. It is composed of cartilage or membrane impregnated with mineral salts, chiefly calcium phosphate and calcium carbonate. This is arranged as an outer hard compact tissue and an inner network of cells (CANCELLOUS tissue), in the spaces of which is red bone marrow. In the shaft of long bones is a medullary cavity containing yellow marrow. Microscopically, the bone tissue is perforated with minute HAVERSIAN CANALS containing blood vessels and lymphatics for the maintenance and repair of the cells (*see* Figure). Bone is covered by a fibrous membrane, the PERIOSTEUM, containing blood vessels and by which the bone grows in girth. *B. age* a measure of skeletal development in assessing physical maturity in children by using X-rays to show how much the bones have grown in a particular body area. *B. graft* transplantation of a healthy piece of bone to replace missing or repair defective bone. *B. marrow* substance which fills the marrow cavities

STRUCTURE OF COMPACT BONE

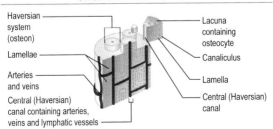

Haversian system (osteon)

Lamellae

Arteries and veins

Central (Haversian) canal containing arteries, veins and lymphatic vessels

Lacuna containing osteocyte

Canaliculus

Lamella

Central (Haversian) canal

of bones. Basically, there are two types: yellow and red marrow. The red marrow consisting mainly of haematopoietic tissue is responsible for producing red blood cells, platelets and most white blood cells. The yellow is mostly fatty connective tissue. *B. marrow transplantation* a procedure used to treat aplastic anaemia, acute leukaemia, lymphoma, myeloma and some rare congenital disorders, with varying success. Healthy stem cells are taken from the donor and given to the recipient whose own bone marrow is no longer able to produce healthy blood cells. Histocompatibility between the donor (usually a sibling) and recipient is essential.

bong a water pipe used for smoking cannabis and other drugs.

borborygmus a rumbling sound caused by gas in the intestines.

Bordetella a genus of bacteria. *B. pertussis* the causal agent of whooping cough.

Bornholm disease an epidemic myalgia with pleural pain and fever due to Coxsackie virus infection. It is named after the Danish island of Bornholm where there was an outbreak in 1930.

botulism a rare but extremely severe form of food poisoning due to a neurotoxin (botulin) produced by *Clostridium botulinum*, sometimes found in improperly canned or preserved foods. The symptoms include vomiting, abdominal pain, headache, weakness, constipation and nerve paralysis, which causes difficulty in seeing, breathing and swallowing. Death is usually due to paralysis of the respiratory organs.

bougie a flexible cylindrical instrument used to dilate a stricture, as in the oesophagus or urethra.

bovine relating to the cow or ox. *B. tuberculosis* that caused by infection from infected cows' milk, usually affecting glands and bones.

bowel the intestine.

Bowen's disease a very early form of skin cancer affecting the squamous cells. The main symptom is a red, scaly patch on the skin.

bowleg deformity where there is an outward curvature of one or both legs near the knee. This results in a gap between the knees on standing. Also known as genu varum.

Bowman's capsule *Sir W.P. Bowman, British physician, 1816–1892.* The expanded end of the kidney tubule, which surrounds the glomerulus.

brace 1. a support used in orthopaedics to hold parts of the body in their correct positions. 2. an orthodontic appliance to correct the alignment of teeth.

brachial relating to the arm. *B. artery* the continuation of the axillary artery along the inner side of the upper arm. *B. plexus* a network of nerves at the root of the neck supplying the upper limb.

brachytherapy radiotherapy delivered into or adjacent to a tumour by means of an intracavitary or interstitial radioactive source.

Braden scale *See* PRESSURE ULCER ASSESSMENT SCALES.

bradycardia abnormally low rate of heart contractions and consequent slow pulse.

bradycephaly a common condition affecting babies, also known as flat-head syndrome where the back of the head is flattened as a result of spending a lot of time lying on their backs. The head widens and the forehead may bulge. The head shape will generally improve over time. *See also* PLAGIOCEPHALY.

bradykinesia excessive slowness of voluntary movements and speech; a characteristic of Parkinsonism and some other nervous system disorders.

bradykinin peptide formed from the degradation of protein by enzymes. It is a powerful vasodilator that also causes contraction of smooth muscle.

braille a method of printing developed by *Louis Braille (1809–1852)* for the blind. Letters of the alphabet are represented by patterns of raised dots. These dots are read by passing the fingertips over them.

brain that part of the central nervous system contained in the skull. It consists of the cerebrum, midbrain, cerebellum, medulla oblongata and pons Varolii.

brainstem the lower part of the brain which links with the spinal cord and controls the automatic functions of the body, e.g., heart and respiratory rate. This consists of the midbrain, pons Varolii and medulla oblongata.

brainstorming or 'thought showering' is an approach to problem solving through the encouragement of intensive discussion in a group, generating ideas and solutions about an issue.

bran the husk of grain, i.e., the coarse outer coat of cereals. High in roughage and vitamins of the B complex, bran is frequently recommended as a dietary component both for those with alimentary disorders and for those in normal health.

branchial relating to the clefts (branchia) that are present in the neck and pharynx in the developing embryo. Normally they disappear. *B. cyst* a cystic swelling arising from a branchial remnant in the neck. *B. sinus* (*lateral cervical sinus*) a tract leading from the posterior cervical region which opens in the lower neck in front of the sternomastoid muscle.

Braun's frame *H.F.W. Braun, German surgeon, 1862–1934.* A metal frame which incorporates one or more pulleys and is used to elevate the lower limb and to apply skeletal traction for a compound fracture of tibia and fibula.

Braxton Hicks contractions *J. Braxton Hicks, British gynaecologist, 1823–1897.* Painless uterine contractions occurring during pregnancy, becoming increasingly rhythmic and intense during the third trimester. Sometimes called 'false labour'.

BRCA genes (BRCA1 and BRCA2) genes that produce tumour-suppressor proteins. When either gene is faulty, DNA damage may not be repaired properly and cells are more likely to develop additional alterations that can lead to cancer, particularly of the breast and ovary. Mutations can be inherited and account for around 5%–10% of breast cancers and 15% of ovarian cancers.

breast 1. the anterior or front region of the chest. 2. the mammary gland. *B. abscess* formation of pus in the mammary gland. *B. bone* the sternum. *B. cancer* the breast is a common site of cancer in women and occurs occasionally in men. In the UK one in eight women will develop this disease and although the survival rates for breast cancer continue to increase, the incidence of the disease in the Western world is also increasing. Improvement in these survival rates has come from increased public awareness, breast self-examination, breast screening programmes and improved methods of treatment. Women should train themselves to perform a simple self-examination of the breasts (*see* Figure on p. 54). The best time for this is just after menstruation when the breasts are normally soft but should also be continued after the menopause on a regular basis. If any lump in the breast can be felt, a doctor should be consulted immediately. More than 90% of breast cancers are discovered by the patients themselves. *B. feeding* the method of feeding a baby with milk directly from the mother's breasts. Midwives and paediatricians agree that breast feeding is better for the baby and the mother, both physically and emotionally (*see* Table). *B. pump* an apparatus for removal of milk from the breast with a vacuum created by either hand pressure or an electrical pump—known as expressed breast milk or EBM. *See* MILK.

breath the air taken in and expelled by the expansion and contraction of the thorax. *B. holding* when a young child

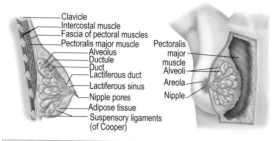

Clavicle
Intercostal muscle
Fascia of pectoral muscles
Pectoralis major muscle
Alveolus
Ductule
Duct
Lactiferous duct
Lactiferous sinus
Nipple pores
Adipose tissue
Suspensory ligaments
(of Cooper)

Pectoralis major muscle
Alveoli
Areola
Nipple

Ten steps to successful breast feeding
1. Have a breast-feeding policy available that is routinely communicated to all health care staff.
2. Train all health care staff in skills necessary to implement this policy.
3. Inform all pregnant mothers about the benefits and management of breast feeding.
4. Help mothers initiate breast feeding within half an hour of birth.
5. Show mothers how to breast feed and how to maintain lactation even if they should be separated from their infants.
6. Give newborn infants no food or drink other than breast milk unless medically indicated.
7. Practice rooming-in—that is, allow mothers and infants to remain together—24 hours a day.
8. Encourage breast feeding on demand.
9. Give no artificial teats or pacifiers (also called dummies and soothers) to breast-feeding infants.
10. Foster the establishment of breast-feeding support groups and refer mothers to them on discharge from hospital or clinic.

Source: WHO/UNICEF Baby Friendly Initiative.

cries, holds its breath and goes blue. *B. sounds* the sounds heard when a stethoscope is placed over the lungs during respiration. *B. test* using a Breathalyser to analyse a person's breath in order to determine the level of alcohol consumed within a certain period of time. Used to test drivers to assess if the person is within or above the legal limit of alcohol consumption. **breathing** the alternate inspiration and expiration of air into and out of the lungs (*see also* RESPIRATION).

breech the buttocks. *B. presentation* a position of the fetus in the uterus such that the buttocks present.

bregma the anterior fontanelle. The membranous junction between the coronal and sagittal sutures.

bridge in dentistry, an irremovable prosthesis carrying false teeth that bridges gaps left when natural teeth are extracted.

British National Formulary (BNF) a publication produced twice a year by the British Medical Association and the

Pharmaceutical Society of Great Britain, containing details of nearly all the drugs currently available on prescription in the UK. Also available electronically. The Nurse Prescribers' formulary is published as an addendum to the BNF. *See also* Appendix 4.

British Pharmacopoeia (BP) the official publication containing the list of drugs and other medicinal substances in use in the UK. The book gives details of how these substances are obtained or prepared, and their dosages and methods of administration. Also available electronically. It is compiled under the auspices of the Medicines and Healthcare Products Regulatory Authority and is regularly revised and brought up to date.

broad ligaments folds of peritoneum extending from the uterus to the sides of the pelvis, and supporting the blood vessels to the uterus and uterine tubes.

Broca's area of speech *P.P. Broca, French surgeon, 1824–1880.* The motor centre associated with speech, situated in the left cerebral hemisphere. Damage to the nerve cells contained in it can impair speech.

Brodie's abscess *Sir B.C. Brodie, British surgeon, 1783–1862.* See ABSCESS.

bromhidrosis offensive and fetid sweat.

bronchi plural of bronchus.

bronchiectasis chronic dilatation of the bronchi and bronchioles with secondary infection, usually involving the lower lobes of the lung. The condition may occur as a congenital malformation of the alveoli with resultant dilatation of the terminal bronchi and is associated with cystic fibrosis. Most often it is an acquired disease secondary to partial obstruction of the bronchi with necrotizing infection. The symptoms include a chronic cough and purulent sputum. May lead to respiratory failure.

bronchiole one of the smallest of the subdivisions of the bronchi.

bronchiolitis inflammation of the bronchioles.

bronchitis inflammation of the bronchi. *Acute b.* a short-lived infection, common in young children and the elderly. It is a descending infection from the common cold, influenza and other upper respiratory conditions. *Chronic b.* a daily productive cough that lasts for 3 months of the year and for at least 2 years in a row. It is one of a number of lung conditions, including emphysema, that are collectively known as chronic obstructive pulmonary disease (COPD).

bronchography radiography of the bronchial tree after introduction of a radio-opaque medium.

bronchomycosis A general term used to cover a variety of fungal infections of the bronchi: aspergillosis and pulmonary candidiasis.

bronchophony resonance of the voice as heard in the chest over the bronchi on auscultation.

bronchopneumonia a descending infection starting around the bronchi and bronchioles. *See also* PNEUMONIA.

bronchopulmonary relating to the lungs, bronchi and bronchioles. *B. dysplasia (BPD)* a chronic respiratory condition occurring in babies who have been ventilated for long periods or have needed prolonged oxygen therapy. It results in serious disruption of lung growth. Examination of radiographs and lung specimens reveals patches of collapse and fibrosis. Following ventilation, these babies usually require supplementary oxygen for several weeks or even months to keep the arterial oxygen tension above 55 kPa.

bronchorrhoea an excessive discharge of mucus from the bronchi.

bronchoscope an endoscope that enables the operator to see inside the bronchi. It can also be used to remove foreign bodies or to take a biopsy.

bronchoscopy examination of the bronchi by means of a bronchoscope.

bronchospasm difficulty in breathing caused by the sudden constriction of plain muscle in the walls of the bronchi. This may arise in asthma or chronic bronchitis.

bronchospirometer an instrument used to measure the capacity of one lung or of one lobe of the lung, or of each lung separately.

bronchotracheal relating to both the trachea and the bronchi. *B. suction* the removal of mucus with the aid of suction.

bronchus *pl.* bronchi. any of the larger passages conveying air to (right or left principal bronchus) and within (lobar and segmental bronchi) the lungs.

brow the forehead. *B. presentation* a position of the fetus such that the forehead appears at the cervix first.

brown fat special type of adipose tissue found in the newborn infant, and which is widely distributed throughout the body. The tissue is highly vascular and owes its colour to the large number of mitochondria found in the cytoplasm of its cells. It allows the infant to increase its metabolic rate and thus its heat production when subjected to cold. At the same time the fat itself is used up.

browser a computer program used to access the internet.

Brucella a genus of bacteria primarily pathogenic in animals but which may affect humans.

brucellosis a rare generalized infection involving primarily the reticuloendothelial system, marked by remittent undulant fever (*see* later), malaise, headache and anaemia, which has been wiped out in most developed countries due to animal vaccination and pasteurization of milk. It is still a problem globally and is the most common bacterial infection spread from animals to humans worldwide. It is caused by various species of *Brucella* and is transmitted to humans from domestic animals such as pigs, goats and cattle, especially through infected milk or contact with the carcass of an infected animal. The disease is also

called undulant fever because one of the major symptoms in humans is a fever that fluctuates widely at regular intervals. Prevention is best accomplished by the pasteurization of milk and a programme of testing, vaccination and elimination of infected animals. Also called Malta fever, abortus fever and Mediterranean fever.

Brudzinski's sign *J. Brudzinski, Polish physician, 1874–1917.* 1. passive flexion of one thigh causing spontaneous flexion of the opposite thigh. 2. flexion of the neck causing bilateral flexion of the hips and knees. These signs are indicative of meningeal irritation.

Brugada syndrome a rare but serious inherited condition resulting in cardiac arrhythmias that can be life threatening.

bruise a superficial injury to tissues produced by sudden impact in which the skin is unbroken. A contusion.

bruit [Fr.] an abnormal sound or murmur heard on auscultation of the heart and large vessels.

bruxism teeth clenching, particularly during sleep. The causes are not completely understood and headaches may result from muscle fatigue and tooth damage.

bubo inflammation of the lymphatic glands of the axilla or groin. Typical of bubonic plague (*see* PLAGUE) and sexually transmitted infections.

buccal pertaining to the cheek or to the mouth.

Budd–Chiari syndrome *G. Budd, British physician, 1808–1882; H. Chiari, Austrian pathologist, 1851–1916.* A rare condition in which thrombosis of the hepatic veins causes vomiting, jaundice, enlargement of the liver and ascites.

Buerger's disease *L. Buerger, American physician, 1879–1943.* Thromboangiitis obliterans.

buffer 1. a physical or physiological system that tends to oppose change within that system, e.g., the reflexes involved in blood pressure homeostasis.

2. a chemical system that acts to prevent change in the concentration of another chemical substance. Sodium bicarbonate is the chief buffer of the blood and tissue fluids. 3. anything that is used to reduce shock or jarring upon contact.

buggery anal intercourse, either heterosexual or homosexual. In law, the term also includes sexual contact with an animal (bestiality). Also known as sodomy.

bulbar pertaining to the medulla oblongata. *B. paralysis see* PARALYSIS.

bulbourethral relating to the bulb of the urethra (bulb of the penis). *B. glands* small glands opening into the male urethra. Cowper's glands.

bulimia abnormal increase in the sensation of hunger. *B. nervosa* a pattern of 'binge eating' controlled by self-induced vomiting or use of laxatives or episodes of uncontrolled and compulsive overeating occurring in response to stress. Bulimic 'binges' often occur in anorexia nervosa.

bulk-forming agent an antidiarrhoeal agent that makes the faeces less fluid by absorbing water.

bulla a large, fluid-containing blister.

bullying the tormenting of others through repeated verbal harassment, physical assault or other subtle methods of coercion such as manipulation or sending hurtful or scary messages or phone calls, SMS text, emails or other social media messages. Bullying is widespread and occurs in settings where people interact. This includes schools and workplaces. These settings have a responsibility to create an environment where children and adults feel safe. In recent years steps have been taken to develop policies against bullying. *See also* HARASSMENT.

bundle a collection of nerve fibres all running in the same direction. *B. branch block* the delay in conduction along either branch of the atrioventricular bundle of the heart. The abnormality is detected by an ECG recording.

bundle of His *L. His Jr, Swiss physiologist, 1863–1934.* The band of neuromuscular fibres which, passing through the spectrum of the heart, divides at the apex into two parts, these being distributed into the walls of the ventricles. The impulse of contraction is conducted through the structure. Atrioventricular bundle.

bunion a prominence of the head of the metatarsal bone at its junction with the great toe, caused by inflammation and swelling of the bursa at that joint. Usually due to shoes that distort the natural shape of the foot. Also known as HALLUX VALGUS.

buphthalmos abnormal enlargement of the eyes in congenital GLAUCOMA.

burden of proof the duty to establish the facts; usually associated with litigation including insurance claims and criminal proceedings.

Burkitt's lymphoma *D.P. Burkitt, Irish surgeon, 1911–1993.* African lymphoma. A cancer of the lymphatic system, frequently in the jaw, occurring almost exclusively in children living in low-lying moist areas. Occurs in New Guinea and Central Africa. The Epstein–Barr virus (EB virus), a herpes virus, has been isolated from Burkitt's lymphoma cells in culture, and has been implicated as a causative agent.

burn an injury to tissues caused by: (a) physical agents, the sun, excess heat or cold, friction, nuclear radiation; (b) chemical agents, acids or caustic alkalis; (c) electrical current. Burns are described as being partial thickness (involving only the epidermis) or full thickness (involving the dermis and underlying structures) or first degree, second degree and third degree. Clinically, emphasis is placed on the percentage of the body affected by the burn. The treatment of shock and prevention of infection and malnutrition need special attention. *B. chart see* LUND AND BROWDER CHART.

burnout a term used to describe a state of emotional, mental and physical exhaustion as a result of excessive and prolonged stress amongst workers and commonly in members of the helping professions. Burnout is characterized by chronic low energy, defensiveness and emergence of manoeuvres designed to create distance between helper and patient/client. Dissatisfaction and tension may be carried over from the work situation into the personal one and self-esteem and confidence may suffer badly.

burr a bit for a surgical drill, used for cutting bone or teeth. *B. hole* a circular hole drilled in the cranium to permit access to the brain or to release raised intracranial pressure.

bursa a small sac of fibrous tissue, lined with synovial membrane and containing synovial fluid. It is situated between parts that move upon one another at a joint to reduce friction.

bursitis inflammation of the bursa. It produces pain and may impede movement of the joint. *Prepatellar b.* housemaid's knee.

buttock either of the two fleshy prominences formed by the gluteal muscles at either side of the lower spine.

bypass diversion of flow. Formation of a shunt. *Aortocoronary b.* diversion of flow from the aorta to the coronary arteries via a saphenous vein or artificial graft. *Femoropopliteal b.* diversion of flow from the femoral to the popliteal artery to overcome an occlusion.

byssinosis an industrial disease caused by inhalation of cotton or linen dust in the workplace. A type of pneumoconiosis.

byte the storage space in the memory of a computer allocated to one character or letter, usually composed of a sequence of eight bits.

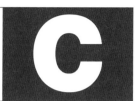

C symbol for *carbon*; *centigrade* or *Celsius*; *cytosine*.

© symbol for *copyright*.

Ca symbol for *calcium*.

cachexia a condition of extreme debility. The patient is emaciated, the skin being loose and wrinkled from rapid wasting, but shiny and tense over bone. The eyes are sunken, the skin yellowish, and there is a grey 'muddy' complexion. The mucous membranes are pale and anaemia is extreme. The condition is typical of the late stages of chronic diseases.

cadaver a corpse. The dead body used for dissection.

caecum the blind pouch forming the beginning of the large intestine. The vermiform appendix is attached to it.

caesarean section delivery of a fetus by an incision through the abdominal wall and uterus. Performed for the safety of either the mother or the infant. Tradition has it that Julius Caesar was born in this way.

caesium *symbol* Cs. A metallic element. *C.-137* radioactive caesium; a fission product from uranium.

CAFCASS an independent service which supports and represents children in family court cases. Stands for Children and Family Court Advisory and Support Service.

café-au-lait spot pigmented macules of a distinctive light-brown colour, like coffee with milk, as in neurofibromatosis and Albright's syndrome.

caffeine an alkaloid of tea and coffee which acts as a nerve stimulant and diuretic.

caffeinism an agitated state due to the excessive ingestion of caffeine.

caisson disease decompression sickness. *See* BENDS.

calcaneum the heel bone. Calcaneus.

calcareous chalky. Containing lime.

calciferol the chemical name for vitamin D.

calcification 1. the deposit of lime in any tissue, e.g., in the formation of callus. 2. the deposit of lime salts in cartilage as part of the normal process of bone formation. *Dystrophic c.* the deposition of calcium in abnormal tissue, such as scar tissue or atherosclerotic plaques, without abnormalities of blood calcium.

calcitonin a polypeptide hormone, produced by the parafollicular or C cells of the thyroid gland, which regulates blood calcium levels.

calcium *symbol* Ca. A metallic element necessary for the normal development and functioning of the body. Calcium is the most abundant mineral in the body; it is a constituent of bones and teeth. Deficiency or excess of serum calcium causes nerve and muscle dysfunctions and abnormalities in blood clotting. The correct concentration is regulated by hormones. *C. carbonate* chalk. *C. gluconate* used as an antacid. A compound that is easily absorbed and can be given by intramuscular or intravenous route to raise the blood calcium. *C. lactate* a compound that increases the coagulability of blood; used orally as a calcium supplement.

calculus 1. a stony concretion which may be formed in any of the secreting organs of the body or their ducts. 2. a calcified deposit that forms on the surface of the teeth leading to tooth decay and gum disease.

Caldicott guardian all NHS organizations must appoint a Caldicott guardian to safeguard the confidentiality of patient information, as do all local councils with a social services responsibility. They must be either: a member of the organization's management board or a senior health professional with responsibility for promoting clinical governance in the organization. The Caldicott principles apply in addition to the requirements of DATA PROTECTION LEGISLATION.

calibrator 1. an instrument for measuring the size of openings. 2. an instrument used to dilate a tube, e.g., in urethral stricture.

caliper a two-pronged instrument that may be used to exert traction on a part. *Walking c.* an appliance fitted to a boot or shoe to give support to the lower limb. It may be used when the muscles are paralysed or in the repair stage of fractures.

calipers compasses for measuring diameters and curved surface. *Skinfold c.* an instrument used in nutritional assessment for determining the amount of body fat. A fold of skin and subcutaneous tissue, usually over the triceps muscle, is pinched away from the underlying muscle using the thumb and forefinger.

callisthenics mild gymnastics for developing the muscles and producing a graceful carriage.

callosity the plaques of thickened skin often seen on the soles of the feet or the palms of the hand, areas subject to friction.

callous hard and thickened.

callus 1. a callosity. 2. the tissue that grows round fractured ends of bone and develops into new bone to repair the injury.

calor [L.] *heat*; one of the signs of inflammation.

caloric pertaining to heat or calories.

calorie A unit of heat. Used to denote physiological values of various food substances, estimated according to the amount of heat they produce on being oxidized in the body. *See* OXIDIZATION. A large calorie (or kilocalorie, *symbol* Cal or kcal) represents the heat required to raise 1 kg (1000 g) of water by 1°C. A small calorie (*symbol* cal) equals the heat produced in raising 1 g of water by 1°C. In the SI system the calorie is replaced by the joule (1 cal = 4.18 J).

calorific heat-producing.

calorimeter an apparatus for measuring the heat that is produced or lost during a chemical or physical change.

calyx any cup-shaped vessel or part. *C. of kidney* the cup-like terminations of the ureter in the renal pelvis surrounding the pyramids of the kidney.

Campylobacter a genus of bacteria, family Spirillaceae, made up of gram-negative, non-spore-forming, motile, spirally curved rods. Causes an acute intestinal illness lasting several days. Usually associated with unpasteurized milk, partially cooked meat and poultry.

canal a tubular passage. *Alimentary c.* the passage along which the food passes on its way through the body. *C. of Schlemm* that which drains the aqueous humour. *Cervical c.* that through the cervix of the uterus. *Semicircular c.* one of the three canals in the middle ear responsible for maintenance of balance.

canaliculus a small channel or canal.

cancellous being porous or spongy. Applied to the honeycomb type of bone tissue in the ends of long bones and in flat and irregular bones.

cancer a general term to describe malignant growths in tissue, of which

CARCINOMA is of epithelial and SARCOMA of connective tissue origin, as in bone and muscle that is parasitic and flourishes at the expense of the host. The basic aetiology of cancer remains unknown but many potential causes are now recognized, e.g. cigarette smoking, ionizing radiation, exposure to certain chemicals and overexposure to the sun. Hereditary factors also play an important part in its development. A cancerous growth is one that is not encapsulated, but infiltrates surrounding tissues, the cells of which it replaces by its own. It is spread by the lymph and blood vessels and causes metastases in other parts of the body. Death is caused by destruction of organs to a degree incompatible with life, by extreme debility and anaemia, or by haemorrhage. For early warning signs of cancer, *see* Table. *C. centre* these centres provide services for patients with more common cancers and will have a range of additional specialist services including radiotherapy, complex chemotherapy and care of rare cancers to ensure adequate specialization. *C. phobia* an irrational fear of cancer. *C. staging* is a measure of how much a cancer has grown and spread. A common method of cancer staging is based on the measurement of the primary tumour (T), any spread to lymph nodes (N) and rate of metastases (M), and is known as the TNM classification. There are also other staging systems and some use a number system such as stage 1, 2, 3 or 4 (or stage I, II, III or IV). *C. screening See* SCREENING. *C. units* specialist wards and clinics in district general hospitals with a full range of supportive services for people with more common cancers and rapid referral patterns for patients with symptoms indicating a high risk of a diagnosis of malignancy.

cancrum oris gangrenous stomatitis. An ulceration of the mouth which is a rare complication of measles particularly in debilitated African children. Noma.

Candida a genus of small fungi, formerly called *Monilia*. *C. albicans* the species that causes candidiasis.

Early warning signs of cancer
• Any lump or thickening, especially in the breast, testicle, lip or tongue.
• Any irregular or unexplained bleeding or discharge. Blood in the urine or bowel movements. Blood or bloody discharge from the nipple or any body opening. Unexplained vaginal bleeding or discharge, or any bleeding after the menopause. Coughing up blood.
• A sore that does not heal, particularly around the mouth, tongue or lips, or anywhere on the skin.
• Noticeable changes in the colour, shape, thickness or size of a wart, mole or mouth sore.
• Continual indigestion or difficulty in swallowing.
• Persistent hoarseness or cough.
• Persistent change in normal elimination (bowel or bladder habits).
• Persistent headache.
• Persistent fatigue, nausea or vomiting.
• Unexplained loss of weight or appetite.
• Repeated instances of infection or persistent low-grade fever (constant or intermittent).
• Persistent pain in bone.

candidiasis infection by the *Candida* fungus. Occurs particularly in moist areas, such as mouth, vagina and skin-folds. Popularly known as thrush. Candidiasis can occur as a result of a debilitating illness or immunosuppressive therapy and/or cytotoxic drugs. The infection may also occur as a result of disturbed intestinal flora, and in pregnancy. Oral infection may be due to poor hygiene, carious teeth or badly fitting dentures.

canine 1. pertaining to a dog. 2. an 'eye tooth'. There are two in each jaw between the incisors and the molars. *See* DENTITION.

cannabis an illegal drug (class B) which may be swallowed or smoked. It produces hallucinations and a temporary sense of wellbeing, followed by extreme lethargy. Alternative terms for cannabis include marijuana, spliff, hashish, blow, hash, grass, pot, weed, ganja and dope.

cannula a hollow tube for insertion into the body by which fluids are introduced or removed. Usually a trocar is fitted into it to facilitate its introduction.

canthus the angle formed by the junction of the upper and lower eyelids.

CAPD continuous ambulatory peritoneal dialysis.

capillarity the action by which a liquid will rise upwards in a fibrous substance or in a fine tube. Capillary attraction.

capillary 1. hair-like. 2. a minute vessel connecting an arteriole and a venule. 3. a minute vessel of the lymphatic system.

capsular relating to a capsule. *C. ligaments* those that completely surround a movable joint, forming a capsule which loosely encloses the bones and is lined with synovial membrane which secretes a fluid for lubrication of the articular surfaces. Also called articular capsule.

capsule 1. a fibrous or membranous sac enclosing an organ. 2. a small soluble case of gelatin in which a nauseous medicine may be enclosed. 3.

the gelatinous envelope which surrounds and protects some bacteria.

capsulotomy the incision of a capsule, particularly that of a joint or of the lens of the eye.

caput head. *C. succedaneum* a transient soft swelling on an infant's head, due to pressure during labour, which disappears within the first few days of life.

carbaminohaemoglobin a compound of carbon dioxide and haemoglobin, present in the blood.

carbohydrate a compound of carbon, hydrogen and oxygen. Carbohydrates are classified into mono-, di-, tri-, poly- and heterosaccharides. In food they are an important and immediate source of energy for the body; 1 g of carbohydrate yields 17 kJ (4 kcal). They are synthesized by all green plants. In the body they are absorbed immediately or stored in the form of glycogen.

carbon *symbol* C. A non-metallic element. *C. dioxide* a gas which, dissolved in water, forms weak carbonic acid. As a product of metabolism by the oxidation of carbon, it leaves the body via the lungs. It can be compressed until it freezes, and then forms a solid (carbon dioxide snow, also known as dry ice) used as an escharotic in various skin conditions. Inhalations of the gas in a 5–7% mixture with oxygen are useful for stimulating the depth of respiration. *C. monoxide* a colourless gas that is very poisonous. It is a major constituent of coal gas and is usually present in the exhaust gases from petrol and diesel engines. In poisoning there is vertigo, flushed face with very red lips, loss of consciousness, and convulsions. The blood is bright red because of the formation of carboxyhaemoglobin.

carbonic anhydrase an enzyme that catalyses the decomposition of carbonic acid into carbon dioxide and water, facilitating transfer of carbon dioxide from tissues to blood and from blood to alveolar air.

carboxyhaemoglobin the combination of carbon monoxide with haemoglobin in the blood in carbon monoxide poisoning.

carbuncle an acute staphylococcal inflammation of subcutaneous tissues, which causes local thrombosis in the veins and death of tissue with several discharging sinuses. In appearance it resembles a collection of boils.

carcinogen any substance or agent that can produce a cancer.

carcinogenic pertaining to substances or agents that produce or predispose to cancer.

carcinoid syndrome a rare condition associated with certain bowel tumours, which spread to other parts of the body. Marked by attacks of severe cyanotic flushing of the skin and by diarrhoea, bronchoconstrictive attacks, pain, serious heart damage, sudden drops in blood pressure, oedema and ascites. Symptoms are caused by serotonin, prostaglandins and other biologically active substances secreted by the tumour.

carcinoma a malignant growth of epithelial tissue. Microscopically the cells resemble those of the tissue in which the growth has arisen. *Adenoic c.* adenocarcinoma. *Basal cell c.* a rodent ulcer (*see* ULCER). *Epithelial c.* epithelioma. *Squamous cell c.* one arising from the squamous epithelium of the skin.

carcinomatosis the condition in which a carcinoma has given rise to widespread metastases.

cardia the cardiac orifice of the stomach.

cardiac 1. pertaining to the heart. 2. pertaining to the cardia. *C. arrest* the cessation of the heart beat. *C. asthma* see ASTHMA. *C. atrophy* fatty degeneration of the heart muscle. *C. catheterization* a procedure whereby a catheter is passed to the heart usually from the femoral or radial arteries, jugular or femoral veins. Its passage through the heart can be watched on a screen. Blood pressure readings and specimens can also be taken, thus aiding diagnosis of heart abnormalities. Once in place, the catheter can be used to perform a number of procedures including coronary angiography and cardiac ablation. *C. cycle* the sequence of events, lasting about 0.8 seconds, during which the heart completes one contraction. *C. massage* rhythmic compression of the heart performed in order to re-establish circulation of the blood in cardiac arrest. *C. monitor* equipment used to monitor and visually record the cardiac cycle. *C. pacemaker* an electrical device that stimulates the heart muscle to maintain myocardial contractions. *See* PACEMAKER. *C. stimulant* a pharmacological agent that increases the action of the heart. Cardiac glycosides, e.g., digoxin and digitalis, increase myocardial contractions and decrease the heart rate and conduction velocity, thus allowing more time for the ventricles to relax and fill with blood.

cardialgia pain in the region of the heart.

cardice a solid form of carbon dioxide used primarily as a coolant. Also known as dry ice.

cardiodynia pain in the heart.

cardiogenic originating in the heart. *C. shock* shock caused by disease or failure of heart action.

cardiography the recording of the force and movements of the heart producing a tracing on paper (a cardiogram) or monitor.

cardiologist a medically qualified person skilled in the diagnosis of heart disease.

cardiology the study of the heart: how it works and its diseases.

cardiomyopathy a chronic disorder of the heart muscle not resulting from atherosclerosis.

cardiopulmonary relating to the heart and lungs. *C. bypass (CPB)* the use of the heart–lung machine to oxygenate and pump the blood round the body while the surgeon operates on the heart. *C. resuscitation (CPR)* whereby life-saving measures are commenced to maintain the respiration and circulation of a patient who has sustained a cardiac arrest. *See* Appendix 2 Resuscitation.

cardioscope a flexible instrument with a lens and illumination attachment; used for examining the inside of the heart.

cardiospasm spasm of the sphincter muscle at the cardiac end of the stomach. It may result in dilatation of the oesophagus, difficulty in swallowing solids and liquids, and regurgitation of undigested food. Achalasia.

cardiothoracic pertaining to the heart and thoracic cavity. A specialized branch of surgery.

cardiotocography the simultaneous recording of the fetal heart rate, fetal movements and uterine contractions in order to discover possible lack of oxygen (hypoxia) to the fetus. Fetal monitoring.

cardiotomy surgical incision into the heart or the cardia. *C. syndrome* an inflammatory reaction after heart surgery. There is pyrexia, pericarditis and pleural effusion.

cardiotoxic anything that has a deleterious or poisonous effect on the heart.

cardiovascular concerning the heart and blood vessels. *C. system* the heart together with the two chief networks of blood vessels: the systemic circulation and the pulmonary circulation.

cardioversion a method of restoring an abnormal heart rhythm to normal (as in atrial fibrillation) by means of an electric shock.

carditis inflammation of the heart.

care the provision of welfare and protection to children, the elderly in need, the sick and other vulnerable people. An important component of nursing practice (and that of other health care professionals) that extends the concept to include psychosocial and physical care interventions. *C. certificate* a set of introductory skills, knowledge and behaviours that enable entrants new to health and social care to provide compassionate, safe and high-quality care and support. The care certificate is based on 15 standards which must all be completed before the care certificate can be awarded. *C. contact time* part of the safer-staffing initiative developed by the Chief Nursing Officer for England providing guidance for organizations about the amount of time nurses spend in direct contact with patients, and the capacity and capability of their workforce. *C. hours per patient day (CHPPD)* measures the hours of direct care given per patient by nurses and health care support workers in acute settings. *C. pathway* an integrated approach or pathway which determines and utilizes locally agreed multidisciplinary practice based on guidelines and evidence for a specific patient or client group. *C. plan* an individualized plan for the care of a patient. Nursing information in this document includes data from the patient assessment regarding the patient's needs and nursing diagnosis, the specific nursing interventions are outlined, the desired goals stated and the priorities set. *See* NURSING (CARE PLAN).

Care Programme Approach (CPA) a way that services are assessed, planned, co-ordinated and reviewed for someone with mental health problems or a range of related complex needs.

Care Quality Commission (CQC) the regulator of health and adult social care in England. It monitors, inspects and rates care services to ensure they are safe, caring, effective, responsive and well led on an on-going basis. This includes services provided by the NHS, local authorities, private companies and voluntary organizations—whether in hospitals, GP surgeries, clinics, care homes or people's own homes.

Caregiver Strain Index (CSI) measure used by community and mental health nurses to assess caregiver strain for those carers who are providing care for a family member or partner in the home. The results of the questionnaire answered by the caregiver provide a crude analysis of how well the carer is coping in the care situation.

care in the community policy whereby patients with continuing medical and social care needs are cared for in a community or domestic, rather than institutional, setting. Care in the community is part of the UK Government agenda to give patients and clients more right to choose and be involved in their care.

carer someone who cares, unpaid, for a friend or family member in need who cannot cope without support due to illness or disability.

Care Act 2014 gives people in England, who provide substantial care on a regular basis, the right to ask for an assessment from social services. Local councils have a duty to promote the wellbeing of carers. In Wales, Scotland and Northern Ireland there is country-specific legislation to cover carers' rights.

caries suppuration and subsequent decay of bone, corresponding to ulceration in soft tissues. In caries, the bone dissolves; in necrosis it separates in large pieces and is thrown off. *Dental c.* decay of the teeth due to penetration of bacteria through the enamel to the dentine. *Spinal c.* tuberculosis of the spine. Pott's disease.

Caring about Carers a national strategy supporting an estimated 6 million carers in England and Wales. Its main features are: (a) grants to allow English local authorities to help carers take a break; (b) credits towards a second pension; (c) council tax reductions for more disabled people and their carers; (d) more carer-friendly employment policies; and (e) support for young carers including those at school.

carminative an aromatic drug that relieves flatulence and associated colic. Cloves, ginger, cardamom and peppermint are examples.

carneous fleshy. *C. mole* a tumour of organized blood clot surrounding a dead fetus in the uterus. *See* ABORTION.

carotene the colouring matter in carrots, tomatoes and other yellow foods and in fats. It is a provitamin capable of conversion into vitamin A in the liver.

carotid the principal artery on each side of the neck. *C. bodies* chemoreceptors in the bifurcation of both carotid arteries which monitor the oxygen content of the blood. *C. sinuses* dilated portions of the internal carotids containing the baroreceptors that monitor blood pressure.

carpal relating to the carpus or wrist. *C. tunnel syndrome* compression of the median nerve at the wrist causing numbing and tingling in the fingers and thumb.

carpopedal relating to the wrist and foot. *C. spasm* spasm of the hands and feet such as occurs in tetany.

carpus the eight bones forming the wrist and arranged in two rows: (a) scaphoid, lunate, triquetral, pisiform; (b) trapezium, trapezoid, capitate, hamate.

Carr-Hill formula a resource formula used to distribute funding to general practices based on costs of delivering routine primary care services to a practice population.

carrier 1. a person who harbours the microorganisms of an infectious disease but is not necessarily affected by it, although that person may infect others. 2. one who carries and passes on a hereditary abnormality.

cartilage a specialized, fibrous connective tissue present in adults and forming most of the temporary skeleton in the embryo. The three most important types are hyaline cartilage, elastic cartilage and fibrocartilage. Also, a general term for a mass of such tissue in a particular site in the body. *Elastic c.* cartilage containing elastic fibres and forming the pinna of the ear, the epiglottis and part of the nasal septum. *Fibro-c.* cartilage in which bundles of white fibres predominate, forming the intervertebral discs and costal cartilages. *Hyaline c.* flexible, somewhat elastic, semitransparent cartilage with an opalescent bluish tint, composed of a basophilic fibril-containing substance with cavities in which the chondrocytes occur.

cartilaginous of the nature of cartilage.

caruncle a small fleshy swelling. *Lacrimal c.* a small reddish body situated at the medial junction of the eyelids. *Urethral c.* a small fleshy growth occurring at the urinary orifice in females and giving rise to great pain on micturition.

case a particular instance of disease, as in a case of leukaemia; sometimes used incorrectly to designate the patient with the disease. *C. conference* a meeting of professionals involved in the care of a particular person (often a child), to agree patterns of action and to monitor progress. *C.–control study* an epidemiological study in which the characteristics of cases of disease are compared with a matched control group of persons without the disease. Also called retrospective study, case referent study. *C. fatality rate* the number of persons dying of a particular disease expressed as a proportion of the total contracting the disease; usually expressed as a percentage. *C. history* the collected data concerning an individual and that person's family and environment, including the medical history and any other information that may be useful in analysing and diagnosing the health issues or for instructional or research purposes. *C. load* a system of care whereby a nurse, midwife or health visitor is responsible for a group of patients or clients. *C. mix* 1. mix of patients seen by a consultant/hospital/

region. 2. classification of patient care and treatment into groups which provides a useful measure for audit and performance comparisons. 3. national office designs and refines classifications used to describe NHS healthcare activity in England.

caseation degeneration of diseased tissue into a cheesy mass.

casein the chief protein of milk. It forms a curd from which cheese is made. *C. hydrolysate* a predigested concentrated protein; a useful supplement for a high-protein diet.

cast 1. a positive copy of an object, e.g., a mould of a hollow organ (a renal tubule, bronchiole, etc.), formed of effused plastic matter and extruded from the body, as in a urinary cast; named, according to constituents, as epithelial, fatty, waxy, etc. 2. a positive copy of the tissues of the jaws, made in an impression, over which denture bases or other restorations may be fabricated. 3. to form an object in a mould. 4. a stiff dressing or casing, usually made of plaster of Paris, used to immobilize body parts. 5. strabismus.

castor oil a vegetable oil now rarely used internally as it is a purgative. Externally it is protective and soothing and may be used in zinc ointment to protect the skin from excoriation.

castration the removal of the testes in the male or the ovaries in the female.

cat-scratch disease (fever) a benign, subacute, regional lymphadenitis with fever, resulting from a scratch or bite of a cat or a scratch from a surface contaminated by a cat. Three quarters of all cases occur in children.

catabolism the chemical breakdown of complex substances in the body to form simpler ones, with a release of energy. *See* METABOLISM.

catalase an enzyme found in body cells, including red blood cells and liver cells.

catalyst a substance that hastens or brings about a chemical change without itself undergoing alteration; for example, enzymes act as catalysts in the process of digestion.

cataract opacity of the crystalline lens of the eye causing partial or complete blindness. It may be congenital or may be due to degenerative changes, injury or diabetes.

catarrh chronic inflammation of a mucous membrane accompanied by an excessive discharge of mucus.

catatonia a syndrome of motor abnormalities occurring in schizophrenia, but less commonly in organic cerebral disease, characterized by stupor and the adoption of strange postures, or outbursts of excitement and hyperactivity. The patient may change suddenly from one of these states to the other.

catchment area a specific geographical area for which an NHS Trust or health centre is responsible for providing the health care services.

catecholamines a group of compounds that have the effect of sympathetic nerve stimulation. They have an aromatic and an amine portion and include dopamine, adrenaline and noradrenaline.

catgut a substance used in surgery for sutures and ligatures.

catharsis 1. a cleansing or purgation. 2. the bringing into consciousness and the emotional reliving of a forgotten (repressed) painful experience as a means of releasing anxiety and tension.

catheter a tubular, flexible instrument, passed through body channels for withdrawal of fluids from (or introduction of fluids into) a body cavity. Catheters are made of a variety of materials including plastic, metal, rubber and gum-elastic. *Angiographic c.* one through which a contrast medium is injected for visualization of the vascular system of an organ. *Arterial c.* one inserted into an artery and utilized as part of a catheter–transducer–monitor system to continuously observe the BLOOD PRESSURE of critically ill patients. An arterial catheter also may be inserted for radiological studies of the arterial system and for delivery of chemotherapeutic agents directly into the arterial supply of malignant tumours. *Cardiac c.* a long, fine catheter especially designed for passage, usually through a peripheral blood vessel, into the chambers of the heart under fluoroscopic control. *Central venous c.* a long, fine catheter inserted into a vein for the purpose of administering, through a large blood vessel, parenteral fluids (as in parenteral NUTRITION), antibiotics and other therapeutic agents. This type of catheter is also used in the measurement of central venous pressure (*see* CENTRAL (VENOUS PRESSURE)). *Self-retaining c.* a catheter made in such a way that after introduction the blind end expands so that it can remain in the bladder. Useful for continuous or intermittent drainage or where frequent specimens are required. *Ureteric c.* a fine gum-elastic catheter passed up the ureter to the renal pelvis and used to insert a contrast medium in retrograde urography.

catheterization the insertion of a catheter into a body cavity.

cation an ion or group of ions having a positive charge and moving towards the negative electrode in electrolysis.

cauda a tail-like appendage. *C. equina* the bundle of coccygeal, sacral and lumbar nerves with which the spinal cord terminates.

caudal referring to a cauda. *C. block* a local anaesthetic agent injected into the sacral canal so that operations may be carried out in the peritoneal area without a general anaesthetic.

caul the amnion, which occasionally does not rupture but envelops the infant's head at birth.

causalgia an intense burning pain which persists after peripheral nerve injuries.

caustic a substance, usually a strong acid or alkali, capable of burning organic tissue. Silver nitrate (*lunar c.*) and carbon dioxide snow are those most commonly used, e.g., silver nitrate to destroy warts.

cauterization the destruction of tissue with cautery.

cautery 1. the application of searing heat by a hot instrument, an electric current or other means such as a laser. 2. an agent so used. *Cold c.* cauterization by carbon dioxide, called also cryocautery.

cavernoma a cluster of abnormal blood vessels usually found in the brain or spinal cord resembling a raspberry. They often cause no symptoms but can bleed or press on other parts of the brain leading to various problems depending on the location.

cavernous having caverns or hollows. *C. breathing* sounds heard on auscultation over a pulmonary cavity. *C. sinus* a venous channel lying on either side of the body of the sphenoid bone through which pass the internal carotid artery and several nerves. *C. sinus thrombosis* a serious complication of any infection of the face, the veins from the orbit draining into the sinus and carrying the infection into the cranium.

cavitation the formation of cavities, e.g., in the lung in tuberculosis.

cavity a confined space or hollow or potential hollow within the body or one of its organs, e.g., the abdominal cavity or a decayed hollow in a tooth.

CCG clinical commissioning group.

CCU coronary care unit.

cell 1. the basic structural unit of living organisms (*see* Figure). A microscopic mass of protoplasm, consisting of a nucleus surrounded by cytoplasm and enclosed in a cell membrane, from which all organic tissues are constructed. Each cell can reproduce itself by mitosis. 2. a small, more or less enclosed, space. *C. division* the

processes by which cells multiply. *See* MITOSIS and MEIOSIS.

cellulitis a diffuse inflammation of connective tissue, especially of subcutaneous tissue, which causes a typical brawny, oedematous appearance of the part; local abscess formation is not common.

cellulose a carbohydrate forming the covering of vegetable cells, i.e., vegetable fibres. Not digestible in the alimentary tract of humans but gives bulk and, as 'roughage', stimulates peristalsis.

Celsius scale *A. Celsius, Swedish astronomer, 1701–1744.* A temperature scale with the melting point of ice set at 0° and the boiling point of water at 100°. The normal temperature of the human body is 36.9°C. Formerly known as the centigrade scale. *See* FAHRENHEIT SCALE.

cementum cement. Connective tissue with a bone-like structure which covers the root of a tooth and supports it within the socket.

censor 1. a member of a committee on ethics or for critical examination of a medical or other society. 2. the psychic influence that prevents unconscious thoughts and wishes coming into consciousness.

censorship in psychiatry, the process of selecting, accepting or rejecting conscious ideas, memories and impulses arising from the individual's subconscious.

census enumeration of a population. The national census was first introduced in England and Wales in 1801 and has since been repeated every 10 years (except in 1941). It usually records name, address, age, sex, occupation, marital status and other social information.

Centers for Disease Control and Prevention (CDC) an agency of the US Department of Health and Human Services, located in Atlanta, Georgia, which serves as a centre for the control, prevention and investigation of diseases. A

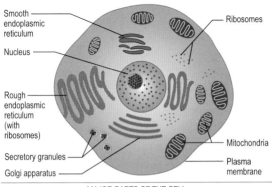

Smooth endoplasmic reticulum

Ribosomes

Nucleus

Rough endoplasmic reticulum (with ribosomes)

Secretory granules

Golgi apparatus

Mitochondria

Plasma membrane

MAJOR PARTS OF THE CELL

similar function is performed in England by the Centre of Infectious Disease Surveillance and Control, in Wales by the Public Health Wales Communicable Diseases Surveillance Centre, in Northern Ireland by the Public Health Agency and in Scotland by Health Protection Scotland.

centigrade *see* CELSIUS SCALE.

centile *see* PERCENTILE.

central pertaining to the centre or midpoint. *C. nervous system (CNS)* the brain and spinal cord. *C. sulcus* a deep groove in each of the hemispheres of the brain separating the frontal and parietal lobes. *See* FONTANELLES. *C. venous pressure* the pressure recorded by the introduction of a catheter into the right atrium in order to monitor the condition of a patient after a major operative procedure, such as heart surgery.

Central Sterile Supplies and Disinfection Unit (CSSD) a hospital sterilization and disinfection unit or department.

central venous catheter/line a special catheter that is inserted into a large central vein either through a peripheral vein or a skin tunnel for the administration of drugs, the infusing of hypertonic fluids and to measure pressures. The catheter/line also allows long-term access for the administration of medications, nutritional support and blood products.

centrifugal conveying away from a centre, such as from the brain to the periphery. Efferent; the reverse of centripetal.

centrifuge an apparatus that rotates at high speed. If a test tube, for example, is filled with a fluid such as blood or urine and rotated in a centrifuge, any bacteria, cells or other solids in it are precipitated.

centripetal conveying from the periphery to the centre. Afferent; the reverse of centrifugal.

centromere the region(s) of the chromosomes which become(s) allied with the spindle fibres at mitosis and meiosis.

centrosome a body in the cytoplasm of most animal cells, close to the nucleus. It divides during mitosis, one half migrating to each daughter cell.

centrosphere the cell centre, in an area of clear cytoplasm near the nucleus.

cephalhaematoma a swelling beneath the pericranium, containing blood, which may be found on the head of the newborn infant. Caused by pressure during labour. Gradually reabsorbed within the first few days of life.

cephalocele cerebral hernia. *See* HERNIA.

cephalography radiographic examination of the contours of the head.

cephalometry measurement of the dimensions of the head of a living person either directly or by radiography. *See also* PELVIMETRY.

cerclage [Fr.] encircling of a part with a ring or loop, as for correction of an incompetent cervix uteri or fixation of the adjacent ends of a fractured bone. *See* SHIRODKAR'S SUTURE.

cerebellum the portion of the brain below the cerebrum and above the medulla oblongata. Its functions include the coordination of fine voluntary movements and posture.

cerebral relating to the cerebrum. *C. cortex* the outer layer of the cerebrum, composed of neurones. *C. haemorrhage* rupture of a cerebral blood vessel. Likely causes are aneurysm and hypertension. *See* APOPLEXY. *C. hernia see* HERNIA. *C. irritation* a condition of general nervous irritability and abnormality, often with photophobia, which may be an early sign of meningitis, tumour of the brain, etc. It is also associated with trauma. *C. palsy* a condition caused by injury to the brain during or immediately after birth. Coordination of movement is affected, and may cause the child to be flaccid or athetoid, in which condition there is constant random and uncontrolled movement.

cerebration mental activity.

cerebrospinal relating to the brain and spinal cord. *C. fluid (CSF)* the fluid made in the choroid plexus of the ventricles of the brain and circulating from them into the subarachnoid space around the brain and spinal cord.

cerebrovascular pertaining to the arteries and veins of the brain. *C. accident* a disorder (also called stroke) arising from an embolus, thrombus or haemorrhage in the cerebrum; may vary in severity from a transient weakness or tingling in a limb to profound paralysis, coma and death. *C. disease* any disorder of the blood vessels of the brain and its meninges.

cerebrum the largest part of the brain, occupying the greater portion of the cranium and consisting of the right and left hemispheres divided by the longitudinal fissure (*see* Figure). Each hemisphere contains a lateral ventricle. The internal substance is white and the convoluted surface is grey. The centre of the higher functions of the brain.

cerumen a waxy substance secreted by the ceruminous glands of the auditory canal. Earwax.

cervical pertaining to the neck or the constricted part of an organ, e.g., uterine cervix. *C. canal* the passage through the uterine cervix. *C. cancer* cancer of the uterine cervix. *C. cerclage*

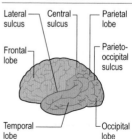

CEREBRUM

Lateral sulcus
Central sulcus
Parietal lobe
Frontal lobe
Parieto-occipital sulcus
Temporal lobe
Occipital lobe

a stitch placed in the cervix to prevent pre-term labour due to an incompetent cervix. *C. collar* a rigid or semirigid immobilizing support for the neck. *C. rib* a short, extra rib, often bilateral, which sometimes occurs on the seventh cervical vertebra and may cause pressure on an artery or nerve. *C. smear* a test for disorders of the cervical cells; material is scraped from the uterine cervix and examined microscopically. *C. spondylosis* a degenerative disease of the intervertebral joints and discs of the neck. *C. vertebra* one of the seven bones forming the neck portion of the spinal column.

cervicitis inflammation of the neck of the uterus.

cervix a constricted portion or neck. *C. uteri* the neck of the uterus; it is about 2 cm long and projects into the vagina. Capable of wide dilatation during childbirth.

CESDI Confidential Enquiry into Stillbirths and Deaths in Infancy. Function is now taken on by MBRRACE-UK (Mothers and Babies: Reducing Risk through Audits and Confidential Enquiries across the UK). *See* CONFIDENTIAL ENQUIRY.

cestode tapeworm.

chafe irritation of the skin as caused by the friction between skinfolds. Occurs particularly in moist areas.

chalazion a meibomian or tarsal cyst. A swollen sebaceous gland in the eyelid. A small, hard tumour may develop.

chancre 1. the initial lesion of syphilis developing at the site of inoculation. 2. a papular lesion occurring at the site of infection in tuberculosis or in sporotrichosis.

chancroid soft chancre. A venereal ulceration, due to *Haemophilus ducreyi*, accompanied by inflammation and suppuration of the local glands.

character 1. the combination of traits and qualities distinguishing the unique nature of the individual. 2. a letter, mark or numeral seen on a computer

screen or printed. *C. change* indicates alteration in a person's recognized behaviour to one alien to the person's normal manner of conduct. *C. disorder* a chronic state in which the person exhibits maladaptive and unacceptable forms of behaviour and social response.

Charcot's disease or joint *J.M. Charcot, French neurologist, 1825–1893.* A chronic progressive, degenerative disease of the stress-bearing portion of one or more joints. The disease is the result of an underlying neurological disorder, e.g., diabetic neuropathy, or tabes dorsalis from syphilis, or leprosy.

Charcot's triad nystagmus, intention tremor and scanning speech. A trio of signs of disseminated sclerosis.

chart a record in graphic or tabular form. *Genealogical c.* a graph showing various descendants of a common ancestor, used to indicate those affected by genetically determined disease. *Reading c.* a chart with material printed in gradually increasing type sizes, used in testing acuity of near vision. *Snellen's c.* a chart printed with block letters in gradually decreasing sizes, used in testing visual acuity.

charting the keeping of important facts about a patient and the progress of their illness. Patient records will normally include a range of charts depending on the diagnosis, and the observations and treatments deemed to be necessary.

cheilosis maceration at the angles of the mouth; fissures may also occur. It may be associated with general debility or riboflavin deficiency.

chelating agent a drug that has the power of combining with certain metals and so aiding excretion, to prevent or overcome poisoning. *See* DIMERCAPROL and PENICILLAMINE.

chemical change this differs from physical change in that a profound alteration in properties results, usually permanently and usually accompanied by use of energy in a new substance, e.g., hydrogen (two atoms) plus oxygen produces water.

chemical compound any substance produced by chemical change which may then be broken up into its components only by chemical means, unlike a mixture, which can usually be separated mechanically.

chemistry the science that deals with the elements, the atoms which compose them and the compounds that they form.

chemoprophylaxis the prevention of an acute or recurrent attack of a specific disease by the administration of chemotherapeutic agents, e.g., antibiotics to treat infections or the use of antitubercular drugs for tuberculosis.

chemoreceptor a sensory nerve ending or group of cells that is sensitive to chemical stimuli in the blood.

chemosis swelling of the conjunctiva due to the presence of fluid; an oedema of the conjunctiva.

chemotaxis the reaction of living cells to chemical stimuli. These are either attracted (*positive c.*) or repelled (*negative c.*) by acids, alkalis or other substances.

chemotherapy the specific treatment of disease by the administration of chemotherapeutic agents prescribed to delay or arrest growth of cancer cells. Administered by the oral, intramuscular and intravenous routes and occasionally directly into a body cavity, e.g., the bladder. Used to arrest the progress of or eradicate a specific pathological condition in the body without causing irreversible harm to healthy tissue.

chest the thorax. *Barrel c.* one more rounded than usual, with raised ribs and, usually, kyphosis. It is often present in emphysema. *C. leads* leads applied to the chest during the course of an electrocardiographic recording. *Flail c.* one where part of the chest wall moves in opposition to respiration as a result of multiple fractures of the ribs. *Pigeon c.* a chest with the sternum protruding forwards.

Cheyne–Stokes respiration *J. Cheyne, British physician, 1776–1836; W. Stokes, British physician, 1804–1878*. Tidal respiration. A form of irregular but rhythmic breathing with temporary cessations (apnoea). It is likely to be present in cerebral tumour, in narcotic poisoning and in advanced cases of arteriosclerosis and uraemia.

Chiari malformations structural defects in the cerebellum sometimes causing hydrocephalus as a result of obstruction of the cerebral spinal fluid. These malformations can also cause headaches, difficulty in concentrating and thinking and a range of other symptoms.

chiasma a crossing point. *Optic c.* the crossing point of the optic nerves.

chickenpox *see* VARICELLA.

chilblain a condition resulting from defective circulation when exposure to cold causes localized swelling and inflammation of the hands or feet, with severe itching and burning sensations.

child the human young, from infancy to puberty. *C. abuse* physical, sexual or emotional mistreatment or neglect or the non-accidental act of omission by a parent or other custodian responsible for the care of a child. Child abuse encompasses malnutrition and other kinds of neglect through ignorance, as well as deliberate withholding from the child of the necessary and basic physical care, including the medical and dental care necessary for the child to grow. Examples of physical abuse range from burns and exposure to extreme cold, to beating, poisoning, strangulation, withholding food and water and fabricating illness so that the child is subject to unnecessary medical intervention (also known as Munchausen syndrome by proxy or fabricated or induced illness (FII)). If a child is seen to be in danger of suffering significant harm, from physical, sexual, emotional or neglectful causes, the child may be registered on the Child Protection Register. If a nurse, health visitor or midwife has reasonable cause to suspect the abuse of a child, appropriate action must be taken in order to protect that child. *See also* CHILDREN ACT 2004. *Deprived c.* a vague term usually implying that the child in question has been raised in a situation lacking in love, affection and consistent parenting responses from adults. Sometimes used to suggest that the child has experienced a generalized deficit of life opportunities, both interpersonal and social. *C. protection* the Children Act emphasizes that the needs of the child are paramount in any decision making and that policies encourage families to stay together where possible, replacing parents' rights with one of parental responsibility. *C.p. register* a record of children at risk of, or suspected of being at risk of abuse; the key worker, usually a social worker, ensures that a Child Protection Plan is carried out. Access to the register of named children is restricted to those with direct dealings with children. *C. sexual abuse* the subjection of a child to sexual activity likely to cause physical or psychological harm. Sexual abuse can occur with or without physical contact taking place. Non-contact child sexual abuse includes grooming, exploitation, persuading children to perform sexual acts over the internet and flashing. *C. surveillance* the assessment of a (usually preschool) child's progress at defined ages by a health visitor, general practitioner or a community paediatrician to identify any developmental or physical concerns.

child care any matter associated with the upbringing and welfare of children, both familial and in relation to welfare and social services. *C.c. officer* a social worker who has a responsibility to investigate any situation where a child is thought to be at risk of harm due to neglect, injury or desertion, and in those situations where the child is considered 'beyond control' by the parents/guardians or is offending.

child development the stages of physical, psychological and social growth and attainment that occur from birth to adulthood.

child health clinic a centre which infants and preschool children attend on a regular basis to ensure normal progress and development. Immunizations against infectious diseases, screening and health promotion information are also provided.

childbirth the act or process of giving birth to a child. Parturition. *Natural c.* the act of giving birth without medical intervention. Relaxation and other complementary techniques are used to minimize pain and discomfort, allowing the mother and her partner to remain in control of events which are allowed to progress naturally.

childminder a person who is registered with Ofsted in England, the Care Inspectorate in Scotland, the local Health and Social Care Trusts in Northern Ireland or with the Care and Social Services Directorate Inspectorate in Wales and who is approved to mind an agreed number of children aged from birth to 5 years during the day.

Children Act 2004 Act of Parliament bringing together comprehensive law relating to children defining their rights, identifying parental responsibilities and detailing procedures to protect them. The Children Act is responsible for promoting awareness of views and interests of children, having regard to the United Nations Convention on the Rights of the Child. Agencies involved in children's services have a duty to cooperate to improve wellbeing of children and young people. Children's services authorities must establish Local Safeguarding Children Boards to protect children from harm; local authorities must ascertain feelings of children when making decisions about services for children in need, and providing accommodation for children under the Act.

Children's Centres responding to local community needs, providing child and family health services, childcare advice and early learning specialist services.

Chinese medicine a traditional system based on the principles of Yin and Yang, combining acupuncture with a range of medications from herbal and animal sources.

Chinese restaurant syndrome transient arterial dilatation due to ingestion of monosodium glutamate, which is used in seasoning Chinese food; marked by throbbing head, light-headedness, tightness of the jaw, neck and shoulders, and backache.

chiropody podiatry, the study and care of the feet and the treatment of minor foot complaints.

chiropractic a system of treatment employing manipulation of the spine and other bony structures.

chi-squared test a statistical test to determine whether two or more groups of observations differ significantly from one another, i.e., more than would be expected by chance.

Chlamydia and *Chlamydophila*. Genus of bacteria comprising various species and serotypes which cause many illnesses including Chlamydia pneumonia (especially in children and in young adults); pneumonia acquired through maternal transmission; acute and chronic conjunctivitis (e.g., adult and neonatal inclusion conjunctivitis); trachoma; and adult pharyngitis. Several serotypes of *C. trachomatis* are the most common cause of sexually transmitted diseases in the UK, many EU countries and the USA, including non-gonococcal urethritis and epididymitis in men, cervicitis, urethritis and pelvic inflammatory disease in women, Reiter's syndrome, and lymphogranuloma venereum. In England, it is recommended that sexually active young people under the age of 25 years are tested each year for Chlamydia.

chloasma a condition in which there is brown, blotchy discoloration of the skin of the face, especially during pregnancy.

chlorine *symbol* Cl. A yellow, irritating poisonous gas. A powerful disinfectant, bleach and deodorizing agent. Used in hypochlorites for sterilization purposes.

cholangiography radiography of the hepatic, cystic and bile ducts after the insertion of a radio-opaque contrast medium.

cholangitis inflammation of the bile ducts.

cholecystectomy excision of the gallbladder.

cholecystitis inflammation of the gallbladder.

cholecystoduodenostomy an anastomosis between the gallbladder and the duodenum.

cholecystography radiography of the gallbladder after administration of a radio-opaque contrast medium.

cholecystolithiasis the presence of stones in the gallbladder.

cholecystotomy an incision into the gallbladder, usually to remove gallstones.

choledocholithiasis the presence of stones in the bile duct.

cholelithiasis presence of gallstones in the bladder or bile ducts.

cholera an acute, notifiable, infectious enteritis endemic and epidemic in Asia and also in Africa. Caused by *Vibrio cholerae*, associated with faecal contamination of water supplies, overcrowding and unhygienic conditions. It is marked by profuse diarrhoea, muscle cramp, suppression of urine with severe dehydration; it is often fatal but with the early administration of rehydration together with salts and sugar solution as early as possible affected people make a full recovery. Oral cholera vaccination is available to travellers to areas where cholera is endemic. For travellers the local drinking water should be boiled or sterilized and uncooked foods avoided.

cholestasis arrest of the flow of bile due to obstruction of the bile ducts.

cholesteatoma a rare small tumour containing cholesterol. It may occur in the middle ear or in the meninges, central nervous system or bones of the skull.

cholesterol a sterol found in nervous tissue, red blood corpuscles, animal fat and bile. It is a precursor of bile acids and steroid hormones, and occurs in the most common type of gallstone, in atheroma of the arteries, in various cysts and in carcinomatous tissue. Most of the body's cholesterol is synthesized, but some is obtained in the diet. Blood cholesterol levels are influenced by diet, weight, heredity and metabolic diseases, e.g., diabetes mellitus, and can be measured by blood tests. Dietary measures to lower cholesterol include reducing the saturated fat intake and increased exercise.

choline an essential amine, found in the blood, cerebrospinal fluid and urine, which aids fat metabolism. Formerly classified as a vitamin of the B complex.

cholinergic pertaining to nerves that release acetylcholine as the chemical stimulator at their nerve endings. *C. drugs* drugs that inhibit cholinesterase and so prevent the destruction of acetylcholine.

cholinesterase an enzyme that rapidly destroys acetylcholine.

chondroblast an embryonic cell that forms cartilage.

chondroma a benign new growth arising in cartilage.

chondromalacia a condition of abnormal softening of cartilage.

chorda a sinew or cord.

chordee downward curvature of the penis caused by congenital anomaly (common in hypospadias) or urethral infection.

chorditis inflammation of the vocal or spermatic cords.

chordotomy an operation on the spinal cord to divide the anterolateral nerve pathways for relief of intractable pain. Cordotomy.

chorea a symptom of disease of the basal ganglia when the individual suffers from spasmodic, involuntary, rapid movements of the face, shoulders and hips. Chorea may also be a side effect of certain drugs. *Huntington's c.* (or Huntington's disease) a rare hereditary disorder which manifests itself in early middle age. The individual also suffers from progressive dementia, which often precedes a premature death. *Sydenham's c.* May occur in childhood. Characterized by rapid, irregular voluntary movement. Recovery may take some time but most children will recover completely.

choreiform resembling chorea.

choriocarcinoma formerly known as chorioepithelioma. A highly malignant neoplasm usually arising from the trophoblast of a hydatidiform mole (see HYDATIDIFORM MOLE). It may develop after an abortion or the evacuation of a hydatidiform mole or even in normal pregnancy. Metastases usually develop rapidly but the disease normally carries a good prognosis if early treatment is given.

chorion the outer membrane enveloping the fetus; the placenta.

chorionic pertaining to the chorion. *C. gonadotrophin* human chorionic gonadotrophin (HCG). *C. villi* small protrusions on the chorion from which the placenta is formed. They are in close association with the maternal blood and, by diffusion, interchange of nutriment, oxygen and waste matters is effected between the maternal and the fetal blood. *C. villus sampling* tissue removed from the gestational sac early in pregnancy so that chromosomal and other inherited disorders can be identified. Can be carried out at an earlier stage than amniocentesis.

chorioretinitis inflammation of the choroid and retina of the eye. Choroidoretinitis.

choroid the pigmented and vascular coat of the eyeball, continuous with the iris and situated between the sclera and retina. It reduces the amount of light that falls upon the retina. *C. plexus* specialized cells in the ventricles of the brain that produce cerebrospinal fluids. There is one choroid plexus in each ventricle.

choroiditis inflammation of the choroid.

Christmas disease a hereditary bleeding disease similar to haemophilia but is due to a deficiency of clotting factor IX; also called haemophilia B. The name is derived from that of the first patient to be studied.

chromatography a method of chemical analysis by which substances in solution can be separated as they percolate down a column of powdered absorbent or ascend an absorbent paper by capillary traction. A definite pattern is produced and substances may be recognized by the use of appropriate colour reagents. Amino acids can be identified in this way.

chromatometry the measurement of colour perception.

chromosome in animal cells, a structure in the nucleus, containing a linear thread of DEOXYRIBONUCLEIC ACID (DNA), which transmits genetic information and is associated with RIBONUCLEIC ACID (RNA) and histones. During cell division the material composing the chromosome is compactly coiled. Each organism of a species is normally characterized by the same number of chromosomes in its somatic cells, 46 being the number usually present in humans: 22 pairs of autosomes, and two sex chromosomes (XX or XY), which determine the sex of the organism. In the mature GAMETE (ovum or spermatozoon) the number of chromosomes is halved as a result of MEIOSIS.

chronic of long duration; the opposite of acute. *C. fatigue syndrome* extreme fatigue for the patient over a long period, often years. The cause of this condition is not fully understood, although some cases have been reported following recovery from a viral infection. Most commonly affects women between 25 and 45 years age. The main symptom is constant tiredness but other symptoms may include poor concentration, sore throat, tender lymph nodes, muscle and joint pain. Also known as myalgic encephalomyelitis (ME). *C. kidney disease (CKD)* progressive loss of kidney function over a period of months or years. *C. obstructive pulmonary disease (COPD)* a combination of chronic bronchitis and emphysema in which there is disruption of air flow into or out of the lungs. Dyspnoea, wheezing and cough predominate, often made worse by any exertion or pollution in the environment. Patients may be severely disabled and require oxygen for long periods.

chronological the recording of a number of events starting with the earliest and following the order in which they occurred. *C. age* the age of an individual expressed as a period of time that has elapsed since birth. In infants, this may be given in hours, days or weeks but for children and adults it is expressed in years.

Churg–Strauss syndrome also known as eosinophilic granulomatosis with polyangiitis. A type of vasculitis that mainly affects adults aged 30–45 years.

Chvostek's sign *F. Chvostek, Austrian surgeon, 1835–1884.* A spasm of the facial muscles which occurs in tetany. It can be elicited by tapping the facial nerve.

chyle digested fats which, as a milky fluid, are absorbed into the lymphatic capillaries (lacteals) in the villi of the small intestine.

chylothorax the presence of effused chyle in the pleural cavity.

chyme the semiliquid acid mass of food that passes from the stomach to the intestines.

chymotrypsin an enzyme secreted by the pancreas. It is activated by trypsin and aids in the breakdown of proteins.

Ci symbol for *curie* a measure of radioactivity.

cicatrix the scar of a healed wound (*see* KELOID).

cilia 1. the eyelashes. 2. microscopic filaments projecting from some epithelial cells, known as ciliated membranes, as in the bronchi, where cilia wave the secretion upwards.

ciliary hair-like. *C. body* a structure just behind the corneosclceral margin, composed of the ciliary muscle and processes. *C. muscle* the circular muscle surrounding the lens of the eye. *C. processes* the fringed part of the choroid coat arranged in a circle in front of the lens.

Cimex a genus of blood-sucking bugs. *C. lectularius* the common bedbug.

CINAHL *see* CUMULATIVE INDEX TO NURSING AND ALLIED HEALTH LITERATURE.

cineangiocardiography angiography using a cine camera to show the movements of the heart and blood vessels.

circadian denoting a period of 24 hours. *C. rhythm* the rhythm of certain biological activities that take place daily.

circinate having a circular outline. *Tinea circinata* is ringworm.

circle of Willis *T. Willis, British physician and anatomist, 1621–1675.* An anastomosis of arteries at the base of the brain, formed by the branches of the internal carotid and the basilar arteries.

circulation movement in a circular course, as of the blood (*see* Figures on pp. 78–79). *Collateral c.* enlargement of small vessels establishing adequate blood supply when the main vessel to the part has been occluded. *Coronary c.* the system of vessels that supplies the heart muscle itself. *Extracorporeal c.* 1. removal of the blood by intravenous cannulae, passing it through a machine to oxygenate it, and then pumping it back into circulation. 2. the 'heart–lung' machine or pump respirator, used in cardiac surgery. *Lymph c.* the flow of lymph through lymph vessels and glands. *Portal c.* the passage of blood from the alimentary tract, pancreas and spleen, via the portal vein and its branches through the liver and into the hepatic veins. *Pulmonary c.* passage of the blood from the right ventricle via the pulmonary artery through the lungs and back to the heart by the pulmonary veins. *Systemic c.* the flow of blood throughout the body. The direction of flow is from the left atrium to the left ventricle and through the aorta, with its branches and capillaries. Veins then carry it back to the right atrium, and so into the right ventricle.

circumcision excision of the prepuce or foreskin of the penis. An operation performed for religious reasons, or sometimes for phimosis or paraphimosis. *Female c.* excision of the labia minora and/or labia majora, and sometimes the clitoris; still performed ritualistically in certain countries, the extent of the surgery varying from one culture to another. Prior to pregnancy it may cause problems with micturition and intercourse. Special care may be required during labour and delivery, and excision and separation of the tissues may be needed; alternatively a caesarean section may be considered. Gynaecological complications include bladder-wall necrosis, urinary or vesico-vaginal fistulae. Female circumcision is illegal in most countries but the laws are poorly enforced. Also known as female genital mutilation.

circumduction moving in a circle, e.g., the circular movement of the upper limb.

circumoral around the mouth. *C. pallor* a pale area around the mouth contrasting with the flushed cheeks, e.g., in scarlet fever.

cirrhosis a degenerative change that can occur in any organ, but especially in the liver. May be due to viruses, microorganisms or toxic substances (*portal c.*). Fibrosis results and interferes with the working of the organ. In the liver it causes portal obstruction,

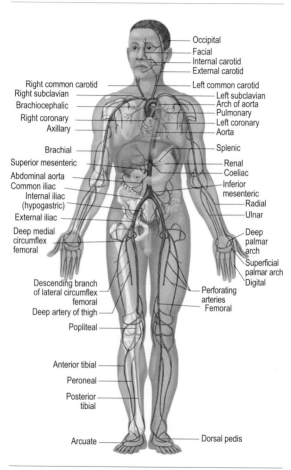

ARTERIAL CIRCULATION

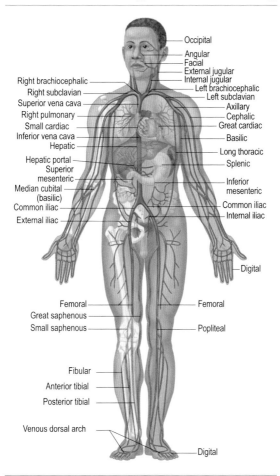

VENOUS CIRCULATION

with fatigue, muscle cramps and weight loss. Consequent developments may include ascites, jaundice, splenomegaly, oesophageal varices and episodes of bleeding and bruising. Clinical features may vary considerably. Digital clubbing may be present.

cisterna a space or cavity containing fluid. *C. chyli* the dilated portion of the thoracic duct containing chyle. *C. magna* the subarachnoid space between the cerebellum and medulla oblongata.

cisternal concerning the cisterna. *C. puncture* insertion of a hollow needle into the cisterna magna to withdraw cerebrospinal fluid.

citric acid acid found in the juice of lemons, limes, etc. An antiscorbutic.

CJD *See* CREUTZFELDT–JAKOB DISEASE.

Cl symbol for *chlorine*.

clairvoyance extrasensory perception. The act or power of knowing about objects or events without the use of the senses.

clang association rhyming speech. A way of speaking where words are associated that are similar in sound. Observed in some mental disorders.

clapping in physiotherapy, rhythmic beating with cupped hands. Frequently used over the chest to aid expectoration.

class 1. a system that divides members of a society into sets based upon social or economic status and is based upon cultural characteristics in common. 2. a group of objects that have a common characteristic.

claudication lameness. *Intermittent c.* limping, accompanied by severe pain in the legs on walking, which disappears with rest. A sign of occlusive arterial disease.

claustrophobia fear of confined spaces, such as small rooms.

clavicle the collar bone. A long bone, part of the shoulder girdle.

clawfoot a deformity in which the longitudinal arch is abnormally raised. Pes cavus.

clawhand a deformity in which the fingers are bent and contracted, giving a claw-like appearance.

cleft a fissure or longitudinal opening. *C. lip* a congenital fissure in the upper lip, often accompanied by cleft palate. *C. palate* a congenital defect in the roof of the mouth due to failure of the medial plates of the palate to meet. Often associated with cleft lip.

client 1. a recipient of a professional service. 2. a recipient of health care, regardless of the person's state of health and where the service is delivered. 3. a patient.

climacteric the period of the menopause in women. Also used to denote the decline in sexual drive in men.

climax 1. the stage when a disease is at its greatest intensity. 2. the stage in sexual intercourse when orgasm occurs.

clinic 1. instruction of students at the bedside. 2. a department of a hospital devoted to the treatment of a particular type of disease or a place which patients attend for a consultation with a medical or nurse practitioner.

clinical relating to bedside observation and the treatment of patients. *C. audit* a cyclical measurement and evaluation by health professionals of the clinical standards they are achieving. *C. commissioning groups (CCGs)* created in 2013 and responsible in England for the planning and commissioning of local health services. They are clinically led by GPs and are responsible for most of the total NHS budget in England. They originally were not able to commission GP services but are now able to take on this function. *C. governance* a framework through which NHS organizations are accountable for continuously improving the quality of their services and for safeguarding high standards of care by creating an environment in which excellence in care will flourish. *C. nurse specialist* a qualified nurse who has acquired advanced knowledge and skills in a specific area of clinical nursing. *C. risk index for babies (CRIB)* a professional scoring tool used in assessing the initial neonatal risks for babies, and also for comparing the performance of one neonatal intensive care unit with another. *C. risk management* the means by which adverse events occurring in organizations and usually related to the delivery of patient care are systematically assessed and reviewed in order to seek ways for prevention of future incidents. *C. senates* established in England to provide independent clinical advice to commissioners to help them make the best decisions about health care. *C. skills* skills required by clinicians (doctors, nurses, dentists and other clinical professions). Clinical skills vary depending on specialty but core skills remain constant, e.g., communication skills, history-taking skills, record-keeping, basic physical examination, etc. *C. supervision* an exchange between practising professionals to enable the development of professional skills. Has a vital role in sustaining and developing professional practice in nursing and midwifery. *See* Appendix 13. *C. trial* a research investigation designed to provide objective information on the therapeutic efficacy of a particular drug or therapy.

clip a metal device for holding the two edges of a wound together or for controlling the flow of liquid through a tube.

clitoridectomy excision of the clitoris. *See* CIRCUMCISION (FEMALE).

clitoris a small organ, formed of erectile tissue, situated at the anterior junction of the labia minora in the female.

clone cells which are genetically identical to each other and have descended by asexual reproduction from the parent cell, to which they are also genetically identical.

clonic having the character of clonus. The second stage of a tonic–clonic seizure (formerly known as a grand mal fit). *See* EPILEPSY.

clonus muscle rigidity and relaxation which occurs spasmodically. *Ankle c.* spasmodic movements of the calf muscles when the foot is suddenly pushed upwards, the leg being extended.

Clostridium a genus of anaerobic spore-forming bacteria, found as commensals of the gut of animals and humans and saprophytes of the soil. Pathogenic species include *C. botulinum* (botulism), *C. tetani* (tetanus) and *C. perfringens* (also known as *C. welchii*) (gas gangrene).

Clostridium difficile (C. difficile) a spore-forming bacterium that is present in the gut of some adults and children and normally does not cause any problems in healthy people. However, sometimes antibiotics are given to a patient to treat an infection which can interfere with the balance of the 'good bacteria' present in the gut. When this happens, *C. difficile* bacteria can multiply and cause symptoms such as diarrhoea and pyrexia. Most cases occur in a health care environment such as a hospital or care home. Generally, people with *C. difficile* infection make a full recovery, but the infection can sometimes be fatal especially in the elderly or very young. The risks of transmitting *C. difficile* amongst patients during health care episodes can be minimized by prudent antimicrobial prescribing, the isolation of those with *C. difficile* diarrhoea with enhanced environmental cleansing, and especially hand hygiene. Care should be taken not to rely on alcohol hand gels, which do not destroy bacterial spores. *See* Appendix 11.

clot a semisolid mass formed in a liquid, such as blood or lymph, by coagulation.

clotting coagulation. The formation of a clot (*see* BLOOD CLOTTING). *C. time* coagulation time. The length of time taken for shed blood to coagulate.

clubbing broadening and thickening of the tips of the fingers (and toes) due to bad circulation. It occurs in chronic diseases of the heart and respiratory system, such as congenital cardiac defect and tuberculosis.

clubfoot talipes.

clumping the collecting together into clumps. The reaction of bacteria and blood cells when agglutination occurs.

cluster headaches severe attacks of pain in one side of the head and often felt around the eye. The exact cause is unknown but they tend to start in adulthood and run in families. Typically, they will occur every day for several weeks at a time and will then subside and a period of remission follows. Although they are not life threatening, they significantly affect the quality of life of people who suffer from them.

Co symbol for *cobalt.*

coaching a form of non-directive interaction in which the coach supports the coachee to identify goals and solutions to challenges. The coachee might be a professional but increasingly professionals are encouraged to adopt a coaching style in conversations with patients particularly about self-management of long-term conditions.

coagulase an enzyme formed by pathogenic staphylococci that causes coagulation of plasma. Such bacteria are termed *c. positive.*

coagulation clotting. *See* BLOOD CLOTTING.

coagulation factor concentrate 1. effective against the bleeding tendency in haemophilia. 2. an agent that counteracts the bleeding tendency in haemophilia. Factor VIII is one of the clotting factors, deficiency of which causes the more frequent, classic, sex-linked haemophilia. It is available in a recombinant (manufactured rather than from humans) preparation for preventive and therapeutic use.

coagulum the mass of fibrin and cells formed when blood clots; the mass formed when other masses coagulate, e.g., milk curd.

coal tar a by-product obtained in the destructive distillation of coal; used in ointment or solution in the treatment of eczema and psoriasis.

coarctation a condition of contraction or stricture. *C. of aorta* a congenital malformation characterized by deformity of the aorta, causing narrowing, usually severe, of the lumen of the vessel. Surgical resection of the stricture may be performed.

cobalt *symbol* Co. A metallic element, traces of which are necessary in the diet to prevent anaemia. *Radioactive c.* cobalt-60, used as a source of gamma irradiation in radiotherapy prior to lineal accelerators.

cocaine a colourless alkaloid, obtained from coca leaves, which has a powerful but brief stimulant action. Formerly used as a local anaesthetic, cocaine has been replaced by less addictive preparations like procaine, lignocaine and amethocaine, also known as tetracaine. It is a Class A controlled drug. It is now a major 'recreational' drug, producing euphoria with many undesirable behavioural and social effects. It is highly addictive and usually taken by snorting. Regular inhaling of the drug can damage the lining of the nose. Overdose can cause seizures and cardiac arrest. Also known, in its various forms, as 'crack', 'coke', 'snow', 'flake', 'nose candy' or 'rocks'.

cocainism addiction to cocaine. Longterm abuse is associated with a toxic psychosis.

coccus a bacterium of spheroidal shape.

coccydynia persistent pain in the region of the coccyx.

coccyx the terminal bone of the spinal column, in which four rudimentary vertebrae are fused together to form a triangle.

cochlea the spiral canal of the internal ear.

cochlear implant a surgically implanted electronic device that can help to provide a sense of sound to a person who is profoundly deaf.

Cochrane library *A. Cochrane, 1909–1988.* Collection of systematic reviews of published research. An international multidisciplinary collaboration of health professionals, consumers and researchers who review randomized controlled clinical trials.

cod liver oil purified oil from the liver of the codfish; valuable source of vitamins A and D.

code 1. a set of rules governing one's conduct. 2. a system by which information can be communicated. *Genetic c.* the arrangement of nucleotides in the DNA of the chromosomes and in the RNA of the protein transcription apparatus in the cell. *C. for nurses and midwives* a code of professional conduct for the nurse and midwife. Revised periodically, this code is intended to provide definite standards of practice and conduct that are essential to the ethical discharge of the nurse's and midwife's responsibility and to inform the public, other professions and employers of the standard of professional conduct expected of a registered practitioner. Many other professional groups have their own standards of conduct, performance and ethics. Some of these groups are regulated by the Health and Care Professions Council and include arts therapists, biomedical scientists, chiropodists and podiatrists, clinical scientists, dieticians, occupational therapists, orthoptists, paramedics, physiotherapists, prosthetists, orthotists, radiographers and speech and language therapists. *See* Appendix 5.

coeliac relating to the abdomen. *C. disease* an inflammatory condition of the gastrointestinal tract due to a hypersensitivity to gluten (found in barley, wheat, oats and rye) in the diet. Damage to the gut causes malabsorption leading to weight loss and vitamin and mineral deficiencies that may cause anaemia and ill health. Diagnosis is made by blood, urine and faecal testing together with jejunal biopsies. Treatment involves a lifelong gluten-free diet. Coeliac disease can affect all ages and runs in some families. The incidence in the UK is 1:1000 *C. plexus* nerve complex that supplies the abdominal organs.

coenzyme an organic molecule activator to a larger protein enzyme.

cognition the action of knowing. Cognitive function of the conscious mind in contrast to the effective (feeling) and conative (willing). *C. behavioural therapy (CBT)* a method of treating psychological disorders based on the approach that the client's problems arise from their way of looking at the world and oneself. In cognitive therapy the client is helped to identify negative or false cognitions and then encouraged to try out new thought strategies in daily living. *Mild c. impairment* a brain function disorder that is more serious than the normal cognitive decline that occurs with ageing but not significant enough to interfere with activities of daily living. It may occur as a transitional stage between normal ageing and dementia.

cohabit 1. to live together and have a sexual relationship without being married. 2. to coexist.

cohort a group of people possessing a common characteristic, such as being born in the same year or of the same sex, used in research to make generalizations derived from quantitative data. *C. study* concerning a specific group or subpopulation in a research study.

coil *see* INTRAUTERINE DEVICE.

coitus sexual intercourse between male and female. *C. interruptus* a method of contraception in which the erect penis is removed from the vagina before ejaculation occurs.

cold 1. of low temperature. 2. a viral infection affecting the membranes of the nose and throat and the bronchial tubes. *C. sore* herpes simplex. *See* HERPES.

colic acute paroxysmal abdominal pain. *Biliary c.* pain due to the presence of a gallstone in a bile duct. *Infantile c.* excessive crying due to pain and distress. Most common in the first 3 months of life. The infant may pull up its legs and expel gas from the anus or 'belch'. May be due to air swallowing, milk intolerance or natural hyperactivity. *Intestinal c.* severe griping spasmodic abdominal pain which may be a symptom of food poisoning or of intestinal obstruction. *Renal c.* pain due to the presence of a stone in the ureter. *Uterine c.* spasmodic pain originating in the uterus, as in dysmenorrhoea.

coliform resembling the bacillus *Escherichia coli.*

colitis inflammation of the colon. It may be due to a specific organism, as in dysentery, but the term *ulcerative c.* denotes a chronic disease, often of unknown cause, in which there are attacks of diarrhoea, with the passage of blood and mucus.

collagen a fibrous structural protein that constitutes the protein of the white (collagenous) fibres of skin, tendon, bone, cartilage and all other connective tissues. It also occurs dispersed in a gel to provide stiffening, as in the vitreous humour of the eye. *C. diseases* a group of diseases having in common certain clinical and histological features that are manifestations of involvement of connective tissues (*see* CONNECTIVE (TISSUES)).

collapse 1. a state of extreme prostration due to defective action of the heart, severe shock or haemorrhage. 2. falling in of a structure.

collar bone the clavicle.

collateral accessory to. *C. circulation see* CIRCULATION.

Colles' fracture *A. Colles, Irish surgeon, 1773–1843.* Fracture of the lower end of the radius at the wrist following a fall on the outstretched hand. Typically, it produces the 'dinner fork' deformity.

colloid 1. glue-like. 2. the translucent, yellowish, gelatinous substance resulting from colloid degeneration. 3. a chemical system composed of a continuous medium of small particles which do not settle out under the influence of gravity and will not pass through a semipermeable membrane, as in DIALYSIS.

coloboma a congenital fissure of the eye affecting the choroid coat and the retina.

colon the large intestine, from the caecum to the rectum. *Ascending c.* that part rising up to the right of the abdomen in front of the liver. *Descending c.* that part running down from in front of the spleen to the sigmoid colon. *Giant c.* megacolon. *Irritable c. see* IRRITABLE (BOWEL SYNDROME). *Pelvic c., sigmoid c.* that part lying in the pelvis and connecting the descending colon with the rectum. *Transverse c.* that part lying across the upper abdomen connecting the ascending and descending portions (*see* Figure on p. 85).

colonic pertaining to the colon. *C. irrigation* colonic LAVAGE.

colonoscope a fibreoptic instrument, passed through the anus, for examining the interior of the colon.

colony a mass of bacteria formed by multiplication of cells when bacteria are incubated under favourable conditions.

colostomy an artificial opening (stoma) in the large intestine brought to the surface of the abdomen for the purpose of evacuating the bowel.

colostrum the fluid secreted by the breasts in the last few weeks of pregnancy and for the first 3 or 4 days after delivery, until lactation begins. Colostrum is high in protein and initially low in lactose; its fat content is equivalent to breast milk. It is an important source of passive antibody.

colour index an index of the amount of haemoglobin in red blood cells. In normal blood the figure is 1, in iron deficiency anaemia it is less than 1

Enlarged detail of the large intestine, rectum and anus shows the junction between the large and small intestines and the valve-like entry of the ileum into the caecum.

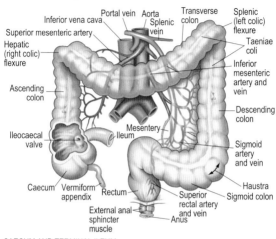

CAECUM AND TERMINAL ILEUM

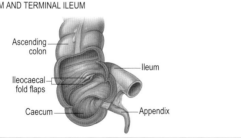

COLON

and in megaloblastic anaemia it is more than 1. *See* BLOOD.

colour vision deficiency any abnormality in colour vision that causes difficulty distinguishing between certain colours. The most common types of colour vision deficiency are reduced discrimination between red and green. A total absence of colour vision is very rare.

colpocele a hernia of either bladder or rectum into the vagina. Vaginocele.

colpohysterectomy removal of the uterus through the vagina.

colpoperineorrhaphy the repair by suturing of an injured vagina and torn perineum.

colpopexy suture of a prolapsed vagina to the abdominal wall.

colporrhaphy repair of the vagina. *Anterior c.* repair for cystocele. *Posterior c.* repair for rectocele.

colposcope a speculum for examining the vagina and cervix by means of a magnifying lens; used for the early detection of malignant changes.

coma a state of unconsciousness from which the patient cannot be aroused. Characterized by an absence of both spontaneous eye movements and response to painful stimuli. *See* GLASGOW COMA SCALE.

comatose in the condition of coma.

comedo a blackhead. A plug of keratin and sebum within the dilated orifice of a hair follicle.

comfort to provide relief of or freedom from pain, depression or anxiety. *C. eating* eating at inappropriate times or eating unusual amounts for the relief of distress or anxiety. *C. measure* a specific action taken to promote the comfort of the patient, e.g., rearranging pillows or providing a change of position.

comforter a baby's dummy or pacifier.

commensal living on or within another organism, and deriving benefit without harming or benefiting the host individual.

comminuted broken into small pieces, as in a comminuted FRACTURE.

Commission on Human Medicines established in 2005 to advise ministers and the licensing authority about the safety, quality and efficacy of human medicines; promotes the collection and investigation of information about adverse drug reactions; and considers representation from applicants or licence holders. *See* YELLOW CARD REPORTING.

commissioning the process by which health needs of the population are delivered and priorities determined. It is a strategic, long-term activity that frames service development within the NHS. Commissioning is a cyclical process involving: assessment of health need, auditing of current service provision, setting priorities, service and practice development, with contracting and the evaluation of services. The commissioning process is undertaken in partnership with other agencies and is led in England by CLINICAL COMMISSIONING GROUPS (CCGs).

commissure a site of union of corresponding parts, as the angle of the lips or eyelids.

commode a bedside chair with a cutaway seat that allows a receptacle to be fitted underneath for the collection of urine and faeces. Used by a patient who is unable to reach the lavatory.

communicable disease an infectious disease caused by microorganisms that may be transmitted from a person, animal or the environment to susceptible persons, either directly or indirectly.

communication skills in the broadest sense involve listening, speaking, writing and reading. In the context of health care, they generally focus on listening and giving information to patients. Communication skills cover both verbal and non-verbal forms of communication. Communication skills may extend to communicating with other clinicians, communicating at conferences or formal meetings, and presenting material in class settings.

community a group of individuals living in an area, having a common interest, or belonging to the same organization. *C. care* the care of individuals within the community, by health care professionals and carers as an alternative to institutional or long-stay residential care. *C. health services* services provided in the community by staff other than those employed by general practices. Staff groups involved include district nurses, health visitors, physiotherapists, speech therapists, podiatrists and school nurses. *C. nurse* a nurse who is based within the community with a responsibility for providing nursing services within the patient's own home or environment and may come from a variety of specialized backgrounds, e.g., psychiatry. All community nurses have a strong commitment towards health promotion and the prevention of ill health. *C. safety partnership* aims to create safer places for people to live, work and visit. Involves different agencies to tackle issues such as antisocial behaviour, domestic violence, crime, and reducing accidents and injuries. *Therapeutic c.* any treatment setting (usually psychiatric) which provides a living–learning situation through group processes emphasizing social, environmental and personal interactions.

compartment syndrome a painful and potentially serious condition caused by a bleeding or swelling within an enclosed bundle of muscles known as a muscle compartment causing damage to the muscles and nearby nerves.

compatibility mutual suitability. The mixing together of two substances without chemical change or loss of power. *See* BLOOD GROUPS.

compensation 1. making good a functional or structural defect. 2. mental mechanism (unconscious) by which a person covers up a weakness by exaggerating a more desirable characteristic.

compensatory techniques assistance for patients/clients in developing new skills to compensate for a recognized disability or deficit.

competence a set of professionally agreed deliverables, outputs and roles that the health care professional must be able to perform in a particular post.

competency a set of behaviour patterns, knowledge and skill that the holder needs to bring to a position in order to perform the required role and functions with competence.

complaint an act of expressing dissatisfaction with a service or individual; may be written or verbal. *C. management* the policies and procedures in place within an NHS organisation to respond to and learn from complaints received from patients, their families and members of the public regarding care, treatment and services.

complement a substance present in normal serum which combines with the antigen–antibody complex to destroy bacteria. *C. fixation test* measurement of the amount of complement with antigen–antibody complex. Complement fixation tests are used to detect antibodies for infectious diseases.

complement system a series of small inactive plasma proteins that are an important part of the innate immune response to infection. When stimulated by the presence of either an antibody–antigen complex or certain microbial products or antigens, complement proteins act as a biochemical cascade, with one protein activating the next. This results in the formation of activated complement which, by various means, attacks and destroys invading microorganisms, dissolves and removes immune complexes.

complementary pertaining to that which completes or makes perfect. *C. feed* feed given to infants to supplement breast feeding when the mother has insufficient milk. *C. therapies* a range of treatments, including yoga, reflexology, homeopathy, acupuncture and others, which may be combined with traditional medicine. *See also* ALTERNATIVE MEDICINE.

complete androgen insensitivity syndrome a condition that affects sexual development before birth and during puberty. People with the condition are genetically male but do not respond to male hormones and as a result have female external genitalia and breasts.

Also known as testicular feminization syndrome.

complex a grouping of various things, as of signs and symptoms, forming a syndrome. In psychology, a grouping of ideas of emotional origin which are completely or partially represented in the unconscious mind. *Inferiority c.* a compensation by assertiveness or aggression to cover a feeling of inadequacy. *See* ELECTRA COMPLEX and OEDIPUS COMPLEX. *C. regional pain syndrome* a poorly understood condition in which the patient experiences persistent severe and debilitating pain often triggered by an injury but which persists after healing has taken place.

compliance the degree to which a patient follows professional advice regarding their therapy.

complication an accident or second disease process arising during the course of or following the primary condition; may be fatal.

compos mentis [L.] *of sound mind.*

compound composed of two or more parts or substances. *C. fracture* a fracture in which a wound through to the skin has also occurred.

comprehension mental grasp of the meaning of a situation.

compress folded material, e.g., lint (wet or dry), applied to a part of the body for the relief of swelling and pain.

compression 1. the act of pressing upon or together; the state of being pressed together. 2. in embryology, the shortening or omission of certain developmental stages.

compression bandages are used in the treatment of leg ulcers to improve venous return and reduce venous hypertension. Following successful healing of the leg ulcer compression hose are worn to prevent reoccurrence.

compression garments these may be fitted and used following burns or for a patient with lymphoedema. They work by exerting pressure on the tissues thus preventing the build up of fluid in the tissues.

compulsion an overwhelming urge to perform an irrational act or ritual.

computed tomography (CT) the utilization of a computerized technique to examine a cross-section of the entire body. The CT scanner produces an image of tissue density in a complete cross-section of the part of the body being scanned.

computerized records health records are now held on computer systems which are required by law to be secure and to maintain confidentiality, usually achieved by limiting access and controlling data sharing. *See also* DATA PROTECTION ACT.

conation a striving in a certain direction. *See* COGNITION.

concept an image or idea held in the mind.

conception 1. the act of becoming pregnant, by the fertilization of an ovum. 2. a concept.

conceptual framework a group of concepts that are broadly defined and organized to provide a rationale or structure for the interpretation of information.

concussion a violent jarring shock. *C. of the brain* temporary loss of consciousness produced by a fall or a blow on the head. There may be amnesia, slow respiration and a weak pulse.

conditioned response a response that does not occur naturally but may be developed by regular association of some physiological function with an unrelated outside event, such as the ringing of a bell or flashing of a light. Soon the physiological function starts whenever the outside event occurs. Also called conditioned reflex. *See also* UNCONDITIONED RESPONSE.

conditioning a form of learning in which a response is elicited by a neural stimulus that had previously been repeatedly presented in conjunction with the stimulus that originally elicited the response. Also called classical and respondent conditioning.

condom a contraceptive sheath worn during sexual intercourse and affording some protection for both partners against sexually transmitted diseases, available for both males and females.

conductive deafness deafness caused by the faulty conduction of sound from the outer to the inner ear.

conductor 1. a substance through which electricity, light, heat or sound can pass. 2. any part of the nervous system that conveys impulses.

condyle a rounded eminence occurring at the end of some bones, and articulating with another bone.

condylomata *sing.* condyloma. An elevated wart-like lesion of the skin. *C. acuminata* small, pointed papillomas of viral origin, usually occurring on the skin or mucous surfaces of the external genitalia or perianal region. *C. lata* wide, flat, syphilitic condylomata occurring on most skin, especially about the genitals and anus.

cone a solid figure with a rounded base, tapering upwards to a point. *C. biopsy* the removal of a cone-shaped section from the cervix of the uterus. It is performed for confirmation of the diagnosis when a cervical smear test result suggests the presence of pre-cancerous cells. *Retinal c.* the cone-shaped end of a light-sensitive cell in the retina, used for acute vision and for distinguishing colours.

confabulation the production of fictitious memories, and the relating of experiences which have no relation to truth, to fill in the gaps due to loss of memory. A symptom of Korsakoff's syndrome.

confidence self-assurance arising from a belief in one's own ability to achieve. *C. interval* in statistics, a range of values that has some specified probability. By convention 95% and 99% confidence intervals are the most used. *C. limits* the bounds of the confidence interval.

confidential enquiry a unique form of audit in which case notes are scrutinized by relevant professionals to identify substandard care and make recommendations for future practice. The Confidential Enquiry into Maternal Deaths and the Confidential Enquiry into Stillbirths and Deaths in Infancy (CESDI), functions now combined under MBRRACE (Mothers and Babies: Reducing Risk through Audits and Confidential Enquiries across the UK), is directly related to maternity care, and midwives may be involved in providing appropriate information. The enquiry includes enquiries into maternal, stillbirths and deaths in infancy. The National Confidential Enquiry into Patient Outcome and Death (NCEPOD) is also available.

confidentiality spoken, written or given in confidence.

conflict a mental state arising when two opposing wishes or impulses cause emotional tension and often cannot be resolved without repressing one of the impulses into the unconscious. Conflict situations may be associated with an anxiety neurosis.

confluent running together.

confusion disturbed orientation in regard to time, place or person, sometimes accompanied by disordered consciousness.

congenital existing and present at the time of birth. Often genetically determined. *C. cataracts* cataracts present at birth seen in children with certain genetic conditions or following infection during pregnancy. *C. dislocation of the hip* failure in position of the head of the femur and development of the acetabulum. *C. heart defect* a structural defect of the heart or great vessels or both. *C. hyperthyroidism* a condition in which not enough thyroxine is secreted at birth. All newborn babies are screened at birth and if diagnosis is confirmed with be treated with thyroxine containing medication. *C. infection* an infection which takes place in utero. The most important congenital infections are rubella, cytomegalovirus, herpes simplex, human immunodeficiency virus (HIV), syphilis and toxoplasmosis.

Congenital Disabilities (Civil Liabilities) Act 1976 this Act is applicable in England, Wales and Northern Ireland and provides for a child to be entitled to recover damages where the child has suffered as a result of a breach in a duty of care owed to the mother or the father unless that breach of duty of care occurred before the child was conceived and either or both parents knew of the occurrence. In Scottish law the same provisions are made. The accuracy and preservation of records is therefore essential. *See* RECORDS.

congestion an abnormal accumulation of blood in any part. *Pulmonary c.* congestion of the lung, as in pneumonia and congestive heart failure.

conjugate to join or yoke together as, in the liver, bilirubin is combined with albumin by the activity of glucuronyl transferase to render it water-soluble so that it may be excreted via the gut. *See also* ICTERUS and JAUNDICE.

conjunctiva the mucous membrane covering the front of the eyeball and lining the eyelids.

conjunctivitis inflammation of the conjunctiva. 'Pink eye' ophthalmia. *Catarrhal c.* a mild form, usually due to cold or irritation. *Granular c.* trachoma. *Phlyctenular c.* marked by small vesicles or ulcers on the membrane. *Purulent c.* caused by virulent organisms, with discharge of pus.

connective joining together. *C. tissues* those that develop from the mesenchyme and are formed of a matrix containing fibres and cells. Areolar tissue, cartilage and bone are examples.

consanguinity blood relationship.

conscious the state of being awake or aware. Levels of consciousness are loosely defined states of awareness of and response to stimuli, essential for the assessment of an individual's neurological status. The level of consciousness is an accurate indicator of the degree of brain (dys)function.

consent in law, voluntary agreement with an action proposed by another. Consent is an act of reason; the person giving consent must be of sufficient mental capacity and in possession of all essential information in order to give valid and informed consent. It is a legal requirement that doctors or researchers inform patients about to undergo surgery or invasive tests or to be a subject involved in a clinical trial of the risks and probable outcomes of the treatment or research. *C. forms* in non-emergency situations, written informed consent is generally required before many clinical procedures, such as surgery (including biopsies), endoscopy and radiographic procedures involving catheterization. The doctor or the health professional concerned must explain to the patient the diagnosis, the nature of the procedure, including the risks involved and the chances of success, and the alternative methods of treatment that are available. A signed declaration that the doctor has explained the nature of the procedure to the patient in non-technical words should be included. Nurses or other members of the health care team may be involved in filling out the consent form and witnessing the signature of the patient. If the patient is a minor, or incapable of giving informed consent, the next-of-kin or guardian must sign the consent form. *Informed c.* a process whereby patients, parents or guardians and research participants are kept fully informed of the procedures that they will be undertaking; enabling them to make an informed choice for consent. Ensuring informed consent is a moral and legal duty for all health care professionals.

conservative treatment the use of non-radical methods to restore health and preserve function.

consolidation a state of becoming solid. *C. of lung* in pneumonia the infected lobe becomes solid with exudate.

constipation incomplete or infrequent action of the bowels, with consequent filling of the rectum with hard faeces. *Atonic c.* constipation due to lack of muscle tone in the bowel wall. *Spastic c.* a form of constipation where spasm of part of the bowel wall narrows the canal. Also known as irritable bowel syndrome.

Consultant in Public Health Medicine Responsible for functions such as promoting health, preventing disease and fostering cooperation between the health and social services.

consumer in health care, may be the user, client, patient or carer, in terms of the services being provided.

consumption 1. the act of consuming, or the process of being consumed. 2. a wasting away of the body; once applied to pulmonary tuberculosis.

contact 1. a mutual touching of two bodies or persons. 2. an individual known to have been in association with an infected person or animal or a contaminated environment. *C. dermatitis* a skin rash marked by itching, swelling, blistering, oozing and scaling. It is caused by direct contact between the skin and a substance to which the person is allergic or sensitive. (*See* LATEX) *C. lens* a glass or plastic lens worn under the eyelids in the front of the eye. It may be worn for therapeutic or for cosmetic reasons. *C. tracing* a public health measure taken to limit the spread of infectious disease, e.g., sexually transmitted diseases, tuberculosis.

contagion 1. the communication of disease from one person to another by direct contact. 2. an infectious disease.

containment a term used in communicable disease control, meaning prevention of spread of disease from a focus of infection. *C. isolation* a patient suspected of having or suffering from a communicable disease is separated from others to prevent the spread of the infection.

content analysis a research technique for the objective, systematic and quantitative description of communications and documentary evidence.

continent 1. able to control urination and defaecation. 2. exercising self-restraint, especially abstaining from sexual activity.

continuing healthcare refers to a package of ongoing care for patients outside of the hospital setting who have been assessed as having a primary health need which might be a long-term condition or other chronic incapacitating illness.

continuing education also known as continuing professional development (CPD) further study and learning after the attainment of basic qualifications. This is vital for all professional practitioners so that they may keep up to date within their field and is accomplished in the form of organized study days or courses, or by individual reading and study. The Nursing and Midwifery Council regulations require nurse and, midwives to undertake periodic revalidation (*see* Appendix 12) which includes updating and refreshment in order to provide research-based care to their patients and clients. The Health and Care Professions Council (HCPC) requires all its registered health care professionals to regularly update their practice. *See* Appendix 5.

continuity of care the concept of a health care provider (general practitioner, nurse or midwife, etc.) being continually involved with a patient throughout treatment over a period which may extend over years.

continuous ambulatory peritoneal dialysis (CAPD) treatment in which the patient is ambulant while receiving peritoneal dialysis.

continuous positive airway pressure (CPAP) medical gas is delivered to the patient at positive pressure to hold open alveoli that would normally close at the end of expiration, thereby increasing oxygenation and reducing the work of breathing.

contraception the prevention of conception and pregnancy.

contraceptive an agent used to prevent conception, e.g., condom, cap that occludes the cervix, spermicidal pessary or cream, hormone skin patches, injections, subdermal implants, intrauterine device (IUD) and oral contraceptives (hormone pills).

contract 1. to make or to enter into an agreement with a person, authority or company to deliver services or goods. 2. in health care, an agreement, usually written, between two people with differing interests and concerns.

contraction a shortening or drawing together, especially applied to muscle action. *Uterine c's* those occurring during labour.

contracture fibrosis causing permanent contraction. *Dupuytren's c.* contraction of the palmar fascia causing permanent bending and fixation of one or more fingers. *See* DUPUYTREN'S CONTRACTURE and Figure on p. 121. *See* VOLKMANN'S ISCHAEMIC CONTRACTURE. *Volkmann's ischaemic c.* contraction resulting from impairment of the blood supply in upper limbs.

contraindication any condition that makes a particular line of treatment impracticable or undesirable.

contralateral occurring on the opposite side.

contrast medium a substance used in radiography to make visible or more visible certain organs.

contrecoup [Fr.] an injury occurring on the opposite side or at a distance from the site of the blow, e.g., brain damage on the opposite side of the skull to the blow.

control 1. restraint or command of objects or events. 2. a standard for testing where the procedure is identical in all respects to the experiment but the factor being studied is absent. *Birth c.* contraception. *C. group* a group of subjects who in the course of an experimental research project do not experience the factor under consideration.

This enables the researcher to make a comparison with the effects produced on the experimental group. *C. of infection* standards and procedures within the health care service that provide guidelines for all staff to control infection within hospitals and in all health care facilities, e.g., ambulances and the community. *See* INFECTION.

Control of Substances Hazardous to Health (COSHH) regulations that require the assessment of risk and action to be taken regarding the use of substances that may be hazardous to health within the workplace.

controlled-dose transdermal absorption of drugs application of a drug patch to the skin: gradual absorption gives a constant level in the blood. Examples of drugs used in this way include analgesics, some types of hormone and nicotine to assist a smoker to cease smoking.

controlled drugs preparations subject to the regulatory control of prescribing and dispensing of psychoactive drugs, including narcotics, hallucinogens, depressants and stimulants.

controlled trial a research method in which one group of subjects in a trial are not exposed to the experimental treatment or investigation, in an attempt to decrease the possibility of error and increase the possibility that the findings of the study are an accurate reflection of reality.

contusion a bruise.

convalescence period of recovery following illness, injury or operation. Also referred to as REHABILITATION.

convection a method of transmission of heat by the circulation of warmed molecules of a liquid or a gas.

conversion 1. the act of changing into something of different form or properties. 2. the transformation of emotions into physical manifestations. 3. manipulative correction of malposition of a fetal part during labour.

convolution a fold or coil, e.g., of the cerebrum or renal tubules.

convulsion involuntary contractions of the voluntary muscles. Convulsive seizures are symptomatic of some neurological disorders; they are not in themselves a disease entity. *Clonic c.* a convulsion marked by alternative contracting and relaxing of the muscles. *Febrile c.* a convulsion occurring almost exclusively in children aged 6 months to 5 years of age, and associated with a fever of 40°C or higher. *Tonic c.* prolonged contraction of the muscles, as a result of an epileptic discharge. *See* EPILEPSY.

Coombs' test *R.R.A. Coombs, British immunologist, 1921–2006.* A test to detect the presence of any antibody on the surface of the red blood cell. Used to detect rhesus incompatibility in maternal or fetal blood and in the diagnosis of haemolytic anaemia.

coordination harmony of movement between several muscles or groups of muscle so that complicated manoeuvres can be made.

coping the process of contending with life difficulties in an effort to overcome or work through them. *C. mechanisms* conscious or unconscious strategies or mechanisms that a person uses to cope with stress or anxiety.

copper *symbol* Cu. A metallic element, traces of which are present in all human tissues.

coprolalia the uncontrolled use of obscene speech. *See* TOURETTE'S SYNDROME.

coprolith a mass of hard faeces in the rectum or colon.

copulation coitus. Sexual intercourse between male and female.

cord a long cylindrical flexible structure. *Spermatic c.* that which suspends the testicle in the scrotum, and contains the spermatic artery and vein and vas deferens. *Spinal c.* the part of the central nervous system enclosed in the spinal column (*see* Figure on p. 365). *Umbilical c.* the connection between the fetus and the placenta, through which the

fetus receives nourishment. *Vocal c's* folds of mucous membrane in the larynx, which vibrate to produce the voice.

corn a local hardening and thickening of the skin from pressure or friction, occurring usually on the feet.

cornea the transparent portion of the anterior surface of the eyeball continuous with the sclerotic coat.

corneal pertaining to the cornea. *C. graft* a means of restoring sight by grafting healthy transparent cornea from a donor in place of diseased tissue. Keratoplasty.

corneoscleral relating to both the cornea and sclera. *C. junction* the point where the edge of the cornea joins the sclera. The limbus.

cornu a horn. *C. of the uterus* one of the two horn-shaped projections where the uterine tubes join the uterus at the upper pole on either side.

coronal relating to the crown of the head. *C. suture* the junction of the frontal and parietal bones.

coronary encircling. Crown-like. *C. arteries* the vessels that supply the heart. *C. artery bypass graft* (CABG) an operation carried out to bypass a coronary artery narrowed by atheroma using a graft from a healthy blood vessel usually from the leg, arm or chest. *C. care unit* a ward or unit within a hospital which provides for the monitoring and intensive care by a specialist team of staff of patients who have suffered an attack of coronary thrombosis and of those who are in the immediate postoperative period following heart surgery. *C. circulation see* CIRCULATION. *C. thrombosis see* THROMBOSIS.

coronaviruses members of a family (Coronaviridae) of large, enveloped, positive-stranded RNA viruses. Human coronaviruses (HCoVs) are a major cause of acute respiratory illnesses, e.g., the common cold (coryza). They can occasionally cause serious infections of the lower respiratory tract in children and adults and necrotizing enterocolitis in newborns.

coroner a public official (e.g., a barrister or solicitor with some medical knowledge) who holds inquests concerning unexpected, sudden, violent or suspicious deaths.

corporate governance the accountability of an NHS Trust to meet standards in corporate management working within the need to meet statutory financial objectives and targets.

corporate working system in which managers and practitioners work within a team ethos, sharing a designated workload and providing an equity of service.

corpse a dead body; cadaver.

corpulent obese.

corpus a body. *C. albicans* the scar tissue on the surface of the ovary which replaces the corpus luteum before the recommencement of menstruation. *C. callosum* the mass of white matter that joins the two cerebral hemispheres together. *C. cavernosum* either of the two columns of the erectile tissue forming the body of the clitoris or the penis. *C. luteum* the yellow body left on the surface of the ovary and formed from the remains of the Graafian follicle after the discharge of the ovum. If it retrogresses, menstruation occurs, but it persists for several months if pregnancy supervenes. *C. striatum* a mass of grey and white matter in the base of each cerebral hemisphere.

corpuscle a small protoplasmic body or cell, as of blood or connective tissue.

cortex [L.] an outer layer, as the bark of the trunk or root of a tree, or the outer layer of an organ or other structure, as distinguished from its inner substance. *Adrenal c.* the tissue surrounding the medulla or core of the adrenal gland. *Cerebral c.* the grey matter covering the two cerebral hemispheres. *Renal c.* the outer covering of the kidney.

corticospinal relating to the cerebral cortex and the spinal cord. *C. tract* the pyramidal tract. The nerve fibres making up the main pathway for rapid voluntary movement.

corticosteroid any of the hormones produced by the adrenal cortex or their synthetic substitutes. Glucocorticoids are responsible for carbohydrate, fat and protein metabolism. They have powerful anti-inflammatory properties. Mineralocorticoids, e.g., aldosterone, are responsible for salt and water regulation.

corticotrophin Adrenocorticotrophic hormone (ACTH).

cortisol the naturally occurring hormone of the adrenal cortex. Hydrocortisone.

cortisone a naturally occurring corticosteroid. Inactive in humans until converted into cortisol.

Corynebacterium a genus of slender, rod-shaped, gram-positive and non-motile bacteria. *C. diphtheriae* Klebs–Löffler bacillus, the causative agent of diphtheria.

coryza acute infection of the upper respiratory tract, characterized by perfuse discharge from nasal mucous membranes, sneezing and watering of the eyes. Highly contagious. The medical name for the common cold.

cosmetic 1. improving something outwardly. 2. relating to treatment intended to improve a person's appearance. *C. dentistry* treatment to improve the appearance of the teeth or to prevent further damage to teeth or gums, e.g., the whitening of teeth or fitting a crown to a damaged tooth. *C. surgery* an operation to improve a person's appearance, e.g., mammoplasty to reduce or enhance the breasts or the removal of skin blemishes or excess body fat and tissue.

cost effectiveness a concept which relates cost to the effectiveness of a service and thus provides value for money, e.g., screening programmes to detect cervical cancer, rate of detection, and cost of the service and of treatment.

costal relating to the ribs. *C. cartilages* those that connect the ribs to the sternum directly or indirectly.

costochondritis inflammation of the cartilage that joins the ribs to the sternum. It will usually resolve after a few weeks.

cot death *see* SUDDEN INFANT DEATH SYNDROME.

cotyledon A cup-shaped depression. Applied to the subdivisions of the placenta.

cough voluntary or reflex explosive expulsion of air from the lungs. Its purpose is usually to expel a foreign body or accumulations of mucus. *Dry c.* one where no expectoration occurs. *Wet c.* one where expectoration of mucus or foreign body occurs. *Whooping c.* infectious disease caused by *Bordetella pertussis*.

counselling a process of consultation and discussion in which one individual (the counsellor) listens actively and offers guidance to another who is experiencing difficulties (the client). The counsellor does not direct or make decisions for the client. The general aim is to solve problems and increase awareness. The emphasis is on clients finding their own solutions. *Disaster c.* specialized counselling offered to victims of a major disaster, e.g., an aircraft crash or terrorist attack, or a natural event, e.g., an earthquake. The survivors of such disasters often experience psychological problems and post-traumatic stress disorder resulting in ill health.

counterextension 1. the holding back of the upper fragment of a fractured bone while the lower is pulled into position. 2. the raising of the foot of the bed in such a way that the weight of the body counteracts the pull of the extension apparatus on the lower part of the limb. Used especially for fracture of the femur.

counterirritant a substance that produces mild inflammation of the skin when applied to it, but relieves pain and congestion.

countertraction the reduction of fractures by traction from two opposing directions at once.

coupling in cardiology, the frequent occurrence of a normal heart beat followed by an extraventricular beat. May be found as a result of digitalis overdose.

couvade the experiencing of the symptoms of pregnancy and childbirth by the father.

coxa the hip joint. *C. valga* a deformity of the hip in which there is an increase in the angle between the neck and the shaft of the femur. *C. vara* a deformity in which the angle between the neck and the shaft of the femur is smaller than normal.

Coxiella a genus of microorganisms of the order Rickettsiales. *C. burnetii* the causative agent of Q fever.

Coxsackie virus one of a group of enteroviruses that may give rise to a variety of illnesses, including meningitis, pleurodynia, acute myocarditis and acute pericarditis.

crab louse *Phthirus pubis*. See LOUSE.

crack purified form of cocaine, produced by a technique known as 'freebasing'. *See* COCAINE.

cradle 1. a frame placed over the body or limb of a bed patient for protecting injured parts and preventing them from coming into contact with the bedclothes. 2. infant's bed with protective sides and, in the past, often on rockers. 3. to support, hold, comfort in the arms. *C. cap* an oily crust sometimes seen on the scalp of infants; also called milk crust (crusta lactea). Caused by excessive secretion of the sebaceous glands in the scalp.

cramp a painful spasmodic muscular contraction which may result from fatigue.

cranial relating to the cranium. *C. nerves* the 12 pairs of nerves arising directly from the brain (see Figure).

craniopharyngioma a cerebral tumour arising in the craniopharyngeal pouch just above the sella turcica.

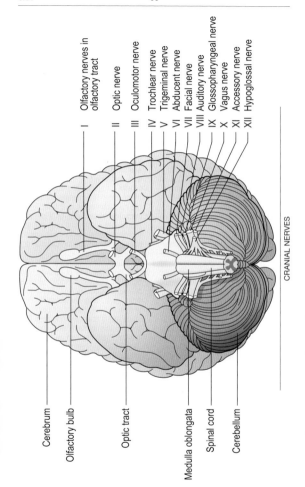

CRANIAL NERVES

I — Olfactory nerves in olfactory tract
II — Optic nerve
III — Oculomotor nerve
IV — Trochlear nerve
V — Trigeminal nerve
VI — Abducent nerve
VII — Facial nerve
VIII — Auditory nerve
IX — Glossopharyngeal nerve
X — Vagus nerve
XI — Accessory nerve
XII — Hypoglossal nerve

Cerebrum
Olfactory bulb
Optic tract
Medulla oblongata
Spinal cord
Cerebellum

craniosacral therapy a form of osteopathic treatment in which very gentle manipulation of the cranium attempts to release tensions within the skull which are thought to be the cause of various problems. The therapy has been successfully used to treat babies fractious after difficult forceps or vacuum extraction deliveries, colic and hyperactivity in older infants.

craniostenosis premature closure of the suture lines of the skull in an infant. Surgery may be required to relieve raised intracranial pressure.

craniosynostosis premature closure of the cranial sutures.

craniotabes a patchy thinning of the bones of the vault of the skull of an infant; associated with RICKETS and OSTEOGENESIS IMPERFECTA (brittle bones).

craniotomy a surgical opening of the skull made to relieve pressure, arrest haemorrhage or remove a tumour.

cranium 1. the skull. 2. the bony cavity that contains the brain.

creatine a nitrogenous compound present in muscle. It is also found in the urine in conditions in which muscle is rapidly broken down, e.g., acute fevers and starvation. *C. phosphate* a high-energy phosphate store in muscle.

creatinine a normal constituent of urine; a product of protein metabolism.

creatinuria increased concentration of creatine in the urine.

credentialing review and examination of the credentials of health care professionals to ensure that they have training and the qualifications necessary to deliver care and support to the patient and the family.

credibility a criterion for evaluating the data of qualitative research study, referring to the amount of confidence in the truth of the given information.

Credit Accumulation and Transfer System (CATS) learning points or credits awarded by an academic institution to an individual for prior academic learning and/or evidence of the acquisition of professional expertise demonstrated, e.g., through a personal professional profile, contributing towards academic or professional awards. Originally developed to provide flexibility between academic institutions. *See* APEL and APL.

crepitation 1. the grating sound caused by friction of the two ends of a fractured bone or on movement of an arthritic joint. 2. a similar sound heard in the lungs through a stethoscope. *See* RALE.

crepitus 1. *see* CREPITATION. 2. the noisy discharge of flatus from the bowels.

cretinism congenital hypothyroidism. An obsolete term.

Creutzfeldt–Jakob disease *H.G. Creutzfeldt, German physician, 1885–1964; A. Jakob, German physician, 1884–1931.* Abbreviated CJD. A progressive dementia transmissible through prion protein. A new variant of CJD has been reported in younger adults with a shorter incubation period and usually fatal.

cribriform perforated like a sieve. *C. plate* part of the ethmoid bone. *See* ETHMOID.

cricoid ring-shaped. *C. cartilage* the ring-shaped cartilage at the lower end of the larynx.

cri du chat syndrome a hereditary congenital syndrome characterized by hypertelorism, microcephaly, severe mental deficiency, and a plaintive cat-like cry; due to the deletion of part of the short arm of chromosome 5. Also known as Chromosome 5p deletion syndrome.

crisis 1. a decisive point in acute disease; the turning point towards either recovery or death. *See* LYSIS. 2. a sudden paroxysmal intensification of symptoms in the course of a disease. 3. life crisis; a period of disorganization that occurs when a person meets an obstacle to an important life goal, such as the sudden death of a family member or a difficult family conflict. *Addisonian c., adrenal c.* symptoms of fatigue, nausea and vomiting and collapse accompanying an acute attack of adrenal failure. *Blast c.* a sudden, severe change in the course of chronic myelocytic leukaemia. The clinical picture resembles that seen in acute myelogenous leukaemia, with an increase in the proportion of myeloblasts. *C. intervention* counselling or psychotherapy for patients in a life crisis that is directed at supporting the patient through the crisis and helping the patient to cope with the stressful event that precipitated it. *Identity c.* usually occurring during adolescence, manifested by a loss of the sense of the sameness and historical continuity of one's self, and inability to accept the role the individual perceives as being expected by society.

criterion the basis on which a decision is made, e.g., for drug dosage, treatment plans, research trials, etc.

critical 1. arising from a crisis. 2. implying serious risk or uncertainty as to outcome. *C. appraisal* an analysis of a research project using the parameters of research design, methodology, examination of results and relevance, e.g., relating the findings to practice. *C. care outreach team* a team of specialist critical care practitioners based in hospital, whose main role is to share specialist skills and support ward staff in order to prevent admissions to the critical care facilities, and to facilitate appropriate discharges and transfers from the critical care unit. *C. care unit* a unit within a hospital that supports and treats patients with critical disorders or diseases of the vital physiological systems. May also be called intensive care unit. *See* INTENSIVE CARE UNIT. *C. path analysis* in project management tasks and actions are considered to be independent with the timing of each action crucial to the overall completion of the project. In clinical care a schedule or pathway of procedures, or diagnostic tests for a patient is designed to ensure an efficient coordinated programme of treatment. *C. thinking* a purposeful,

goal-directed approach based upon scientific evidence rather than assumption or memorization. Critical thinking is an organized approach to discovery that involves reflection and assimilation of information which enables the nurse or health care provider to arrive at an informed decision or to make a judgement.

Crohn's disease *B.B. Crohn, American physician, 1884–1983.* Regional ileitis. *See* ILEITIS. Crosby capsule a device for obtaining biopsies of small bowel mucosa.

cross-matching a test of the compatibility of donor blood to be transfused to a patient. *See* BLOOD GROUPS.

cross-sectional study a non-experimental research design that looks at data at one point in time, that is, in the immediate present.

croup a condition resulting from acute obstruction of the larynx caused by allergy, foreign body, infection or new growth; occurs chiefly in infants and children. There is spasmodic dyspnoea, a harsh cough and stridor.

crown that part of the tooth that appears above the gum.

crowning the stage in labour when the top of the infant's head becomes visible at the vulva.

cruciate resembling a cross. *C. ligament see* LIGAMENT.

'crush' syndrome the oedema, oliguria and other symptoms of acute renal failure that follow crushing of a part, especially a large muscle mass, causing the release of myoglobin into the circulation.

crutch appliance usually in the form of a light, tubular metal rod with hand grips and plastic loops for the forearms, to aid walking when the patient must not weight-bear (as in fractures of lower limbs) or when a lower limb is missing.

cryaesthesia abnormal sensitivity to cold.

cryoanalgesia the relief of pain by application of cold by cryoprobe to peripheral nerves.

cryobank a facility for freezing and preserving semen at low temperatures (usually −196.5°C) for future use.

cryoprecipitate any precipitate that results from cooling. Of particular therapeutic value is the cryoprecipitate from fresh plasma, which is rich in factor VIII and is used to treat haemophilia.

cryopreservation maintenance of the viability of excised tissue or organs by storing at very low temperatures.

cryosurgery the use of extreme cold to destroy tissue.

cryotherapy therapeutic use of cold.

cryptococcosis infection caused by the yeast *Cryptococcus neoformans*, having a predilection for the brain and meninges but also invading the skin, lungs and other parts. It particularly affects persons immunocompromised by disease or therapy.

cryptorchidism failure of the testicles to descend into the scrotum; cryptorchism.

CT computerized tomography.

Cu symbol for *copper*.

cubitus 1. the forearm. 2. the elbow. *C. valgus* deformity of the elbow where the palm of the hand is abducted and thus turns outwards. *C. varus* deformity where there is adduction of the forearm.

cue something that gives a hint or idea of something else. A cue is a verbal or non-verbal signal in communication from one person to another. It is a remembered item which connects with further information or meaning.

cued recall retrieval of information from memory with the help of cues, perhaps using the first letter of the word or name to be remembered.

culdoscope an endoscope used in culdoscopy.

culdoscopy direct visual examination of the female viscera through an endoscope introduced into the pelvic cavity through the posterior vaginal fornix.

culture 1. the propagation of microorganisms or of living tissue cells in special media conducive to their growth. 2. a collective noun for the symbolic and acquired aspects of human society, including convention, custom and language. 3. a singular noun for the customs and features of an ethnic (racial, religious or social) group. 4. in the NHS refers to the way that the values and beliefs of an organization are put into practice. *C. shock* A feeling of alienation often accompanied by feelings of depression and rejection that results from a radical change in culture, e.g., as a result of migration from one country to another.

cumulative adding to. *C. action* occurs when a dose of a slowly released drug is given too frequently and accumulates in the system leading to the development of toxic symptoms, e.g., with some barbiturates and digoxin.

Cumulative Index to Nursing and Allied Health Literature (CINAHL) a computerized database of English language nursing and allied health literature.

cupping 1. the formation of a cup-shaped concavity with the hand: (a) to produce a skin erythema, thereby improving local circulation; and (b) to loosen excessive secretions from air passages, and perhaps induce coughing. 2. the use of a cupping glass to stimulate skin blood flow.

curative anything which promotes healing by overcoming disease.

curettage [Fr.] the scraping of a surface with a curette for therapeutic purposes or to obtain biopsy material.

curette a spoon-shaped instrument used for the removal of unhealthy tissues by scraping.

Curling's ulcer *T.B. Curling, British surgeon, 1811–1888.* An ulcer of the duodenum developed after severe burns of the body.

cursor on the computer screen, a blinking character that indicates where the next character will appear.

curvature the curving of a line, whether normal or abnormal. *Spinal c.* abnormal deviation of the vertebral column.

Cushing's disease *H.W. Cushing, American surgeon, 1869–1939.* A condition of oversecretion by the adrenal cortex due to an adenoma of the pituitary gland. Symptoms include obesity, abnormal distribution of hair and atrophy of the genital organs. A rare disorder.

cushingoid referring to symptoms resembling those of Cushing's disease, e.g., the side effects of steroid therapy.

cusp a pointed or rounded projection, such as on the crown of a tooth, or a segment of a cardiac valve.

cutaneous pertaining to the skin.

cutdown an incision into a vein with insertion of a catheter for intravenous infusion. It is performed when an infusion cannot be started by venepuncture. Also used with hyperalimentation therapy when concentrated solutions need to be given into the superior vena cava.

cuticle the narrow band of epidermis extending from the nail wall on to the nail surface; also called eponychium.

cyanocobalamin vitamin B_{12} (anti-anaemic factor) found in liver, eggs and fish. It combines with the intrinsic factor secreted in gastric juice for absorption and is essential for erythrocyte maturation. Administered by injection in the treatment of pernicious anaemia.

cyanosis a bluish appearance of the skin and mucous membranes, caused by imperfect oxygenation of the blood. It indicates circulatory failure and is common in respiratory diseases. It is also seen in 'blue babies'.

cyberstalking internet harassment, for example, repetitive unsolicited and/or inappropriate emails, including hate, obscene or threatening mail or live chat harassment. *See* BULLYING and HARASSMENT.

cyclamate a non-nutritive sweetener.

cycle a series of recurring events. *Cardiac c.* the events occurring between one heart beat and the next. *Menstrual c.* the changes that occur each month in the female reproductive system.

cyclic pertaining to or occurring in a cycle.

cyclodialysis an operation used in glaucoma to improve drainage from the anterior chamber of the eye at the corneoscleral junction.

cyclodiathermy a treatment for glaucoma without penetration of the eyeball. Diathermy is applied to the sclera to cause fibrosis around the ciliary body, so allowing the aqueous humour to drain.

cycloplegia paralysis of the ciliary muscle of the eye.

cyclopropane a gas used for general anaesthesia. It is not irritating to the respiratory tract but is highly inflammable and is therefore potentially dangerous.

cyclothymia the alteration of mood seen in bipolar disorder.

cyesis pregnancy. *Pseudo-c.* signs and symptoms suggestive of pregnancy arising when no fertilization has taken place. 'Phantom pregnancy'.

cyst 1. a cavity or sac with epithelium, containing liquid or semi-solid matter. 2. a stage in the life cycle of certain protozoan parasites when they acquire tough protective coats. *Branchial c.* one formed in the neck from non-closure of the branchial cleft during development. *Chocolate c.* an ovarian cyst occurring in endometriosis. *Daughter c.* a small cyst that develops from a large one. *Dermoid c.* a congenital type containing skin, hair, teeth, etc. It is due to abnormal development of embryonic tissue. *Hydatid c.* the larval cyst stage of the tapeworm, usually found in the liver. *Meibomian c.* a swelling of a meibomian gland caused by obstruction of its duct. *Multilocular c.* a cyst that is divided into compartments or locules. *Ovarian c.* a cyst of the ovary, usually non-malignant, but sometimes becoming very large and requiring surgical removal. *Retention* *c.* any cyst caused by blockage of a duct. *Sebaceous c.* a retention cyst caused by the blockage of a duct from a sebaceous gland so that the sebum collects. *Sublingual c.* a ranula. *Thyroglossal c.* one in the thyroglossal tract near the hyoid bone at the base of the tongue.

cystathioninuria a hereditary disorder of cystathionine metabolism, marked by increased concentrations in the urine. May be associated with learning difficulties.

cysteine a sulphur-containing amino acid formed by the ingestion of dietary proteins.

cystic fibrosis mucoviscidosis. An autosomal inherited disorder associated with accumulation of excessively thick and tenacious mucus and abnormal secretion of sweat and saliva. The disease occurs particularly frequently in Caucasians. One person in 25 is a carrier and, in Britain, one person in 2500 is affected. The severity of cystic fibrosis varies widely. Although inherited it may not manifest itself during the early weeks of life, or it may cause meconium ileus in the newborn. Most cases are detected soon after birth through newborn screening. Therapeutic management is long term, initially centring on replacement of pancreatic enzymes, physiotherapy and antibiotics. Even with prompt and vigorous treatment permanent lung damage may occur. Lung or heart/lung transplants offer good results with an improved quality of life. Gene therapy is currently being developed. In those families with a history of the condition amniocentesis can be used to determine if a fetus is affected. Diagnosis is by the serum immune reactive trypsin (IRT) test. Early diagnosis and treatment improves the long-term prognosis and life expectancy.

cysticercosis a disease caused by infestation with the cysticercus of *Taenia solium* (pork tapeworm). Has been eliminated from pig herds in the UK but may be found in immigrants or travellers who have ingested infected pork.

cysticercus the cystic or larval form of the tapeworm.

cystine an amino acid closely related to cysteine. Sometimes excreted in urine in the form of minute crystals (cystinuria).

cystinosis an inherited metabolic disorder in which cystine is deposited in the tissues.

cystitis inflammation of the urinary bladder.

cystocele a prolapse of the bladder into the vagina.

cystodiathermy the application of a high-frequency electric current to the bladder mucosa, usually for the removal of papillomas.

cystography radiography of the urinary bladder after the introduction of a radio-opaque contrast medium. *Micturating c.* radiographic examination during the act of passing urine.

cystoscope an endoscope for examining the interior of the urinary bladder.

cystostomy the operation of making a temporary or permanent opening into the urinary bladder.

cystotomy incision of the urinary bladder for removal of calculi, etc. *Suprapubic c.* incision above the pubis.

cystourethrography radiography of the urinary bladder and urethra.

cytogenetics the study of cells during mitosis in order to examine the chromosomes and the relationship between chromosome abnormality and disease.

cytology the microscopic study of the form and functions of the cells of the body. *Exfoliative c.* an aid to the early diagnosis of malignant disease. Secretions or surface cells are examined for premalignant changes.

cytolysin a substance that causes cytolysis. *See* BACTERIOLYSIN and HAEMOLYSIN.

cytolysis the destruction of cells.

cytomegalic inclusion disease an infection due to cytomegalovirus. In the congenital form, there is hepatospleno-megaly with cirrhosis, and microcephaly with learning difficulties and develop-mental delay. Acquired disease may cause a clinical state similar to infectious mononucleosis.

cytomegalovirus a virus belonging to the herpes simplex group.

cytopheresis a technique to remove specific cellular components from the blood, e.g., white blood cells or plate-lets needed to treat a patient, or to remove abnormal constituents.

cytoplasm the protoplasmic part of the cell surrounding the nucleus.

cytosine one of the pyrimidine bases found in DEOXYRIBONUCLEIC ACID (DNA). *C.*

arabinoside an antimetabolite used in the treatment of acute leukaemia. Cytarabine.

cytotoxic 1. having a deleterious effect upon cells. 2. an agent or drug that damages or destroys cells. Used to treat various forms of cancer and sometimes other conditions. The handling of cytotoxic drugs is a health and safety issue. Health care workers should follow local guidelines and pol-icies regarding administration of these drugs.

cytotoxins antibodies which are toxic to cells.

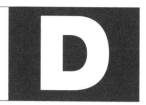

D   symbol for *deuterium*.

dacryolith   a calculus in a lacrimal duct.

dacryoma   a benign tumour which arises from the lacrimal epithelium.

dactyl   a finger or toe; a digit.

dactylology   communication between individuals by signs made with the fingers and hands. Finger spelling.

daltonism   colour blindness; inability to distinguish red from green. *See* COLOUR VISION.

dander   small scales from the hair or feathers of animals, which may be a cause of allergy in sensitive persons.

dandruff   white scales shed from the scalp. If moist from serous exudate they have a greasy appearance.

Darwinism   *C.R. Darwin, British naturalist, 1809–1882.* The theory of the evolution of species through natural selection.

data   *sing.* datum; a collection of facts. *Continuous d.* data that have a continuous set of values, e.g., for variables such as height, weight and antibody titres in response to vaccination. *D. processing* the storage and analysis of data to produce statistical tabulations, often by computer. **Data Protection Legislation** from 25 May 2018 data protection within Europe will be governed by the General Data Protection Regulation (GDPR). It will be directly applicable in all Member States of the European Union although EU Member States may maintain or introduce further conditions, including limitations, with regard to the processing of genetic data, biometric data or data concerning health. The GDPR treats health data as a 'special category' of personal data which is considered to be sensitive by its nature. Processing is prohibited unless exceptions apply (for example, obtaining an individual's explicit consent, where processing is necessary for archiving purposes in the public interest, scientific or historical research purposes or statistical purposes or where Member States have inserted further conditions or limitations). *D. set* a collection of information made on a group and related to certain variables that are being investigated. *Discrete d.* data with a single value or characteristic, e.g., colour of hair.

database   information collected, stored, reviewed and updated, and used for evaluation and audit.

day care   a specialized service for pre-school children, either as a substitute for or as an extension to family life. A similar service may be provided for the elderly needing care and support and to provide respite for family carers. *See* DAY CENTRE.

day centre   a specialized facility that offers care, treatment and a respite service for the elderly or the mentally ill.

day nursery   a centre for the care, during the daytime, of children up to school age. Provided by the local authority, voluntary agencies and the private sector. Funding is available for all children from 3 years or from 2 years if certain criteria are met.

day patient care a service provided either in a specialized ward or in a hospital ward for treatment/investigation/minor surgery. The patient is admitted and discharged on the same day. See AMBULATORY CARE.

dB symbol for *decibel.*

DBS Disclosure and Barring Service. The DBS provides criminal record checks for applicants to certain professions or roles in England and Wales. Different systems apply in Scotland and Northern Ireland.

DDT dichlorodiphenyltrichloroethane; dicophane. A powerful insecticide banned in some countries as classified as probably carcinogenic to humans but approved by the World Health Organization for the control of MALARIA.

deafness complete or partial loss of hearing affecting about 10% of adults and more than 50% of people over 65 years of age. May be called 'hearing impairment' or 'hearing loss' especially when there is only partial loss of hearing. *Conduction or middle ear d.* deafness due to the sound wave failing to reach the cochlea. *Perceptive or nerve d.* deafness due to damage to the cochlea or auditory nerve.

deamination a process of hydrolysis, taking place in the liver, by which amino acids are broken down and urea is formed.

death the cessation of all physical and chemical processes that occur in all living organisms or their cellular components. *Brain d.* the diagnosis of clinical brain stem death is governed, in the UK, by a set of guidelines ratified by the Medical Royal Colleges and their Faculties. The testing procedure is performed twice by two different doctors to eliminate any observer error. The time interval between testing is not specified. For medicolegal purposes

the time of death is that time when the second examination has been completed and the patient fulfils the criteria. Performance of the brain death criteria under the appropriate circumstances allows the patient a dignified death, reduces the agony of the relatives and releases scarce resources for other seriously ill patients. *Clinical d.* the absence of heart beat (no pulse can be felt) and cessation of breathing. *Cot d.* sudden infant death syndrome (SIDS). *D. certificate* certificate issued by the registrar for deaths after receipt of a preliminary certificate completed and signed by an attending doctor, indicating the date and probable cause of death. Only after issue of this certificate, indicating that the death has been registered, can the body be disposed of. *D. instinct* a concept, introduced by Freud, proposing a self-destructive drive opposed by the sexual instinct, which perpetually seeks a renewal of life. May manifest itself as a repetition compulsion with the aim of annihilating oneself. *D. rate* the number of deaths per stated number of persons (100 or 10 000 or 100 000) in a certain region in a certain period.

debility a condition of weakness and lack of physical tone.

debridement the removal of foreign substances and injured tissues from a traumatic wound. Part of the immediate treatment to promote healing.

decalcification removal of calcium salts, e.g., from bone in disorders of calcium metabolism.

decapsulation removal of a fibrous capsule.

decay 1. the gradual decomposition of dead organic matter. 2. the process or stage of ageing of living matter. *Radioactive d.* the process by which an unstable atom loses energy by the emission of gamma rays or beta or alpha particles and is transformed to a more stable atom.

decerebrate a person with brain damage whose neurological reactions are severely impaired and in whom cerebral functioning has ceased. A state of deep coma.

decibel *symbol* dB. A unit of intensity of sound, used particularly in estimating the degree of deafness.

decidua the thickened lining of the uterus for the reception of the fertilized ovum to protect the developing embryo. It is shed when pregnancy terminates.

deciduous falling off; subject to being shed, as deciduous teeth.

decision-making the act or process of choosing a preferred option or course of action from a set of alternatives. It forms the basis of almost all deliberate or voluntary behaviour. *D. rule* a formal or mechanical formula or principle for deciding on a course of action in response to input data. *D. theory* any theory that attempts to explain how decisions are reached. Most often applied to theories that use mathematical models to analyse human decision processes.

decompensation failure to compensate. In particular, failure of the heart to overcome disability or increased work load.

decompression return to normal environmental pressure after exposure to greatly increased pressure. *Cerebral d.* removal of a flap of the skull and incision of the dura mater for the purpose of relieving intracranial pressure. *D. sickness* a disorder characterized by joint pains, respiratory manifestations, skin lesions and neurological signs, occurring as a result of rapid reduction in air pressure. Aviators flying at high altitudes and persons breathing compressed air in caissons and diving apparatus are particularly susceptible to this disorder. Formerly known as 'bends'.

decongestant 1. reducing congestion or swelling. 2. an agent that reduces congestion or swelling, usually of the nasal membranes. Decongestants may be inhaled, taken as spray or nose drops, or used orally in liquid or tablet form.

decontamination the freeing of a person or an object of some contaminating substance such as nerve gas, infective or radioactive material, etc. Decontamination involves a combination of processes including cleaning, disinfection and sterilization. It is an important issue for public health in the prevention of hospital-acquired infection and minimizing the risk of the iatrogenic transmission of other organisms.

decortication an operation to strip the outer layer of an organ, e.g., the removal of the thickened pleura in the treatment of chronic empyema.

decrudescence diminution or abatement of the intensity of symptoms.

decubitus the position assumed when lying down. *D. ulcer* an ulcer due to interference with the local circulation from prolonged or severe pressure on the surface body tissue resulting in tissue anoxia and cell death; also called bedsore and pressure ulcer. See PRESSURE.

decussation a crossing, particularly of nerve fibres. A chiasma. *Pyramidal d.* the crossing of the pyramidal nerve fibres in the medulla oblongata.

deep vein thrombosis abbreviated DVT. A blood clot that forms in the deep veins of the lower leg; may be symptomless or can cause redness, swelling, tenderness and fever. The clot can travel and lodge in the heart or lungs (see PULMONARY EMBOLISM) resulting in sudden death. The so-called 'economy class syndrome' is the formation of a clot occurring during or just after a long journey in an aeroplane, where the lack of space restricts leg movements. Other risk factors are: obesity, smoking, previous DVT, pregnancy and being >40 years of age.

defecation elimination of waste and undigested food, as faeces, from the rectum.

defence behaviour directed to protection of the individual from injury.

Character d. any character trait, e.g., a mannerism, attitude or affectation, which serves as a DEFENCE MECHANISM. *D. mechanism* in psychology, an unconscious mental process or coping pattern that lessens the anxiety associated with a situation or internal conflict and protects the person from mental discomfort. *Insanity d.* a legal concept that a person cannot be convicted of a crime if lacking criminal responsibility by reason of insanity at the time of commission of the crime.

defervescence the period of abatement of fever.

defibrillation the restoration of normal rhythm to the heart in ventricular or atrial fibrillation.

defibrillator equipment by which normal rhythm is restored in the heart ventricular or atrial fibrillation by the application of a high-voltage electric current.

defibrination the removal of fibrin from blood plasma to prevent clotting. Used in the preparation of sera.

deficiency disease a condition caused by dietary or metabolic deficiency, including all diseases due to an insufficient supply of essential nutrients.

deficit a deficiency or variation from that which is considered to be normal.

defined daily dose abbreviated DDD. The measure of the standard daily therapeutic dose of a drug. The World Health Organization publishes a list of DDDs for various drugs.

deglutition the act of swallowing.

dehiscence splitting open, as of a wound.

dehydration excessive loss of fluid from the body by persistent vomiting, diarrhoea or sweating, or from the lack of intake. Severe dehydration is a serious condition that may lead to fatal shock, acidosis and the accumulation of waste products in the body, as in uraemia.

déjà vu [Fr.] an illusion that a new experience is a repetition of a previous experience.

deleterious harmful; injurious.

delinquency criminal or antisocial conduct, especially among juveniles.

delirium acute confusional state. A common condition in high fever. It is marked by an irregular expenditure of nervous energy, incoherent talk and delusions. Delirium is common in patients in Intensive Care and is associated with poor outcomes in this group of patients. *D. tremens* an acute psychosis common in chronic alcoholism, usually following abstinence from alcohol. *Traumatic d.* a possible occurrence after severe head injury. There is much confusion and disorientation.

delivery childbirth; parturition.

Delphi technique a long-range forecasting technique in which qualitative value judgements are made about information. Judgements are made independently and anonymously, pooled and summarized before being fed back to the contributors for another round of opinion.

deltoid triangular. *D. muscle* the triangular muscle of the shoulder arising from the clavicle and scapula, with insertion into the humerus.

delusion a false idea or belief held by a person which cannot be corrected by reasoning. *D. of grandeur* erroneous belief in one's own greatness, wealth or position. *D. of persecution* paranoia. *Depressive d.* a sense of unworthiness or sinfulness.

dementia a global and progressive deterioration of the mental faculties which is irreversible and affects memory, intellect, judgement, personality and emotional control. Dementia is a syndrome associated with an ongoing decline of the brain and its abilities as a result of disease such as ALZHEIMER'S DISEASE or STROKE. *D. with Lewy bodies* is a type of dementia which involves tiny abnormal structures (Lewy bodies) forming inside brain cells. They disrupt the chemistry of the brain and lead to the death of brain cells. *Frontotemporal d.* (including PICK'S

DISEASE) dementia where the front and side parts of the brain are damaged. Clumps of abnormal proteins form inside brain cells, causing them to die. *Incipient d. see* MILD COGNITIVE IMPAIRMENT. *Mixed d.* defines when someone has more than one type of dementia, and a mixture of the symptoms of those types. It is common for someone to have both Alzheimer's disease and vascular dementia together. *Vascular d.* dementia occurring when the oxygen supply to the brain is reduced because of narrowing or blockage of blood vessels, resulting in some brain cells becoming damaged or dying.

demography the statistical science dealing with populations, including matters of health, disease, births and mortality.

De Morgan's spots red or purplish raised spots in the skin consisting of a cluster of minute blood vessels. Found in middle-aged and older people, the spots becoming more numerous with increasing age. The spots may bleed if damaged but treatment is unnecessary. *See* AGE SPOTS.

demulcent an agent that soothes and allays irritation, especially of sensitive mucous membranes.

demyelination destruction of the medullary or myelin sheaths of nerve fibres, such as occurs in disseminated and multiple sclerosis. Demyelinization.

dendrite one of the protoplasmic filaments of a nerve cell by which impulses are transmitted from one neurone to another. Dendron.

dendritic 1. appertaining to a dendrite. 2. branching. *D. ulcer* a corneal ulcer caused by the virus of herpes simplex. It has a branching appearance as it spreads.

denervation severance or removal of the nerve supply to a part.

dengue a painful viral haemorrhagic fever spread by mosquitoes that occurs in tropical countries throughout the world. The dengue flavivirus that causes the disease, one of four types of a group B arbovirus, is carried by *Aedes* mosquitoes which breed in stagnant water. No existing antivirals are effective. Prevention is based on public health measures to eliminate the breeding grounds of the *Aedes* mosquitoes until a vaccine is developed. Because of the intense pain in the bones, dengue is also known as breakbone fever.

denial a defence mechanism in which the existence of intolerable actions, ideas, changed circumstances, terminal illness, etc. is unconsciously denied.

dental relating to dentistry or to the teeth. *D. hygienist* a trained person carrying out dental procedures such as scaling of the teeth and oral cleansing, who works with the assistance of the dentist in providing preventative dental health care. *D. implants* replace teeth. The roots provide a foundation for fixed replacement teeth that are made to match natural teeth. *D. nurse* a member of the dental health team, recognized and registered, who assists the dentist at the patient's side in passing instruments, preparing materials and generally assisting the dentist. *D. plaque* a sticky rough coating on the teeth formed by food deposits, bacteria and dead cells. It is the chief cause of dental decay if not removed regularly by good dental hygiene. *D. pulp* the tissue within the dental cavity containing nerves, blood and lymph vessels.

dentine the calcified substance forming the bulk of a tooth between the pulp and the enamel.

dentist a person qualified to practise dentistry.

dentistry the art and science of the teeth, mouth and associated tissues and bone. Dentistry also includes preventative dental care and education concerned with preserving the health of the teeth and gums as well as the supplying and fitting of dentures.

dentition the process of teething. *Primary d.* cutting of the temporary or milk teeth, beginning at the age of 6

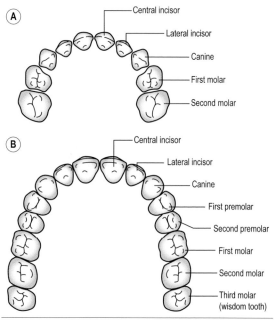

(A) PRIMARY DENTITION, (B) SECONDARY DENTITION

A
- Central incisor
- Lateral incisor
- Canine
- First molar
- Second molar

B
- Central incisor
- Lateral incisor
- Canine
- First premolar
- Second premolar
- First molar
- Second molar
- Third molar (wisdom tooth)

or 7 months and continuing until the end of the second year. A full set consists of eight incisors, four canines and eight premolars: 20 teeth in all. Deciduous dentition. *Secondary d.* cutting of the permanent teeth, beginning in the sixth or seventh year, and being complete by the 12th to 15th year except for the posterior molars or 'wisdom teeth'. There are 32 permanent teeth: eight incisors, four canines, eight premolars or bicuspids and 12 molars. Permanent dentition. (*See* Figure.)

dentoid tooth-like.

denture a removable dental prosthesis, which may contain one artificial tooth, or several or a full set of teeth.

deodorant a substance that destroys or masks an offensive odour. *See* ANTIPERSPIRANT.

deoxygenated deprived of oxygen. *D. blood* that which has lost much of its oxygen in the tissues and is returning to the lungs for a fresh supply.

deoxyribonucleic acid abbreviated DNA. A nucleic acid of complex molecular structure occurring in cell nuclei as the basic structure of the genes. It is responsible for the control and passing on of hereditary characteristics, and is present in all body cells of every species, including unicellular organisms and DNA viruses. DNA molecules are linear polymers of small molecules called *nucleotides*, each of which consists of one molecule of the five-carbon sugar *deoxyribose*, bonded to a *phosphate* group and to one of the four *bases* twisted into a double helix. The four bases are two purines, *adenine* (A) and *guanine* (G), and two pyrimidines, *cytosine* (C) and *thymine* (T). The structure of DNA was described in 1953 by J.D. Watson and F.H.C. Crick.

Department of Health is the national headquarters of the NHS, negotiating funding with the Treasury and leading and shaping health and care provision in England. It also provides strategic leadership to the NHS and social care organizations in England, setting their overall direction and establishing and monitoring standards. Its key responsibilities are: creating national policies and legislation, providing the long-term vision and ambition to meet current and future challenges; providing funding, assuring the delivery and continuity of services and accounting to Parliament in a way that represents the best interests of the patient, public and taxpayer; supporting research and technology, promoting honesty, openness and transparency, and instilling a culture that values compassion, dignity and the highest quality of care; learning from the experiences of patients. Similar government departments perform this role in Scotland, Wales and Northern Ireland. The Department makes reciprocal arrangements with other countries and represents the UK on health matters in the European Union, the World Health Organization and other international bodies.

dependence 1. addiction; the total psychophysical state of a user in which the usual or increasing quantities of the drug or activity (e.g., internet games or gambling) are required to prevent the onset of withdrawal symptoms. 2. the level of reliance a person has on others for carrying out the activities of daily living.

dependency a state of relying on another person for love, affection, mothering, comfort, security, food, warmth, shelter, protection, etc. *D. studies* the measurement of the need for care required by a patient based on the ability to carry out self-care. The main self-care activities measured are the ability to feed, the ability to carry out toilet requirements, including dressing, and the level of mobility.

depersonalization a condition in which patients feel that their personality has changed so that they become onlookers observing their own actions. It may occur in almost any mental illness.

depilatory an agent that will remove hair temporarily. Preoperative depilation reduces the risk of wound infection and, unlike shaving of the skin, is non-abrasive.

depressant a drug that reduces functional activity of an organ. Anaesthetics, sedatives, tranquillizers and alcohol are depressants.

depression 1. a hollow or depressed area. 2. a lowering or decrease of functional activity. 3. in psychiatry, a morbid sadness, dejection or melancholy, distinguished from grief, which is realistic and proportionate to a personal loss. Profound depression may be symptomatic of a mental health disorder when feelings of sadness, hopelessness, helplessness, combined with a loss of interest in the social activities of life, are experienced for weeks or months rather than just a few days. Symptoms vary with the severity of the depression, but commonly include loss of appetite or overeating, sleep disturbances, lack of sex drive, poor concentration with overall a low mood and poor self-esteem. Clinical depression may or may not be associated with stressful events or trauma. Risk factors include genetic and social issues, for example, poverty, social isolation, substance abuse and previous history. The severely depressed may also have suicidal thoughts. Treatment is with the use of medication and/or cognitive behavioural therapy/talking therapy and lifestyle changes. Seasonal affective disorder is depression that occurs when the person's mood changes according to the season due to reduced levels of sunlight. Sufferers feel low in winter and better in spring. *See* SEASONAL AFFECTIVE DISORDER SYNDROME.

deprivation loss or absence of parts, organs, powers, or things that are needed. *D. indices* national variables that are used to assess the economic and social wellbeing within the population of England based on 37 indicators. These include income, employment, education, health, crime, housing and environmental indicators. *Emotional d.* deprivation of adequate and appropriate interpersonal or environmental experience in the early developmental years. *Maternal d. syndrome* a group of symptoms, including delayed emotional and physical development, arising in infants who have been deprived of care and love provided by a mother or mothering figure according to *John Bowlby, 1907–1990.* Deprivation of maternal care during the first 3 years of life is thought to be particularly critical as this is the optimal period for the forming of social attachments. *Sensory d.* deprivation of the usual external stimuli and the opportunity for perception.

Derbyshire neck *see* GOITRE.

derealization loss of a sense of reality. Surroundings and events seem unreal.

dereism mental activity in which fantasy runs unhampered by logic and experience; describes autistic thinking.

dermal filler injections used to fill out wrinkles and creases in skin used for cosmetic reasons.

dermatillomania a compulsion to pick at skin to the point where there are visible wounds. An impulse-control disorder.

dermatitis inflammation of the skin. *Contact d.* that arising from touching a substance to which the person is sensitive. *Exfoliative d.* widespread scaling and itching of the skin, sometimes occurring as a reaction to treatment with certain drugs. *Industrial d., occupational d.* that caused by exposure to chemicals or other substances met with at work. *Sensitization d.* dermatitis due to an allergic reaction. *Traumatic d.* inflammation due to injury. *Varicose d.* dermatitis, usually of the lower portion of the leg, due to varicosities of the smaller veins. *X-ray d.* radiodermatitis; inflammatory reaction of the skin to radiotherapy.

dermatoglyphics study of the patterns of ridges of the skin of the fingers, palms, toes and soles. Of interest in anthropology and law enforcement as a means of establishing identity, and in medicine, both clinically and as a genetic indicator, particularly of chromosomal abnormalities.

dermatographia a condition in which urticarial weals occur on the skin if a blunt instrument or fingernail is lightly drawn over it.

dermatology the science of skin diseases.

dermatomycosis a fungal infection of the skin.

dermatomyositis a rare collagen disease producing inflammation of the voluntary muscles with necrosis of the muscle fibres.

dermatosis any skin disease, especially one which does not produce inflammation.

dermis the skin, especially the layer under the epidermis.

dermoid pertaining to the skin. *D. cyst see* CYST.

desensitization 1. the prevention or reduction of immediate hypersensitivity reactions by the administration of graded doses of allergen; hyposensitization. *See also* IMMUNOTHERAPY. 2. in behaviour therapy, the treatment of phobias and related disorders by intentionally exposing the patient, in imagination or in real life, to emotionally distressing stimuli.

designer drugs used to describe synthetic variants (drug analogues) of potent controlled drugs (including narcotics and stimulants) that are not themselves controlled. These substances currently circumvent existing drug legislation and many are relatively easy to synthesize from common industrial chemicals. Many designer drugs are extremely potent (some synthetic analogues of heroin are 1000 times as potent as heroin) and are consequently extremely dangerous.

desquamation peeling of the superficial layer of the skin, either in flakes or in powdery form.

detachment separation from or state of indifference to other people, one's surroundings or environment leading to social isolation. *D. of the retina* separation of the retina, or a part of it, from the choroid.

detergent a cleansing and antiseptic agent.

deterioration progressive impairment of function; worsening.

detoxification the process of neutralizing toxic substances; detoxication.

detritus debris; material that has disintegrated.

detrusor muscle of the urinary bladder, the action of which is to push down.

detumescence 1. the subsidence of a swelling. 2. the subsidence of an erect penis after ejaculation.

development the process of growth and differentiation. *Cognitive d.* the development of intelligence, conscious thought and problem-solving ability that begins in infancy. *Psychosexual d.* the development of the psychological aspects of sexuality from birth to maturity. *Psychosocial d.* the development of the personality, including the acquisition of social attitudes and skills, from infancy through to maturity.

developmental pertaining to development. *D. anomaly* absence, deformity or excess of body parts as the result of faulty development of the embryo. *D. milestones* significant behaviours used to mark the process of development (*see* AGE (ACHIEVEMENT)). Walking is a developmental milestone in locomotor development, conversation in cognitive development.

deviance generally any pattern of behaviour that violates prevailing standards of morality or behaviour within a society. The term is usually qualified to indicate the specific form of deviance.

deviation variation from the normal. In ophthalmology, lack of coordination of the two eyes. *Standard d.* in research, a method of grouping data on either side of the mean of a graph. In a normal distribution curve around 68% of the data will be covered in one standard deviation above and below the mean. A measure of dispersion of scores around the mean value. It is the square root of variance.

devitalized devoid of vitality or life; dead.

DEXA scan a special type of X-ray that measures bone mineral density. Also known as dual X-ray absorptiometry, DXA or bone density scan.

dextran a plasma volume expander, formed of large glucose molecules, which, given intravenously, increases the osmotic pressure of blood.

dextrocardia location of the heart in the right side of the thorax.

dextrose D-glucose (dextrose), an important energy source for all tissues and the sole energy source for the brain. Commonly used in intravenous infusion solutions and may also be used orally in rehydration solutions to replace electrolytes and fluids.

diabetes a disease characterized by excessive excretion of urine. *See* POLYURIA. Diabetes is a group of metabolic diseases characterized by hyperglycaemia resulting from defects in insulin secretion, insulin action or both. The chronic hyperglycaemia of diabetes is associated with long-term damage, dysfunction and failure of various organs, primarily the eyes, kidneys, nerves, heart and blood vessels. Because insulin is involved in the metabolism of carbohydrates, proteins and fats, diabetes is not limited to a disturbance of glucose metabolism. Polyuria, thirst and debility are common presenting symptoms. Type 1 diabetes, formerly known as insulin-dependent diabetes mellitus, is the less common form and results from the destruction of the insulin-producing cells of the pancreas occurring most commonly in childhood or adolescence. Type 2 diabetes, formerly known as non-insulin-dependent diabetes mellitus or maturity onset diabetes, is due to an insufficiency of insulin and usually occurs over the age of 40 years and individuals are often obese. The goal of treatment is to maintain blood glucose and lipid levels within normal limits and to prevent complications. In both types of diabetes, treatment is aimed at promoting a sense of health and wellbeing. The diet must be controlled with adequate carbohydrate and the body weight stabilized. Type 1 is always treated with insulin. Type 2 may be treated with weight reduction, diet, the use of oral medications which promote the production of insulin by the pancreas and by insulin. All insulin has to be given by injection, usually subcutaneously. Pump systems to deliver continuous insulin under the skin are available. Ongoing problems occur with reduced sensitivity of nerve endings causing patients to acquire infections, often on the feet. *See* DIABETIC. *Brittle d.* the patient's diabetic condition is difficult to control because of alternating episodes of hyperglycaemia and hypoglycaemia. Also known as *unstable d.* or *labile d. D. insipidus* a disease resulting from insufficient secretion of

the antidiuretic hormone by the pituitary gland, and which may follow injury, infection or be congenital, resulting in dehydration of the patient, polydipsia and polyuria.

diabetic 1. relating to diabetes. 2. a person affected with diabetes. *D. gangrene*, *d. retinopathy* and *d. cataract* are complications of diabetes mellitus.

diabetogenic inducing diabetes. Some drugs or physical conditions, such as pregnancy or disease, precipitate the symptoms of diabetes in those prone to the disease.

diagnosis determination of the nature of a disease. *Clinical d.* diagnosis made by the study of signs and symptoms. *Differential d.* the recognition of one disease among several presenting similar symptoms. *Nursing d.* a stage in the nursing process. A statement of a health care problem, or the potential for one in the health status of the patient/client which the nurse is competent to intervene in and treat based on data obtained during the nursing assessment.

dialysate the material passing through the membrane in dialysis.

dialyser 1. the membrane used in dialysis. 2. the machine or 'artificial kidney' used to remove waste products from the blood in cases of renal failure.

dialysis the process by which crystalline substances will pass through a semipermeable membrane, whereas colloids will not. In medicine this process is employed to remove waste and toxic products from the blood in cases of renal insufficiency. *Peritoneal d.* use of the peritoneum as the semipermeable membrane. A dialysing solution is infused into the abdominal cavity and allowed to run out again when sufficient time has elapsed for dialysis to have occurred. Waste products are thus removed from the blood. *See* HAEMODIALYSIS.

diameter a straight line passing through the centre of a circle to opposite points on the circumference.

Differences between hyperglycaemia and hypoglycaemia in patients with diabetes mellitus	
Hypoglycaemia	**Hyperglycaemia**
• Heart palpitations • Fatigue • Pale skin • Shakiness • Anxiety • Sweating • Hunger • Irritability • Tingling sensation around the mouth • Crying out during sleep • Confusion, abnormal behaviour or both, such as the inability to complete routine tasks • Visual disturbances, such as blurred vision • Seizures • Loss of consciousness	• Increased thirst • Headaches • Trouble concentrating • Blurred vision • Frequent urination • Fatigue (weak, tired feeling) • Weight loss • Vaginal and skin infections • Slow-healing cuts and sores • Worse vision • Nerve damage causing painful cold or insensitive feet, loss of hair on the lower extremities, or erectile dysfunction • Stomach and intestinal problems such as chronic constipation or diarrhoea • Damage to eyes, blood vessels, or kidneys

Cranial d's measurement of the fetal head at term. If these are abnormal, delivery through the vagina may not be possible. *Pelvic d's* measurements between the bones and joints of the pelvis made in women to determine whether the fetus can pass through at the time of childbirth.

diapedesis the passage of white blood cells through the walls of blood capillaries.

diaphoresis perspiration; particularly profuse perspiration.

diaphragm 1. the muscular dome-shaped partition separating the thorax from the abdomen. 2. any separating membrane or structure. *Contraceptive d.* a rubber cap which occludes the cervix.

diaphragmatic hernia a protrusion of any or part of an abdominal organ through the diaphragm into the thoracic cavity.

diaphysis the shaft of a long bone.

diarrhoea rapid movement of faecal matter through the intestine resulting in poor absorption of water, nutritive elements and electrolytes. Commonest causes of diarrhoea include bacterial or viral infections, food sensitivity, laxatives, the use of antibiotics and dietary indiscretion. Other causes include irritable bowel syndrome and systemic diseases. Diarrhoea that persists for more than a week or is recurring requires medical investigation. *Tropical d.* sprue.

diarthrosis a freely moving articulation, e.g. ball and socket joint. A synovial joint.

diastole the phase of the cardiac cycle in which the heart relaxes between contractions; specifically, the period when the two ventricles are dilated by the blood flowing into them. *See* SYSTOLE.

diathermy production of heat in a body tissue by a high frequency electric current. *Medical d.* sufficient heat is used to warm the tissues but not to harm them. *Short-wave d.* used in physiotherapy to relieve pain or treat infection. *Surgical d.* of very high frequency; used to coagulate blood vessels or to dissect tissues. Cautery.

DIC disseminated intravascular coagulation.

dichromatic pertaining to colour blindness when there is ability to see only two of the three primary colours. *See* COLOUR VISION DEFICIENCY.

dicrotic having a double beat. *D. pulse* a small wave of distension following the normal pulse beat; occurring at the closure of the aortic valve.

diet 1. the customary amount and kind of food and drink taken by a person from day to day. 2. a diet planned to meet the specific requirements of the individual, including or excluding certain foods. *Bland d.* one that is free from any irritating or stimulating foods. *Elimination d.* one for diagnosis of food allergy, based on omission of foods that might cause symptoms in the patient. *High-calorie d.* one that furnishes more calories than needed to maintain weight, often more than 3500–4000 kcal/day. *High-fibre d.* one relatively high in dietary fibre, which decreases bowel transit time and relieves constipation. *High-protein d.* one containing large amounts of protein, consisting largely of meats, fish, milk, peas, beans and nuts. *Liquid d.* a diet limited to liquids or to foods that can be changed to a liquid state (*see also* LIQUID (DIET)). *Low-calorie d.* one containing fewer calories than needed to maintain weight. *Low-fat d.* one containing limited amounts of fat. *Low-residue d.* one with a minimum of cellulose and fibre and restriction of the connective tissue found in certain cuts of meat. It is prescribed for irritations of the intestinal tract, after surgery of the large intestine, in partial intestinal obstruction, or when limited bowel movements are desirable, as in colostomy patients. Also called low-fibre diet. *See* Appendix 1.

dietary chaos syndrome a syndrome in which patients believe that control of eating and body weight is the key to good health and wellbeing. A variety of approaches are used which include bulimia and periods of abstinence from food, the use of laxatives or prolonged chewing of food without swallowing. *See* ANOREXIA and BULIMIA.

dietetics the science of applying the principles of nutrition to the feeding of individuals or groups.

dietary reference values abbreviated DRV. Published values (Department of Health) for most nutrients that provide for a range of intakes related to age, gender and activity required to maintain health. These values are based upon the nutritional requirements of groups living in the UK.

dietitian a person qualified in the principles of nutrition who applies these to the feeding of an individual or of a group of people usually in a shared setting, e.g., hospitals or residential homes. May also work in the commercial sector, e.g., food processing industry.

differential making a difference. *D. blood count* see BLOOD COUNT. *D. diagnosis* see DIAGNOSIS.

differentiation 1. the distinguishing of one thing from another. 2. the act or process of acquiring completely individual characteristics, such as occurs in the progressive diversification of cells and tissues in the embryo. 3. increase in morphological or chemical heterogeneity.

diffuse scattered or widespread, as opposed to localized.

diffusion 1. the spontaneous mixing of molecules of liquid or gas so that they become equally distributed. 2. dialysis.

digestion 1. the act or process of converting food into chemical substances that can be absorbed into the blood and utilized by the body tissues.

2. the subjection of a substance to prolonged heat and moisture, so as to disintegrate and soften it. (*See* Figure.)

digit a finger or toe. *Accessory d., supernumerary d.* an additional digit occurring as a congenital abnormality.

digital coded in simple 'on–off' binary units such as in computers and the traditional view of the activation of neurones.

digitalization the administration of digitalis (digoxin) in a dosage schedule designed to produce and then maintain optimal therapeutic concentrations of its cardiotonic glycosides.

dilatation, dilation 1. the act of dilating or stretching. 2. the condition, as of an orifice or tubular structure, of being dilated or stretched beyond normal dimensions. *D. and curettage* expanding of the opening of the womb to permit scraping of the walls of the uterus; also called D & C. *D. of the heart* compensatory enlargement of the cavities of the heart, with thinning of the walls.

dilator 1. an instrument used for enlarging an opening or cavity such as the rectum, the male urethra or the cervix. 2. a muscle that causes dilatation. 3. a drug that causes dilatation, e.g., a vasodilator. *Hegar's d's* a series of dilators used to widen the cervical canal before examination of the uterus under anaesthesia.

diluent 1. diluting. 2. an agent that dilutes or renders less potent or irritant.

dimercaprol a colourless, oily liquid used to treat acute poisoning by mercury, gold and lead.

dimethyl phthalate abbreviated DIMP. An insect repellent in liquid or ointment form that is effective for several hours when applied to the skin.

Diogenes syndrome gross self-neglect, usually in the elderly.

dioptre the unit used in measuring lenses for spectacles. When parallel

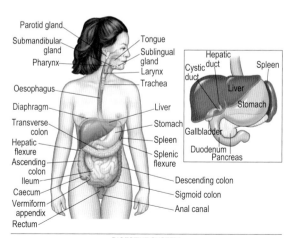

Parotid gland
Submandibular gland
Pharynx
Tongue
Sublingual gland
Larynx
Trachea
Oesophagus
Diaphragm
Liver
Transverse colon
Stomach
Hepatic flexure
Spleen
Ascending colon
Splenic flexure
Ileum
Caecum
Descending colon
Vermiform appendix
Sigmoid colon
Rectum
Anal canal

Hepatic duct
Cystic duct
Spleen
Liver
Stomach
Gallbladder
Duodenum
Pancreas

DIGESTIVE SYSTEM

light enters a lens and focuses at a distance of 1 m, the refractive power of the lens is 1 dioptre, and from this basis abnormalities are calculated.

diphtheria a severe, notifiable, infectious disease, characterized by the formation of membranes in the throat and nose and rarely the skin (in an open wound), and toxic neurological and cardiac complications; caused by the bacillus *Corynebacterium diphtheriae*. Primary prevention is provided by the routine immunization of the population in childhood. *See* Appendix 10.

Diphyllobothrium a genus of large tapeworm. *D. latum*, the broad or fish tapeworm, grows up to 10 m long and may infest humans after the consumption of uncooked infected fish.

diplegia paralysis of similar parts on either side of the body.

diplococcus 1. any of the spherical, lanceolate or coffee-bean-shaped bacteria occurring, usually in pairs, as a result of incomplete separation after cell division in a single plane. 2. any organism of the genus *Diplococcus*.

diploid 1. having a pair of each chromosome characteristic of a species (in humans, 46 chromosomes). 2. a diploid individual or cell.

diplopia double vision, in which two images are seen in place of one, due to lack of coordination of the external muscles of the eye.

dipsomania a morbid craving for alcohol, which occurs in bouts.

disability any restriction or lack (resulting from an impairment) of ability to perform an activity in the manner or within the range considered normal for a human being. *Developmental d.* a substantial disability of indefinite duration, with onset before the age of 18 years, and attributable to intellectual disability, autism, cerebral palsy, epilepsy or other neuropathy.

disaccharide any of a class of sugars, e.g., maltose, lactose, each molecule of which yields two molecules of monosaccharide on hydrolysis. *D.*

intolerance the inability to absorb disaccharides owing to an enzyme deficiency.

disarticulation separation; amputation at a joint.

disc a flattened circular structure. *Intervertebral d.* a fibrocartilaginous pad that separates the bodies of two adjacent vertebrae. *Optic d.* a white spot in the retina. It is the point of entrance of the optic nerve.

discharge 1. a setting free, or liberation; used for the release of a patient from hospital, clinic or therapy programme. 2. material or force set free. 3. an excretion or substance evacuated. *D. planning* the preparation required for the return of a patient/client to the usual life at home.

disciplinary action taken by the employer when a member of staff has made a serious error, acted unprofessionally or negligently or has been convicted of a criminal offence. The process follows an agreed disciplinary procedure. *See* Appendix 5.

disclosing solution a topically applied preparation which reveals plaque and other deposits on teeth by staining them. May also be given as a tablet to be chewed; any plaque is stained red.

discography radiographic examination after the injection of a radio-opaque contrast medium into an intervertebral disc.

discoid eczema a long-term skin condition causing itchy, reddened, swollen and cracked patches on the skin.

discrete composed of separate parts that do not become blended.

disease a definite pathological process having a characteristic set of signs and symptoms. It may affect the whole body or any of its parts, and its aetiology, pathology and prognosis may be known or unknown. (For separate diseases, *see* under individual names.)

disengagement the process by which an individual, usually elderly, gradually withdraws from the community and obligations towards friends and family. The effect of this process is to lead to social isolation for the individual with alienation and disregard for the community. This situation may be compounded by physiological deficits and disabilities. *D. theory* a psychosocial theory of ageing by which both society and the individual prepare for death by gradually reducing all social contacts which leads to poor relationships, egocentricity and sometimes depression.

disimpaction reduction of an impacted fracture.

disinfect to destroy microorganisms, but not usually bacterial spores, reducing the number of microorganisms to a level that is not harmful to health.

disinfectant an agent that destroys infection-producing organisms. Heat and certain other physical agents, such as steam, can be disinfectants, but in common usage the term is reserved for chemical substances such as glutaraldehyde, sodium hypochlorite or phenol. Disinfectants are usually applied to inanimate objects because they are too strong to be used on living tissues. Chemical disinfectants are not always effective against spore-forming bacteria.

disinfection the act of disinfecting. *Terminal d.* disinfection of a sick room and its contents at the termination of a disease.

disinfestation destruction of insects, rodents or pests present on the person or the clothes or in the surroundings, and which may transmit disease.

dislocation the displacement of a bone from its natural position upon another at a joint; luxation.

dismemberment the amputation of a limb or a part of it.

disorientation loss of proper bearings, or a state of mental confusion as to time, place or identity.

displacement removal to an abnormal location or position. *D. activity* in psychology, unconscious transference of an emotion from its original object on to a more acceptable substitute.

disposition a tendency to suffer from certain diseases.

dissect 1. to cut carefully in the study of anatomy. 2. during an operation, to separate according to natural lines of structure.

disseminated widely scattered or dispersed. *D. intravascular coagulation* abbreviated DIC. Widespread formation of thromboses in the capillaries. It is a secondary complication of a diverse group of obstetric, surgical, haemolytic, infection and neoplastic disorders.

dissociation separation. 1. the splitting up of molecules of matter into their component parts, e.g., by heat or electrolysis. 2. in psychology, the separation of ideas, emotions or experiences from the rest of the mind, giving rise to a lack of unity of which the patient is not aware.

distal situated away from the centre of the body or point of origin. The opposite of proximal.

distension enlargement. *Abdominal d.* enlargement of the abdomen by gas in the intestines or fluid in the abdominal cavity.

distractibility inability to focus or maintain attention on any one subject.

distraction 1. any thing that diverts a person's attention. 2. the location of joint surfaces caused by extension but without injury to the parts involved. 3. mental or emotional distress, anguish or confusion. *D. therapy* diverting the focus of attention on one activity, object or person to another. Used in the management of pain.

distribution 1. the sharing out or spreading of an agent, object or population within an area. 2. in research, the relative frequencies with which scores of a different size occur.

diuresis increased excretion of urine.

diuretic 1. increasing urine excretion or the amount of urine. 2. an agent that promotes urine secretion. Diuretic drugs are classified by chemical structure and pharmacological action, although a diuretic medication may contain drugs from one or more groups, e.g., loop diuretics, osmotic and potassium-sparing diuretics, and thiazides.

diurnal occurring during daytime or period of light. Diurnal animals have one period of rest and one of activity in 24 hours.

diverticulitis inflammation of a diverticulum. It is most common in the colon; lower abdominal pain with colic and constipation may occur. Intestinal obstruction or abscesses may develop as a result of collections of bacteria and irritating agents being trapped in small blind pouches formed in the intestinal walls.

diverticulosis the presence of diverticula in the colon without inflammation.

diverticulum a pouch or pocket in the lining of a hollow organ, as in the bladder, oesophagus or large intestine. *Meckel's d.* a small sac occurring in the ileum as a congenital abnormality.

dizygotic, dizygous pertaining to or derived from two separate zygotes (fertilized ova); said of non-identical twins.

dizziness a feeling of unsteadiness or haziness, accompanied by anxiety. *See* VERTIGO.

DNA deoxyribonucleic acid.

Döderlein's bacillus *A.S.G. Döderlein, German obstetrician and gynaecologist, 1860–1941.* A lactobacillus occurring normally in vaginal secretions.

dolor [L.] pain.

dominant in genetics, capable of expression when carried by only one of a pair of homologous chromosomes. The opposite to recessive. *D. gene* one which will produce its characteristics when it is present in either a hetero- or homozygous state, i.e., it may be inherited from one parent only.'

'domino' booking a plan of maternity care whereby a mother has her baby in a consultant unit, cared for by the community midwife. They return home following delivery after an interval of

at least 6 h. The name derives from *domi*ciliary midwife *in* and *out*.

donor 1. an organism that supplies living tissue to be used in another body, such as a person who furnishes blood for transfusion or an organ for transplantation. 2. a substance or compound that contributes part of itself to another substance (acceptor). *Universal d.* a person with group O blood; such blood is sometimes used in emergency transfusion. Transfusion of blood cells rather than whole blood is preferred.

dopa the precursor of dopamine and an intermediate product in the biosynthesis of noradrenaline and adrenaline. It is used in Parkinson's disease and manganese poisoning. Also called L-dopa and levodopa.

dopamine a substance allied to noradrenaline and used in the treatment of cardiogenic shock. Also occurs naturally in the adrenal medulla and the brain, where it functions as a transmitter of nervous impulses.

Doppler effect the relationship of the apparent frequency of waves, as of sound, light and radio waves, to the relative motion of the source of the waves and the observer.

Doppler ultrasound flowmeter a device for measuring blood flow that transmits sound at a frequency of several megahertz along a blood vessel. Rapid pulsatile changes in flow as well as steady flow can be recorded; hence, it is helpful in assessing intermittent claudication, thrombus obstruction of deep veins and other abnormalities of blood flow in the major arteries and veins.

dorsal relating to the back or posterior part of an organ.

dorsiflexion bending backwards of the fingers or toes, i.e., upwards.

dorsum 1. the back. 2. the upper or posterior surface.

dose the amount of a drug taken at a given time or the amount of irradiation given to a patient. Drug dose can be expressed in terms of the weight of its active ingredient, the volume of liquid to be drunk or its effects upon the body tissues. The amount of radiation absorbed during a session of radiotherapy is expressed in units called millisieverts. *See* RADIATION.

dosimeter one of various devices used to detect and measure exposure to radiation; worn by personnel near to radiation sources.

double-blind trial a test for the real effect of a new drug or treatment in clinical practice. Neither the patient nor the staff administering the treatment knows which of two apparently identical treatments is the new one being tested.

douche a stream of fluid directed to flush out a cavity of the body.

doula from the Greek word meaning 'woman who serves other women'. In maternity terms, one who provides emotional and practical support throughout pregnancy, and labour and postnatally.

download an action that is designed to transfer a file from a computer on the internet to your own computer by means of a modem and telephone line.

Down's syndrome *J.L.H. Down, British physician, 1828–1896.* A chromosomal abnormality, the commonest type having 47 instead of 46 chromosomes. The extra one is a third copy of chromosome 21, so that the condition is also called trisomy 21. This condition is associated with increasing maternal age. In the other form of Down's syndrome a translocation occurs, usually between chromosomes 14 and 21, as a structural rearrangement originating in the child, although the parents have normal chromosomes. Alternatively the translocations may occur as a result of a similar translocated chromosome in the parents; this increases the risk of the condition recurring in further pregnancies by 10%. The child exhibits certain features which include slanting

eyes with specked iris, broad hands with a single palmar crease, short neck with loose skin and hypotonia. Other abnormalities may also occur, e.g., congenital heart disease. Learning difficulties are also present but the range of ability is wide.

dracontiasis a tropical disease caused by infestation with the guinea-worm; acquired by drinking contaminated water.

Dracunculus a genus of roundworms; includes the guinea-worm.

drain 1. to withdraw liquid generally. 2. any device by which a channel or open area may be established for exit of fluids or purulent material from a cavity, wound or infected area.

dramatherapy the therapeutic use of drama, in which clients are encouraged to act out their feelings in order to overcome problems.

dream mental activity that occurs during deep (*see* REM) sleep, usually in the form of vivid images, emotions and imagined events. Often rapidly forgotten on waking.

dreaming the activity of engaging in fantasies or speculation during quiescent waking periods. Also called daydreaming. Some research suggests that this activity helps to promote positive mental health for the individual concerned.

dressing material applied to cover a wound or a diseased surface of the body. *See* WOUND DRESSING.

drive in psychology, an urge or motivating force.

droplet infection infection due to inhalation of respiratory pathogens suspended in liquid particles exhaled from someone already infected.

dropsy an old-fashioned term used to describe excess fluid in the tissues (oedema).

drug 1. any medicinal substance. 2. a narcotic. 3. to administer a drug. *D. addiction* a state of periodic or chronic intoxication produced by the repeated consumption of a drug, characterized by: (a) an overwhelming desire or need (compulsion) to continue use of the drug and to obtain it by any means; (b) a tendency to increase the dosage; (c) a psychological and usually a physical dependence on its effects; and (d) a detrimental effect on the individual and on society. *D. idiosyncrasy* an individual response to a drug that is unique to that person and quite different from what is expected. *D. interaction* modification of the potency of one drug by another (or others) taken concurrently or sequentially. Some medication interactions are harmful and some may have therapeutic benefits. Present knowledge of these interactions is limited. Drugs may also interact with various foods. In general, these interactions fall into three categories: (a) food malabsorption; (b) nutritional status; and (c) alteration of drug response by nutrients. In teaching patients self-care in the taking of prescribed medications, one should explain the need for meticulously following directions related to the intake of food and drink while the medication regimen is being followed. *D. misuse* the use of drugs for purposes other than those for which they are prescribed or recommended. The major groups of drugs and medicines generally considered to be most commonly misused are stimulants ('uppers'), depressants ('downers'), psychedelics and narcotics. *D. tolerance* a progressive reduction in the effect of a drug following repeated use. To achieve the desired effect increasingly larger doses of the medication are needed. *D. trial* the testing undertaken of any new drug before it becomes available for medical use.

dry eye syndrome a common condition in which the eyes do not make sufficient tears. Also known as KERATO-CONJUNCTIVITIS SICCA or dry eyes.

dry socket infection of the soft tissues of a tooth socket, occurring 2 or 3 days after tooth extraction, often a lower molar. It is a painful condition

requiring dental treatment with socket irrigation and local and/or systemic antibiotics.

DSH deliberate self-harm. *See* PARASUICIDE.

Dubowitz score a method used to assess gestational age in a low-birth-weight infant.

Duchenne dystrophy *G.B.A. Duchenne, French neurologist, 1806–1875.* Progressive muscular dystrophy occurring in childhood. *See* DYSTROPHY.

duct a tube or channel for the passage of fluid, particularly one conveying the secretion of a gland.

ductless without an excretory duct. *D. glands* ENDOCRINE glands.

ductus a duct. *D. arteriosus* a passage connecting the pulmonary artery and aorta in intrauterine life, which normally closes at birth. When it remains open it is called persistent ductus arteriosus. *See also* PATENT (DUCTUS ARTERIOSUS).

dumping the rapid evacuation of the contents of an organ. *D. syndrome* a feeling of fullness, weakness, sweating and dizziness which may occur after meals following a partial gastrectomy.

duodenal pertaining to the duodenum. *D. intubation* the use of a special tube which is passed via the mouth and stomach into the duodenum. Used for withdrawal of duodenal contents for pathological examination. *D. ulcer* a peptic ulcer occurring in the duodenum near the pylorus.

duodenostomy the formation of an artificial opening into the duodenum, through the abdominal wall, for purposes of feeding in cases of gastric disease.

duodenum the first 20–25 cm of the small intestine, from the pyloric opening of the stomach to the jejunum. The pancreatic and common bile ducts open into it.

Dupuytren's contraction or contracture *Baron G. Dupuytren, French surgeon, 1777–1835.* Contracture of the palmar fascia, causing permanent

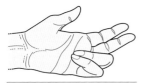

DUPUYTREN'S CONTRACTURE

bending and fixation of one or more fingers (*see* Figure).

dura mater a strong fibrous membrane forming the outer covering of the brain and spinal cord.

duty of candour a contractual duty imposed on all providers of care to NHS patients to provide to the service user and any other relevant personal necessary support and all relevant information in the event of a reportable patient safety incident.

duty of care 1. the legal responsibility in the law of negligence that a person must take reasonable care to avoid causing harm. 2. a nurse, midwife or medical practitioner has an accepted duty to a patient or client irrespective of any contractual agreement existing between the parties. The law has developed a set of rules on the expected standard of care to assist in determining whether or not a professional has neglected their duty of care, based on the standards prevailing at the time of any case questioning the issue. *See* Appendix 5.

duty of partnership duty placed on NHS bodies and local government to develop joint local delivery plans involving other parts of the NHS, local voluntary organizations and businesses.

dwarfism the state of being short in stature. Arrest of growth and development, e.g., due to renal rickets, congenital iodine deficiency syndrome or deficient pituitary function.

dysarthria difficulty speaking caused by brain damage which is either developmental due to birth disorder or acquired in later life due to neurological disorders or head injury.

dysarthrosis a deformed, dislocated or false joint.

dyschondroplasia a rare condition in which cartilage is deposited in the shaft of some bones. The affected bones become shortened and deformed.

dyscrasia a morbid condition, usually referring to an imbalance of component elements. *See also* BLOOD DYSCRASIA.

dysdiadochokinesis a sign of cerebellar disease in which the ability to perform rapid alternating movements, such as rotating the hands, is lost.

dysentery inflammation of the intestine, especially of the colon, with abdominal pain, tenesmus and frequent stools, often containing blood and mucus. The causative agent may be chemical irritants, bacteria, protozoa, viruses or parasitic worms. *Amoebic d.* common in tropical countries; caused by the protozoon *Entamoeba histolytica.* Spread is decreased in places with high standards of hygiene and sanitation. A notifiable disease in the UK. Also called amoebiasis. *Bacillary d.* the most common and acute form of the disease, caused by bacteria of the genus *Shigella. S. sonnei* is the most frequent cause in the UK. A notifiable disease. Also called shigellosis.

dysfunction impairment of function.

dysgammaglobulinaemia an immunological deficiency state marked by selective deficiencies of one or more, but not all, classes of immunoglobulin, resulting in heightened susceptibility to infectious diseases.

dysgerminoma a tumour that is usually malignant derived from germinal cells that have not been differentiated to either sex, occurring in either the ovary or the testicle.

dyshidrosis a disturbance of the sweat mechanism in which an itching vesicular rash may be present.

dyskinesia impairment of voluntary movement.

dyslalia impairment of speech, caused by a physical disorder.

dyslexia difficulty in reading or learning to read; accompanied by difficulty in writing and spelling correctly.

dysmaturity the condition of being small or immature for gestational age; said of fetuses that are the product of a pregnancy involving placental insufficiency or dysfunction. Also called small for dates, or light for gestational age.

dysmenorrhoea painful menstruation. *Primary (spasmodic) d.* painful menstruation occurring without apparent cause. The onset is usually shortly after puberty and occurs with each subsequent period. May be helped by hormonal therapy. *Secondary (congestive) d.* painful menstruation occurring in a woman who has previously had normal periods for some years. Often due to endometritis. The condition tends to worsen as the local congestion increases.

dysostosis abnormal development of bone.

dyspareunia painful or difficult coitus in women.

dyspepsia indigestion. There may be abdominal discomfort, flatulence, nausea and sometimes vomiting. *Nervous d.* dyspepsia in which anxiety and tension aggravate the symptoms.

dysphagia difficulty in swallowing.

dysphasia difficulty in speaking as the result of a brain lesion. There is a lack of coordination and an inability to arrange words in their correct order.

dysplasia abnormal development of tissue.

dyspnoea difficult or laboured breathing. *Expiratory d.* difficulty in expelling air. *Inspiratory d.* difficulty in taking in air.

dyspraxia partial loss of ability to perform coordinated movements. Also known as developmental co-ordination disorder (DCD).

dysrhythmia disturbance of a regularly occurring pattern. Often applied to an abnormality of rhythm of the brain waves, as shown in an electroencephalogram.

dystaxia difficulty in controlling voluntary movements.

dystonia a lack of tonicity in a tissue, often referring to the muscles.

dystrophia dystrophy. *D. myotonica* a rare hereditary disease of early adult life in which there is progressive muscle wasting and gonadal atrophy.

dystrophy a disorder of an organ or tissue caused by faulty nutrition of the affected part. Dystrophia. *Muscular d.* a group of hereditary diseases in which there is progressive muscular weakness and wasting.

dysuria difficult or painful micturition.

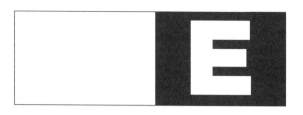

ear the organ of hearing and of equilibrium (*see* Figure on p. 124). It consists of three parts: (a) the *external e.*, made up of the expanded portion, or pinna, and the auditory canal, separated from the middle ear by the drum, or tympanum; (b) the *middle e.*, an irregular cavity containing three small bones (incus, malleus and stapes) that link the tympanic membrane to the internal ear; it also communicates with the pharyngotympanic tube and the mastoid cells; (c) the *internal e.*, which consists of a bony and a membranous labyrinth (the cochlea and semicircular canals).

eating disorders a general term for disturbed behaviour involving food, eating and body weight. *See* ANOREXIA, BULIMIA and DIETARY CHAOS SYNDROME.

EB virus Epstein–Barr virus.

EBM expressed breast milk. *See* EXPRESSION.

Ebola haemorrhagic fever (EHF) a severe and acute, fatal, haemorrhagic viral disease, also known as Ebola virus disease, principally seen in central and west African countries, caused by the Ebola virus, of the family *Filoviridae*. Death occurs in up to 90% of cases. Ebola virus can be transmitted in several ways, the most significant being person-to-person through direct contact with body fluids (e.g., blood, semen, vaginal fluid) of an infected person. *See* MARBURG VIRUS DISEASE.

ecchymosis a bruise; an effusion of blood under the skin causing discoloration.

eccrine secreting externally. Applied particularly to the sweat glands, which are generally distributed over the body. *See* APOCRINE.

ECG electrocardiogram.

Echinococcus a genus of tapeworm. *E. granulosus* infests dogs and may also infect humans. The larval form develops into cysts (hydatids), which occur in the liver, lung, brain and other organs.

echocardiography a method of studying the movements of the heart by the use of ultrasound.

echoencephalography a method of brain investigation by ultrasonic echoes.

echolalia the pathological involuntary repetition of phrases or words spoken by another person.

echopraxia the automatic repetition of the movements of others.

echovirus a group of viruses (enteroviruses), the name of which was derived from the first letters of the description 'enteric cytopathogenic human orphan'. At the time of the isolation of the viruses the diseases they caused were not known, hence the term 'orphan'. It is now known that these viruses produce many types of human disease, especially aseptic meningitis, diarrhoea and respiratory diseases.

e-cigarette a handheld electronic device that mimics the effects of smoking tobacco cigarettes by heating a

External ear (not to scale)   Middle ear   Inner ear

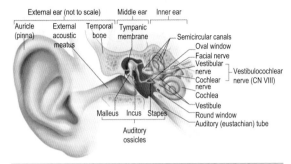

Auricle | External | Temporal | Tympanic
(pinna) | acoustic | bone | membrane
| meatus

Semicircular canals
Oval window
Facial nerve
Vestibular nerve
Cochlear nerve
Vestibulocochlear nerve (CN VIII)
Cochlea
Vestibule
Round window
Auditory (eustachian) tube

Malleus   Incus   Stapes

Auditory
ossicles

THE EAR

liquid to generate an aerosol, called a vapour, that is inhaled. Also known a vaping.

eclampsia a severe condition in which convulsions may occur as a result of an acute toxaemia of pregnancy.

ecology the study of the relationship between living organisms and the environment.

economy the management of money or domestic affairs. *Token e.* in behaviour therapy, a programme of treatment in which the patient earns tokens, exchangeable for tangible rewards, by engaging in appropriate personal and social behaviour, and loses tokens for antisocial behaviour. *E. class syndrome See* DEEP VEIN THROMBOSIS.

ecstasy 1. a feeling of exaltation. It may be accompanied by sensory impairment and lack of activity but with an expression of rapture. 2. an illegal drug. It is widely used as an accompaniment to modern dance music culture. Has resulted in several fatalities in young people. Causes intense thirst leading to the drinking of large quantities of water resulting in fatal damage to the body's fluid balance, kidney failure and coma. Also known as 'MDMA' or 'E'.

ECT electroconvulsive therapy.

ectoderm the outer germinal layer of the developing embryo from which the skin and nervous system are derived.

ectogenous produced outside an organism. *See* ENDOGENOUS.

ectoparasite a parasite that spends all or part of its life on the external surface of its host, e.g., a louse.

ectopia displacement or abnormal position of any part. *E. cordis* congenital malposition of the heart outside the thoracic cavity. *E. vesicae* a defect of the abdominal wall in which the bladder is exposed.

ectopic 1. pertaining to or characterized by ectopy. 2. located away from the normal position. 3. arising or produced at an abnormal site or in a tissue where it is not normally found. *E. pregnancy* pregnancy in which the fertilized ovum becomes implanted outside the uterus instead of in the wall of the uterus. Also called extrauterine pregnancy.

ectopy displacement or malposition, especially if congenital.

ectropion eversion of an eyelid, often due to contraction of the skin or to paralysis. It causes a persistent overflow of tears and hypertrophy of exposed conjunctiva.

eczema 1. a general term for any superficial inflammatory process involving primarily the epidermis, marked early by redness, itching, minute papules and vesicles, weeping, oozing and crusting, and later by scaling, lichenification and often pigmentation. 2. atopic dermatitis. Eczema is a common allergic reaction in children but it also occurs in adults. Childhood eczema often begins in infancy, the rash appearing on the face, neck and folds of elbows and knees. It may disappear by itself when an offending food is removed from the diet, or it may become more extensive and in some instances cover the entire surface of the body. Severe eczema can be complicated by skin infections. The cause of eczema can be either exogenous (due to external or traumatic factors) or endogenous (due to internal or constitutional factors).

edentulous without natural teeth.

Edwards' syndrome also known as trisomy 18, a serious genetic condition caused by an additional copy of chromosome 18. Babies born with Edwards' syndrome tend to be very small and will have serious complications. They will rarely live for more than a few weeks and if they survive are likely to have severe physical and learning disabilities.

EEG electroencephalogram.

effacement taking up of the cervix. The process by which the internal os dilates, so opening out the cervical canal and leaving only a circular orifice, the external os. This process precedes cervical dilatation, particularly in a primigravida, while both occur simultaneously in a multigravida during labour.

effective 1. the extent to which something succeeds. 2. a result produced by agent, action or force, e.g., resources to achieve desired outcomes. Cost effectiveness. *E. dose* the amount of a drug given to a patient to achieve the required treatment result.

effector a motor or sensory nerve ending in a muscle, gland or organ.

efferent conveying from the centre to the periphery. *See also* AFFERENT. *E. nerves* nerves coming from the brain to supply the muscles and glands.

effleurage [Fr.] stroking movement in massage. In NATURAL CHILDBIRTH, a light circular stroke of the lower abdomen, done in rhythm to control breathing, to aid in relaxation of the abdominal muscles, and to increase concentration during a uterine contraction. The stroking is accomplished by moving the wrist only.

effort syndrome a rare condition characterized by breathlessness, palpitations, chest pain and fatigue, associated with abnormal anxiety for which no pathological explanation has been found.

effusion the escape of blood, serum or other fluid into surrounding tissues or cavities.

ego in psychoanalytical theory, that part of the mind which the individual experiences as 'self'. The ego is concerned with satisfying the unconscious primitive demands of the 'id' in a socially acceptable form.

egocentrism a type of thinking in which a person has difficulty in seeing another's point of view. This self-centring is normal in young children but in adults may indicate delayed cognitive development.

Ehlers-Danlos syndrome (EDS) a group of rare inherited disorders that affect connective tissue. There are several types of EDS, some which will give mild symptoms and others which may be life threatening.

eidetic having the ability to visualize exactly objects or events that have previously been seen. Having a photographic memory.

ejaculation 1. the act of ejecting semen, a reflex action that occurs as the result of sexual stimulation. 2. a sudden utterance or exclamation, which may be out of context.

elastic capable of stretching. *E. bandage* one that will stretch and will exert continuous pressure on the part bandaged. *E. stocking* a woven rubber stocking worn to prevent deep vein thrombosis. *E. tissue* connective tissue containing yellow elastic fibres.

elation in psychiatry, a feeling of well-being or a state of excitement. It occurs to a marked degree in hypomania and to an intense degree in mania. *See* EUPHORIA.

elbow the joint between the upper arm and the forearm. It is formed by the humerus above and the radius and ulna below.

elder abuse *see* ABUSE.

elective usually pertaining to a surgical procedure that is performed by choice, as opposed to an emergency life-saving procedure. Timing of the procedure may also be arranged to be mutually convenient for the patient and surgeon.

Electra complex libidinous fixation of a daughter towards her father. The female version of the Oedipus complex.

electrocardiogram abbreviated ECG. A tracing made of the various phases of the heart's action by means of an electrocardiograph. The normal electrocardiogram is composed of a P wave, Q, R and S waves (known as the QRS COMPLEX, or QRS wave), and a T wave. The P wave occurs at the beginning of each contraction of the atria. The QRS wave occurs at the beginning of each contraction of the ventricles. The T wave seen in a normal electrocardiogram occurs as the ventricles recover electrically and prepare for the next contraction. There is a refractory period between these waves.

electrocardiograph an instrument that records the electrical potential of the heart from electrodes on the chest and limbs.

electrocautery an instrument for the destruction of tissue by means of an electrically heated needle or wire loop.

electrocoagulation a method of coagulation using a high-frequency current. A form of surgical diathermy.

electroconvulsive therapy abbreviated ECT. Electroplexy. The passage of an electric current through the frontal lobes of the brain, which causes a convulsion. It is used in the treatment of severe depression. A general anaesthetic and muscle relaxant are given before treatment.

electrocorticography electroencephalography with the electrodes applied directly to the cortex of the brain during surgery to locate a small lesion, e.g., a scar.

electrode the terminal of a conducting system or cell of a battery, through which electricity enters or leaves the body; may be in the form of a plate or pad.

electroencephalogram abbreviated EEG. A tracing of the electrical activity of the brain. Abnormal rhythm is an aid to diagnosis in epilepsy and cerebral tumour.

electroencephalograph an instrument for recording the electrical activity of the cortex of the brain. The electrodes are applied to the scalp.

electrolysis 1. chemical decomposition by means of electricity, e.g., an electric current passed through water decomposes it into oxygen and hydrogen. 2. the destruction of tissue by means of electricity, e.g., the removal of surplus hair.

electrolyte a compound which, when dissolved in a solution, will dissociate into ions. These ions are electrically charged particles and will thus conduct electricity. *E. balance* the maintenance of the correct balance between the different elements in the body tissues and fluids.

electron a negatively charged particle revolving round the nucleus of an atom. *E. microscope* a type of microscope employing a beam of electrons rather than a beam of light, which allows very small particles such as viruses to be identified.

electronic health record abbreviated EHR. Longitudinal record of a patient's health and health care which combines information from primary health care with periodic care from other institutions.

electronic patient record abbreviated EPR. A computerized record of the care provided for a patient both in primary and secondary settings. *See also* SUMMARY CARE RECORD.

electrophoresis a method of analysing the different proteins in blood serum by passing an electric current through the serum to separate the electrically charged particles. The particles gradually separate into bands as a result of the difference in rate of movement according to the electrical charge on the particles.

electroretinography a method of examining the retina of the eye by means of electrodes and light stimulation for assessment of retinal damage.

element 1. any of the primary parts or constituents of a compound. 2. in chemistry, a simple substance that cannot be decomposed by ordinary chemical means; the basic 'stuff' of which all matter is composed.

elephantiasis a chronic disease of the lymphatics producing excessive thickening of the skin and swelling of the parts affected, usually the lower limbs. It may be due to filariasis in tropical and subtropical climates.

elimination the removal of waste matter, particularly from the body. Excretion.

ELISA abbreviation for enzyme-linked immunosorbent assay (also called enzyme immunoassay; EIA), a laboratory technique to identify the presence of an antibody or an antigen in a sample, such as blood or saliva. It is the principal technique used in testing for human immunodeficiency virus (HIV) infection. It is a highly accurate test, but positive results are always confirmed by additional testing.

emaciation excessive wasting of body tissues. Extreme thinness.

email an electronic method of exchanging digital messages between people using digital devices such as computers and mobile phones. Email operates primarily across the internet. *E. address* a series of characters that precisely identifies the location of an individual electronic mail box.

emasculation the removal of the penis or testicles; castration.

embolectomy surgical removal of an embolus, frequently arterial emboli that are cutting off the blood supply to the limbs.

embolism obstruction of a blood vessel by a travelling blood clot or particle of matter. *Air e.* the presence of gas or air bubbles, usually sucked into the large veins from a wound in the neck or chest. *Cerebral e.* obstruction of a vessel in the brain. *Coronary e.* the blockage of a coronary vessel with a clot. *Fat e.* globules of fat released into the blood from a fractured long bone. *Infective e.* detached particles of infected blood clot from an area of inflammation which, obstructing small vessels, result in abscess formation, i.e., pyaemia. Also known as pyaemic embolism. *Pulmonary e.* blocking of the pulmonary artery or one of its branches by a detached clot, usually due to thrombosis in the femoral or iliac veins. *Retinal e.* blockage, due to air or a blood clot, of the central retinal artery, resulting in loss of vision.

embolus a substance carried by the bloodstream until it causes obstruction by blocking a blood vessel. *See* EMBOLISM.

embrocation a liquid applied to the body by rubbing to treat strains. A liniment.

embryo the fertilized ovum in its earliest stages, i.e., until it shows human characteristics during the second month. After this it is termed a fetus.

embryology the study of the growth and development of the embryo from the unicellular stage until birth.

emergency a sudden crisis requiring urgent intervention. *E. planning* plan outlining how to deal with a serious incident, such as a major transport accident, extreme weather, terrorist incident, major fire, outbreak of infectious disease or chemical spill. Each level and part of the NHS has an emergency plan, which must relate to the emergency plans of other agencies, such as local authorities, police and fire services. EPRR stands for emergency preparedness, resilience and response and emergency plans are requirement of the NHS under the Civil Contingencies Act (2004). *E. protection order* a court order whereby a child is removed from the care of the parents in the interests of the child's safety.

emesis vomiting.

emetic an agent that can induce vomiting.

emic perspectives that are shared and understood by members of a group, community or culture; 'the insiders'. These views may contrast to those of 'outsiders' (*see* ETIC). Used in ethnographic and qualitative research.

eminence a projection, usually rounded, from a surface, e.g., of a bone.

emission involuntary ejection (of semen).

emollient any substance used to soothe or soften the skin.

emotion feeling or affect; a state of arousal characterized by alteration of feeling tone and by physiological behavioural changes. The physical form of emotion may be outward and evident to others, as in crying, laughing, blushing or a variety of facial expressions; however, emotion is not always reflected in the appearance and actions even though psychic changes are taking place. Joy, grief, fear and anger are examples of emotions.

emotional 1. relating to the emotions. 2. arousing emotions or readily showing the emotions. *E. bias* situation in which emotional attitudes affect logical judgement. An emotional reaction. *E.*

deprivation a lack of loving attention during a child's early years when there has been a failure to achieve a psychological and emotional tie between parent and child. This may lead to impulsive behaviour and an inability to sustain trusting relationships in later life. *See* BONDING. *E. disorders* characterized by swings in mood ranging from extreme excitement to one of depression. Emotional lability. *E. intelligence* the ability to recognize own and others' emotions to guide thinking and behaviour. *E. maturity* the achievement of maximum emotional control.

empathy the power of projecting oneself into the feelings of another person or into a situation.

emphysema the abnormal presence of air in tissues or cavities of the body. *Pulmonary e.* a chronic disease of the lungs. Distension of alveoli causes intervening walls to be broken down and bullae to form on the lung surface. It also causes distension of the bronchioles and eventual loss of elasticity so that inspired air cannot be expired, making breathing difficult. Included in a group of diseases referred to as chronic obstructive pulmonary disease (COPD). *Surgical e.* the presence of air or any other gas in the subcutaneous tissues, introduced through a wound and evidenced by crepitation on pressure. Also known as tissue emphysema.

empirical based on experience and not on scientific reasoning.

empowerment the capacity to empower, to give power or authority, e.g., to patients to take control over their own care and to work in partnership with care providers.

empyema a collection of pus in a cavity, most commonly referring to the pleural cavity.

en face [Fr.] 1. a position in which the mother's face and that of her infant are on the same plane and approximately 20 cm apart; a position usually held during breast feeding. 2. en face imaging is a technique used to provide a view of any given layer within the retina and choroid within the eye.

enable 1. To provide a person with the authority, power, means or the opportunity to develop and achieve what is important to them as an individual or as a member of a community or organization. 2. To make possible or easy.

enamel the hard outer covering of the crown of a tooth.

enarthrosis ball and socket joint, the most freely moving type of joint.

encanthis a small fleshy growth at the inner canthus of the eye, which may form an abscess.

encapsulated enclosed in a capsule.

encephalin (**enkephalin**) an opiate-like substance produced by the pituitary which has analgesic effects. This substance may also be produced synthetically. *See* ENDORPHIN.

encephalitis inflammation of the brain. There are many causes of encephalitis, most usually viral but may be bacterial. At first the symptoms may be mild, with headache, general malaise and muscle ache similar to that associated with influenza. The more acute and serious symptoms may include fever, delirium, convulsions and coma, and in a significant number of patients result in death. *See* JAPANESE ENCEPHALITIS.

encephalocele herniation of the brain through the skull.

encephalography examination of the brain.

encephalomalacia softening of the brain.

encephalomyelitis inflammation of the brain and spinal cord.

encephalomyelopathy any disease condition of the brain and spinal cord.

encephalopathy cerebral dysfunction with diffuse disease or damage of the brain. Especially chronic degenerative conditions of toxic, nutritional or metabolic aetiology.

encephalotrigeminal angiomatosis *see* STURGE-WEBER SYNDROME.

encopresis incontinence of faeces not due to organic defect or illness.

end of life care care pathway for people nearing the end of life. Also incorporates planning for future care, making wishes and preferences known in advance.

endarterectomy the surgical removal of the lining of an artery, usually because of narrowing of the vessel by atheromatous plaques. *Thrombo-e.* removal of a clot with the lining.

endarteritis inflammation of the innermost coat of an artery. *E. obliterans* a type that causes collapse and obstruction in small arteries.

endemic pertaining to a disease prevalent in a particular locality. *See* EPIDEMIC.

endemiology the study of all the factors pertaining to endemic disease.

endocarditis inflammation of the endocardium characterized by vegetations on the endocardium and heart valves. Due to infection by microorganisms, fungi or *Rickettsia*, or to rheumatic fever. Can affect all ages.

endocardium the membrane lining the heart.

endocervicitis inflammation of the mucous membrane lining the uterine cervix.

endocrine secreting within. Applied to those glands whose secretions (hormones) flow directly into the blood and not outwards through a duct. The chief endocrine glands are the thyroid, parathyroids, suprarenals and pituitary (*see* Figure on p. 130). The pancreas, stomach, liver, ovaries and testes also produce internal secretions. *See* EXOCRINE.

endocrinology the science of the endocrine glands and their secretions.

endoderm entoderm.

endogenous produced within the organism; *see* EXOGENOUS. *E. depression* one in which the disease derives from internal causes.

endolymph the fluid inside the membranous labyrinth of the ear.

endometriosis the presence of endometrium in an abnormal situation, e.g., in the ovaries, the intestines or the urinary bladder. The ectopic tissue

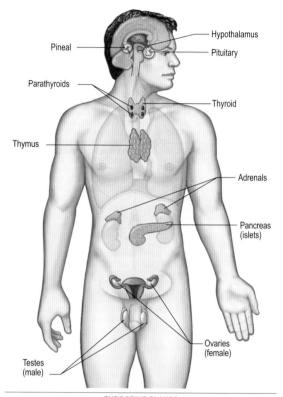

ENDOCRINE GLANDS

undergoes the same hormonal changes as normal endometrium (*see* Figure on p. 243). As there is no outlet for bleeding when menstruation occurs, the woman suffers considerable pain.

endometritis inflammation of the endometrium.

endometrium the mucous membrane lining the uterus.

endomyocarditis inflammation of the lining membrane and muscles of the heart.

endoparasite a parasite that lives within the body of its host.

endophthalmitis   inflammation of the ocular cavity and adjacent structures.

endorphin   one of a group of opiate-like peptides produced naturally by the body at neural synapses at various points in the central nervous system, where they modulate the transmission of pain perceptions. Endorphins raise the pain threshold and produce sedation and euphoria; the effects are blocked by naloxone, a narcotic antagonist. Also known as enkephalins.

endoscope   fibreoptic endoscopes are in general use for visualization of tubular structures and cavities within the body. Light is carried by very fine glass fibres along a flexible tube that can 'see' around corners. This allows for examination, photography, biopsy and treatment of body cavities or organs in a conscious, relaxed (sometimes sedation is given) patient. Older style endoscopes are rigid and made of metal.

endospore   *see* SPORE.

endosteoma   a neoplasm in the medullary cavity of a bone.

endosteum   the lining membrane of bone cavities.

endothelioma   a malignant growth originating in the endothelium.

endothelium   the membranous lining of serous, synovial and other internal surfaces.

endotoxin   a poison produced by and retained within a bacterium, e.g., *Salmonella typhi*, which is released only after the destruction of the bacterial cell. *See* EXOTOXIN.

endotracheal   within the trachea. *E. tube* an airway catheter which is inserted into the trachea when a patient requires ventilatory support. It also allows for the removal of secretions by suction.

enema   1. introduction of fluid into the rectum. 2. a solution introduced into the rectum to promote evacuation of faeces or as a means of administering nutrient or medicinal substances. 3. introduction of a radio-opaque material in a radiological examination of the colon (*barium e.*), or via a tube inserted into the jejunum in a radiological examination of the small bowel (*small bowel e.*).

energy   the ability to do work or effect a physical change in status. Energy has many forms including light, heat and sound. Food through its breakdown within the body provides energy for human activity, strength, growth and vitality and this is measured in calories or joules. Carbohydrates provide 4 kcal/g and fats provide 9 kcal/g. *E. conservation* an occupational therapy technique that seeks to assist patients/clients in maximizing the use of limited physical energy to maintain quality of daily life. This approach is also used by nurses and other health care workers working with the elderly and physically disabled in the community. *E. requirements* the amount of energy that is required by a person for cell metabolism, growth and activity. This is influenced by age, gender, activity and health. *See* METABOLISM. UK Department of Health Estimated Average Requirements (EAR): a daily calorie intake of around 2000 calories per day for a woman and 2500 for a man. Excess energy foods are stored as fat. This fat provides a supplementary source of energy if the diet is inadequate.

enervation   1. general weakness and loss of strength. 2. removal of a nerve.

engagement   the entry of the presenting part of the fetus, normally the head, into the true pelvis. Occurs in the last stage of pregnancy.

enhanced supportive care (ECS)   an initiative to fully meet the needs of patients on active anti-cancer treatment and to prevent and manage adverse physical and psychological effects of cancer and its treatment.

enkephalin   either of two naturally occurring pentapeptides isolated from the brain, which have potent opiate-like effects and probably serve as neurotransmitters. They are classified as endorphins. *See* ENDORPHINS.

enophthalmos a condition in which the eyeball is abnormally sunken into its socket.

ensiform xiphoid; sword-shaped. *E. cartilage* the lowest portion of the sternum.

Entamoeba a genus of protozoa, some of which are parasitic in humans. *E. histolytica* the cause of amoebic dysentery.

enteral within the gastrointestinal tract. *E. diets* or *e. feeding* provides nutrition for those patients who are unable to ingest sufficient nutrients orally but who are able to utilize them in the body to provide for energy requirements and for healing. Feeding may be through nasogastric, gastrostomy or jejunostomy tubes by bolus, gravity or pump assisted. *See* PARENTERAL FEEDING.

enteric pertaining to the intestine. *E. coated* a special coating applied to tablets or capsules which prevents release and absorption of their contents until they reach the intestine.

enteritis inflammation of the small intestine.

Enterobacteriaceae a family of gram-negative, rod-shaped bacteria, many of which are normally found in the human intestine.

enterobiasis infestation by threadworms.

Enterobius a genus of nematode worms. *E. vermicularis* the threadworm or pinworm, a small white worm parasitic in the upper part of the large intestine. Gravid females migrate to the anal region to deposit their eggs, sometimes causing severe itching. Infection and re-infection is frequent in children. Treatment is with an anthelmintic drug.

enterococcus any streptococcus of the human intestine. An example is *Streptococcus faecalis*, only harmful out of its normal habitat, when it may cause a urinary infection or endocarditis.

enterocolitis inflammation of both the large and the small intestine.

enterokinase an intestinal enzyme that converts trypsinogen into trypsin; enteropeptidase.

enterostomy the formation of an external opening into the small intestine. It may be (a) temporary, to relieve obstruction, or (b) permanent, in the form of an ileostomy in cases of total colectomy.

enterotomy any incision of the intestine.

enterotoxin a toxin that is produced by one of the many organisms that cause food poisoning. Such toxins frequently prove more resistant to destruction than the bacteria themselves.

enterovirus a virus that infects the gastrointestinal tract and then attacks the central nervous system. This subgroup includes Coxsackie, polio and echoviruses, which are now known, together with rhinoviruses, as picornaviruses.

entoderm the innermost of the three germ layers of the embryo along with the mesoderm (intermediate) and ectoderm (outer) layers. It gives rise to the lining of most of the respiratory tract and to the intestinal tract and its glands.

entropion inversion of an eyelid, so that the lashes rub against the eyeball.

enucleation removal of an organ or other mass intact from its supporting tissues, as of the eyeball from the orbit.

enuresis involuntary passing of urine, usually during sleep at night (bed-wetting).

environment the surroundings of an organism which influence its development and behaviour.

environmental health the concept that an individual's living and working environment has an impact upon health and well-being. Factors that can influence health include housing, food hygiene, refuse collection, infestation, and air and noise pollution.

enzyme a protein that will catalyse a biological reaction. *See* CATALYST.

enzyme-linked immunosorbent assay *see* ELISA.

eosin a red dye used to stain biological specimens. A derivative of bromine and fluorescein.

eosinophil a cell having an affinity for eosin. A type of white blood cell containing eosin-staining granules.

eosinophilia excessive numbers of eosinophils present in the blood.

ependyma the membrane lining the cerebral ventricles and the central canal of the spinal cord.

ependymoma a neoplasm arising from the lining cells of the ventricles or central canal of the spinal cord. It gives rise to signs of hydrocephalus and is treated by surgery and radiotherapy.

epiblepharon a congenital condition in which an excess of skin of the eyelid folds over the lid margin so that the eyelashes are pressed against the eyeball.

epicanthus a vertical fold of skin on either side of the nose, sometimes covering the inner canthus; a normal characteristic in persons of certain races, but anomalous in others.

epicardium the visceral layer of the pericardium.

epicondyle a protuberance on a long bone above its condyle.

epicondylitis also known as tennis elbow caused by strenuous overuse of the muscles and tendons of the forearm.

epicritic pertaining to sensory nerve fibres in the skin which give the appreciation of touch and temperature.

epidemic the presence in a population of disease or infection in excess of that usually expected.

epidemiology the study of the distribution of diseases in populations. It includes the attack rate (incidence), risk factors, other influences and the numbers affected at any one time (prevalence).

epidermis the non-vascular outer layer or cuticle of the skin. It consists of layers of cells which protect the dermis.

epidermoid pertaining to certain tumours which have the appearance of epidermal tissue.

Epidermophyton a genus of fungi that attack skin and nails, but not hair. The cause of ringworm and athlete's foot.

epididymis [Gr.] an elongated, cord-like structure along the posterior border of the testis, whose coiled duct provides for the storage, transport and maturation of spermatozoa.

epididymitis inflammation of the epididymis.

epididymo-orchitis inflammation of the epididymis and the testis.

epidural outside the dura mater. *E. analgesia* also known as extradural or peridural anaesthesia. A form of pain relief for childbirth and chronic pain, obtained by a single injection of a local analgesic or intermittently via a catheter into the epidural space in order to block the spinal nerves. It may be approached by two routes: (a) caudal, through the sacrococcygeal membrane covering the sacral hiatus; or (b) lumbar, through the intervertebral space and ligamentum flavum.

epigastrium that region of the abdomen situated over the stomach.

epiglottis a cartilaginous structure which covers the opening from the pharynx into the larynx during swallowing and prevents food from passing into the trachea.

epilation removal of hairs with their roots. It may be effected by pulling out the hairs, by electrolysis or the application of an epilatory cream/ointment.

epilatory an agent that produces epilation.

epilepsy the epilepsies, a group of conditions characterized by convulsive attacks due to disordered electrical activity of the brain cells. In a major attack the patient falls to the ground unconscious, following an aura or unpleasant sensation. There are first tonic and then clonic contractions, from which stage the patient passes into a deep sleep. A minor attack is a momentary loss of consciousness only. Both these types of epilepsy are idiopathic and are not caused by any damage to the brain. *Focal* or *Jacksonian e.* a symptom of a cerebral lesion. The convulsive movements are often localized and close observation of the onset and course of the attack may greatly assist diagnosis. *Temporal lobe e.* characterized by hallucinations of sight, hearing, taste and smell, paroxysmal disorders of memory and automatism. Caused by temporal or parietal lobe disease.

epileptiform resembling an epileptic fit.

epiloia tuberous sclerosis. A congenital disorder with areas of hardening in the cerebral cortex and other organs, characterized clinically by learning disability and epilepsy.

epinephrine adrenaline.

epineurium the sheath of tissue surrounding a nerve.

epiphora persistent overflow of tears, often due to obstruction in the lacrimal passages or to ectropion.

epiphysis the end of a long bone, developed separately from but attached by cartilage to the diaphysis (the shaft), with which it eventually unites. Growth in length takes place from the line of junction.

episcleritis inflammation of the outer coat of the eyeball. It is seen as a slightly raised bluish nodule under the conjunctiva.

episiotomy an incision made in the perineum when it will not stretch sufficiently during the second stage of labour.

epispadias a malformation in which there is an abnormal opening of the urethra on to the dorsal surface of the penis. *See* HYPOSPADIAS.

epistaxis bleeding from the nose.

epithelioma any tumour originating in the epithelium.

epithelium the surface layer of cells of the skin or lining tissues.

epithelization development of epithelium. The final stage in the healing of a surface wound. Epithelialization.

Epstein–Barr virus *M.A. Epstein, British pathologist, b. 1921; Y. Barr, Irish pathologist, 1932–2016.* A herpes virus that causes infectious mononucleosis. It has been isolated from cells cultured from Burkitt's lymphoma, and has been found in certain cases of nasopharyngeal cancer. Also called EB virus.

Equality and Human Rights Commission (EHRC) launched in 2007 the Commission is an independent statutory body established under the Equality Act 2006 and 2010. The EHRC has statutory remit to promote and monitor human rights; and to protect, enforce and promote equality across the nine 'protected grounds: age, disability, gender, race, religion and belief, pregnancy and maternity, marriage and civil partnership, sexual orientation and gender reassignment.

Erb's palsy *W.H. Erb, German physician, 1840–1921.* Paralysis of the arm, often due to birth injury causing pressure on the brachial plexus or lower cervical nerve roots. Also known as Erb-Duchenne Palsy.

erectile having the power of becoming erect. *E. tissue* vascular tissue which, under stimulus, becomes congested and swollen, causing erection of that part. The penis consists largely of erectile tissue.

erection the enlarged and rigid state of the sexually aroused penis. Erection can also occur in the clitoris and the nipples of the female.

erepsin the enzyme of succus entericus, secreted by the intestinal glands, which splits peptones into amino acids.

ergonomics the scientific study of human beings in relation to their work and the effective use of human energy.

ergosterol a sterol occurring in animal and plant tissues which, on ultraviolet irradiation, becomes a potent antirachitic substance, vitamin D$_2$ (ergocalciferol).

erogenous arousing erotic feelings. *E. zones* areas of the body, stimulation of which produces erotic desire, e.g., the oral, anal and genital orifices and the nipples.

erosion the breaking down of tissue, usually by ulceration. *Cervical e.* a covering of columnar epithelium on the vaginal part of the uterine cervix, arising from erosion of the squamous epithelium, which normally covers it.

erotic pertaining to sexual love or lust.

eroticism, erotism a sexual instinct or desire; the expression of one's instinctual energy or drive, especially the sex drive.

eructation belching; the escape of gas from the stomach through the mouth.

eruption a breaking out, e.g., of a skin lesion, or the cutting of teeth.

erysipelas a febrile disease characterized by inflammation and redness of the skin and subcutaneous tissues, and caused by group A haemolytic streptococci.

erysipeloid an infective dermatitis or cellulitis due to infection with *Erysipelothrix insidiosa*; it usually begins in a wound (often the result of a prick by a fish bone) and remains localized, rarely becoming generalized and septicaemic.

erythema redness of the skin caused by congestion of the capillaries in its lower layers. It occurs with any skin injury, infection or inflammation. *E. induratum* a manifestation of vasculitis. *E. multiforme* an acute eruption of the skin and sometimes of the mucous membranes, which may be due to an allergy or to drug sensitivity. *E. nodosum* a painful disease in which bright-red, tender nodes occur below the knee or on the forearm; it may be associated with tuberculosis.

erythematous characterized by erythema.

erythrasma a skin disease due to infection by *Corynebacterium minutissimum*, attacking the armpits or groins. It causes no irritation but is contagious.

erythroblast originally, any nucleated erythrocyte, but now more generally used to designate the nucleated precursor from which an erythrocyte develops.

erythroblastosis the presence of erythroblasts in the blood. *E. fetalis* a severe haemolytic anaemia with an excess of erythroblasts in the newly born. Due to rhesus incompatibility between the child's and the mother's blood.

erythrocyte a mature red blood cell. The cells contain haemoglobin and serve to transport oxygen. They are developed in the red bone marrow found in the cancellous tissue of all bones (*see* Figure). The haemopoietic factor vitamin B$_{12}$ is essential for the change from proerythroblast to normoblast, and iron, thyroxine and vitamin C are also necessary for its perfect structure. *E. sedimentation rate* abbreviated ESR. The rate at which the cells of citrated blood form a deposit in a graduated 200 mm tube (Westergren method). The normal is less than 10 mm of clear plasma in 1 hour. This

ERYTHROCYTE DEVELOPMENT IN BONE MARROW

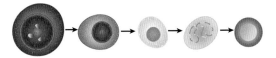

Proerythroblast   Erythroblast   Normoblast   Reticulocyte   Erythrocyte

is much increased in severe infection and acute rheumatism.

erythrocythaemia increase in numbers of red blood cells due to over-activity of the bone marrow; Vaquez' disease; polycythaemia vera.

erythrocytopenia erythropenia; deficiency in numbers of red blood cells.

erythrocytosis erythrocythaemia.

erythroderma abnormal redness of the skin, usually over a large area.

erythropoiesis the manufacture of red blood corpuscles.

erythropoietin a hormone, produced by the kidney, which stimulates the production of red blood cells in the bone marrow. *E. therapy* the use of erythropoietin to promote new blood formation in the treatment of anaemia.

erythropsia a defect of vision in which all objects appear red. May occur after a cataract operation.

eschar a slough or scab which forms after the destruction of living tissue by gangrene, infection or burning.

Escherichia a genus of Enterobacteriaceae. *E. coli* an organism normally present in the intestines of humans and other vertebrates. Although not generally pathogenic, it may set up infections of the gallbladder, bile ducts, and urinary and intestinal tracts. Strain O157, normally found in the gut of cattle, occasionally has been responsible for serious outbreaks of food poisoning in humans.

esophoria latent convergent strabismus. The eyes turn inwards only when one is covered up.

esotropia convergent strabismus. One or other eye turns inwards, resulting in double vision.

ESP extrasensory perception.

ESR erythrocyte sedimentation rate.

ESRD end-stage renal disease. *See* RENAL.

essence 1. an indispensable part of anything. 2. a volatile oil dissolved in alcohol.

essential indispensable. *E. amino acids* those amino acids that must be

obtained in the diet and are necessary for the maintenance of tissue growth and repair. *See* AMINO ACID. *E. drugs* a concept developed by the World Health Organization as a scheme to extend the range of drugs to populations who have poor access because of the existing supply structure. A core drug list based on local health needs was developed. The World Health Organization perceives essential drug lists as an indication of those drugs needed to meet common national requirements in poorer countries. The lists are updated on a two-yearly basis with an emphasis on local ownership and the involvement of national policies in implementation. *E. fatty acids* unsaturated fatty acids that are necessary for body growth. *E. oils* specially prepared aromatic oils which are obtained from the different parts of plants including flowers, leaves, seeds, wood, roots and bark. Used in aromatherapy.

ester a compound formed by the combination of an acid and an alcohol, with the elimination of water.

esterase an enzyme that causes the hydrolysis of esters into acids and alcohol.

ethanol alcohol.

ethanolamine an intravenous sclerosing agent used to inject haemorrhoids.

ether a volatile inflammable liquid formerly used as a general anaesthetic agent.

ethics a code of moral principles. Each practitioner, upon entering a profession, is invested with the responsibility to adhere to the standards of ethical practice and conduct set by that profession. *E. committee* a group of lay people with professional health care practitioners, nurses, doctors and other experts. They consider and discuss ethical issues and monitor research projects that involve the use of human subjects.

ethmoid a sieve-like bone separating the cavity of the nose from the cranium. The olfactory nerves pass through its perforations.

ethnic pertaining to a social group, members of which share cultural bonds or physical (racial) characteristics. *E. minority* a social grouping of people who share cultural or racial factors but who constitute a minority within the greater culture or society.

ethnocentrism the belief that one's own group, community, society or even way of doing things is superior to those of others, leading to mistrust or doubt about others' values and beliefs.

ethnography a qualitative research approach developed by anthropologists with the purpose of describing an aspect of a culture, but also aimed at learning about the culture or factor being studied.

ethnology the science dealing with the human races, their descent, relationship, etc.

ethnomethodology a sociological theory which concentrates on the case study using participant or non-participant observation.

ethyl chloride a volatile liquid used as a local anaesthetic. When sprayed on intact skin it causes local insensitivity, through freezing.

ethylene oxide a gas that is sporicidal and viricidal and capable of penetrating relatively inaccessible parts of an apparatus during sterilization. It is used for equipment which is too delicate to be sterilized by other methods.

etic the perspectives of a group, community or culture held by observers who are 'outsiders' or non-participants. *See* EMIC.

etiolation paleness of the skin due to lack of exposure to sunlight.

etiology *see* AETIOLOGY.

eucalyptus oil an oil derived from the leaves of the eucalyptus tree; it has mild antiseptic properties and is used in the treatment of nasal catarrh.

eugenics the study of measures that may be taken to improve future generations, both physically and mentally.

eugeria the state of a high quality of life in old age. Eugeria should be the normal state for the elderly but may be affected by physical or mental illness.

eunuch a castrated male.

euphoria an exaggerated feeling of wellbeing, often not justified by circumstances. Less extreme than ELATION.

eurhythmics gentle body exercises performed to music.

European Health Insurance Card (EHIC) gives access to health care across the European Economic Area and Switzerland.

European Medicines Agency authorizes the use of medicinal products in the European Union. Works with national medicines regulatory bodies and aims to protect and promote the health of the citizens of European Member States (*see also* MEDICINES AND HEALTHCARE PRODUCTS REGULATORY AGENCY).

European Pressure Ulcer Advisory Panel (EPUAP) set up to find best evidence to prevent and treat pressure ulcers. Guidelines from EPUAP includes an international pressure ulcer classification system (*see* Table on pp. 316–318).

European Union Nursing Directives the EU directives seek to ensure that nurses and midwives from the member states of the EU receive similar educational programmes which meet defined standards to facilitate free movement of nursing personnel between the member states.

eustachian tube *B. Eustachio, Italian anatomist, 1520–1574.* The pharyngotympanic tube.

eustachitis inflammation of the eustachian tube.

euthanasia 1. an easy or good death. 2. the deliberate ending of the life of a person suffering from an incurable disease painlessly in order to relieve suffering. Euthanasia is illegal in the UK.

euthyroid having a normally functioning thyroid gland.

evacuant 1. promoting evacuation. 2. an agent that promotes evacuation.

evacuation 1. an emptying or removal, especially the removal of any material from the body by discharge through a natural or artificial passage. 2. material discharged from the body, especially the discharge from the bowels.

evacuator an instrument that produces evacuation, e.g., one designed to wash out small particles of stone from the bladder after lithotripsy.

evaluation a critical appraisal or assessment; a judgement of the value, worth, character or effectiveness of that which is being assessed. In the health care field this includes assessment of the patient's position on the health/illness continuum, and of the effectiveness of patient care activities in bringing about a change in the patient's position. Accepted as the last phase of the nursing process. All nurses must evaluate their care, to improve clinical decision making, quality and outcomes, using a range of methods and amending the plan of care if necessary.

eventration 1. the protrusion of the intestines through the abdominal wall. 2. removal of abdominal viscera.

eversion turning outwards. *E. of the eyelid* ectropion. The upper eyelid may be everted for examination of the eye or for the removal of a foreign body.

evidence-based practice systematically appraising clinical situations and then using up-to-date research findings as a basis for decisions by the nursing or other health-related professions. An approach to clinical practice first developed at McMaster University (Canada) which is based on the following four principles: (a) clinical and other health care decisions should be based on the best evidence available from patients and populations as well as from the laboratory; (b) the patient's problem determines the nature and source of evidence to be sought,

rather than habit, protocol or tradition; (c) identifying the best evidence calls for the integration of epidemiological and biostatistical ways of thinking with those derived from pathophysiology and clinical experience; (d) the conclusions of this search and critical appraisal of evidence are worthwhile only if they are translated into actions that affect patients.

evisceration removal of internal organs. *E. of the eye* removal of the contents of the eyeball, but not the sclera.

evolution the development of living organisms which change their characteristics during succeeding generations.

evulsion extraction by force.

Ewing's tumour *J. Ewing, American pathologist, 1866–1943.* A rare form of sarcoma usually affecting the shaft of a long bone in young adults.

exacerbation an increase in the severity of the symptoms of a disease.

exanthem an infectious disease characterized by a skin rash.

exanthematous pertaining to any disease associated with a skin eruption.

excavation scooping out. *Dental e.* the removal of decay from a tooth before inserting a filling.

exception in health care the justification for clinical variance made by a practitioner and usually peer-reviewed by others.

excision the cutting out of a part.

excitation the act of stimulating.

excitement a physiological and emotional response to a stimulus.

excoriation an abrasion of the skin.

excrement faecal matter; waste matter from the body.

excrescence abnormal outgrowth of tissue, e.g., a wart.

excreta the natural discharges of the excretory system: faeces, urine and sweat.

excretion the discharge of waste from the body.

exercise performance of physical exertion for improvement of health or correction of physical deformity. *Active e.* motion imparted to a part by voluntary contraction and relaxation of its controlling muscles. *Isometric e.* active exercise performed against stable resistance, without change in the length of the muscle. No movement occurs at any joints over which the muscle passes. *Passive e.* motion imparted to a segment of the body by another individual, or a machine or other outside force, or produced by voluntary effort of another segment of the patient's own body. *Range of movement (ROM) e's* exercises that move each joint through its full range of movement, that is, to the highest degree of movement of which each joint is normally capable.

exfoliation the splitting off from the surface of dead tissue in thin flaky layers.

exhalation 1. the giving off of a vapour. 2. the act of breathing out.

exhibitionism 1. showing off; a desire to attract attention. 2. exposing the genitals to others in socially unacceptable circumstances.

exocrine pertaining to those glands that discharge their secretion by means of a duct, e.g., salivary glands. *See* ENDOCRINE.

exogenous of external origin.

exomphalos 1. hernia of the abdominal viscera into the umbilical cord. 2. congenital umbilical hernia.

exophthalmometer an instrument for measuring the extent of protrusion of the eyeball.

exophthalmos abnormal protrusion of the eyeball which results in a marked stare. May be due to injury or disease and is often associated with thyrotoxicosis.

exostosis a bony outgrowth from the surface of a bone.

exotoxin a poison produced by a bacterial cell and released into the tissues surrounding it. *See* ENDOTOXIN.

exotropia divergent strabismus; the eyes turn outwards.

expected or estimated date of delivery abbreviated EDD. Used in midwifery and obstetrics to calculate the date of delivery of a baby. This is calculated by counting forwards 9 months and adding 7 days from the first day of the last normal menstrual period or counting back 3 months and adding 7 days.

expected outcome in a nursing care plan the rationale for a statement regarding a nursing intervention and what it is expected to achieve.

expectorant a remedy that promotes and facilitates expectoration.

expectoration sputum; secretions coughed up from the air passages. Its characteristics are a valuable aid in diagnosis and note should be taken of the quantity ejected, its colour and the amount of effort required. Frothiness denotes that it comes from an air-containing cavity; fluidity indicates oedema of the lung.

experiential learning learning from experiencing a situation. May also be facilitated with the use of role play or of a simulated situation and reflecting upon the experience.

expiration 1. the act of breathing out. 2. termination or death.

exploration the operation of surgically investigating any part of the body.

expression 1. the aspect or appearance of the face as determined by the physical or emotional state. 2. the act of squeezing out or evacuating by pressure, e.g., the removal of breast milk by hand or breast pump. 3. the manifestation of a heritable trait in an individual carrying the gene or genes that determine it.

exsanguination extensive blood loss due to internal or external haemorrhage.

extended family one that includes aunts, uncles, cousins and grandparents. *See* FAMILY.

extension 1. the straightening out of a flexed joint, such as the knee or elbow. 2. the application of traction to a fractured or dislocated limb by means of a weight.

extensor a muscle that extends or straightens a limb.

exterior on the outside.

exteriorize 1. to bring an organ or part of one to the outside of the body by surgery. 2. in psychiatry, to turn one's interests outwards.

extra- prefix denoting outside, additional or beyond.

extracapsular outside the capsule. May refer to a fracture occurring at the end of the bone but outside the joint capsule, or to cataract extraction.

extracellular outside the cell. *E. fluid* tissue fluid that surrounds the cells.

extracorporeal membrane oxygenation abbreviated ECMO. This is a life support procedure using an extracorporeal technique providing both cardiac and respiratory oxygen to patients whose heart and lungs are severely diseased or damaged. Blood is taken from the patient, directed through a machine (artificial kidney or 'heart-lung') for oxygenation and removal of carbon dioxide, and it is returned to the general circulation.

extraction 1. the process or act of pulling or drawing out. 2. the preparation of an extract. *Breech e.* extraction of an infant from the uterus in cases of breech presentation. *Vacuum e.* removal of the uterine contents by application of a vacuum. An alternative to the forceps method of delivering a baby.

extrapyramidal outside the pyramidal (cerebrospinal) tract. *E. system* the nerve tracts and pathways that are not within the pyramidal tracts.

extrasensory outside or beyond any of the known senses. *E. perception* abbreviated ESP. Appreciation of the thoughts of others or of current or future events without any normal means of communication.

extrasystole premature contraction of the atria or ventricles. *See* SYSTOLE.

extrauterine occurring outside the uterus. *E. pregnancy* ectopic gestation; development of a fetus outside the uterus.

extravasation effusion or escape of fluid from its normal course into surrounding tissues. *E. of blood* a bruise.

extremity distal part; a hand or foot.

extrinsic originating externally. *E. factor* a substance present in meat and other foodstuffs. Also called cyanocobalamin (vitamin B_{12}), it is necessary for the manufacture of red blood cells. The intrinsic factor produced in the stomach is necessary for the absorption of vitamin B_{12}. *E. muscle* a muscle originating away from the part that it controls, such as those controlling the movements of the eye.

extroversion turning inside out, e.g., of the uterus, as sometimes occurs after labour, or in psychology the turning of thoughts to the external environment.

extrovert a person who is sociable, a good mixer, outgoing and interested in what is going on in the social environment. A personality type first described by Jung. *See* INTROVERT.

extubation removal of a tube used in intubation.

exudation the slow discharge of serous fluid through the walls of the blood cells and its deposition in or on the tissues.

eye the organ of sight. A globular structure with three coats. The nerve tissue of the retina receives impressions of images via the pupil and lens. From this the optic nerve conveys the impressions to the visual area of the cerebrum (*see* Figure on p. 141). *E. contact* two people making direct contact in the vicinity of the other's eyes. Also called mutual gaze. Forms an important component of non-verbal communication in many cultures between people although the health care professional will need to be sensitive to the cultural background of the person as some cultures consider direct eye contact inappropriate. *E. strain* fatigue of the eye(s) from overuse and tiredness; often

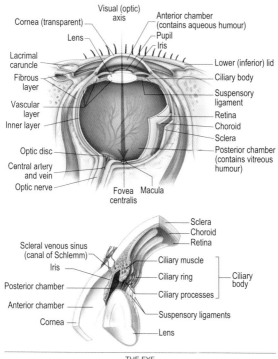

THE EYE

associated with headaches. May be due to poor lighting or an uncorrected defect in focusing.

eyelid a protective covering of the eye, composed of muscle and dense connective tissue covered with skin, lined with conjunctiva and fringed with eyelashes. Eyelids contain the Meibomian glands.

eye tooth an upper canine tooth.

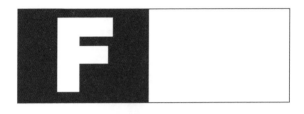

F symbol for *Fahrenheit* and *fluorine*.

fabricated or induced illness *see* MUNCHAUSEN SYNDROME and MUNCHAUSEN SYNDROME BY PROXY.

face the front of the head from the forehead to the chin. *F. lift* also known as rhytidectomy. Cosmetic surgery to lift and pull loose skin to remove wrinkles. *F. presentation* the appearance of the face of the fetus first at the cervix during labour.

facet a small flat area on the surface of a bone. *F. syndrome* a slight dislocation of the small facet joints of the vertebrae giving rise to pain and muscle spasm.

facial pertaining to the face or lower anterior portion of the head. *F. nerve* the seventh cranial nerve, which supplies the salivary glands and superficial face muscles. *F. paralysis see* PARALYSIS.

facies facial expression; it often gives some indication of the patient's condition. *Adenoid f.* the open mouth and vacant expression associated with mouth breathing and nasal obstruction. *Parkinson f.* fixed expression, due to paucity of movement of facial muscles, characteristic of Parkinsonism.

factor V Leiden *see* THROMBOPHILIA.

faeces waste matter excreted by the bowel, consisting of indigestible cellulose, food which has escaped digestion, bacteria (living and dead) and water.

Fahrenheit scale *G.D. Fahrenheit, German physicist, 1686–1736.* A scale of heat measurement. It registers the freezing point of water at 32°, the normal heat of the human body at 98.4°, and the boiling point of water at 212°. Symbol F. *See* CELSIUS.

failure inability to perform or to function properly. *F. to thrive* delay in normal growth and development in an infant. There are many causes but malnutrition or difficulty in absorbing essential nutrients is a main factor, as well as those that are psychosocial in origin, e.g., emotional deprivation. *Heart f.* inability of the heart to maintain a circulation sufficient to meet the body's needs. *Kidney f., renal f.* inability of the kidney to excrete metabolites at normal plasma levels under normal loading, or inability to retain electrolytes when intake is normal; in the acute form, marked by uraemia and usually by oliguria, with hyperkalaemia and pulmonary oedema. *Respiratory f., ventilatory f.* a life-threatening condition in which respiratory function is inadequate to maintain the body's needs for oxygen supply and carbon dioxide removal while at rest.

fainting *see* SYNCOPE.

faith healing an attempt to cure disease or disability with the use of spiritual powers or by the influence of the personality of the healer.

falciform sickle-shaped. *F. ligament* a fold of peritoneum which separates the two main lobes of the liver and connects it with the anterior abdominal wall and the diaphragm.

fall moving downwards quickly and without control. The tendency to fall to the ground increases with age when reflex actions are slower. Various conditions of the elderly, e.g., poor sight or walking disorders, increase the risk of falls as does the taking of sleeping pills or tranquillizer drugs. Broken bones are a common complication, most usually in women, who are more prone to osteoporosis. A fall or the fear of falling can have an adverse psychological effect on an elderly person, who may become reluctant to leave the home. Community care staff as falls specialist nurses or other practitioners can provide practical advice and support to prevent or minimize further falls, e.g., ensuring that floor coverings and wiring are made safe, suitable footwear is worn, good lighting is available and hand rails are secure and safe.

fallopian tube *G. Fallopius, Italian anatomist, 1523–1563.* Uterine tube. One of a pair of tubes, about 10–14 cm long, arising out of the upper part of the uterus. The distal end of each tube is fimbriated and lies near an ovary. The tubes' function is to conduct the ova from the ovaries to the interior of the uterus. An oviduct.

Fallot's tetralogy abbreviated TOF *E.L.A. Fallot, French physician, 1850–1911.* A congenital cyanotic heart disease with four characteristic defects: (a) pulmonary stenosis; (b) interventricular defect of the septum; (c) overriding of the aorta, i.e., opening into both right and left ventricles; (d) hypertrophy of the right ventricle.

falx a sickle-shaped structure. *F. cerebri* the fold of dura mater that separates the two cerebral hemispheres.

familial occurring in or affecting members of a family more than would be expected by chance.

family 1. a group of people who reside together and who may be related by blood or marriage, especially a husband, wife and their children. 2. a taxonomic category below

an order and above a genus. *Blended f.* a family unit composed of a couple and their offspring, including some from previous relationships. Also known as a reconstituted family. *Extended f.* a nuclear family and their close relatives, such as the children's grandparents, aunts and uncles. *Extended nuclear f.* a nuclear family who nevertheless make frequent social contacts with the extended family group despite geographical distance. *F. planning* the arrangement, spacing and limitation of the children in a family, depending upon the wishes and social circumstances of the parents. *F. centred care* a nursing approach to care and treatment of children which recognizes the needs of the family and their circumstances in the planning and delivery of services being provided for the child. *F. therapy* a therapeutic process whereby the psychotherapist uses family group therapy to resolve problems for one member of the family. *Nuclear f.* a couple and their children, by birth or adoption, who are living together and are more or less isolated from their extended family. *Single parent f.* a lone parent and offspring living together as a family unit.

Fanconi's syndrome *F. Fanconi, Swiss paediatrician, 1892–1979.* A rare inherited disorder of metabolism in which reabsorption of phosphate, amino acids and sugar by the renal tubules is impaired. The kidneys fail to produce acid urine, and resulting features are thirst, polyuria and rickets, leading to chronic renal failure.

fang the root of a tooth.

fantasy an imagined sequence of events or mental images that serves to satisfy unconscious wishes or to express unconscious conflicts.

farmer's lung extrinsic allergic alveolitis, a disease occurring in those in contact with mouldy hay. Due to a hypersensitivity pneumonitis, with widespread reaction in the lung tissue. It causes excessive breathlessness.

FAS fetal alcohol syndrome.

fascia a sheath of connective tissue enclosing muscles or other organs.

fasciculation isolated fine muscle twitching which gives a flickering appearance.

fasciculus a small bundle of nerve or muscle fibres; a fascicle.

fat 1. the adipose or fatty tissue of the body. 2. neutral fat; a triglyceride which is an ester of fatty acids and glycerol. *F. soluble vitamins* those vitamins that are soluble in fat, i.e., vitamins A, D, E and K. *Wool-f.* lanolin. *See also* BROWN FAT.

fatigue a state of weariness which may range from mental disinclination for effort to profound exhaustion after great physical and mental effort. *Muscle f.* may occur during prolonged effort owing to oxygen lack and accumulation of waste products.

fatty containing or similar to fat. *F. acid see* ESSENTIAL. *F. degeneration* a degenerative change in tissue cells due to the invasion of fat and consequent weakening of the organ. The change occurs as a result of incorrect diet, shortage of oxygen in the tissues or excessive consumption of alcohol. *F. liver disease* non-alcoholic fatty liver disease (NAFLD) includes a range of conditions caused by the build up of fat in the liver usually seen in obese people.

fauces the opening from the mouth into the pharynx. *Pillars of the f.* the two folds of muscle covered with mucous membrane that pass from the soft palate on either side of the fauces. One fold passes into the tongue, the other into the pharynx, and between them is situated the tonsil.

favism an acute haemolytic anaemia caused by ingestion of fava beans or inhalation of the pollen of the plant, usually occurring in certain individuals as a result of a genetic abnormality with a deficiency in an enzyme, glucose-6-phosphate dehydrogenase, in the erythrocytes. Called also fabism.

favus a type of ringworm infection rare in the UK, with formation of scabs, in appearance like a honeycomb. It usually affects the scalp and is due to a fungus infection (*Trichophyton schoenleinii*).

Fe symbol for iron.

fear a normal emotional response, in contrast to anxiety and phobia, to consciously recognized external sources of danger; it is manifested by alarm, apprehension or disquiet. *Obsessional f.* a recurring irrational fear that is not amenable to ordinary reassurance; a phobia.

febrile characterized by or relating to fever. *F. convulsion* a convulsion which occurs in early childhood and is associated with pyrexia. Also known as *F. seizures*.

fecundation fertilization.

fecundity the ability to produce offspring frequently. In demography, the physiological ability to reproduce, as opposed to fertility.

federations groups of general practices that formally work together to provide services for their practice populations.

feedback a method of homeostatic control where some of the output is returned as input for monitoring purposes. Feedback mechanisms are important in the regulation of such physiological processes as hormone and enzyme reactions. *F. treatment see* BIOFEEDBACK. *Negative f.* a rise in the output of a substance is detected and further output is thus inhibited. *Positive f.* a rise in output causes either a direct or indirect rise in the output of another substance.

Felty's syndrome *A.R. Felty, American physician, 1895–1963.* The triad of rheumatoid arthritis, splenomegaly and leukopenia. Often associated with anaemia, lymphadenopathy and vasculitic cutaneous ulceration.

female a person with two X chromosomes and normally having a vagina and uterus and the ability to reproduce after puberty. *F. genital mutilation*

(FMG) the cutting of female genitals carried out on young girls before puberty where there is no medical indication that this is necessary. It is also known as female circumcision. It is illegal in the UK.

feminization 1. the normal induction or development of female sexual characteristics. 2. the induction or development of female secondary sexual characteristics in the male. *Testicular f. syndrome* now called COMPLETE ANDROGEN INSENSITIVITY SYNDROME is a condition in which the subject is phenotypically female, but lacks nuclear sex chromatin and is of XY chromosomal sex.

femoral pertaining to the femur. *F. artery* that of the thigh from groin to knee. *F. canal* the opening below the inguinal ligament through which the femoral artery passes from the abdomen to the thigh.

femur the thigh bone.

fenestra a window-like opening. *F. ovalis* the oval opening between the middle and the internal ear.

ferritin a complex formed of an iron and protein molecule; one of the forms in which iron is stored in the body.

ferrous containing iron. *F. fumarate, f. gluconate, f. succinate* and *f. sulphate* are iron salts which are given orally to treat iron-deficiency anaemia.

ferrule a rubber cap used on the end of walking sticks, frames and crutches to prevent slipping.

fertilization the impregnation of the female sex cell, the ovum, by a male sex cell, a spermatozoon. *In vitro f.* artificial fertilization of the ovum in laboratory conditions. The timing and conditions for implantation into a uterus have to be perfect if successful pregnancy is to ensue.

fester to become superficially inflamed and to suppurate.

festination an involuntary tendency to take short accelerating steps in walking; seen in conditions such as Parkinson's disease.

fetal pertaining to the fetus. *F. alcohol syndrome* abbreviated FAS. Physical and mental abnormalities due to excessive maternal alcohol intake during pregnancy. Abnormalities may include microcephaly, growth deficiencies, learning disabilities, hyperactivity, heart murmurs, skeletal malformation and diminished growth. The exact amount of alcohol consumption that will produce fetal damage is unknown, but the periods of gestation during which the alcohol is most likely to result in fetal damage are 3–4.5 months after conception and during the last trimester. *F. assessment* determination of the wellbeing of the fetus. Assessment techniques and procedures include: (a) medical and family histories and physical examination of the mother; (b) ULTRASONOGRAPHY; (c) assessment of fetal activity with the mother recording fetal movements over a given period of time. Usually used in conjunction with other fetal wellbeing tests; (d) chemical assessment of placental function; (e) assays of amniotic fluid obtained by AMNIOCENTESIS; and (f) electronic and ultrasonic fetal heart rate monitoring. *F. distress* the clinical manifestation of fetal hypoxia which may be due to maternal or fetal causes. *F. position* a position resembling that of the fetus in the womb, sometimes adopted by a child or adult in a state of distress or depression.

fetishism a state in which an object is regarded with an irrational fear, or an erotic attraction which may be so strong that the object is necessary for achieving sexual excitement.

fetor an offensive smell.

fetoscope an endoscope for viewing the fetus in utero.

fetus the developing baby between the eighth week and the end of pregnancy.

fever 1. an abnormally high body temperature; pyrexia. 2. any disease characterized by marked increase of body temperature.

fibre a thread-like structure.

fibreoptics the transmission of light rays along flexible tubes by means of very fine glass or plastic fibres. Use is made of this in endoscopic instruments. In dentistry, commonly used as a light source attached to a handpiece.

fibrescope an endoscope in which fibreoptics are used.

fibrillation a quivering, vibratory movement of muscle fibres. *Atrial f.* rapid contractions of the atrium causing irregular contraction of the ventricles in both rhythm and force. *Ventricular f.* fine rapid twitchings of the ventricles leading to circulatory arrest. Rapidly fatal unless it can be controlled.

fibrin an insoluble protein that is essential to clotting of blood, formed from fibrinogen by action of thrombin.

fibrinogen a soluble protein which is present in blood plasma and is converted into fibrin by the action of thrombin when the blood clots.

fibrinolysin a proteolytic enzyme that dissolves fibrin.

fibrinolysis the dissolution of fibrin by the action of fibrinolysin. The process by which clots are removed from the circulation after healing has taken place.

fibrinopenia a deficiency of fibrinogen in the blood. There is a tendency to bleed as the coagulation time is increased.

fibroadenoma a benign tumour of glandular and fibrous tissue. *See* ADENOMA.

fibroangioma a benign tumour containing both fibrous and vascular tissue.

fibroblast a connective tissue cell.

fibrocartilage cartilage with fibrous tissue in it.

fibrochondritis inflammation of fibrocartilage.

fibrocystic disease of the pancreas an inherited disease. Cystic fibrosis, mucoviscidosis.

fibroid 1. having a fibrous structure. 2. a fibroma or a fibromyoma, usually one occurring in the uterus.

fibroma a benign tumour of connective tissue.

fibromyoma a tumour consisting of fibrous and muscle tissue; frequently found in or on the uterus.

fibroplasia the formation of fibrous tissue when a wound heals. *Retrolental f.* a condition characterized by the presence of fibrous tissue behind the lens, leading to detachment of the retina and blindness, attributed to use of excessively high concentrations of oxygen in the care of preterm infants. Now known as RETINOPATHY OF PREMATURITY.

fibrosarcoma a malignant tumour arising in fibrous tissue.

fibrosis fibrous tissue formation, such as occurs in scar tissue or as the result of inflammation. It is the cause of adhesions of the peritoneum or other serous membranes. *F. of the lung* condition that may precede bronchiectasis and emphysema.

fibrositis inflammation of fibrous tissue. The term is loosely applied to pain and stiffness, particularly of the back muscles, for which no other cause can be found.

fibula the slender bone from knee to ankle, on the outer side of the leg.

field of vision the area within view, as for the fixed eye or a camera, or in an operation.

fifth disease also known as slapped cheek syndrome or parvovirus; a mild but contagious viral infection that gives bright red cheeks which normally clears up without treatment. Most common in children.

fight or flight response activation of the sympathetic nervous system in response to danger or stress.

filament a small thread-like structure.

Filarioidea a genus of nematode worms which may be found in the connective tissues and lymphatics, having been transmitted to humans by mosquitoes. Found mainly in the tropics and subtropics.

filariasis an infection by filaria, particularly by *Wuchereria bancrofti*, resulting in blockage of the lymphatics, which causes swelling of the surrounding tissues. Elephantiasis may occur.

filiform thread-like. *F. papillae* the fine thread-like processes that cover the anterior two-thirds of the tongue.

filter a device for eliminating certain elements, such as (a) particles of a certain size from a solution, or (b) rays of a certain wavelength from a stream of radiant energy.

filtrate the fluid that passes through a filter.

filtration 1. the removal of precipitate from a liquid by means of a filter. 2. the removal of rays of a certain wavelength from an electromagnetic beam. *F. angle* the angle of the anterior chamber of the eye through which the aqueous humour drains; blockage of this channel gives rise to glaucoma.

fimbria a fringe. *F. of the uterine tube* the thread-like projections that surround the pelvic opening of the uterine tube.

finger a digit of the hand. *Clubbed f.* one with enlargement of the terminal phalanx with constant osseous changes; occurs in many heart and lung diseases. *F. spelling* SEE SIGN LANGUAGE. *Hammer f., mallet f.* permanent flexion of the distal phalanx of a finger due to avulsion of the extensor tendon. *Trigger f.* temporary flexion of a finger which is overcome in a sudden jerk by active or passive extension of the finger. It is caused by thickening of the flexor tendon in a narrowed tendon sheath. *Webbed f's* fingers more or less united by strands of tissue; syndactyly.

fingerprint the impression left upon a surface of the ridged pattern of the skin of the fingertips. Loops, whorls, arches and combinations of these form distinct patterns for each human individual and not even identical twins have the same fingerprint pattern.

first aid emergency care and treatment of an injured person before complete medical and surgical treatment can be secured. *See* Appendix 3.

fission a form of asexual reproduction by dividing into two equal parts, as in bacteria. *Binary f.* the splitting in two of the nucleus and the protoplasm of a cell, as in protozoa. *Nuclear f.* the splitting of the nucleus of an atom, with the release of a great quantity of energy.

fissure a narrow slit or cleft. *Anal f.* a painful crack in the mucous membrane of the anus. *F. of Rolando* a furrow in the cortex of each cerebral hemisphere, dividing the sensory from the motor area; the central sulcus.

fistula an abnormal passage between two epithelial surfaces, usually connecting the cavity of one organ with another or a cavity with the surface of the body. *Anal f.* the result of an ischiorectal abscess where the channel is from the anus to the skin. *Biliary f.* a leakage of bile to the exterior, following operation on the gallbladder or ducts. *Blind f.* one which is open at only one end. *Faecal f.* one in which the channel is from the intestine through the wound caused by an operation on the intestines when sepsis is present. *Rectovaginal f.* fistula from the rectum to the vagina which may result from a severe perineal tear during childbirth. *Tracheo-oesophageal f.* an opening from the trachea into the oesophagus; a congenital deformity. *Vesicovaginal f.* an opening from the bladder to the vagina, either from error during operation or from ulceration, as may occur in carcinoma of the cervix.

fit a commonly used term for paroxysmal motor discharges leading to sudden convulsive movements, as in epilepsy, eclampsia and hysteria. *F. note* a statement of fitness to work issued by medical practitioners.

fitness associated with a sense of well-being, and the ability to undertake sustained physical exertion without undue breathlessness. Fitness needs to be maintained on a regular basis by the person taking regular physical exertion or exercise.

fixation 1. the process of rendering something immovable, such as a joint or a fractured bone. 2. in psychology, a term used to describe a failure to progress wholly or in part through the normal stages of psychological development to a fully developed personality. 3. in optics, directing the sight straight at an object.

flaccid soft, flabby. *F. paralysis see* PARALYSIS.

flail exhibiting abnormal or pathological mobility. *F. chest* a loss of stability of the chest wall due to multiple rib fractures or detachment of the sternum from the ribs as a result of a severe crushing chest injury. The loose chest segment moves in a direction that is the reverse of normal. *F. joint* an unusually movable joint.

flap a mass of tissue, used for grafting in plastic surgery, which is left attached to its blood supply and used to repair defects either adjacent to it or at some distance from it.

flare the response of the skin to an allergic or hypersensitivity reaction. Reddening of the skin that spreads outwards.

flatfoot a condition due to absence or sinking of the medial longitudinal arch of the foot, caused by weakening of the ligaments and tendons.

flatulence excessive formation of gases in the stomach or intestine.

flatulent suffering from flatulence. *F. distension* swelling due to gas in the stomach or intestines. It is a common complication after abdominal operations and is caused by intestinal stasis.

flatus gas in the stomach or intestine.

flea a small, wingless blood-sucking insect parasite. The common human flea, *Pulex irritans,* rarely transmits disease. Cat and dog fleas, *Ctenocephalides,* are also relatively harmless. The rat fleas *Xenopsylla* and *Nosopsyllus* are the vectors of bubonic plague.

flexion bending; moving a joint so that the two or more bones forming it draw towards each other. *Plantar f.* bending the fingers or toes downwards.

Flexner's bacillus *S. Flexner, American bacteriologist, 1863–1946.* One of the group of pathogenic bacteria which cause bacillary dysentery; *Shigella flexneri.*

flexor any muscle causing flexion of a limb or other part of the body.

flexure a bend or curve.

flight of ideas the rapid movement of ideas and speech from one fragmentary topic to another that occurs in mania.

floaters wisps or strands within the eye that are visible to the patient. Usually caused by detachment and collapse of the vitreous humour and the normal ageing process.

flooding 1. excessive loss of blood from the uterus. 2. a form of desensitization for the treatment of phobias and related disorders. The patient is repeatedly exposed, in imagination or real life, to emotionally distressing aversive stimuli of high intensity. Also called exposure therapy.

florid having a flushed facial appearance.

flowmeter an instrument used to measure the flow of liquids or gases.

fluctuation a wave-like motion felt on palpation of the abdomen.

fluid 1. a liquid or gas; any liquid of the body. 2. composed of molecules which freely change their relative positions without separation of the mass. *Amniotic f.* the fluid within the amnion that bathes the developing fetus and protects it from mechanical injury. *Body f's* the fluids within the body, composed of water, electrolytes and non-electrolytes. The volume and distribution of body fluids vary with age, sex and amount of adipose tissue. *Cerebrospinal f.* the fluid contained within the ventricles of the brain, the subarachnoid space and the central canal of the spinal cord. *Extracellular f.* fluid outside the cell, constituting one-third of the total body fluid. *F. chart* a chart used to record the daily intake and output of fluids for a patient. The amount of intake and output is usually totalled every 24 hours. The chart provides a crude indicator for the patient's fluid balance status. *Interstitial f.* the extracellular fluid bathing most tissues, excluding the fluid within the lymph and blood vessels. *Intracellular f.* fluid within the cell, constituting two-thirds of the total body fluid.

fluid balance a state in which the volume of body water and its solutes (electrolytes and non-electrolytes) is within normal limits and there is normal distribution of fluids within the intracellular and extracellular compartments. The total volume of body fluids should be about 60% of the body weight.

fluke one of a group of parasitic flatworms (Trematoda). Different varieties may affect the blood, the intestines, the liver and the lungs.

fluorescein a dye used to detect corneal ulceration. When it is dropped on the eye the ulcer stains green.

fluorescence the property of reflecting back light waves, usually of a lower frequency than those absorbed so that invisible light (e.g., ultraviolet) may become visible.

fluorescent capable of producing fluorescence. *F. screen* a screen that becomes fluorescent when exposed to X-rays. *F. treponemal antibody test* a serological test for syphilis; the first to become positive after infection.

fluoridation the adding of fluorine to water, in those areas where it is lacking, in order to reduce the incidence of dental caries. Fluorine may also be added to tooth paste as a caries preventative.

fluorine symbol F.

fluoroscope an instrument for the study of moving internal organs and contrast medium using X-rays.

flush a redness of the face and neck. *Hectic f.* one occurring in conditions such as septic poisoning and pulmonary tuberculosis. *Hot f.* one occurring during the menopause, accompanied by a feeling of heat.

flutter an irregularity of the heart beat.

focus 1. the point of convergence of light or sound waves. 2. the local seat of a disease. *F. group* small group led by a leader, with the aim of generating data on a designated topic through discussion and interaction. A research technique.

focusing the ability of the eye to alter its lens power to focus correctly at different distances.

folic acid one of the VITAMINS of the B complex. Folic acid is involved in the synthesis of amino acids and DNA; its deficiency causes megaloblastic anaemia. Green vegetables, liver and yeast are major sources. *F. a. antagonist* any antimetabolite cytotoxic drug that inhibits the action of the folic acid enzyme.

folie à deux [Fr.] the occurrence of identical psychoses simultaneously in two closely associated persons.

follicle a very small sac or gland. *Hair f.* the sheath in which a hair grows. *F.-stimulating hormone* abbreviated FSH. A hormone, produced by the anterior pituitary gland, which controls the maturation of the GRAAFIAN FOLLICLES in the ovary.

follicular pertaining to a follicle. *F. conjunctivitis* inflammation occurring in the lower conjunctival fornix. *F. tonsillitis* tonsillitis arising from infection of the tonsillar follicles.

folliculosis an abnormal increase in the number of lymph follicles. *Conjunctival f.* a benign non-inflammatory overgrowth of follicles of the conjunctiva of the eyelids.

fomentation treatment by warm, moist applications; also, the substance thus applied.

fomites inanimate objects or material on which disease-producing agents may be conveyed.

fontanelle a soft membranous space between the cranial bones of an infant (see Figure). *Anterior f.* that between the parietal and frontal bones, which closes at about the age of 18 months. Rickets causes delay in this process. *Posterior f.* the junction of the occipital and parietal bones, at the sagittal suture, which closes within 3 months of birth.

food anything which, when taken into the body, serves to nourish or build up

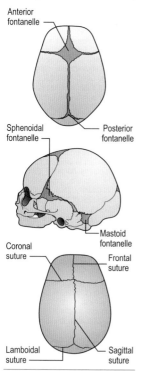

Anterior fontanelle

Sphenoidal fontanelle — Posterior fontanelle

Mastoid fontanelle

Coronal suture

Frontal suture

Lambdoidal suture — Sagittal suture

THE FONTANELLES

the tissues or to supply body heat. *F. additives see* ADDITIVES. *F. allergy* sensitivity to one or more of the components of a normal diet, e.g., peanuts, cow's milk or eggs. The reaction to the allergen usually occurs within a short period of ingesting the trigger food and includes lip swelling, vomiting, abdominal distension and diarrhoea. Serious allergies can cause anaphylactic shock requiring a self-administered injection of adrenalin. The only effective treatment is total avoidance of the offending food. *See* ANAPHYLAXIS. *F. intolerance* an adverse reaction to a food or to a specific food ingredient that occurs each time the substance is ingested that is not due to food poisoning or involves the immune system. The specific cause of food intolerance may be difficult to trace, others are more recognizable, e.g., lactose intolerance is due to a genetic deficiency of the enzyme lactase needed for the digestion of lactose in milk. *F. poisoning* a group of notifiable acute illnesses caused by ingestion of contaminated food. It may result from toxaemia from foods, such as those inherently poisonous or those contaminated by poisons, foods containing poisons formed by bacteria, or food-borne infections. Food poisoning usually causes inflammation of the gastrointestinal tract (gastroenteritis). This may occur quite suddenly, soon after the food has been eaten. The symptoms are acute, and include tenderness, pain or cramps in the abdomen, nausea, vomiting, diarrhoea, weakness and dizziness. *See* BOTULISM.

Food Standards Agency organization charged with protecting health in relation to food, with powers to act throughout the food chain to develop policies. Advises consumers, ministers and the food industry on all aspects of food safety and standards. In Scotland this function is carried out by Food Standards Scotland.

foot the terminal part of the lower limb. *Athlete's f.* ringworm of the foot; tinea pedis. *F. drop* inability to keep the foot at the correct angle owing to paralysis of the flexors of the ankle. *F. presentation* the presentation of one or both legs instead of the head during labour.

foramen an opening or hole, especially in a bone. *F. magnum* the hole in the occipital bone through which the spinal cord passes. *F. ovale* the hole between the left and right atria in the fetus. *Obturator f.* the large hole in the innominate bone. *Optic f.* the opening in the posterior part of the orbit through which the optic nerve and the ophthalmic artery pass.

forceps surgical instruments with two opposing blades used for lifting or compressing an object. *Artery f. (Spencer Wells f.)* compress bleeding points during an operation. *Cheatle f.* long forceps for lifting utensils. *Obstetric f.* various patterns are used in difficult labour to facilitate delivery. *Vulsellum f.* have claw-like ends for exerting traction.

forensic pertaining to or applied in legal proceedings. *F. medicine* the branch that is concerned with the law and has a bearing on legal problems. It includes the investigation of unexplained death or injury. *F. psychiatry* the consideration of current mental health laws and their relationship to mental health care and the consideration of issues such as diminished responsibility and fitness to stand trial. Mental health nurses work closely with the justice system and courts for offenders with mental health problems.

foreskin the prepuce.

forgetfulness the inability to remember or recall events, appointments, objects, etc. that make for daily life. Failure to retrieve memories may occur as a normal result of inattention although it is a common difficulty that develops with increasing age. In the elderly worsening forgetfulness may be associated with the development of dementia.

formaldehyde a gaseous compound with strongly disinfectant properties. It is used in solution for disinfection of excreta and utensils and also in the preparation of toxoids from toxins.

formula 1. an expression, using numbers or symbols, of the composition of, or of directions for preparing, a compound, such as a medicine; or of a procedure to follow to obtain a desired result; or of a single concept. 2. a mixture for feeding an infant, composed of milk and/or other ingredients.

formulary a prescriber's handbook of drugs. *See* BRITISH NATIONAL FORMULARY (BNF) and NURSE PRESCRIBERS' FORMULARY (NPF).

fornix an arch. *Conjunctival f.* the reflection of the conjunctiva from the eyelids on to the eyeball. *F. cerebri* an arched structure at the back and base of the brain. *F. of the vagina* the recesses at the top of the vagina in front (anterior f.), back (posterior f.) and sides (lateral f.) of the cervix uteri.

fossa a small depression or pit. Usually applied to fossae in bones. *Cubital f.* the triangular depression at the front of the elbow. *Iliac f.* the depression on the inner surface of the iliac bone. *Pituitary f.* the depression in the sphenoid bone. *See* SELLA TURCICA.

foster children children in the care of foster parents as a short- or long-term measure. The objective is to provide the child with the security of a home environment and to reunite the child with their own natural family as soon as possible.

foster parents persons who undertake for reward the care of children who are not related to them within the meaning of the Children Act (1989) and the Children and Families Act (2014).

Fothergill's operation *W.E. Fothergill, British gynaecologist, 1865–1926.* Amputation of the cervix, with anterior and posterior colporrhaphy for prolapse of the uterus. Also known as the MANCHESTER OPERATION.

foundation doctor junior doctors in their first two years following graduation from medical school. Abbreviated to F1 for first-year foundation doctors and F2 for second-year doctors.

Foundation NHS Trusts Foundation Trusts are subject to the same standards, performance ratings and systems of inspection as other NHS organizations, although they are free from the direction of the Secretary of State for Health. NHS foundation trusts are not-for-profit, public benefit corporations. They are part of the NHS and currently provide over half of all NHS hospital, mental health and ambulance services in England and Wales. NHS foundation trusts were created to devolve decision making from central government to local organizations and communities. They provide and produce health care according to core NHS principles—free care based on need and not the ability to pay. The foundation trusts are accountable to their local communities through their members and governors, their commissioners through contracts and also to Parliament and the Care Quality Commission through the legal requirement to register and to meet the required standards of the care provided. Monitor, now part of NHS IMPROVEMENT, is the independent regulator. Anyone who lives in the area which the foundation trust serves or who works for a foundation trust, or has been a patient or service user can become a member of the trust.

fourchette [Fr.] the fold of membrane at the perineal end of the vulva.

fovea a fossa; a small depression, particularly that of the retina which contains a large number of cones, giving form and colour, and is therefore the area of most accurate vision.

fracture 1. to break a part, especially a bone. 2. a break in the continuity of bone. The signs and symptoms are pain, swelling, deformity, shortening of the limb, loss of power, abnormal mobility, and crepitus. Fractures are generally caused by trauma, by either a direct or an indirect force on the bone. Fractures may also be caused by muscle spasm or by disease that results in decalcification of the bone. The different types and classification of fractures are shown in the figure. *March f.* a hairline crack in the long bone of the foot caused by repeated trauma associated with long marches and with jogging. Also known as fatigue or stress fracture. *Pathological f.* one due to weakening of the bone structure by pathological processes, such as neoplasia, osteomalacia or osteomyelitis. *Pott's f.* a fracture dislocation of the ankle involving the lower end of the fibula and sometimes the internal malleolus of the tibia. *Spontaneous f.* one that occurs as a result of little or no violence, usually of a bone weakened by disease.

frailty a distinctive health state related to the ageing process in which multiple body systems gradually become diminished. *F. score* the assessment of people who are frail to quantify their level of frailty in order to provide a consistent approach to management.

frame a rigid supporting structure or a structure for immobilizing a part. *Braun f.* a metal frame used to elevate the lower limb in fractures of the tibia and fibula. *Quadriplegic standing f.* a device for supporting in the upright position a patient whose four limbs are paralysed. *Stryker f.* one consisting of canvas stretched on anterior and posterior frames, on which the patient can be rotated around the longitudinal axis. *Walking f.* a walking aid with three or four legs.

freckle a brown pigmented spot on the skin. *Hutchinson's melanotic f.* a non-invasive malignant melanoma which occurs mainly on the faces of middle-aged women.

free association in psychoanalysis a spontaneous mental process whereby words used in a non-logical chain

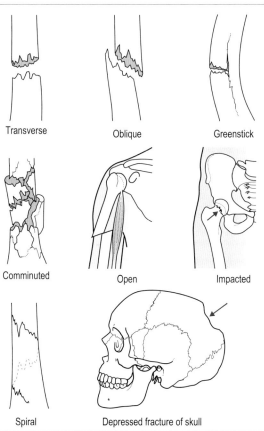

FRACTURES OF BONE

suggest ideas, thoughts or feelings without selection or repression.

free-floating anxiety generalized and pervasive anxiety with no link to a specific situation or object creating a feeling of unease and dread for the patient.

Freedom of Information Act all NHS organizations are required to have a publication scheme which sets out the type of information that it publishes or intends to publish, the form in which the information is published and details of any changes. NHS organizations must answer requests for information within the terms of the individual right of access given by the Act. This applies to all types of recorded information held by the organization regardless of its date, although the Act does include some specific exemptions.

Freiberg's disease *A.H. Freiberg, American surgeon, 1868–1940.* Osteochondritis of the second metatarsal bone, in which there is pain on walking and standing.

frenotomy the cutting of the frenulum of the tongue to cure tongue-tie.

frenulum frenum; a fold of mucous membrane which limits the movement of an organ. *F. of the tongue* the fold under the tongue.

Freudian *S. Freud, Austrian psychiatrist, 1856–1939.* Relating to the theories of Freud, who was the originator of psychoanalysis and the psychoanalytical theory of the cause of neurosis.

friable easily crumbled or torn.

friction the act of rubbing one object against another. *F. massage* a circular or transverse pressure applied by fingertip or thumb to a localized area. Used for the relief of pain. *F. murmur* the grating sound heard in auscultation when two rough surfaces rub together, as in dry pleurisy.

Friedländer's bacillus *K. Friedländer, German pathologist, 1847–1887.* The cause of a rare form of pneumonia. *Klebsiella friedländeri.*

Friedreich's ataxia or disease *N. Friedreich, German physician, 1825–1882.* A rare form of hereditary ataxia.

friends and family test gives patients opportunity through the completion of a short questionnaire to provide feedback on services they have used. Services receive this feedback and can take actions in real-time to address feedback.

frigidity an absence of normal sexual desire; usually refers to women.

Fröhlich's syndrome *A. Fröhlich, Austrian neurologist, 1871–1953.* A group of symptoms associated with disease of the pituitary body: increased adiposity, atrophy of the genital organs, and development of feminine characteristics. Also known as ADIPOSOGENITAL DYSTROPHY.

frontal 1. relating to the forehead. 2. relating to the front or anterior aspect of a structure.

frostbite impairment of circulation, chiefly affecting the fingers, the toes, the nose and the ears, due to exposure to severe cold. The first stage is represented by chilblains. Advanced cases show thrombosis and dry gangrene.

frottage [Fr.] 1. a rubbing movement in massage. 2. sexual gratification by rubbing against another person's body.

frozen shoulder a stiff and painful shoulder; adhesive capsulitis. Treatment may include stretching under anaesthesia, combined with exercises and pain relief. The cause is unknown.

frozen watchfulness the state of a young child who is unresponsive to its surroundings, but is clearly aware of them. The state of frozen watchfulness is usually a marker of child abuse.

fructose fruit sugar, a monosaccharide.

FSH follicle-stimulating hormone.

fugue a period of altered awareness during which a person may wander for hours or days and perform purposive actions although memory for the period may be lost. It may follow an epileptic fit or occur in hysteria or schizophrenia.

fulguration the destruction of tissue by diathermy.

fulminating sudden in onset and rapid in course.

fumigation disinfection by exposure to the fumes of a vaporized germicide.

function 1. the natural action or intended purpose of a person, organ or structure. 2. to perform special work or an action.

fundus the base of an organ or the part farthest removed from the opening. *F. of the eye* the posterior part of the inside of the eye as shown by the ophthalmoscope. *F. of the stomach* that part above the cardiac orifice. *F. of the uterus* the top of the uterus; that part farthest from the cervix.

fungal nail infection infection affecting the finger nail, toe nail or nail bed. It is not usually serious but can be difficult to treat and nails can become thickened and unsightly. Also known as ONYCHOMYCOSIS.

fungate to grow rapidly and produce fungus-like growths. Often occurs in the late stages of malignant tumours.

fungicide a preparation that destroys fungal infection.

fungiform shaped like a fungus or mushroom.

fungus a member of the group of eukaryotic organisms that include microorganisms, such as yeast and moulds. Some varieties cause diseases, such as otomycosis or ear fungus, and candidiasis, commonly known as thrush.

funnel chest a developmental deformity in which there is a depression in the sternum and an inward curvature of the ribs and costal cartilages.

furor a state of intense excitement during which violent acts may be performed. This may occur after an epileptic fit.

furuncle a boil.

furunculosis a staphylococcal infection represented by many, or crops of, boils.

furunculus a furuncle. *F. orientalis* a protozoal infection, mainly of the tropics, which causes a chronic ulceration. Cutaneous leishmaniasis.

fusiform shaped like a spindle.

fusion 1. the union between two adjacent structures. 2. the coordination of separate images of the same object in the two eyes into one image.

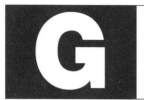

g symbol for *gram*.

G symbol for *guanine*.

Ga symbol for *gallium*.

gag 1. an instrument placed between the teeth to keep the mouth open. 2. the reflex action that occurs when the back of the throat is stimulated.

gait manner of walking. *Ataxic g.* the foot is raised high, descends suddenly, and the whole sole strikes the ground. *Cerebellar g.* a staggering walk indicative of cerebellar disease. *Four-point g.* a method which may be adopted when using sticks or crutches, which allows maximum stability. *Spastic g.* stiff, shuffling walk, the legs being kept together.

galactorrhoea 1. an excessive flow of milk. 2. secretion of milk after breast feeding has ceased.

galactosaemia an inborn error of metabolism in which there is inability to convert galactose to glucose. The rare genetic disorder becomes manifest soon after birth and is characterized by feeding problems, vomiting, diarrhoea, abdominal distension, enlargement of the liver and learning disabilities. Treatment consists of exclusion from the diet of milk and all foods containing galactose or lactose. It is particularly prevalent within the Irish traveller population.

galactose a monosaccharide derived from lactose. D-Galactose is found in lactose or milk, sugar and cerebrosides of the brain. *G. tolerance test* a laboratory test to determine the liver's ability to convert the sugar galactose into glycogen.

gallbladder the sac under the lower surface of the liver, which acts as a reservoir for bile. (*See* Figure on p. 227.)

gallium *symbol* Ga. A radioisotope of gallium used in detecting some soft-tissue disorders.

gallium scan a radioactive isotope of gallium may be administered intravenously in a total body scan to detect metastatic spread, lymphomas, or a focus of infection.

gallop rhythm heart rhythm that may occur when there is ventricular overload.

gallstone a concretion formed in the gallbladder or bile ducts. Gallstones vary in size and may be multiple and faceted. *G. colic see* BILIARY (COLIC).

gamete a sex cell which combines with another to form a zygote, from which a complete organism develops. A spermatozoon or an ovum.

gamete intrafallopian transfer abbreviated GIFT. A technique for assisting conception. The woman must have at least one patent fallopian tube. Oocytes and spermatozoa are mixed in the laboratory and introduced into a fallopian tube, and the fertilized egg may then become embedded in the uterus. The GIFT procedure is used less nowadays with current advances in in vitro fertilization techniques.

gametocyte a cell that is undergoing gametogenesis.

gametogenesis the production of the gametes by the gonads.

gamma the third letter in the Greek alphabet. *G. camera* an apparatus for depicting a part of the body into which radioactive isotopes emitting gamma rays have been introduced. *G. encephalography* a method of localizing a brain tumour by using radioactive isotopes emitting gamma rays. *G.-globulin* a class of plasma proteins composed almost entirely of IgG, an IMMUNOGLOBULIN protein that contains most antibody activity. *G. rays* electromagnetic rays, of shorter wavelength and with greater penetration than X-rays, which are given off by certain radioactive substances and which are used in radiotherapy. Also used in the sterilization of articles that would be destroyed by the heat and moisture required in autoclaving.

ganglion 1. a collection of nerve cells and fibres, forming an independent nerve centre, as is found in the sympathetic nervous system. 2. a cystic swelling on a tendon.

ganglionectomy excision of a ganglion.

gangrene death of body tissue, generally in considerable mass, due either to loss of blood supply or to the effects of certain infections. *Dry g.* occurs gradually and results from slow reduction of the blood flow in the arteries. There is no subsequent bacterial decomposition; the tissues become dry and shrivelled. It occurs only in the extremities, and can occur with ARTERIOSCLEROSIS and DIABETES (MELLITUS). *Gas g.* a serious wound infection resulting from wounds/lacerations infected by anaerobic bacteria, especially species of *Clostridium*, a soil microbe often found in the intestines of humans and animals. It is an acute, severe, painful condition in which muscles and subcutaneous tissues become filled with gas and a serosanguineous exudate.

Fatal without appropriate antibiotics and supportive therapy. *Moist g.* caused by sudden stoppage of blood, resulting from burning by heat or acid, severe freezing, physical accident that destroys the tissue, or a clot or other embolism. At first, tissue affected by moist gangrene has the colour of a bad bruise, and is swollen and often blistered. The gangrene is likely to spread with great speed. Toxins are formed in the affected tissues and absorbed.

Ganser's syndrome (state) *S.J.M. Ganser, German psychiatrist, 1853–1931.* Amnesia, disturbance of consciousness and hallucinations, associated with senseless answers to questions, and absurd acts. Usually a transient response to a troublesome situation, e.g., prisoners on remand (prison psychosis).

gargle 1. a solution for rinsing the mouth and throat. 2. to rinse the mouth and throat by holding a solution in the open mouth and agitating it by expulsion of air from the lungs.

gargoylism *see* HURLER'S SYNDROME.

gas molecules of a substance very loosely combined; a vapour. A gas does not keep shape or volume on being released. *G. and air analgesia* an authorized form of analgesia using nitrous oxide and air, by which the pains of labour are lessened without affecting uterine contractions. *Laughing g.* nitrous oxide. *Marsh g.* methane. *Sternutatory g.* one that causes sneezing. *Tear g.* one that is irritating to the eyes and causes excessive lacrimation.

Gasser's ganglion *J.L. Gasser, Austrian anatomist, 1723–1765.* The trigeminal ganglion. The ganglion of the sensory root of the fifth cranial nerve.

gastrectomy excision of part or whole of the stomach used in the treatment of stomach cancer and perforation of the stomach wall. Gastrectomy was previously performed frequently for the treatment of PEPTIC ULCERS but with advances in medication are only performed in severe cases. *Sleeve g.* used to treat people with potentially life-threatening obesity. Surgery reduces the stomach size buy up to 75% resulting in an inability to eat large amounts of food, and subsequently resulting in weight loss.

gastric pertaining to the stomach. *G. analysis* analysis of the stomach contents by microscopy and tests to determine the amount of acid present. *G. band* a silicone band placed around the top portion of the stomach reducing the need to eat as much food to feel full. Also known as a lap band or LAGB (laparoscopic adjustable gastric band). Used in the treatment of obesity. *G. bypass* surgical creation of a small gastric pouch that empties directly into the jejunum through a gastrojejunostomy, thereby causing food to bypass the duodenum; performed for the treatment of morbid OBESITY. *G. flu* a popular term for what may be any of several disorders of the stomach and intestinal tract. The symptoms are nausea, diarrhoea, abdominal cramps and fever. *G. juice* the clear fluid secreted by the glands of the stomach to assist digestion. It contains an enzyme called pepsin, which acts upon proteins in the presence of weak hydrochloric acid. *G. lavage* a treatment for some types of poisoning where the stomach contents are washed out through a stomach tube. *G. ulcer* ulceration of the gastric mucosa, associated with hyperacidity and often precipitated by *Helicobacter pylori* organisms. The condition is often aggravated by stress.

gastrin a hormone, secreted by the walls of the stomach, which excites continued secretion of digestive juice while food is in the stomach.

gastritis inflammation of the lining of the stomach.

gastro-oesophagostomy a surgical anastomosis between the stomach and the oesophagus.

gastrocnemius the principal muscle of the calf of the leg. It flexes both the ankle and the knee.

gastrocolic pertaining to the stomach and colon. *G. reflex* after a meal, increased peristalsis causes the colon to empty into the rectum. This gives rise to a desire to defecate.

gastroduodenostomy a surgical anastomosis between the stomach and the duodenum.

gastroenteritis inflammation of the stomach and intestines causing episodes of nausea, vomiting, appetite loss, fever, abdominal pain and diarrhoea. A mild episode usually only lasts a few days but a severe one may cause dehydration, shock and collapse especially in children and the elderly. The illness may be caused by any one of a number of organisms: bacteria, bacterial toxins, viruses and other organisms in food and water.

gastroenterology the study of diseases of the gastrointestinal tract.

gastroenterostomy a surgical anastomosis between the stomach and small intestine.

gastroileac pertaining to the stomach and ileum. *G. reflex* food entering the stomach sets up powerful peristalsis in the ileum and opening of the ileocaecal valve.

gastrointestinal pertaining to the stomach and intestine. *G. tract* the alimentary tract.

gastrojejunostomy a surgical anastomosis between the stomach and the jejunum. gastroparesis a long term condition where the stomach cannot empty properly, caused by damage to nerves and muscle.

gastroscope a fibre optic endoscope especially designed for passage into the stomach to permit examination of its interior.

gastrostomy the creation of an opening into the stomach. This procedure is done to provide for the administration of food and liquids when stricture of the oesophagus or other conditions make swallowing impossible. *See* ARTIFICIAL (FEEDING).

gastrotomy a surgical incision of the stomach.

gastrula an early stage in the development of the fertilized ovum.

gate control theory of pain theory proposing that a neural mechanism in the dorsal horns of the spinal cord acts like a gate which can increase or decrease the flow of nerve impulses from peripheral fibres to the central nervous system. It is the position of the gate that determines how much information is transmitted to the brain and therefore the amount of pain generated. Influences such as anxiety and anticipation cause the gate to open and therefore increase the level of pain experienced, whereas other factors may cause the gate to close, thereby reducing the pain.

gatekeepers the individuals or groups in an organization who regulate access to goods and services.

gateway drug generic name for alcohol, cocaine or cannabis referring to their supposed roles as conduits leading on to the taking of harder drugs.

Gaucher's disease *P.C.E. Gaucher, French physician, 1854–1918.* A rare familial disease in which fat is deposited in the reticuloendothelial cells, causing an enlarged spleen and anaemia.

gauze a thin open-meshed material used for dressing wounds.

gavage [Fr.] forced feeding; the giving of fluids and nourishment by oesophageal or other type of tube directly into the stomach.

gay popular term for a homosexual, usually male.

Geiger counter *H. Geiger, German physicist, 1882–1945.* An instrument for detecting and registering radioactivity. The apparatus is sensitive to the rays emitted.

gelatin an albuminoid, obtained from connective tissue or bone. Used in pharmacy for suppositories and capsules, and in bacteriology as a culture medium. In absorbable film and sponge, it is used in surgical procedures.

gender the perceived differences between the two sexes that generate social differentiation, inequality, discrimination and prejudice. Gender refers to the socially constructed characteristics of men and women. *G. identity* the concept or inner feeling that a person has of being male and masculine or female and feminine. Differentiation of gender identity begins in infancy, continuing through childhood, and reinforced in adolescence. This parental attitudes and expectations as well as psychological and social pressures. *G. identity disorder* also known as gender dysmorphia and gender dysphoria a term used for those disorders marked by a persistent sense of a mismatch between one's experienced gender and assigned gender.

gene one of the biological units of heredity, self-reproducing and located at a definite position (locus) on a particular chromosome. *Dominant g.* one that is capable of transmitting its characteristics irrespective of the genes from the other parent. *G. therapy* the use of 'healthy' genes, the process being known as somatic-gene cell therapy, to cure or treat a hereditary disease. *Recessive g.* one that can pass on its characteristics only if it is present with a similar recessive gene from the other parent. *See* MENDEL'S THEORY. General anaesthesia a drug that brings about a reversible loss of consciousness.

General Medical Council abbreviated GMC. The regulating body of all medical practitioners within the UK. It licenses doctors to practise and is charged with: (a) keeping the register of practising doctors up to date; (b) fostering good medical practice; (c) promoting high standards in medical education; and (d) dealing firmly and fairly with doctors whose fitness for practice is in doubt.

general practitioner abbreviated GP. The role of the general practitioner or primary care physician in the UK is unique. Besides being the first point of contact for most patients, GPs must offer the first treatment or referral for all problems which are presented to them. In addition, GPs give personal and continuing care to their patients and families, often over the course of many years.

generalised anxiety disorder (GAD) a long term condition causing anxiety to a range of situations and issues. Feelings of anxiety are constant and can affect daily living.

generic 1. pertaining to a genus. 2. non-proprietary, relating to a drug name not protected by a trademark, usually descriptive of the drug's chemical structure.

genetic 1. pertaining to reproduction or to birth or origin. 2. inherited. *G. code* the arrangement of genetic material stored in the DNA molecule of the chromosome. *G. counselling* supportive service for prospective parents who can receive advice as to the likelihood of their children being born with a genetically transmitted disorder. *G. engineering* the alteration of a genome of an organism to change its heritable characteristics. In practice this technique currently is used to mass produce a variety of drugs and vaccines used in medical treatment, e.g., growth hormone and human insulin. Further development offers enormous scope for the advancement of medicine in the treatment of disease and genetic disorders. *G. screening* 1. tests used to screen individuals whose genotypes are associated with specific diseases. These individuals may develop the disease itself or pass it on to their offspring. 2. testing a specific population for the presence of a genetic disease—for example, testing neonates for cystic fibrosis.

genetics the study of heredity and natural development.

genital herpes caused by the herpes simplex virus (HSV types 1 or 2) and presents with painful blisters on or around the genitalia and transmitted through sexual contact.

genital warts small fleshy lumps appearing on the genitalia caused by strains of the human papillovirus (HPV) and transmitted through sexual contact.

genitalia the organs of reproduction.

genitourinary referring to both the reproductive organs and the urinary tract.

genome the total amount of genetic information in the chromosomes of an organism, including genes and DNA sequences.

genotype the genetic characteristics of an individual either over the genome as a whole or at one particular locus.

genupectoral relating to the knee and chest. *G. position* the knee–chest position. *See* POSITION.

genus a taxonomic rank used in biological classifications of living organisms.

geriatrics the branch of medicine covering old age and the disorders arising from it.

germ 1. a microbe. 2. that from which something may develop; a seed.

German measles *see* RUBELLA.

germicide an agent capable of destroying pathogenic microorganisms.

germinoma a neoplasm of the testis or ovum.

gerontology the study of the changes associated with old age and the ageing processes. Includes both mind and body and involves many disciplines, e.g., psychology, sociology, pharmacology, biology and social care.

Gessell's developmental chart *A. Gessell, American psychologist, 1880–1961.* A chart in use for many years that showed the expected motor, social and psychological development of children. Use has fallen over the years.

gestaltism a theory of holism in psychology which claims that ideas come as a whole and are not subdivisible.

gestation the period of development of the young in mammals, from the time of fertilization of the ovum to birth.

See also PREGNANCY. *Ectopic g.* fetal development in some part other than the uterus, usually the uterine tube. *G. period* the duration of pregnancy; in the human female about 280 days when measured from the first day of the last menstrual period. *See also* EXPECTED DATE OF DELIVERY.

gestational diabetes high blood sugar occurring in non-diabetic women during pregnancy. It usually disappears after birth but women who have had the condition should be screened annually as they have a greater risk of developing type 2 diabetes.

gestational trophoblastic disease a group of pregnancy-related tumours arising from the tissue that grows to form the placenta during pregnancy.

Ghon focus *A. Ghon, Czechoslovakian pathologist, 1866–1936.* The primary lesion of pulmonary tuberculosis, as seen on chest radiograph, after it has healed by fibrosis and calcification.

giant cell arteritis a condition in which the medium and large arteries in the head and neck become inflamed.

giardiasis *A. Giard, French biologist, 1846–1908.* An infection with *Giardia lamblia*, a pear-shaped protozoon that causes a persistent protracted diarrhoea, often resulting in intestinal malabsorption.

gigantism or giantism; abnormal growth of the body, often due to over-activity of the anterior lobe of the pituitary gland.

Gilbert's syndrome higher levels of bilirubin build up in the blood leading to episodes of mild jaundice.

Gilles de la Tourette's syndrome (disease) abbreviated TS. *G.E.A.B. Gilles de la Tourette, French neurologist, 1857–1904.* Multiple tics, especially of the face and upper part of the body, often associated with involuntary obscene utterances. The condition usually has its onset in childhood and often becomes chronic. The cause is unknown but is believed to be a combination of genetic and environmental factors.

gingiva the gum; connective tissue surrounding the necks of the teeth.

gingivectomy the surgical removal of the gum margins to get rid of pockets and improve the shape of the gums.

gingivitis inflammation of the gums.

ginko or ginkgo extract from the maidenhair tree, used by herbalists and naturopaths and claimed to be helpful in circulatory disorders, reduced circulation in the brain, senility, depression and premenstrual syndrome.

ginseng extract of the root of plants of genus *Panax*, used widely in Chinese medicine; reputed to have the power to cure many diseases and to have properties to improve sexual health and impotence.

gland an organ composed of specialized cells which secrete fluid prepared from the blood, either for use in the body, or for excretion as waste material. *Ductless (endocrine) g.* one that produces an internal secretion but has no canal (duct) to carry the secretion away, e.g., the thyroid gland. *Exocrine g.* one that discharges its secretion through a duct, e.g., the parotid gland. *Lymph g. see* LYMPH (NODES). *Mucous g.* one that secretes mucus.

glanders a disease of horses communicable to humans, and caused by the bacterium *Burkholderia mallei*.

glandular pertaining to a gland. *G. fever see* MONONUCLEOSIS, INFECTIOUS.

glans [L.] *acorn*. An acorn-shaped body, such as the rounded end of the penis or the clitoris.

Glasgow Coma Scale a standardized system for quickly evaluating the level of consciousness in the critically ill. Measures include: eye opening according to four criteria, verbal response against five criteria, and motor response using six criteria. Scores of 3–8 are classified as severe, i.e., 'coma'. COMA is defined as no response and no eye opening.

glass test a simple test for meningitis that involves pressing a clear glass against a rash. If the rash remains visible it may indicate purpura, which occurs in meningitis. *See* MENINGITIS.

glaucoma raised intraocular pressure. *Closed-angle g.* one that occurs when there is a mechanical defect in the drainage angle; may be primary or secondary. It may be acute, when there is pain and blurring of vision, or chronic, when there may be no pain, but a gradual loss of vision. *Open-angle g.* chronic primary glaucoma in which the angle remains open but drainage becomes gradually diminished; tends to run in families. *Primary g.* one that occurs without any previous disease. It is a common cause of blindness, partial or complete, in the elderly. *Secondary g.* one that occurs when some ocular disease is complicated by an increase in intraocular pressure.

gleet chronic gonococcal urethritis marked by a transparent mucous discharge.

glenoid resembling a hollow. *G. cavity* the socket of the shoulder joint.

glia neuroglia; the connective tissue of the brain and spinal cord.

glioblastoma a malignant glioma arising in the cerebral hemispheres.

glioma a malignant tumour composed of neuroglial cells affecting the brain and spinal cord.

globulins a protein group, forming constituents of the blood (*serum g.*) and cerebrospinal fluid.

globus a ball or globe. *G. hystericus* a symptom of hysteria when a patient feels unable to swallow because there is a lump in the throat. *G. pallidus* the pale medial part of the lentiform nucleus of the brain.

glomerulitis inflammation of the glomeruli of the kidney.

glomerulonephritis a bilateral, non-infectious inflammation of the kidneys. The cause is unknown but the condition is associated with immunological disturbance. It may be acute, presenting rapidly but reversibly, or it may be chronic, presenting slowly and irreversibly.

glomerulosclerosis degenerative changes in the glomerular capillaries of the renal tubule, leading to renal failure.

glomerulus the tuft of capillaries within the nephron, which filters urine from the blood.

glossal relating to the tongue.

glossitis inflammation of the tongue.

glossolalia 'speaking in tongues'; unintelligible speech. The patient speaks in an imaginary language.

glossopharyngeal pertaining to the tongue and pharynx. *G. nerve* the ninth cranial nerve.

glossoplegia paralysis of the tongue.

glottis the space between the vocal cords. The term is sometimes used for that part of the larynx which is associated with voice production.

glucagon a polypeptide produced by the pancreas. It aids glycogen breakdown in the liver and raises the blood sugar level.

glucocorticoid any corticoid substance that raises the concentration of liver glycogen and blood sugar, i.e., cortisol (hydrocortisone), cortisone and corticosterone.

gluconeogenesis the production of glucose from the non-nitrogen portion of the amino acids after deamination. It occurs in the liver and kidneys.

glucose dextrose or grape-sugar; a simple sugar, a monosaccharide in certain foodstuffs, especially fruit, and in normal blood; the chief source of energy for living organisms. *See also* DEXTROSE. *G.-6-phosphate dehydrogenase* (G6PD) a red-cell enzyme. Inherited deficiency that occurs most often in males and causes a tendency to haemolytic anaemia. *See* FAVISM. *Oral G. tolerance test* test in which a quantity of glucose is given and the concentration of glucose in the blood is estimated at intervals afterwards.

Used mainly when diabetes mellitus is suspected.

glue ear the accumulation of sticky material in the middle ear resulting in impaired hearing, most common in young schoolchildren. Also known as otitis media with effusion (OME).

glue sniffing solvent abuse.

glutamic acid one of the 22 amino acids formed by the digestion of dietary protein.

glutamic–oxaloacetic transaminase an enzyme found in cardiac muscle and the liver. Raised serum levels (SGOT) may indicate an acute myocardial infarction or the presence of liver disease.

glutamic–pyruvic transaminase an enzyme found in the liver. Measurement of serum levels (SGPT) is used in the study and diagnosis of liver diseases.

glutaraldehyde a disinfectant active against all viruses, fungi, vegetative bacteria and spores. Used in aqueous solution for sterilization of non-heat-resistant equipment.

glutaric aciduria type 1 a rare inherited condition characterized by an inability to process certain amino acids. Babies are tested for the condition as part of NEWBORN BLOOD SPOT SCREENING. The condition can be treated with diet and medication.

gluteal relating to the buttocks. *G. muscles* three muscles that form the fleshy part of the buttocks.

gluten a sticky protein found in wheat and other cereals, e.g., rye and barley. Gluten consists of two proteins: gliadin and glutenin. Some people are sensitive to gluten, which causes in them intestinal malabsorption (gluten-induced enteropathy). *G.-induced enteropathy* see COELIAC DISEASE.

glycaemic index (GI) the classification of carbohydrate foods based on their overall effects on blood glucose levels. Carbohydrates are ranked 1 to 100. Foods with a low GI factor, e.g., wholegrain cereals, raise blood glucose levels a little and are absorbed more slowly and evenly, whereas those with a high GI factor, e.g., refined flours and sugars, raise blood glucose levels sharply and considerably. Low level GI diets have been shown to improve blood glucose and lipid levels in people with type 1 and type 2 diabetes.

glycerin a colourless syrupy substance obtained from fats and fixed oils. It has a hygroscopic action. As an emollient it is an ingredient of many skin preparations. *G. suppository* one composed of glycerin and gelatin, used as an evacuant. *G. of thymol* an antiseptic mouthwash and gargle.

glycine a non-essential amino acid.

glycogen the form in which carbohydrate is stored in the liver and muscles. Animal starch. *G. storage disease* inherited disease in which there is a deficiency in the synthesis of glycogen. This accumulates in the liver, causing enlargement.

glycogenesis the process of glycogen formation from the blood glucose.

glycogenolysis the breakdown of glycogen in the body so that it may be utilized.

glycosuria an excess of glucose in the urine, a symptom of diabetes mellitus. *Renal g.* sugar in the urine, in an otherwise healthy person, due to a rare inherited inability to reabsorb glucose normally.

gnathic pertaining to the jaw.

goal a statement of what a nursing intervention is expected to achieve in either the short or longer term. May also be referred to as an outcome. *See* NURSING.

goblet cell a goblet-shaped cell, found in the intestinal epithelium, which produces mucus.

goitre the thyroid gland may enlarge (without any disturbance of its function) at puberty, during pregnancy, or as a result of taking oral contraceptives. In many parts of the world the main cause of a goitre is a lack of iodine in the diet. *Exophthalmic g.* hyperthyroidism with marked protrusion of the eyeballs (exophthalmos). Graves' disease may lead to thyrotoxicosis and weight loss is often reported.

gold *symbol Au.* A metallic element previously used in treating rheumatoid arthritis. *Radioactive g.* an isotope that gives off beta and gamma rays. Used, in the form of small grains or seeds, in the treatment of some malignant conditions.

Golgi apparatus *C. Golgi, Italian histologist, 1844–1926.* Specialized structures seen near the nucleus of a cell during microscopic examination.

Golgi's organ the sensory end-organs in muscle tendons which are sensitive to stretch.

gonad a reproductive gland; the testicle or ovary.

gonadotrophic having influence on the gonads. *G. hormone* gonadotrophin.

gonadotrophin any hormone having a stimulating effect on the gonads. Two such hormones are secreted by the anterior pituitary: follicle-stimulating hormone (FSH) and luteinizing hormone (LH), both of which are active, but with differing effects, in the two sexes. *Chorionic g.* a gonad-stimulating hormone produced by cytotrophoblastic cells of the placenta; used in the treatment of underdevelopment of the gonads and to induce ovulation in infertile women.

gonioscope an apparatus for examining the angle of the anterior chamber of the eye.

goniotomy an operation for glaucoma; it consists in opening Schlemm's canal under direct vision.

gonococcus *Neisseria gonorrhoeae*, a diplococcus which causes gonorrhoea.

gonorrhoea a common sexually transmitted disease caused by *Neisseria gonorrhoeae* infecting the genital tract and most often transmitted during sexual activity, including anal and oral sex. An infected woman may also transmit the disease to her baby during childbirth. Spread by the bloodstream, it may give rise to iritis or arthritis. Scar tissue formation may bring about urethral stricture or infertility owing to occlusion of the uterine tubes. Gonorrhoea has an incubation period of 2–10 days. In men, symptoms include a discharge from the urethra and dysuria. Many infected women have no symptoms.

gonorrhoeal relating to gonorrhoea. *G. arthritis* intractable infection of joints, causing great pain and disability.

goose-flesh the reaction of the skin to cold and fear. The blood vessels and hair follicles in the skin contract causing the hair to stand up, giving the impression of plucked poultry skin. Also known as goose pimples.

gout a form of arthritis with an excess of uric acid in the blood. It is characterized by painful inflammation and swelling of the smaller joints, especially those of the big toe and thumb. Inflammation is accompanied by the deposit of urates around the joints.

Graafian follicle *R. de Graaf, Dutch physician and anatomist, 1641–1673.* A follicle which is formed in the ovary and contains an ovum. A follicle matures during each menstrual cycle, ruptures and releases the ovum (ovulation), which is then picked up by the fimbriated end of the uterine tube.

graft 1. any tissue or organ for implantation or transplantation. 2. to implant or transplant such tissue. *Allogenic g.* a graft from a compatible donor. *Autogenous g.* a graft taken from and given to the same individual. *Bone g.* a portion of bone transplanted to repair another bone. *Corneal g.* a portion of cornea, usually from a recently dead person, used to repair a diseased cornea. *Homologous g.* tissue obtained from the body of another animal of the same species but with a genotype differing from that of the recipient; a homograft or allograft. *Pedicle g.* a skin graft, one end of which remains attached to its original site until the grafting has become established.

graft-versus-host disease (reaction) abbreviated GvHD. May follow a successful transplant. A condition that occurs when immunologically competent cells or their precursors are transplanted into an immunologically incompetent recipient (host) that is not histocompatible with the donor. Characteristic signs include skin lesions, ulceration, alopecia, painful joints and haemolytic anaemia. GvHD is a frequent complication of bone marrow transplants but risks can be reduced by the giving of immunosuppressant drugs and use of corticosteroid drugs. Human leukocyte antigen (HLA) matching of the donor and recipient reduces the possibility of GvHD disease. GvHD effect can however be good for attacking the original cancer cells.

gram *symbol* g. The fundamental SI unit of weight, equal to one thousandth of a kilogram.

Gram's stain *H. Gram, Danish physician, 1853–1938.* A method of staining bacteria which is used to classify them into gram-negative and gram-positive.

grand mal [Fr.] former name for tonic clonic seizures. *See* EPILEPSY.

grande multipara a woman who has borne four or more children. Increasing parity can lead to an increased risk of problems in pregnancy, labour and the puerperium.

granular containing small particles. *G. casts* the degenerated cells from the lining of renal tubules excreted in the urine in certain kidney disorders.

granulation 1. the division of a hard solid substance into small particles. 2. the growth of new tissue by which ulcers and wounds heal when the edges are not in apposition. It consists of new capillaries and fibroblasts which fill in the space and later form fibrous tissue. The resulting scar is often unsightly.

granulocyte any cell containing granules in its cytoplasm, especially polymorphonuclear leukocytes which contain neutrophilic, basophilic and eosinophilic granules in their cytoplasm.

granulocytopenia a marked reduction in the number of granulocytes in the blood. The condition may precede agranulocytosis.

granuloma a tumour composed of granulation tissue, usually due to chronic infection or invasion by a foreign body.

granulomatosis an infection producing granulomata. *Lipoid g.* xanthomatosis; Hand–Schüller–Christian disease.

gravel small 'sandy' calculi formed in the kidneys and bladder, and sometimes excreted with the urine. They can also form in the gallbladder where they can accumulate or cause low-grade cholecystitis.

Graves' disease *R.J. Graves, Irish physician, 1796–1853.* Exophthalmic goitre; thyrotoxicosis; hyperthyroidism.

gravid pregnant.

gravity weight. *Specific g.* the weight of a substance compared with that of an equal volume of water.

gray *symbol* Gy. The SI unit used to denote the absorbed dose in radiation therapy.

grey syndrome rare potentially fatal condition seen in preterm babies caused by a reaction to the drug chloramphenicol. Characterized by ashen grey cyanosis, vomiting, abdominal distension, hypothermia and shock.

grey-scale display a method to show the texture of tissue on ultrasound display. The amplitude of each echo is represented by varying shades of grey. A bright white outline is seen from specular surfaces, a mottled grey from various tissue areas, and black from collections of fluid, such as the bladder and amniotic sac.

grid a chart with horizontal and vertical lines on which curves may be plotted.

grief *see* BEREAVEMENT.

groin the junction of the upper thigh with the abdomen. The groins slope outwards and upwards from the pubic region.

grounded theory a qualitative research approach which emphasizes the process of theory generation from systematically collected and stored data, the concept being that the theory remains 'grounded in' the data, demonstrating the fit between the theory and the supporting empirical evidence.

group therapy a form of psychotherapy in which a group of 4–12 patients meets regularly with the therapist in order to discuss and share problems, anxieties and fears in a psychotherapeutic setting. The group also provides emotional support for self-revelation and a structured environment for trying out new ways of relating to people.

growing pains recurrent quasi-rheumatic limb pains peculiar to early youth, once believed to be caused by the growing process. It is now recognized that growth does not cause pain and that these pains can be a symptom of many different disorders.

growth 1. the progressive development of a living thing, especially the process by which the body reaches its point of complete physical development. 2. an abnormal formation of tissue, such as a tumour. *G. hormone* a substance that stimulates growth, especially a secretion of the anterior lobe of the pituitary gland that directly influences protein, carbohydrate and lipid metabolism, and controls the rate of skeletal and visceral growth.

guanine a purine base, one of the constituents of all nucleic acids.

guardian *ad litem* a person usually from the local authority social service department, who is appointed by a court to look after the interests of a child before his or her full Adoption Order is granted. Meanwhile the prospective adoptive parents have continuous possession of the child, and are visited and interviewed by the guardian *ad litem* to ensure that the home will be satisfactory. In Scotland the curator *ad litem* is the equivalent term.

guided imagery a complementary therapy that uses pleasant mental images of events, feelings or sensations as a distraction method in coping with pain.

Guillain–Barré syndrome *G. Guillain, French neurologist, 1876–1961; A. Barré, French neurologist, 1880–1967.* Acute infective polyneuritis. After an infection, usually respiratory, there is a general weakness or paralysis which frequently affects the respiratory muscles as well as the peripheral ones.

guilt feelings of self-blame and reproach causing distress to the individual who believes that they have contravened accepted cultural, moral and ethical standards of behaviour. A deep, lasting and sometimes seemingly inappropriate sense of guilt is often a feature of psychiatric disorder.

guinea-worm a nematode worm, *Dracunculus medinensis*, which burrows into human tissues, particularly the legs or feet.

Gulf War syndrome also known as Gulf War illness, experienced by military personnel during the Gulf War and later wars as a variety of symptoms including chronic fatigue, muscle and joint pains, headaches, memory loss, depression and irritability. Possibly due to chemical exposure (e.g., to insecticides or nerve gas) or the interaction of multiple vaccinations and drugs given to protect personnel from the perceived threat of chemical or biological warfare combined with prolonged fatigue and stress.

gumboil the opening on the gum of an abscess at the root of a tooth.

gumma a soft, degenerating tumour characteristic of the tertiary stage of syphilis. It may occur in any organ or tissue.

gustatory relating to taste.

gut the intestine.

Guthrie test 1. a sensitive screening test for PHENYLKETONURIA. 2. test performed on a small amount of blood, usually taken from the heel stab and carried out on a neonate ideally on the 5th day of life as part of the NEWBORN BLOOD SPOT TEST. The newborn blood spot test screens for nine rare but serious conditions: SICKLE CELL DISEASE, CYSTIC

FIBROSIS, CONGENITAL HYPERTHYROIDISM and six inherited metabolic diseases.

gutta a drop. *G. percha* the juice of a tropical tree which, when dried, forms an elastic semisolid substance. Used in dentistry as a root filler.

GvHD disease graft-versus-host disease.

Gy symbol for *gray*.

gynaecologist one who specializes in the diseases of the female genital tract.

gynaecology the science of those diseases that are peculiar to the female genital tract.

gynaecomastia excessive growth of the male breast.

gypsum plaster of Paris (calcium sulphate).

gyrus a convolution, as of the cerebral cortex.

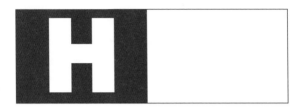

H symbol for *hydrogen*.

H5N1 virus that causes a virulent strain of avian influenza.

habit automatic response to a specific situation acquired as a result of repetition and learning. *Drug h.* drug addiction. *H. forming* drugs that may lead to physiological addiction. *H. retraining* technique used by nurses to retrain patients in the process for control of micturition. The patient is encouraged to void at set times according to an agreed baseline chart but may use the lavatory at other times. *H. training* a method used in psychiatric nursing whereby deteriorated patients can be rehabilitated and taught personal hygiene by constant repetition and encouragement.

habilitation the process of assisting a patient towards achieving the maximum social and physical independence of their potential. The patient/client is usually someone disabled from birth who is learning and not relearning a skill.

habituation gradual adaptation to a stimulus or to the environment. The acquisition of a habit, e.g., a condition resulting from the repeated consumption of a drug, but with little or no tendency to increase the dose; there may be psychic but no physical dependence on the drug.

haemangioma a benign tumour formed by dilated blood vessels. *Strawberry h.* a birthmark, which may become very large, but frequently disappears in a few years.

haemarthrosis an effusion of blood into a joint.

haematemesis vomiting of blood. If it has been in the stomach for some time and become partially digested by gastric juice, it is of a dark colour and contains particles resembling coffee grounds.

haematin the iron-containing part of haemoglobin.

haematocele a swelling produced by effusion of blood, e.g., in the sheath surrounding a testicle or a broad ligament.

haematocrit the volume of red cells in the blood. Usually expressed as a percentage of the total blood volume.

haematology the science dealing with the nature, functions and diseases of blood.

haematoma a swelling containing clotted blood.

haematomyelia an effusion of blood into the spinal cord.

haematuria the presence of blood in the urine, due to injury or disease of any of the urinary organs.

haemochromatosis a condition in which there is high absorption and deposition of iron leading to a high serum level, pigmentation of the skin and liver failure. Bronze diabetes.

haemoconcentration a loss of circulating fluid from the blood resulting in an increase in the proportion of red blood cells to plasma. The viscosity of the blood is increased.

haemodialysis the removal of waste material from the blood of a patient with acute or chronic renal failure by means of a dialyser or artificial kidney. The apparatus is coupled to an artery and dialysis is achieved by the blood and rinsing fluid (DIALYSATE) passing through a semipermeable membrane. Blood is returned through a vein.

haemoglobin (Hb) the complex protein molecule contained within the red blood cells which gives them their colour and by which oxygen is transported.

haemoglobinopathy any one of a group of hereditary disorders, including sickle-cell anaemia and thalassaemia, in which there is an abnormality in the production of haemoglobin.

haemolysin a substance that destroys red blood cells.

haemolysis the disintegration of red blood cells. Excessive haemolysis, which may produce anaemia, may be caused by injection with viruses or bacteria, drugs, chemicals and incompatible blood transfusions.

haemolytic having the power to destroy red blood cells. *H. disease of the newborn* a condition associated with rhesus incompatibility. *See* RHESUS FACTOR.

haemophilia a condition characterized by impaired coagulability of the blood, and a strong tendency to bleed. Over 80% of all patients with haemophilia have haemophilia A (classic haemophilia), which is characterized by a deficiency of clotting factor VIII. Haemophilia B (Christmas disease), which affects about 15% of all haemophiliac patients, results from a deficiency of factor IX. Inherited as an X-linked recessive trait, it is transmitted by females only, to their male offspring. In order to avoid the debilitating and crippling effects of haemophilia, treatment must raise the level of the deficient clotting factor and maintain it in order to stop

local bleeding. The patient must learn to avoid trauma and to obtain prompt treatment for bleeding episodes. Individuals with haemophilia may range from having a mild to severe phenotype (how they are clinically), and before surgery or dental treatment the patient must be given an infusion of the appropriate clotting factor or on occasions tranexamic acid (an anti-fibrinolytic) may suffice.

Haemophilus a genus of gram-negative rod-like bacteria. *H. ducreyi* the cause of soft chancre. *H. influenzae* bacterium that causes various infectious diseases in humans.

haemophthalmia bleeding into the vitreous of the eye, usually the result of trauma; haemophthalmos.

haemopneumothorax the presence of blood and air in the pleural cavity, usually the result of injury.

haemopoiesis the formation of red blood cells, which normally takes place in the bone marrow and continues throughout life. *Extramedullary h.* the formation of blood cells other than in the bone marrow, e.g., in the liver or spleen.

haemopoietic relating to red blood cell formation. *H. factors* those necessary for the development of red blood cells, e.g., vitamin B_{12} and folic acid.

haemoptysis the coughing up of blood from the lungs or bronchi. Being aerated, it is bright red and frothy.

haemorrhage an escape of blood from a ruptured blood vessel, externally or internally. Arterial haemorrhage involves bright-red blood which escapes in rhythmic spurts, corresponding to the beats of the heart. Venous haemorrhage involves dark-red blood which escapes in an even flow. Haemorrhage may also be: *primary*, at the time of operation or injury; *reactionary* or recurrent, occurring later when the blood pressure rises and a ligature slips or a vessel opens up; *secondary*, may be several days after injury, and usually due to sepsis. Special types are as follows. *Antepartum h.* that which occurs before labour starts. See PLACENTA (PRAEVIA). *Cerebral h.* an episode of bleeding into the cerebrum; one of the three main forms of STROKE. *Concealed h.* collection of the blood in a cavity of the body. *Intracranial h.* bleeding within the cranium, which may be extradural, subdural, subarachnoid or cerebral. *Intradural h.* bleeding beneath the dura mater. It may be due to injury and causes signs of compression. The cerebrospinal fluid will be bloodstained. *Postpartum h.* that which occurs within 12–24 hours of delivery, from the genital tract, and which either measures 500 ml or more, or which adversely affects the woman's condition. Secondary postpartum haemorrhage is excessive bleeding more than 24 hours after delivery.

haemorrhagic pertaining to or characterized by haemorrhage. *H. disease of the newborn* a self-limited haemorrhagic disorder of the first days of life, caused by deficiency of vitamin K-dependent blood clotting factors II, VII, IX and X. It should be prevented by the prophylactic administration of vitamin K to all newborn babies. *Viral h. fevers* a group of notifiable virus diseases of diverse aetiology but with similar characteristics of fever, headache, myalgia, prostration and haemorrhagic symptoms. They include dengue haemorrhagic fever, See MARBURG DISEASE, EBOLA VIRUS DISEASE, LASSA FEVER and YELLOW FEVER.

haemorrhoid a 'pile' or locally dilated rectal vein. Piles may be either external or internal to the anal sphincter. Pain is caused on defecation, and bleeding may occur.

haemorrhoidectomy the surgical removal of haemorrhoids.

haemosiderosis iron deposits in the tissues resulting from excessive haemolysis of red blood cells.

haemostasis the arrest of bleeding or the slowing up of blood flow in a vessel.

haemostatic a drug or remedy for arresting haemorrhage; a styptic.

haemothorax blood in the thoracic cavity, e.g., from injury to soft tissues as a result of fracture of a rib.

hair a delicate keratinized epidermal filament growing out of the skin. The root of the hair is enclosed beneath the skin in a tubular follicle. See Figure on p. 171. Erect hair has a minimal role in thermoregulation of the body. If the body is too cold, arrector pili muscles contract in the skin, pulling the hairs upright and trapping an insulating layer of air. See GOOSE-FLESH. *H. analysis* used as an adjunct to other tests in preconception care of women to assess nutritional status and detect the concentration of up to 18 metals. High levels of some metals such as lead may be associated with congenital abnormalities. Deficiencies of substances such as zinc can be treated with dietary advice and/or supplements. *H. ball* see BEZOAR. *H. loss* see ALOPECIA.

half-life 1. the time it takes for a substance to decay to one-half of its original value. 2. in pharmacology, the time it takes for the level of a drug to decrease to one-half in the blood. This is used to determine the dosing level required for therapeutic treatment.

Halal meat from an animal that has been killed according to Islamic law and is therefore lawful to be eaten by Muslims.

halitosis foul-smelling breath.

hallucination a sensory impression (sight, touch, sound, smell or taste) that has no basis in external stimulation. Hallucinations can have psychological causes, as in mental illness, or they can result from drugs, alcohol, or organic illnesses, such as brain tumour or senility. People subjected to sensory deprivation or overwhelming physical stress sometimes suffer from temporary hallucinations.

hallucinations rating scale abbreviated HRS. A scale that uses 11 items to determine auditory hallucinations in

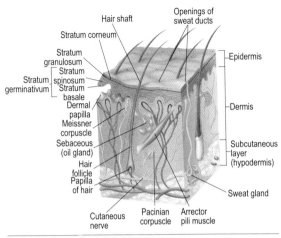

Hair shaft
Openings of sweat ducts
Stratum corneum
Stratum granulosum
Stratum spinosum
Stratum germinativum
Stratum basale
Dermal papilla
Meissner corpuscle
Sebaceous (oil gland)
Hair follicle
Papilla of hair
Cutaneous nerve
Pacinian corpuscle
Arrector pili muscle
Sweat gland
Subcutaneous layer (hypodermis)
Dermis
Epidermis

STRUCTURE OF A HAIR

patients. It also assesses the way in which the hallucinations are experienced and controlled by the patient.

hallucinogen an agent that causes hallucinations, e.g., LSD and cannabis.

hallux the big toe. *H. valgus* a deformity in which the big toe is bent towards the other toes. *H. varus* a deformity in which the big toe is bent outwards away from the other toes.

halo a circular structure, such as a luminous circle seen surrounding an object or light. *Glaucomatous h., h. glaucomatosus* a narrow light zone surrounding the optic disc in glaucoma.

halo effect a beneficial effect noted after a health care intervention, visit or research project. The halo effect cannot be attributed to the content of the interview, visit or project but is the outcome of indefinable factors as a result of the intervention.

halo splint an orthopaedic device used to immobilize the head and neck to assist in the healing of cervical injuries and postoperatively after cervical surgery.

halogen any of the five non-metallic elements chlorine, iodine, bromine, astatine and fluorine.

hamartoma a benign nodule which is an overgrowth of mature tissue.

hammer the malleus. *H. toe* a deformity in which the first phalanx is bent upwards, with plantar flexion of the second and third phalanx.

hamstring the flexors of the knee joint that are situated at the back of the thigh.

hand the terminal part of the arm below the wrist. *Claw h.* a paralytic condition in which the hand is flexed and the fingers contracted, caused by injury to nerves or muscles. *Cleft h.* a congenital deformity in which the cleft between the third and fourth fingers extends into the palm. *H. washing see* Figure and Appendix 11.

Wet hands with water
(warm or cold)

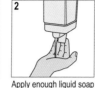

Apply enough liquid soap
to cover hands all over

Rub hands palm to palm

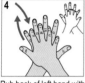

Rub back of left hand with
right palm with fingers
interlaced. Repeat with
the other hand

Rub palms together with
fingers interlaced

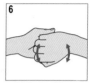

Rub backs of fingers
against palms with
fingers interlocked

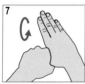

Clasp left thumb with the
right hand and rub in
rotation. Repeat with the
left hand and right thumb

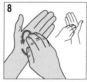

Rub tips of fingers in
opposite palm in a circular
motion going backwards
and forwards. Repeat with
the other hand

Rinse hands with water
(warm or cold)

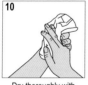

Dry thoroughly with
disposable towel

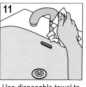

Use disposable towel to
turn off tap

HAND WASHING TECHNIQUE

hand–arm vibration syndrome pain and numbness with blanching in the hand and arm due to the use of vibrating tools, usually in the workplace. The syndrome tends to develop slowly over time and gangrene may develop. Exposure to cold tends to aggravate the condition.

Hand–Schüller–Christian disease *A. Hand, American paediatrician, 1868–1949; A. Schüller, Austrian neurologist, 1874–1958; H.A. Christian, American physician, 1876–1951.* A disease of the reticuloendothelial system in which granulomata containing cholesterol are formed, chiefly in the skull.

hand washing *See* Figure and Appendix 11.

handicap a disadvantage for a given individual, resulting from an impairment or a disability that limits or prevents the fulfilment of a role that is normal (depending on age, sex, and social and cultural factors) for that individual.

Hansen's disease *G.H.A. Hansen, Norwegian physician, 1841–1912.* Leprosy, caused by Hansen's bacillus, *Mycobacterium leprae*. *See* LEPROSY.

haploid having one set of chromosomes after division instead of two.

harassment any repetitive physical or verbal conduct that causes another person alarm or distress, including physically threatening, humiliating, offensive or derogatory acts or utterances. Harassment is unlawful and examples include bullying, workplace violence, sexual harassment, racial, age or gender discrimination and cyberstalking. Harassment can occur in health care settings and this may take many forms, but an example is when a consultant, manager or senior professional repeatedly makes derisory or critical comments to another member of staff in front of patients or colleagues leading to that person losing confidence and feeling powerless in the workplace.

hard drugs an imprecise term used in relation to drugs that are highly addictive, e.g., heroin or cocaine, and therefore prone to misuse.

Harrison's groove or sulcus *E. Harrison, British physician, 1789–1838.* A horizontal groove along the lower border of the thorax corresponding to the costal insertion of the diaphragm; seen in rickets.

Hartmann's solution a saline solution containing sodium lactate used intravenously in treating acidosis.

Hartnup disease a hereditary defect in amino acid metabolism which may produce learning difficulties (named after the first person found to suffer from it).

Hashimoto's disease *H. Hashimoto, Japanese surgeon, 1881–1934.* A lymphoadenoid goitre caused by the formation of antibodies to thyroglobulin. It is an autoimmune condition giving rise to hypothyroidism.

hashish Indian hemp. *See* CANNABIS.

haustration a haustrum, or the process of forming one.

haustrum any one of the pouches formed by the sacculations of the colon.

Haversian canal *C. Havers, British physician and anatomist, 1650–1702.* One of the minute canals that permeate compact bone, containing blood and lymph vessels to maintain its nutrition. *See* BONE.

Hawthorne effect the term given to the usual beneficial effect of a study on the persons participating in the study. It was named after an industrial management study in the USA, where the effect was first identified.

hay fever an atopic ALLERGY characterized by sneezing, itching and watery eyes, running nose and a burning sensation of the palate and throat. It is a localized anaphylactic reaction to an extrinsic allergen, most commonly pollens and the spores of moulds. When the allergen comes in contact with mast-cell-bound IgE immunoglobulin in the tissues of the conjunctiva, nasal mucosa and bronchial tree, the cells release mediators of ANAPHYLAXIS and produce the characteristic symptoms of hay fever. *See* ATOPY.

HCAI a health care associated infection.

HCG human chorionic gonadotrophin. *See* GONADOTROPHIN.

HCl hydrochloric acid.

HCPC *See* HEALTH AND CARE PROFESSIONS COUNCIL.

He symbol for *helium*.

head the anterior or superior part of a structure or organism, in vertebrates containing the brain and the organs of special sense. *H. tilt* or chin lift a method of opening the airway in an unconscious patient. One hand is placed upon the forehead to gently tilt the head back. The fingers of the other hand lift the chin. If head or spinal injury is suspected this manoeuvre should NOT be used. *See* Appendix 3. *H. injury* traumatic injury to the head resulting from a fall or violent blow. Such an injury may be open or closed and may involve a brain CONCUSSION, skull fracture, or contusions of the brain. All head injuries are potentially dangerous because there may be a slow leakage of blood from damaged blood vessels into the brain, or the formation of a blood clot which gradually increases pressure against brain tissue. Long-term effects of head injury may include chronic headache, disturbances in mental and motor function, and a host of other symptoms that may or may not be psychogenic. Organic brain damage and post-traumatic epilepsy resulting from scar formation are possible sequels to head injury. *H. lice see* PEDICULUS.

headache a pain or ache in the head. A symptom rather than a disorder. It accompanies many diseases and conditions, including emotional distress. *See also* CLUSTER HEADACHES and MIGRAINE.

Heaf test *F.G.R. Heaf, British physician, 1894–1973.* A form of tuberculin testing no longer in use. The MANTOUX test is now used instead.

healing the process of return to normal function after a period of disease or injury. *H. by first intention* union of the edges of a clean incised wound without visible granulations, and leaving only a faint linear scar. *H. by second intention* union of the edges of an open wound by the formation of granulations from the bottom and sides. *H. by third intention* union of a wound that is closed surgically several days after the injury.

health the World Health Organization (WHO) states that 'Health is a state of complete physical, mental and social wellbeing and not merely the absence of disease or infirmity.' *H. assessment* an evaluation made by a health care professional of an individual's health status, which takes account of the health history and lifestyle together with the findings of a physical examination. *H. centre* primary health care organization for providing ambulatory health care and coordinating the efforts of all health agencies, commonly focused around the general practitioner's services. *H. culture* a system that attempts to explain and treat health problems and illness and to maintain health. Part of the wider culture to which people belong, it may be a traditional or a biomedical system. *H. food* used to indicate food thought to promote health. *H. lottery* an online game played in the UK to raise money for local health causes. *H. promotion* a process of enabling people to increase control over, and to improve, their health. It moves beyond individual behaviour to focus on a wide range of social and environmental interventions. Supported by the World Health Organization as a process of orientating communities to move health services from a treatment approach to one of prevention. Three key elements defined by WHO which are good governance for health, health literacy and healthy cities. *H. services* the term is usually employed to signify the system or programme by which health care is made available to the population and financed by government or private enterprise, or both. *H. statistics* summated data on any aspect of the health of populations; for example, mortality, morbidity, use of health services, treatment outcome, costs of health care. *Holistic h.* a system of preventive medicine that takes into account the whole individual, and that person's own responsibility for wellbeing, with the total influences (social, psychological, environmental) that affect health, including nutrition, exercise and mental relaxation. *Public h.* the field of medicine that is concerned with safeguarding and improving the health of the community as a whole.

Health and Safety at Work Act 1974 comprehensive legislation that came into force in 1975. It deals with the welfare, health and safety of all employers and employees, except domestic workers in a private house. The Health and Safety Executive (HSE) enforce health and safety law in the UK. The HSE is the independent watchdog for work-related health, safety and illness. It acts in the public interest to reduce work-related deaths and serious injury. It is an executive non-departmental body sponsored by the Department for Work and Pensions.

The Health and Safety Commission (HSC) merged into the HSE in 2008.

health care assistant abbreviated HCA. A support worker in the clinical area who works with the supervision of a registered practitioner who is responsible for the quality of care delivered by the HCA. An HCA should receive training for their role including accessing a clinical healthcare apprenticeship.

health care-associated infection (HCAI; sometimes abbreviated as HAI); also known as nosocomial infections. An infection acquired during an episode of health care in either acute (hospital) or non-acute settings, usually as a result of a clinical intervention, such as urinary catheterization or the insertion of a vascular access device. *See* Appendix 11.

health care system an organized plan of health services. The term is usually employed to denote the system or programme by which health care is made available to the population and financed by government or private enterprise or both.

health education various methods of education aimed at the prevention of disease. All nurses, midwives and health visitors have particular responsibilities and opportunities to promote good health. *Health Education England (HEE)* the organization responsible for ensuring high quality education and training for the health workforce.

Health and Care Professions Council (HCPC) previously the Health Professions Council, is a UK independent body created in 2001 to protect the public by setting and maintaining standards for those health care professionals which it regulates. It currently regulates several professions which include: arts therapists; biomedical scientists; chiropodists/podiatrists; clinical scientists; dietitians; hearing aid dispensers; occupational therapists; operating department practitioners; orthoptists; paramedics; physiotherapists; practitioner psychologists; prosthetists/orthotists; radiographers; social workers (in England) and speech and language therapists. Health Protection Agency (HPA) became part of PUBLIC HEALTH ENGLAND in 2013.

health record is any record of information relating to someone's physical or mental health that has been made by (or on behalf of) a health professional. This could be anything from the notes made by a GP in a local surgery to results of an MRI scan or X-rays. Health records contain personal, sensitive and confidential information. They are usually held electronically or occasionally as paper files by a range of health professionals both in the NHS and the private sector. For the purpose of the Data Protection Act, a registered professional can be one of the following people: registered medical practitioner, dentist, dispensing optician or optometrist, pharmacist or pharmacy technician, child psychotherapist, a scientist employed in a hospital as head of department, registered nurse or midwife, osteopath or chiropractor, any person registered as a member of a profession to which the health and social work professions order extends.

Health Service Commissioner (Health Service Ombudsman UK) appointed to protect the interests of patients in relation to the administration and provision of health care delivered in the NHS. The Commissioner is responsible to Parliament and can investigate complaints and allegations of maladministration by a health authority, NHS Trusts and the clinical practice of medical practitioners. *See* OMBUDSMAN.

health visitor a nurse or midwife who has completed a course in social and preventative medicine leading to a health visiting qualification. The main area of responsibility of health visitors is health education and preventative care families and children under 5 years old. Also known as specialist community public health nurses.

hearing the reception of sound waves and their transmission onwards to the brain in the form of nerve impulses. healthy child programme lead by health visitors, this programme for the early life stages focuses on a universal preventative service, providing families with a programme of screening, immunization, development reviews, supplemented by advice around health, wellbeing and parenting. *H. aid* an apparatus, usually electronic, to amplify sounds before they reach the inner ear. *H. therapy* the support and rehabilitation of people with hearing difficulties, tinnitus or vertigo. It includes the teaching of lip reading, the use of hearing aids and providing tinnitus retraining therapy.

heart a hollow, muscular organ which pumps the blood throughout the body, situated behind the sternum slightly towards the left side of the thorax (*see* Figure on p. 177). *H. attack* myocardial infarction (MI). *H. block* impairment of conduction in heart excitation; often applied specifically to atrioventricular heart block. *H. failure* may be acute, as in coronary thrombosis, or chronic. *H.–lung machine* an apparatus used to perform the functions of both the heart and the lungs during heart surgery. *H. murmur* an abnormal sound heard in the heart, frequently caused by disease of the valves. Occurs when the blood flow through the heart exceeds a certain velocity. *H. rate* the number of heart beats per minute. The normal resting heart rate is 60–100 beats per minute, and should be monitored for rate, strength and rhythm. *H. sounds* the normal heart sounds correspond to the closure of the four valves of the heart. First heart sound = 'LUB', sound corresponding to the closure of the mitral and tricuspid valves. Second heart sound = 'DUP', sound with closure of the aortic and pulmonary valves. *Maximum h. rate* used in sports medicine to assess an individual's heart during exercise. It is equal to 220 minus the age of the person.

heartburn indigestion marked by a burning sensation in the oesophagus, often with regurgitation of acid fluid.

heat warmth. A form of energy, which may cause an increase in temperature or a change of state, e.g., the conversion of water into steam. *H. exhaustion* a rapid pulse, anorexia, dizziness, and cramps in arms, legs or abdomen, sometimes followed by sudden collapse, caused by loss of body fluids and salts under very hot conditions. *Prickly h.* miliaria; heat rash. Acute itching caused by blocking of the ducts of the sweat glands following profuse sweating. *H. stroke* a severe life-threatening condition resulting from prolonged exposure to heat. *See* SUNSTROKE.

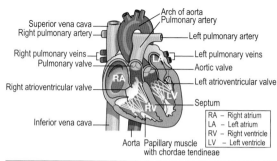

Labels: Superior vena cava, Right pulmonary artery, Right pulmonary veins, Pulmonary valve, Right atrioventricular valve, Inferior vena cava, Arch of aorta, Pulmonary artery, Left pulmonary artery, Left pulmonary veins, Aortic valve, Left atrioventricular valve, Septum, Aorta, Papillary muscle with chordae tendineae

RA	–	Right atrium
LA	–	Left atrium
RV	–	Right ventricle
LV	–	Left ventricle

HEART

hebephrenia a form of schizophrenia characterized by thought disorder and emotional incongruity. Delusions and hallucinations are common.

Heberden's nodes *W. Heberden, British physician, 1710–1801.* Bony or cartilaginous outgrowths causing deformity of the terminal finger joints in osteoarthritis.

hebetude emotional dullness. A common symptom in dementia and schizophrenia.

hectic occurring regularly. *H. fever* a regularly occurring increase in temperature; it is frequently observed in pulmonary tuberculosis. *H. flush* a redness of the face accompanying a sudden rise in temperature.

hedonism excessive devotion to pleasure.

Heimlich manoeuvre *H. Heimlich, Surgeon, 1920–2016.* Now referred to as abdominal thrust. *See* Appendix 2.

Helicobacter a genus of spiral and flagellated gram-negative bacteria. *H. pylori* a species found in the stomach. May cause damage to the prostaglandins protecting the mucosal cells in the stomach wall, leading to progressive gastritis and ulceration.

heliotherapy treatment of disease by exposure of the body to sunlight.

helium *symbol* He. An inert gas sometimes used in conjunction with oxygen to facilitate respiration in obstructional types of dyspnoea and for decompressing deep-sea divers.

helix 1. a spiral twist. Used to describe the configuration of certain molecules, e.g., deoxyribonucleic acid (DNA). 2. the outer rim of the auricle of the ear.

Hellin's law one in about 89 pregnancies ends in the birth of twins; one in 89^2, or 7921, in the birth of triplets; one in 89^3, or 704 969, in the birth of quadruplets. Assisted reproduction techniques have raised the rate of multiple pregnancies; therefore the formula is less indicative of true incidence.

helminthiasis an infestation with worms.

hemeralopia day blindness. The vision is poor in a bright light but is comparatively good when the light is dim. *See* NYCTALOPIA.

hemianopia partial blindness, in which the patient can see only half of the normal field of vision. It arises from disorders of the optic tract and the occipital lobe.

hemicolectomy the removal of the ascending and part of the transverse colon with an ileotransverse colostomy.

hemiparesis paralysis on one side of the body; hemiplegia.

hemiplegia paralysis of one half of the body, usually due to cerebral disease or injury. The lesion is on the side of the brain opposite to the side paralysed.

hemisphere a half sphere. In anatomy, one of the two halves of the cerebrum or cerebellum.

Henle's loop *F.G.J. Henle, German anatomist, 1809–1885.* The U-shaped loop of the uriniferous tubule of the kidney.

Henoch-Schonlein purpura *E.H. Henoch, German paediatrician, 1820–1910.* Allergic PURPURA.

heparin an anticoagulant formed in the liver and circulated in the blood. Injected intravenously it prevents the conversion of prothrombin into thrombin, and is used in the treatment of thrombosis.

hepatectomy excision of a part or the whole of the liver.

hepatic relating to the liver. *H. flexure* the angle of the colon that is situated under the liver.

hepaticojejunostomy the anastomosis of the hepatic duct to the jejunum, usually created after extensive excision for carcinoma of the pancreas.

hepaticostomy a surgical opening into the hepatic duct.

hepatitis inflammation of the liver, characterized by the presence of inflammatory cells in the tissue of the organ. The condition can be self-limiting or can progress to fibrosis and cirrhosis. Hepatitis is acute when it lasts less than 6 months and chronic when it lasts for longer. Worldwide most commonly caused by one of a group of hepatitis viruses, but it can also be due to toxins (alcohol, certain medications, some industrial organic solvents and plants), other infections and autoimmune diseases such as cytomegalovirus infection or Legionnaires' disease. Hepatitis may present with limited or no symptoms, but often leads to jaundice, fever, anorexia and general malaise. *Viral h.* an acute, notifiable, infectious hepatitis caused by one of several different viruses that infect human liver cells, e.g., hepatitis A virus (HAV), hepatitis B virus (HBV), hepatitis C virus (HCV), hepatitis D (Delta virus) and hepatitis E virus (HEV).

hepatization the alteration of lung tissue into a solid mass resembling liver, which occurs in acute lobar pneumonia.

hepatogenous arising in the liver. Applied to jaundice in which the disease arises in the parenchymal cells of the liver.

hepatolenticular pertaining to the liver and the lentiform nucleus. *H. degeneration* Wilson's disease; a progressive hereditary condition, usually occurring between the ages of 10 and 25 years. There are tremors of the head and limbs, pigmentation of the cornea and sometimes defective twilight vision.

hepatoma a primary malignant tumour arising in the liver cells.

hepatomegaly an enlargement of the liver.

hepatosplenomegaly enlargement of the liver and spleen, such as may be found in kala-azar.

hepatotoxic applied to drugs and substances that cause destruction of liver cells, e.g., alcohol.

herbal medicine a form of complementary or alternative medicine in which plants are used for their therapeutic properties.

herd immunity the immunity of a population. When there is a high enough number of persons in a population immune to a particular infection, the infection fails to spread because of the absence of enough susceptibles. For example, in measles this could probably be achieved by vaccination of 90%–95% of the population.

hereditary derived from ancestry; inherited.

heredity the transmission of both physical and mental characteristics to the offspring from the parents. Recessive characteristics may miss one or two generations and reappear later.

hermaphrodite an individual whose gonads contain both testicular and ovarian tissue. These may be combined or there may be a testis on one side and an ovary on the other. The external genitalia may be indeterminate or of either sex. *Pseudo-h.* one whose gonads are histologically of one sex but in whom the genitalia have the appearance of the opposite sex. *True h.* one who possesses both male and female gonads.

hermeneutics the study of meanings in social behaviour and experience. Denotes the art, skill or theory of interpreting human behaviour, speech and writings in terms of intentions and meanings.

hermetic airtight. A wound dressing may be sealed to ensure that the wound is not exposed to air.

hernia a protrusion of any part of the internal organs through the structures enclosing them. *Cerebral h.* a protrusion of brain through the skull. *Diaphragmatic h.* and *hiatus h.* a protrusion of a part of the stomach through the oesophageal opening in the diaphragm. *Femoral h.* a loop of intestine protruding into the femoral canal. More common in females. *Hiatus h. see* DIAPHRAGMATIC H. *Incisional h.* a hernia occurring at the site of an old wound. *Inguinal h.* protrusion of the intestine through the inguinal canal. This may be congenital or acquired, and is commoner in males. A rupture. *Irreducible h.* a hernia that cannot be replaced by manipulation. *Reducible h.* a hernia that can be returned to its normal position by manipulative measures. *Strangulated h.* a hernia of the bowel in which the neck of the sac containing the bowel is so constricted that the venous circulation is impeded, and gangrene will result if not treated promptly. *Umbilical*

h. protrusion of bowel through the umbilical ring. This may be congenital or acquired. *Vaginal h.* rectocele or cystocele.

hernioplasty a plastic repair of the abdominal wall performed after reduction of a hernia.

herniorrhaphy removal of a hernial sac and repair of the abdominal wall.

herniotomy an operation to remove a hernial sac.

heroin a diacetate of morphine used as an analgesic and abused illicitly for its euphoriant effects. The drug readily induces physical dependence and may be sniffed, smoked ('chasing the dragon') or injected subcutaneously or intravenously ('shooting up' or 'mainlining'). Street names for heroin include 'smack', 'H' and 'horse'. *H. baby* a baby that has received regular heroin (morphine) via the placenta before birth and who shows signs of withdrawal after birth. Withdrawal symptoms may persist for 1–4 weeks and include vomiting, abdominal cramps, diarrhoea, sweating, breathing difficulties and hyperactivity.

herpes an inflammatory skin eruption showing small vesicles caused by a herpes virus. *H. simplex* a viral infection which gives rise to localized vesicles in the skin and mucous membranes and is characterized by latency and subsequent recurrence. It is caused by herpes simplex viruses types 1 and 2. Type 1 infection is common in children and is often symptomless. Type 2 infection is common in older age groups and is associated with sexual activity. Recurrent attacks may occur. Lesions appear on the cervix, vulva and surrounding skin in women and on the penis in men. In homosexual men rectal lesions are common. Once the virus enters the body, it stays there for the rest of the person's life. Recurrent attacks are common. To prevent neonatal herpes, Caesarean section is usually recommended for women presenting with clinical genital tract herpes within 2 weeks of delivery to avoid genital herpes being passed on to the baby. *Congenital h. simplex* a serious neonatal condition with a generalized vesicular rash, causing encephalitis and death. *H. zoster* a local manifestation of reactivation of infection of the varicella zoster virus, the causative agent of chickenpox, characterized by a vesicular rash in the area of distribution of a sensory nerve. Called also shingles.

herpes virus one of a group of DNA-containing viruses. They include the causative agents of herpes simplex, herpes zoster, chickenpox, cytomegalic inclusion disease and infective mononucleosis.

heterochromia a difference in colour in the irises of the two eyes or in different parts of one iris. It may be congenital or secondary resulting from inflammation.

heterosexual 1. pertaining to, characteristic of or directed towards the opposite sex. 2. a person with erotic interests directed towards the opposite sex.

heterotropia a marked deviation of the eyes; strabismus or squint.

heterozygous possessing dissimilar alternative genes for an inherited characteristic, one gene coming from each parent. One gene is dominant and the other is recessive. *See* HOMOZYGOUS.

hexachlorophene a detergent and germicidal compound commonly incorporated in soaps and dermatological agents. Topical preparations have been associated with severe neurotoxicity and should not be used on children under 2 years old except on medical advice.

Hg symbol for *mercury*.

hiatus a space or opening. *H. hernia* a protrusion of a part of the stomach through the oesophageal opening in the diaphragm.

Hib an injectable vaccine which protects against *Haemophilus influenzae* type B which causes severe respiratory and ear infections and meningitis. Offered to infants at ages of 2, 3 and 4 months. *See* Appendix 10.

hiccup hiccough; a spasmodic contraction of the diaphragm causing an abrupt inspiratory sound. Also known as myoclonic jerk.

hidrosis the excretion of sweat.

high-altitude sickness the condition resulting from difficulty in adjusting to diminished oxygen pressure at high altitudes. It may take the form of mountain sickness, high-altitude pulmonary oedema or cerebral oedema.

high dependency unit abbreviated HDU. For those patients who do not need intensive care in the clinical situation but require a greater degree of specialist monitoring and observation than in a general ward, nursing and medical care is provided in the high dependency unit.

highly active antiretroviral therapy abbreviated HAART. A treatment regimen that incorporates a combination of different antiviral drugs for human immunodeficiency viral infection. Sometimes also called ART, antiretroviral therapy.

hilum hilus; a recess in an organ by which blood vessels, nerves and ducts enter and leave it.

hindbrain that part of the brain consisting of the medulla oblongata, the pons and the cerebellum.

hip 1. the region of the body at the articulation of the femur and the innominate bone at the base of the lower trunk. These bones meet at the hip joint. Called also *coxa*. 2. loosely, the hip joint. *Total h. replacement* replacement of the femoral head and acetabulum with prostheses that are cemented into the bone; called also *total h. arthroplasty*. The procedure is done to replace a severely damaged arthritic hip joint.

hippus alternate contraction and dilatation of the pupils. This occurs in various diseases of the nervous system, e.g., multiple sclerosis.

Hirschsprung's disease *H. Hirschsprung, Danish physician, 1831–1916.* A rare bowel condition that mainly affects babies where the colon does not function leading to obstruction. A form of MEGACOLON.

hirsute hairy.

hirsutism excessive hairiness.

hirudin the active principle in the secretion of the leech and certain snake venoms that prevents clotting of blood.

Hirudo a genus of leeches. *H. medicinalis* the medical leech.

histamine an enzyme that causes local vasodilatation and increased permeability of the blood vessel walls. Readily released from body tissues, it is a factor in allergy response, greatly increases gastric secretion of hydrochloric acid and increases the heart rate.

histidine one of the ten essential amino acids formed by the digestion of dietary protein. Histamine is derived from it.

histiocyte a stationary macrophage of connective tissue. Derived from the reticuloendothelial cells, it acts as a scavenger, removing bacteria from the blood and tissues.

histiocytosis a group of diseases of bone in which granulomata containing histiocytes and eosinophil cells appear. See HAND–SCHÜLLER–CHRISTIAN DISEASE.

histocompatibility the ability of cells to be accepted and to function in a new situation. Tissue typing reveals this and ensures a higher success rate in organ and tissue transplantation.

histogram a bar-chart. Statistical values are expressed as blocks on a graph.

histology the science dealing with the minute structure, composition and function of tissues.

histolysis the disintegration of tissues.

histoplasmosis infection caused by inhalation of the spores of a yeast-like fungus, *Histoplasma capsulatum.* Usually symptomless, the infection may progress and produce a condition resembling tuberculosis.

HIV human immunodeficiency virus.

HIV disease the entire spectrum of cellular and clinical disease from initial infection and asymptomatic disease to early and late symptomatic disease (AIDS) and death, caused by human immunodeficiency virus (HIV) infection. See HUMAN IMMUNODEFICIENCY VIRUS.

hives urticaria.

Hodgkin's disease *T. Hodgkin, British physician, 1798–1866.* Lymphadenoma, a malignant condition of the reticuloendothelial cells. There is progressive enlargement of lymph nodes and lymph tissue all over the body. Treated by radiotherapy and cytotoxic drugs. This disease has a good prognosis.

holism a philosophy in which the person is considered as a functioning whole rather than as a composite of several systems. May be spelt wholism.

holistic pertaining to holism. *H. health care* a comprehensive approach to health care that implies body–mind–spirit consideration in all actions and interventions for the patient, while recognizing the concept of the uniqueness of the individual and the influence of external and internal environmental factors on health.

Holter monitor *N.J. Holter American biophysicist 1914–1983.* A wearable device used in ambulatory electrocardiography or ECG to record the heart's electrical activity continuously for 24–48 hours or longer. The monitor records by means of electrodes on the chest. The electrodes are placed over bones to minimize artifacts from muscular activity. The extended recording period is useful for noting cardiac arrhythmias which are often difficult to identify in a shorter period of time.

Homans' sign *J. Homans, American surgeon, 1877–1954.* Pain elicited in the calf when the foot is dorsiflexed. Was previously used as being indicative of venous thrombosis.

home the place where a person lives. *H. assessment* made by an occupational therapist to assess the home environment for a patient, in order to determine the need for any adaptations appropriate to the patient's care and needs to maintain independent living at home. *H. birth* the delivery of a baby in the mother's home. Women can choose to deliver their babies and receive care from a community or independent midwife and general practitioner. *H. carers* members of community care teams organized by local authority social services who provide care in the home for older and/or disabled people as part of an agreed care package. *H. help service* provides domestic and housekeeping assistance to those in need contactable through social service departments. It is on either a short-term or long-term basis, and payment is according to means. *H. page* the first page of an internet website.

homeopathy a system of medicine promulgated by C.F.S. Hahnemann (*German physician, 1755–1843*) and based upon the principle that 'like cures like'. Remedies are given which can produce in the patient the symptoms of the disease to be cured, but they are administered in minute doses.

homeostasis a tendency of biological systems to maintain stability while continually adjusting to conditions that are optimal for survival.

homicide murder and manslaughter are two of the offences that constitute homicide. Other specific homicide offences include, for example, infanticide, and causing death by dangerous or careless driving.

homocystinuria a rare but serious inherited condition where the body cannot process the amino acid methionine. Babies are screened for the condition as part of the newborn blood spot screening programme.

homogeneous uniform in character. Similar in nature and characteristics.

homogenize to make homogeneous. To reduce to the same consistency.

homogenous derived from the same source.

homograft a tissue or organ transplanted from one individual to another of the same species. An allograft.

homolateral on the same side; ipsilateral.

homologous 1. in anatomy, having the same embryological origin although performing a different function. 2. in chemistry, possessing a similar structure. *H. chromosomes* those that pair during meiosis and contain an identical arrangement of genes in the DNA pattern.

homologue a part or organ which has the same relative position or structure as another one.

homoplasty surgical replacement of defective tissues with a homograft.

homosexual 1. of the same sex. 2. a person who is sexually attracted to a person of the same sex.

homosexuality sexual and emotional orientation towards persons of the same sex.

homozygous possessing an identical pair of genes for an inherited characteristic. *See* HETEROZYGOUS.

hookworm *see* ANCYLOSTOMA.

hordeolum a stye; inflammation of the sebaceous glands of the eyelashes.

hormone a chemical substance that is generated in one organ and carried by the blood to another, in which it excites activity. *H. replacement therapy* abbreviated as HRT. The giving of prepared hormones orally or by implant, skin patch, gel or nasal spray, as a substitute for those hormones that the body no longer produces or that have been lost as a result of surgery. A combination of oestrogenic hormones is commonly given to women for the relief of menopausal symptoms and the prevention of osteoporosis.

Horner's syndrome *J.F. Horner, Swiss ophthalmologist, 1831–1886.* A rare condition in which there is a lesion on the path of sympathetic nerve fibres in the cervical region. The symptoms include enophthalmos, ptosis, a contracted pupil and a decrease in sweating.

Horton's syndrome *B.T. Horton, American physician, 1895–1980.* Severe headache caused by the release of histamine in the body.

hospice the concept of a hospice is that of a caring community of professional and non-professional people, together with the family. Emphasis is on dealing with emotional and spiritual problems as well as the medical problems of the terminally ill. Of primary concern is control of pain and other symptoms, keeping the patient at home for as long as possible or desirable, and making the remaining days as comfortable and meaningful as possible. After the patient dies, family members are given support throughout their period of bereavement.

hospital an institution for the care, diagnosis and treatment of the sick and injured. *H.-acquired infection* see (HOSPITAL-ACQUIRED) INFECTION. *H. Information System (HIS)* a computerized network of hospitals, laboratories, health care facilities spread throughout Europe meet and collate data relating to the social and health care needs in each area. May also be used to describe the system within an individual NHS Trust or unit.

host the animal, plant or tissue on which a parasite lives and multiplies. *Definitive* or *final h.* one that harbours the parasite during its adult sexual stage. *Intermediate h.* one that shelters the parasite during a non-reproductive period.

hourglass contraction a contraction near the middle of a hollow organ, such as the stomach or uterus, producing an outline resembling an hourglass shape.

housemaid's knee prepatellar bursitis; inflammation of the prepatellar bursa, which becomes distended with serous fluid.

HRT hormone replacement therapy. Hughes syndrome *see* ANTIPHOSPHOLIPID SYNDROME.

human chorionic gonadotrophin see GONADOTROPHIN.

Human Fertilization and Embryology Act 2008 Act which aims to ensure all human embryos outside the body are subject to regulation; ban sex selection of offspring for non-medical reasons; recognize same-sex couples as legal parents through use of donated sperm, eggs or embryos. Monitor collection of data from HFEA to follow up research of infertility treatment. Termination of pregnancy must be performed before 24 weeks of pregnancy by a registered medical practitioner, agreed with a second doctor that the woman or her family would suffer physical, mental or social trauma if the pregnancy were to continue, or if the baby is at risk of gross physical or mental abnormality. Termination of pregnancy may be performed at any time if there is serious risk to the mother's life if the pregnancy were to continue. *See* ABORTION.

Human Fertilization and Embryology Authority (HFEA) a UK Statutory body, its primary purpose is to independently regulate the use of gametes and embryos in fertility treatment and research. It licenses fertility clinics and centres carrying out in vitro fertilization (IVF). HFEA produces a Code of Practice and information for the public. The HFEA also regulates and monitors the storage of sperm, eggs and embryos.

human immunodeficiency virus abbreviated HIV. A lentivirus that belongs to a group of viruses known as retroviruses and causes AIDS in humans. There are two main types of HIV: HIV-1, the predominant AIDS-causing virus in the world, and HIV-2, also an AIDS-causing virus that is found more commonly in countries on the west coast of Africa. HIV is transmitted sexually, parenterally, from mother to child (during pregnancy, at time of birth, or in the postnatal period from breast feeding) and more rarely, iatrogenically. Most people become infected sexually through unprotected penetrative vaginal or anal sexual intercourse. Unprotected means that the male insertive partner has not worn a good-quality, intact rubber latex condom. Parenteral transmission is usually associated with injecting drug users sharing contaminated injection equipment. Blood tests to identify HIV infection detect antibodies to the virus and may not be positive for 8–12 weeks following primary infection. Because it is not possible to detect all HIV-infected patients, all health care workers in direct patient contact should practise universal infection control precautions. *See* UNIVERSAL PRECAUTIONS and Appendix 11. Human Rights Act 1998 incorporates into domestic law the European Convention on Human Rights. The law prohibits any public authority acting in a way that is incompatible with a Convention right, acknowledging the principles and values of fairness together with respect for human dignity as core concepts covered by the Act.

humidity the degree of moisture in the air. *H. therapy* the therapeutic use of water to prevent or correct a moisture deficit in the respiratory tract. The principal reasons for employing humidity therapy are: (a) to prevent drying and irritation of the respiratory mucosa; (b) to facilitate ventilation and diffusion of oxygen and other therapeutic gases being administered; and (c) to aid in the removal of thick and viscous secretions that obstruct the air passages. Another important use of humidity therapy is to aid in obtaining an induced sputum specimen.

humoral immunity an older term for antibody mediated immunity. *See* IMMUNITY.

humour any fluid of the body, such as lymph or blood. *Aqueous h.* the fluid filling the anterior chamber of the eye.

Vitreous h. the jelly-like substance that fills the chamber of the eye between the lens and the retina.

Huntington's disease *G.S. Huntington, American physician, 1851–1927.* A rare, degenerative inherited disorder of the brain in which there is progressive chorea and mental deterioration (dementia).

Hurler's syndrome *G. Hurler, Austrian paediatrician, 1889–1965.* An inherited disorder in which learning difficulties are caused by excess glycosaminoglycans (formerly known as mucopolysaccharides) being stored in the brain and reticuloendothelial system. Also known as gargoylism and mucopolysaccharidosis type 1.

Hutchinson's teeth *Sir J. Hutchinson, British surgeon, 1828–1913.* Typical notching of the borders of the permanent incisor teeth occurring in congenital syphilis.

hyaline resembling glass. *H. degeneration* a form of deterioration that occurs in tumours and is due to deficiency of blood supply. It precedes cystic degeneration. *H. membrane disease see* RESPIRATORY (DISTRESS SYNDROME OF NEWBORN).

hyaluronidase an enzyme that facilitates the absorption of fluids in subcutaneous tissues.

hydatid a cystic swelling containing the embryo of *Echinococcus granulosus*. It may be found in any organ of the body, e.g., in the liver. 'Daughter cysts' are produced from the original. Infection is from contaminated foods, e.g., salads. *H. disease* the result of the presence of hydatids in the lungs, liver or brain.

hydatidiform resembling a hydatid cyst. *H. mole see* MOLE.

hydraemia a modification of the blood in which there is an excess of plasma in relation to the cells. A degree of hydraemia is physiological in pregnancy.

hydramnios an excessive amount of amniotic fluid in the uterus during pregnancy. It is associated with maternal diabetes, congenital abnormalities especially of the central nervous system and with uniovular twins. Sometimes used synonymously with polyhydramnios.

hydrarthrosis a collection of fluid in a joint.

hydrate a compound of an element with water, to combine with water.

hydroa vacciniforme a rare and chronic childhood hypersensitivity of the skin to sunlight, resulting in the formation of a vesicular eruption on the exposed parts, with intense irritation.

hydrocarbon a compound of hydrogen and carbon. Fats are of this type.

hydrocele a swelling caused by accumulation of fluid, especially in the tunica vaginalis surrounding the testicle.

hydrocephalus 'water on the brain'. Enlargement of the skull due to an abnormal collection of cerebrospinal fluid around the brain or in the ventricles. It may be either congenital or acquired from infection, trauma or tumour. The most effective treatment is surgical correction employing a shunting technique.

hydrochloric acid HCl, a colourless compound of hydrogen and chlorine. It is present, in 0.2% solution, in gastric juice and aids digestion.

hydrocolloid dressings absorbent dressings with a soft spongy consistency that are applied to wounds that are subject to pressure, for example those in the sacral area or on heels. They relieve pain from the site, rehydrate and encourage debridement and healing.

hydrogel dressings wound dressings that rehydrate dry necrotic tissue, reduce pain and promote healing.

hydrogen *symbol* H. A combustible gas, present in nearly all organic compounds, which, in combination with oxygen, forms water. *H. ion concentration* the amount of hydrogen in a liquid, which is responsible for its acidity. The degree of acidity is expressed in pH values: the higher the hydrogen ion concentration, the greater the acidity, and the lower the pH value. The concentration in the blood is of importance in acidosis.

hydrolysis the process of splitting up into smaller molecules by uniting with water.

hydrometer an instrument for estimating the specific gravity of fluids, e.g., a urinometer.

hydronephrosis an accumulation of urine in the pelvis of the kidney, resulting in atrophy of the kidney structure, due to an obstruction to the flow of urine from the kidney. The condition may be: (a) congenital, due to malformation of the kidney or ureter; or (b) acquired, due to an obstruction of the ureter by tumour or stone, or to back pressure from stricture of the urethra or an enlarged prostate gland.

hydropathy the treatment of disease by the use of water internally and externally; hydrotherapy.

hydropericarditis inflammation of the pericardium resulting in serous fluid in the pericardial sac.

hydroperitoneum *see* ASCITES.

hydrophobia 1. rabies. 2. irrational fear of water.

hydropneumothorax the presence of fluid and air in the pleural space.

hydrops [L.] abnormal accumulation of serous fluid in the tissues or in a body cavity; previously called dropsy. *Fetal h., h. fetalis* gross oedema of the entire body of the newborn infant, occurring in haemolytic disease of the newborn.

hydrotherapy the treatment of disease by means of water, e.g., douching or bathing.

hydrothorax fluid in the pleural cavity due to serous effusion, as in cardiac, renal and other diseases.

hydroureter an accumulation of urine in a ureter.

hygiene 1. the science of health and its preservation. 2. a condition of practice, such as cleanliness, that is conducive to preservation of health. *Communal h.* the maintenance of the health of the community by the provision of a pure water supply, efficient sanitation, good housekeeping, etc. *Industrial h.* (occupational health) care of the health of workers in an industry. *Mental h.* the science dealing with development of healthy mental and emotional reactions and habits. *Oral h.* the proper care of the mouth and teeth. *Personal h.* individual measures taken to preserve one's own cleanliness and wellbeing.

hygroma a swelling caused by fluid. *Cystic h.* a cystic lymphangioma of the neck. *Subdural h.* a collection of clear fluid in the subdural space.

hygrometer an instrument for measuring the water vapour in the air.

hygroscopic readily absorbing moisture. An example is glycerin, which is used in suppositories as a means of aiding evacuation by moistening the faeces.

hymen a fold of mucous membrane partially closing the entrance to the vagina. *Imperforate h.* a membrane which completely occludes the vaginal orifice.

hyoid shaped like a U. *H. bone* a U-shaped bone above the thyroid cartilage, to which the tongue is attached.

hyperacidity excessive acidity. *Gastric h.* hyperchlorhydria.

hyperactive exhibiting hyperactivity; hyperkinetic.

hyperactivity abnormally increased activity. Developmental hyperactivity of children (hyperkinesia) is characterized by very restless, impulsive behaviour. These children are usually aged between 2 and 4 years, inattentive and have a poor concentration span. Other features that may be associated with hyperactivity include aggression, anxiety, poor eating and sleeping patterns, and social and learning difficulties. Persistent hyperactivity is known as attention deficit hyperactivity disorder, which may require assessment and treatment. *See* ATTENTION DEFICIT SYNDROME.

hyperaemia excess of blood in any part.

hyperaesthesia excessive sensitiveness to touch or to other sensations, e.g., taste or smell.

hyperalimentation a programme of parenteral administration of all nutrients for patients with gastrointestinal dysfunction; also called total parenteral alimentation (TPA) and total parenteral nutrition (TPN). Although the term hyperalimentation is commonly used to designate total or supplementary nutrition by intravenous feedings, it is not technically correct inasmuch as the procedure does not involve an abnormally increased or excessive amount of feeding. *See* NUTRITION (PARENTERAL). *See* Appendix 1.

hyperasthenia extreme weakness.

hyperbaric at a greater pressure than normal; applied to gases under greater than atmospheric pressure. *H. oxygenation* exposure to oxygen under conditions of greatly increased pressure. The patient is placed in a sealed enclosure, called a hyperbaric chamber. Compressed air is introduced; at the same time the patient is given pure oxygen through a face mask. Patients suffering from tetanus and gas gangrene, infections caused by bacteria that are resistant to antibiotics but vulnerable to oxygen, are helped by hyperbaric oxygenation. The technique is also useful in radiotherapy for cancer. When full of oxygen, cancer cells seem more vulnerable to radiation. Carbon monoxide poisoning can be treated by hyperbaric oxygenation. Carbon monoxide molecules, displacing the oxygen in the erythrocytes, usually cause asphyxiation, but hyperbaric oxygenation can often keep the patient alive until the carbon monoxide has been eliminated from the body's system.

hyperbilirubinaemia an excess of bilirubin in the blood.

hypercalcaemia an excess of calcium in the blood. May rarely be caused by over administration of vitamin D, hyperparathyroidism, thyrotoxicosis, prolonged immobility, breakdown of bone by malignant disease, or impaired renal function.

hypercalciuria a high level of calcium in the urine leading to renal stone formation.

hypercapnia an increased amount of carbon dioxide in the blood, causing overstimulation of the respiratory centre. Hypercarbia.

hypercatabolism an excessive rate of catabolism leading to wasting or destruction of a part or tissue.

hyperchloraemia an excess of chloride in the blood.

hyperchlorhydria an excess of hydrochloric acid in the gastric juice.

hypercholesteraemia, hypercholesterolaemia excess of cholesterol in the blood. Predisposes to atheroma and gallstones.

hyperemesis excessive vomiting. *H. gravidarum* an uncommon, serious complication of pregnancy, characterized by severe and persistent vomiting necessitating medical intervention. It is associated with fluid and electrolyte imbalance and a 10% weight loss of the prepregnant weight. The aetiology is not fully understood.

hyperextension the forcible extension of a limb beyond the normal. It is used to correct orthopaedic deformities.

hyperflexion the forcible bending of a joint beyond the normal.

hypergalactia, hypergalactosis excessive secretion of milk.

hyperglycaemia excess of sugar in the blood (normal 4.0–5.9 mmol/litre when fasting); a sign of diabetes mellitus. *See* HYPOGLYCAEMIA; Table on p. 113.

hyperhidrosis excessive perspiration; hyperidrosis.

hyperkalaemia an excess of potassium in the blood. If untreated, this will lead to cardiac arrest.

hyperkeratosis hypertrophy of the horny layers of the skin.

hyperkinesis a condition in which there is excessive motor activity. *See* HYPERACTIVITY.

hyperlipaemia an excess of fat or lipids in the blood.

hypermastia 1. the presence of one or more supernumerary breasts. 2. overdevelopment of one or both breasts.

hypermetropia hyperopia; longsightedness. The light rays entering the eye converge beyond the retina. Clear vision can be obtained by the wearing of spectacles or contact lenses.

hypermobility some or all joints have an unusually large range of movement. *Joint h. syndrome* hypermobility with pain and stiffness of joints and muscles, thin stretchy skin, repeated sprains, strains and dislocations, poor balance and co-ordination, and digestive problems.

hypermotility abnormal or excessive movement usually referring to all or part of the gastrointestinal tract.

hypernatraemia an excess of sodium in the blood, usually diagnosed when the plasma sodium is above 150 mmol/litre. It is the result of loss of water and electrolytes from the body caused by diarrhoea, polyuria, excessive sweating or inadequate fluid intake.

hyperostosis a thickening of bone; a bony outgrowth; exostosis.

hyperparathyroidism excessive activity of the parathyroid glands, causing drainage of calcium from the bones, with consequent fragility and liability to spontaneous fracture.

hyperphasia excessive talkativeness.

hyperpituitarism overactivity of the pituitary gland.

hyperplasia excessive formation of normal cells in a tissue or organ, which increases in size.

hyperpnoea overbreathing; hyperventilation; an abnormal increase in the rate and depth of breathing.

hyperprolactinaemia increased levels of prolactin in the blood; in women, it is associated with infertility and may lead to galactorrhoea. In men it may cause impotence and loss of libido.

hyperpyrexia an excessively high body temperature, i.e., over 41°C.

hypersensitivity abnormal sensitivity, especially to a particular antigen. The reactions include allergies (such as asthma) and anaphylaxis. *Contact h.* produced by contact of the skin with a chemical substance having the properties of an antigen or hapten; it includes contact dermatitis (*see* CONTACT). *Delayed h.* a slowly developing increase in cell-mediated immune response (involving T lymphocytes) to a specific antigen, as occurs in graft rejection, autoimmune disease, etc. *Immediate h.* antibody-mediated hypersensitivity characterized by lesions resulting from release of histamine and other mediators of hypersensitivity from reagin-sensitized mast cells, causing increased vascular permeability, oedema and smooth muscle contraction; it includes anaphylaxis and atopy.

hypersplenism overactivity of an enlarged spleen resulting in the depression of blood cells and platelets.

hypertelorism abnormally increased distance between two organs or parts. *Ocular h., orbital h.* increase in the interocular distance, often associated with craniofacial dysostosis and sometimes with learning disabilities.

hypertension persistently high BLOOD PRESSURE. In adults, it is generally agreed that a blood pressure is abnormally high when the resting, supine arterial systolic pressure is equal to or greater than 140 mmHg and the diastolic pressure is equal to or greater than 90 mmHg. A diagnosis of hypertension should be based on a series of readings rather than a single measurement and will vary with age. Hypertension is very common and usually symptomless but may cause headaches and visual disturbances when severe. Its incidence is highest in men, the middle-aged and the elderly. Associated factors are smoking, high-salt diet, obesity, a family history, lack of exercise and a high degree of stress. Lifestyle changes are recommended, e.g., losing weight, giving up smoking, adopting a low-salt diet. Antihypertensive drugs may be needed to maintain blood pressure readings within reasonable levels. Hypertension is considered to be a risk factor for the development of cardiovascular disease. *Essential h.* high blood pressure without demonstrable change in kidneys, blood vessels or heart.

hyperthermia an exceedingly high body temperature. *Malignant h.* a serious condition, sometimes arising during general anaesthesia.

hyperthyroidism excessive activity of the thyroid gland. See THYROTOXICOSIS.

hypertonic 1. showing excessive tone or tension, as in a blood vessel or muscle. 2. describing a solution that has greater osmotic pressure than normal physiological tissue fluid. *See* HYPOTONIC.

hypertrichosis excessive growth of hair on any part of the body.

hypertrophy an increase in the size of a tissue or a structure caused by an increase in the size of the cells that compose it (as opposed to an increase in the number of cells). *See* HYPERPLASIA.

hyperuricaemia an excess of uric acid in the blood. *See* GOUT.

hyperventilation 1. increase of air in the lungs above the normal amount. 2. abnormally prolonged and deep breathing, usually associated with acute anxiety or emotional tension. Hyperpnoea. Also occurs in uncontrolled diabetes mellitus, kidney failure and in some lung disorders. Symptoms occur as a result of an abnormal loss of carbon dioxide from the blood and include faintness, tetany and a tense feeling of not being able to take a full breath.

hypervitaminosis a condition caused by the intake of an excessive quantity of vitamins.

hypervolaemia abnormal increase in the volume of circulating fluid (plasma) in the body.

hyphaema haemorrhage into the anterior chamber of the eye.

hypnosis an artificially induced passive state in which there is increased amenability and responsiveness to suggestions and commands. In hypnosis, a drowsy phase is followed by a sleep. It may also be used to produce painless childbirth and tooth extraction.

hypnotherapy treatment by hypnosis or by the induction of prolonged sleep.

hypnotic an agent that causes sleep; a soporific.

hypnotism the practice of hypnosis.

hypocalcaemia a deficiency of calcium in the blood.

hypocapnia a deficiency of carbon dioxide in the blood.

hypochloraemia a deficiency of chloride in the blood.

hypochlorhydria a lower than normal amount of hydrochloric acid in the gastric juice.

hypochlorite any salt of hypochlorous acid used in solution to yield chlorine, a disinfecting and germicidal agent.

hypochondria a morbid preoccupation or anxiety about one's health. The sufferer feels that first one part of the body and then another part is the seat of some serious disease.

hypochondriac one affected by hypochondria. *H. region* the hypochondrium.

hypochondrium the upper region of the abdomen on each side of the epigastrium.

hypodermic beneath the skin; applied to subcutaneous injections and to the syringes used for such injections.

hypofibrinogenaemia a lack of fibrinogen in the blood. This may occur in severe trauma or haemorrhage or as an inherited condition.

hypogammaglobulinaemia a deficiency of gamma-globulin in the blood, rendering the person susceptible to infection.

hypogastrium the lower middle area of the abdomen, immediately below the umbilical region.

hypoglossal under the tongue. *H. nerve* the 12th cranial nerve.

hypoglycaemia a condition in which the blood sugar level is less than normal. Usually arising in diabetic patients as a result of insulin overdosage, delay in eating or a rapid combustion of carbohydrate. *See* HYPERGLYCAEMIA; Table on p. 113.

hypokalaemia a low potassium level in the blood. This is likely to be present in dehydration and with the repeated use of diuretics.

hypomania a degree of elation, excitement and activity higher than normal but less severe than that present in mania.

hypometropia myopia; shortsightedness.

hypomotility deficient power of movement in any part.

hyponatraemia a deficiency of sodium in the blood.

hypoparathyroidism a lack of parathyroid secretion, leading to a low blood calcium and tetany.

hypophysis an outgrowth. *H. cerebri* the pituitary gland.

hypopituitarism deficiency of secretion from the anterior lobe of the pituitary gland, causing excessive deposition of fat in children. *See* FRÖHLICH'S SYNDROME. Dwarfism may result. In adults asthenia, drowsiness and adiposity may occur, together with an impairment of sexual activity and premature senility.

hypoplasia imperfect development of a part or organ.

hypopnoea shallow breathing.

hypoproteinaemia a deficiency of serum proteins in the blood.

hypoprothrombinaemia a deficiency of prothrombin in the blood, leading to a tendency to bleed. *See* HAEMOPHILIA.

hyposecretion a deficiency in secretion from any glandular structure or secreting cells.

hyposensitivity a lack of sensitivity, especially to a particular allergen to which the patient may have been exposed over a period.

hypospadias a developmental anomaly in the male in which the urethra opens on the underside of the penis or on the perineum.

hypostasis 1. a sediment or deposit. 2. congestion of blood in a part, due to slowing of the circulation.

hypostatic relating to hypostasis. *H. pneumonia see* PNEUMONIA.

hypotension abnormally low arterial blood pressure; hypopiesis. *Controlled* or *induced h.* an artificially produced lowering of the blood pressure so that an operation field is rendered practically bloodless. *Orthostatic* or *postural h.* temporary hypotension when the patient stands up, producing giddiness and sometimes a faint.

hypotensive producing a reduction in tension, especially pertaining to a drug that lowers the blood pressure.

hypothalamus in the brain a portion of grey matter lying beneath the thalamus at the base of the cerebrum, and forming the floor and part of the lateral wall of the third ventricle. It influences peripheral autonomic mechanisms, endocrine activity and many somatic functions, e.g., a general regulation of water balance, body temperature, sleep, thirst and hunger, and the development of secondary sexual characteristics. It plays an important role in the regulation of protein, fat and carbohydrate metabolism, body fluid volume and electrolyte content, and internal secretion of endocrine hormones.

hypothermia 1. a severe reduction in the core body temperature to below 35°C. The condition usually arises gradually and may prove fatal if untreated.

It is most common among babies and elderly people. 2. artificial cooling of the body to reduce the oxygen requirements of the tissues. Generalized lowering of the body temperature is used in three main situations: (a) to control fever, as in malignant hyperthermia; (b) to enable certain cardiac and neurological operations to be carried out; and (c) to protect the brain from raised intracranial pressure in patients with head injuries or following drowning.

hypothesis a supposition that appears to explain a group of phenomena and is assumed as a basis of reasoning and experimentation. A starting point for further investigations from known facts.

hypothrombinaemia a diminished amount of thrombin in the blood, with a consequent tendency to bleed.

hypothyroidism an insufficiency of thyroid secretion. Hypothyroidism is diagnosed by measuring the level of thyroid hormones in the blood. Babies are screened for the condition shortly after birth as part of the newborn screening programme.

hypotonia 1. deficient muscle tone. 2. deficient tension in the eyeball.

hypotonic describing a solution that has a lower osmotic pressure than another one. *See* HYPERTONIC.

hypoventilation hypopnoea; shallow breathing, usually at a very slow rate. It may cause a build-up of carbon dioxide in the blood.

hypovolaemia a reduction in the circulating blood volume due to external loss of body fluids or to loss from the blood into the tissues, as in shock.

hypoxaemia an insufficient oxygen content in the blood.

hypoxia a diminished amount of oxygen in the tissues. *Anaemic h.* low oxygen content due to deficiency of haemoglobin in the blood.

hysterectomy removal of the uterus. *Abdominal h.* removal via an abdominal incision. *Subtotal h.* removal of the body of the uterus only. *Total h.* removal of the body and cervix.

Vaginal h. removal through the vagina. ***Wertheim's h.*** additional excision of the parametrium, upper vagina and lymph glands. Radical abdominal hysterectomy.

hysteria a psychoneurosis in which the individual converts anxiety created by emotional conflict into physical symptoms, e.g., tics, mutism or paralysis of an arm or leg, that have no organic basis; formerly called conversion reaction or conversion hysteria. The term hysteria is also used to describe a state of tension or excitement in which there is a temporary loss of control over the emotions.

hysterical relating to hysteria.

hystero-oöphorectomy excision of the uterus and the ovaries.

hysterosalpingography radiographic examination of the uterus and uterine tubes after the injection of a radio-opaque dye. Uterosalpingography.

hysterosalpingostomy or an anastomis the operation of forming an anastomosis, or opening, between the distal portion of the uterine tube and the uterus in an effort to overcome infertility when the medial portion is occluded or excised.

hysterotomy incision of the uterus, usually in order to remove a fetus in mid-pregnancy when it is too late to perform a therapeutic abortion.

I symbol for *iodine*.

iatrogenesis additional patient problems, complications or disease brought about by the activities of physicians, surgeons or other health care professionals, including new infections, unwanted effects of drug therapy and psychological distress.

ice water in a solid state, at or below freezing point. *Dry i.* solid form of carbon dioxide also known as cardice. *I. bag* a rubber or plastic bag half-filled with pieces of ice and applied near or to a part to relieve pain or swelling.

ichthyosis a congenital abnormality of the skin in which there is dryness and roughness, the horny layer is thickened and large scales appear.

ICM International Confederation of Midwives. International Council of Nurses.

ICP 1. integrated care pathway. 2. intracranial pressure.

ICSH interstitial cell stimulating hormone.

icterus jaundice. *I. gravis* a rare but fatal form of jaundice occurring in pregnancy. Acute yellow atrophy. *I. gravis neonatorum* haemolytic disease of the newborn. *See* RHESUS FACTOR.

ICU intensive care unit.

id that part of the personality, containing the instinctive drives, which leads to gratification of primitive needs and which exists in the unconscious.

idea a mental impression or conception. *Autochthonous i.* a strange idea that comes into the mind in some unaccountable way, but is not a hallucination. *Compulsive i.* an idea that persists despite reason and will and that drives one to action, usually inappropriate. *Dominant i.* a morbid or other impression that controls or colours every action and thought. *Fixed i.* a persistent morbid impression or belief that cannot be changed by reason. *I. of reference* the incorrect idea that the words and actions of others refer to oneself, or the projection of the causes of one's own imaginary difficulties upon someone else.

identical exactly alike. *I. twins* twins of the same sex developing from a single fertilized ovum. Monozygotic.

identification a mental mechanism by which an individual adopts the attitudes and ideas of another, often admired, person.

identity part of the 'self concept' of being distinguishable and separate from others and who they are in relation to their group or society. People may have several identities, for example: British, midwife, marathon runner and artist. *I. crisis* one in which the individual loses the sense of self-distinctiveness and role in society. Occurs most commonly in the transition from one phase of life to the next, e.g., during adolescence.

ideology 1. the science of the development of ideas. 2. the body of ideas characteristic of an individual or of a social unit.

ideomotion the association of ideas and muscle action, as in involuntary acts.

idiopathic self-originated; applied to a condition the cause of which is not known.

idiosyncrasy 1. a habit or quality of body or mind peculiar to any individual. 2. an abnormal susceptibility to an agent (e.g., a drug) that is peculiar to the individual.

Ig immunoglobulin of any of the five classes: IgA, IgD, IgE, IgG and IgM.

ileal referring to the ileum. *I. conduit* a surgical procedure in which the ureters are transplanted into the ileum, an isolated loop of which is then brought to the surface of the abdomen in order to allow the urine to drain into a bag.

ileitis inflammation of the ileum. *Regional i.* Crohn's disease. A chronic condition of the terminal portion of the ileum in which granulation and oedema may give rise to obstruction.

ileocolitis inflammation of the ileum and colon.

ileocolostomy the making of a permanent opening between the ileum and some part of the colon.

ileoproctostomy surgical anastomosis between the ileum and the rectum; ileorectal anastomosis.

ileorectal referring to the ileum and rectum. *I. anastomosis* ileoproctostomy.

ileosigmoidostomy an operation carried out when most of the colon has to be removed and an anastomosis is made between the ileum and the sigmoid colon.

ileostomy an artificial opening (stoma) created from the ileum and brought to the surface of the abdomen for the purpose of evacuation. Ileostomy is an inevitable part of proctocolectomy. An ileostomy may be temporary or permanent. *I. bags* disposable stoma bags to collect the liquid faecal matter discharged from an ileostomy.

ileum the last part of the small intestine, terminating at the caecum.

ileus failure of peristalsis. Decreased propulsive ability is caused by bowel obstruction or intestinal atony or paralysis. The principal symptoms of ileus are abdominal pain and distension, vomiting (the vomitus may contain faecal material) and constipation. If the intestinal obstruction is not relieved, the patient becomes extremely ill with SHOCK and DEHYDRATION.

iliac pertaining to the ilium. *I. artery* the right and left arteries form the terminal branches of the abdominal aorta and supply blood to the pelvic region and the lower limbs. *I. crest* the crest of the hip bone. *I. fossa* the depression on the concave surface of the iliac bone. *I. vein* the right and left veins join to form the inferior vena cava and drain the blood from the lower limbs and pelvis.

ilium the haunch bone; the upper part of the hip bone.

illness a condition marked by pronounced deviation from the normal healthy state; sickness. *I. behaviour* the way in which ill individuals regard the structure and function of their own body, interpret symptoms and seek treatment for their condition.

illusion a mistaken perception due to a misinterpretation of a sensory stimulus; believing something to be what it is not.

image 1. the mental recall of a former precept. 2. the optical picture transferred to the brain cells by the optic nerve.

imaging diagnostic techniques that are used to produce images of organs or tissues within the body. These may be plain X-rays to view dense structures such as bone, or contrast X-rays used to view internal organs, e.g., barium X-rays to examine the oesophagus, stomach and small intestine. Techniques include ultrasonography. Computerized tomography (CT) uses X-rays and a scanner, other techniques include radionuclide scans and magnetic resonance and positron emission tomography (*see* MAGNETIC RESONANCE IMAGING and RADIONUCLIDE). Techniques use computers to process the data and produce the image.

imago [L.] 1. in psychoanalysis, a childhood memory or fantasy of a loved person that persists in adult life. 2. the adult or definitive form of an insect.

imbalance lack of balance, e.g., of endocrine secretions, between water and electrolytes, or of muscles.

immature unripe; not fully developed, as in a cataract when only a part of the lens is opaque.

immiscible incapable of being mixed, e.g., oil and water.

immobilize to render incapable of being moved, as by a plaster of Paris cast.

immune protected against a particular infection or allergy. *I. response* the (in general) helpful events that follow activation of the immune system, including T lymphocyte activity (cell-mediated responses) and B lymphocyte activity (humoral responses). Immune responses are involved in protecting persons from disease following infection and are also involved in the rejection of transplanted organs and tissues that the body recognizes as foreign, or non-self.

immunity the resistance possessed by the body to infectious diseases, foreign tissues, foreign non-toxic substances and other ANTIGENS. The opposite of susceptibility. Immunological responses in humans can be divided into two broad categories: humoral immunity, which takes place in the body fluids and is concerned with antibody and complement activities; and cell-mediated or cellular immunity, which involves a variety of activities designed to destroy or at least contain cells that are recognized by the body as alien and harmful. Both types of response are instigated by lymphocytes that originate in the bone marrow as stem cells and later are converted into mature cells having specific properties and functions. The two

kinds of lymphocyte that are important to the establishment of immunity are T lymphocytes (T cells), which kill cells infected with viruses and other intracellular parasites, and B lymphocytes (B cells). B lymphocytes mature into plasma cells that are primarily responsible for forming antibodies, thereby providing humoral immunity. Cellular immunity is dependent upon T lymphocytes and is primarily concerned with a delayed type of immune response as occurs in the rejection of transplanted organs, defence against some slowly developing bacterial diseases, allergic reactions and certain autoimmune diseases.

immunization the act of creating immunity by artificial means. *I. schedule* a standard schedule for immunization against infectious diseases (*see* Appendix 10).

immunoassay a quantitative estimate of the proteins contained in the blood serum.

immunodeficiency a deficiency of the immune response, either that mediated by humoral antibody or by cell-mediated responses involving a deficiency of T lymphocytes. *I. disorders* acquired or congenital conditions in which the body's immune system fails to protect against infection, foreign material and some forms of cancer.

immunoglobulin *See* ANTIBODY.

immunology the study of immunity and the body's defence mechanisms.

immunosuppression inhibition of the formation of antibodies to antigens that may be present; used in transplantation procedures to prevent rejection of the transplanted organ or tissue.

immunosuppressive 1. pertaining to or inducing immunosuppression. 2. an agent that induces immunosuppression.

immunotherapy the use of knowledge about immunity to prevent and treat disease. May be used to mean desensitization therapy against specific allergens e.g., snake venom or in therapeutics.

immunotransfusion transfusion of blood from a donor previously rendered immune to the disease affecting the patient.

impaction a state of being wedged. *Dental i.* the condition in which a tooth, usually a molar, is unable to erupt through the gum because it is lodged in position by bone or the other teeth. *Faecal i.* a collection of putty-like or hardened faeces in the rectum or sigmoid colon.

impairment any loss or abnormality of psychological, physiological or anatomical structure or function.

impalpable incapable of being felt by manual examination. May apply to an organ or a tumour.

imperforate without an opening. *I. anus* a congenital defect in which this opening is closed. *I. hymen* complete closure of the vaginal opening by the hymen.

impermeable not permitting the passage of fluid or molecules.

impetigo an acute contagious inflammation of the skin marked by pustules and scabs; of streptococcal or staphylococcal origin. It occurs most commonly on the face and scalp, particularly those of children.

implant any substance grafted into the tissues; may be living cells or inert materials. *Hormone i.* a hormonal pellet which may be implanted subcutaneously. *Intraocular lens i.* a plastic lens which may be implanted in the eye after lens extraction. *Plastic i.* a silicone implant which may be used in plastic surgery, e.g., to reshape the breast.

implantable cardioverter defibrillator (ICD) an implanted device that automatically terminates life-threatening arrhythmias by delivering low energy shocks to the heart, restoring normal rhythm. Some devices have inbuilt pacing capabilities.

implantation the act of planting or setting in. 1. the embedding of the fertilized ovum in the wall of the uterus. 2. the placing of a drug within the tissues. 3. the surgical introduction of healthy tissue to replace tissue that has been damaged.

implementation a phase of the nursing process signifying the giving of care in relation to defined nursing interventions and goals. During this phase the plan of care is put into action.

implosion in behaviour therapy, a form of desensitization used in the treatment of phobias and related disorders. *See* FLOODING.

impotence an outdated term commonly used by the lay person of erectile dysfunction and/or premature ejaculation. The inability in a man to carry out sexual intercourse from either psychological or physical causes.

impregnation insemination; rendering pregnant.

impression an imitation of a person or thing. In dentistry, a mould made of a toothless jaw or of the teeth and surrounding tissues, used in the construction of dentures and dental braces.

impulse 1. a sudden pushing force. 2. a sudden uncontrollable act. 3. nerve impulse. *Cardiac i.* movement of the chest wall caused by the heart beat. *Nerve i.* the electrochemical process propagated along nerve fibres.

IMV intermittent mandatory ventilation.

inaccessibility a state of unresponsiveness characteristic of certain psychiatric patients, e.g., those with schizophrenia.

inarticulate 1. without joints. 2. unable to speak intelligibly.

incarcerated held fast. Applied to (a) a hernia that is immovable, and therefore only curable by operation, and (b) a pregnant uterus held under the sacral brim.

incest sexual intercourse between close blood relatives, e.g., brothers and sisters; marriage between them is legally or culturally prohibited. Some form of incest taboo is found in all known societies, although the relationships prohibited vary.

incidence the number of particular new events which occur in a population in a given period of time. For example, the number of new cases of a disease, such as measles, expressed per 1000 of population per year.

Incident Report a report the completion of which is required of all health care facilities following any accident or untoward incident or near miss involving a patient, visitor or member of staff. These incidents may be clinical, e.g., cardiac arrest or the incorrect administration of a medication, but can also include such issues as the loss of a patient's belongings.

incipient beginning to exist.

incision 1. in surgery, a cut into soft tissue. 2. the act of cutting.

incisor one of the four front teeth in the centre of each jaw.

inclusion something that is enclosed or the act of enclosing. *I. bodies* particles that are temporarily enclosed in the cytoplasm of a cell. For example, in trachoma virus particles can be seen in the conjunctival epithelial cells. Also known as elementary bodies.

incoherent 1. unconnected; inconsistent. 2. uttering speech that is disconnected and rambling.

incompatibility the state of two or more substances being antagonistic, or destroying the efficiency of each other. Applied to mixtures of drugs, and to blood. *See* BLOOD GROUPS.

incompetence inefficiency. *Aortic i.* failure of the aortic valves to regulate the flow of blood. *Mitral i.* failure of the mitral valve to close properly.

incontinence inability to control natural functions or discharges. *Faecal i.* inability to control the movements of the bowels. *Overflow i.* that from an overfull bladder, most common in elderly men with urinary obstruction. *Paralytic i.* loss of control of anal and urethral sphincters due to injury to nerve centres. *Stress i.* that which is due to a defect in the urethral sphincters and is liable to occur when intra-abdominal pressure is increased, as in coughing or lifting heavy weights; most common in women with weak pelvic muscles. *Urinary i.* inability to control the outflow of urine.

incoordination inability to adjust various muscle movements harmoniously.

increment an increase or addition.

incremental to build up as in the contractions of labour or to add in stages.

incrustation the formation of a crust or scab on a wound.

incubation the development and growth of microorganisms and animal embryos. *I. period* the period between the date of infection and the appearance of symptoms of an infectious disease.

incubator 1. an apparatus providing a suitable environment for preterm and ill babies. 2. an apparatus used in a laboratory to develop bacteria at a uniform temperature suitable to their growth.

incus the small anvil-shaped bone of the middle ear. The second auditory ossicle.

indicator 1. the index finger, or the extensor muscle of the index finger. 2. any substance that indicates the appearance or disappearance of a chemical by a colour change or attainment of a certain pH.

indigenous occurring naturally in a certain locality.

indigestion *see* DYSPEPSIA.

indolent slow-growing. Reluctant to heal. Largely painless. *I. ulcer* a chronic ulcer of the skin or mucous membrane.

induction the act of initiating something. *Electromagnetic i.* the production of an electric current in a body because of its nearness to an electrified (or magnetized) body. *I. of abortion* the intentional bringing about of an abortion. *I. of anaesthesia* the start of the administration of a general anaesthetic. *I. of labour* the artificial starting of the process of childbirth.

induration the abnormal hardening of a tissue or organ.

induratio penis plastica (IPP) *see* PEYRONIE'S DISEASE.

industrial referring to industry. *I. or occupational diseases* those that are caused by the nature of the work. *Prescribed i. diseases* those for which Industrial Injuries Disablement benefit is payable.

inebriation the condition of being intoxicated by alcohol; drunkenness.

inert having no action. *I. gas* a gas which does not react with other elements, e.g., neon.

inertia sluggishness; inability to move except when stimulated by an external force. *Uterine i.* lack of muscle contraction during the first and second stages of labour.

infant a child under 1 year of age. Educationally, a child under 7 years of age. *Floppy i., floppy i. syndrome* a congenital myopathy of infants, marked clinically by myotonia and muscle weakness. *I. feeding* the supplying of nutrition to an infant. Breast milk is the ideal food for the baby and if breast feeding is established satisfactorily for the first few months it can aid physical and emotional development. Where it is not possible an infant food formula can be given. *I. mortality rate* the number of deaths of children under 1 year of age per 1000 live births in any one year. *Premature i.* one born before the state of maturity. *See* PRETERM INFANT.

infanticide the killing of a child during the first year of its life.

infantile concerning an infant; childish. *I. paralysis* poliomyelitis.

infantilism persistence of the characteristics of childhood into adult life, marked by underdevelopment of the reproductive organs, and often short stature.

infarct the wedge-shaped area of necrosis in an organ, usually the lung or myocardium, produced by the blocking of an end blood vessel, usually due to an embolism, atheroma or thrombosis.

infarction the formation of an infarct. *Myocardial i.* an infarct of the heart muscle following a coronary thrombosis. *Pulmonary i.* an infarct resulting from obstruction of a branch of the pulmonary artery by embolism or thrombosis.

infection 1. invasion and multiplication of microorganisms in body tissues, especially that causing local cellular injury due to competitive metabolism, toxins, intracellular replication or antigen–antibody response. 2. an infectious disease. *Aerobic i.* infection caused by an aerobe. *Airborne i.* infection by inhalation of organisms suspended in air on water droplets, droplet nuclei or dust particles. *Anaerobic i.* infection caused by an ANAEROBE. *Cross i.* infection transmitted between patients infected with different pathogenic microorganisms. *Droplet i.* infection due to inhalation of respiratory pathogens suspended on liquid particles exhaled by someone already infected. *Health care-associated infections* those acquired during episodes of health care, usually but not exclusively in hospitals. The most common causative agents are *Escherichia coli, Proteus, Pseudomonas* and *Klebsiella* among the gram-negative organisms, and *Staphylococcus, Clostridium difficile* and *Enterococcus* among the gram-positive organisms. *Mixed i.* infection with more than one kind of organism at the same time. *Opportunistic i.* an infection with a microorganism that does not usually cause disease but may do so when the patient's resistance to infection is lowered, e.g., after surgery. *Secondary i.* infection by a pathogen superimposed upon an infection by a pathogen of another kind. *Sexually transmitted i.* an infection transmitted by sexual intercourse or by intimate contact with the genitals, mouth and rectum. *See* SEXUALLY TRANSMITTED INFECTION. *Subclinical i.* infection associated with no detectable symptoms but caused by microorganisms capable of producing easily recognizable diseases, such as poliomyelitis or mumps; it is detected by the production of antibody, or by delayed hypersensitivity exhibited in a skin test reaction to such antigens as tuberculoprotein.

infection prevention and control the utilization of procedures and techniques in the surveillance, investigation and compilation of statistical data in order to reduce the spread of infection, particularly hospital-acquired infections. Practitioners in infection prevention and control are frequently nurses with specialist qualifications who are employed by NHS Trusts and other health care facilities. They have titles such as Director of Infection Prevention and Control (DIPC), Consultants in Infection Prevention and Control, and Infection Prevention and Control Practitioners/ Nurses, and they function as liaison between staff, nurses, doctors, department heads and infection prevention and control committees. Such practitioners also assume some responsibility for teaching patients and their families, as well as employees.

infectious caused by or capable of being communicated by infection. *I. disease* disease caused by a specific, pathogenic microorganism capable of transmission to another individual by direct and indirect contact. *See also* COMMUNICABLE DISEASE. *I. mononucleosis* glandular fever. An acute virus infection, characterized by sore throat and glandular enlargement, caused by the Epstein–Barr (EB) virus. A common infection worldwide, particularly prevalent in older children and young adults in Western countries. The source of infection is human and spread is by oropharyngeal secretions: for example, during kissing. The incubation period is 4–6 weeks and infectivity after the disease may be prolonged.

infective infectious, capable of producing infection; pertaining to or characterized by the presence of pathogens.

inferior lower. *I. vena cava* the lower large vein.

inferiority lesser rank, stature, position or ability. *I. complex see* COMPLEX.

infertility inability of a woman to conceive or of a man to bring about conception.

infestation the presence of animal parasites, e.g., mites, ticks or worms, in or on the body, in clothing or in a house.

infibulation an extensive form of female circumcision performed in some cultures in which the clitoris and labia are removed and the vaginal entrance narrowed. Also known as Type III female genital mutilation according to the WHO classification system. *See* CIRCUMCISION.

infiltration the entrance and diffusion of some substance not usually found there, either fluid or solid, into tissues or cells. *I. analgesia* the injection into tissues of a local analgesic solution.

inflammation a localized protective response elicited by injury or destruction of tissues, which serves to destroy, dilute or wall off both the injurious agent and the injured tissue. The cardinal signs are heat, swelling, pain and redness.

inflammatory bowel disease abbreviated IBD. Collective term for a group of chronic disorders affecting the small and/or large intestines that results in pain, bleeding and diarrhoea. *See* CROHN'S DISEASE.

influenza an acute viral infection of the respiratory tract, occurring in isolated cases, epidemics and pandemics. Also called 'flu'. Transmission is by droplet inhalation and the period of infectivity lasts from 1 day before the onset of symptoms until up to 7 days later. In the UK, most cases occur between December and May, with the peak incidence being in February. There is fever, headache, pain in the back and limbs, anorexia and sometimes nausea and vomiting. The fever subsides in 2–3 days, leaving a feeling of lassitude. There is no specific drug cure for influenza, but an influenza vaccine is available, the formulation of which is changed annually to include recently circulating strains of viruses on recommendation of the World Health Organization. Annual vaccination is advised for persons over 65 years, persons with a serious long-term medical condition, pregnant women, persons living in a residential or nursing home, and children in an at risk group aged 6 months to 2 years. It is routinely given through a nasal spray to children aged 2 and 3 years, children in school years 1, 2, 3 and 4, and older children at risk.

informal patient a patient who has entered hospital voluntarily, i.e., without any statutory requirements for detention.

informatics discipline that integrates science, computer science and information science in systematizing, identifying, collecting, processing and managing data. *Nursing i.* the way in which nurses, managers, researchers and practitioners use information systems in their work, enabling technology to develop a body of readily available knowledge to support the practice of nursing and the delivery of health care.

informed choice in order to make decisions about their own health care and treatment mentally competent patients need to be given information regarding their own condition that is accurate, non-judgemental and valid, in language that is jargon free and understandable. This enables the patient to make an informed choice from the treatment options. In some situations an interpreter may be required.

informed consent *see* CONSENT.

infrared rays of a lower wavelength than those in the visible spectrum. They can produce radiant heat which is used in the treatment of rheumatic conditions. *See* ULTRAVIOLET RAYS.

infusion 1. the process of extracting the soluble principles of substances (especially drugs) by soaking in water. 2. the solution thus produced. 3. the slow therapeutic introduction by gravity of fluid other than blood into a vein.

ingestion the taking in of food and drugs by mouth.

inguinal relating to the groin. *I. canal* the channel through the abdominal wall, above Poupart's ligament, through which the spermatic cord and vessels pass to the testis in the male, and which contains the round ligament of the uterus in the female. *I. ligament* Poupart's ligament; that connecting the anterior superior spine of the ilium to the tubercle of the pubis.

inhalation 1. the drawing of air or other substances into the lungs. 2. any drug or solution of drugs, administered (as by means of nebulizers or aerosols) by the nasal or oral respiratory route.

inhaler a device used for administering an inhalation of a drug in powder or as a vapour. Used mainly in the treatment of respiratory disorders, for example asthma and chronic respiratory disorders.

inherent a characteristic that is innate or natural and essentially a part of the person.

inheritance the acquisition of qualities and characteristics from parents and ancestors.

inhibition arrest or restraint of a process. In psychiatry, the unconscious restraining of an instinctual drive.

injection 1. the forcing of a liquid into a part, as into the subcutaneous tissues, the vascular tree or an organ (*see* Figure on p. 200). 2. a substance so forced or administered; in pharmacy, a solution of a medicament suitable for injection. 3. prominence of small blood vessels on the surface of an organ or tissue, frequently indicating the vascular phase of an inflammatory response. *Depot i.* the giving of a medication by injection, usually intramuscularly, that can be absorbed slowly over a period of time. Many drugs and hormones are given in this way. *Hypodermic i.* that made just below the skin; a subcutaneous injection. *Intramuscular i.* that made into a muscle. *Intrathecal i.* that made into the subarachnoid space of

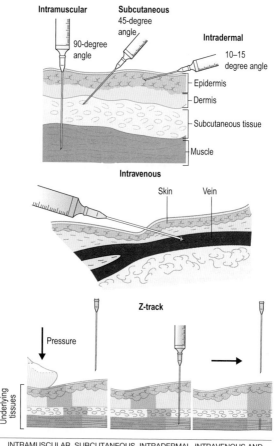

INTRAMUSCULAR, SUBCUTANEOUS, INTRADERMAL, INTRAVENOUS AND
Z-TRACK INJECTIONS

the spinal cord. *Intravenous i.* that made into a vein. *Subcutaneous i.* that made into the subcutaneous tissues; a hypodermic injection.

inlay material inserted to replace a defect in a tissue: for example, a bone graft or a filling cast in metal to fit a hole in a tooth.

innate inborn; present in the individual at birth.

innervation nerve supply to a part.

innocent as applied to a tumour, benign or non-malignant.

innocuous harmless.

innominate unnamed. *I. artery* a branch of the aorta, now termed the brachiocephalic trunk. *I. bone* the hip bone, formed by the union of the ilium, ischium and pubis.

inoculation 1. introduction of pathogenic microorganisms, injected material, serum or other substances into tissues of living organisms or into culture media. 2. introduction of a disease agent (usually a live infectious agent) into a healthy individual to produce a mild form of the disease, followed by IMMUNITY.

inorganic of neither animal nor vegetable origin.

inotropic affecting the force or energy of muscular contractions, particularly the heart muscle. Beta-blocking drugs are said to be inotropic.

inquest a legal inquiry held by a coroner, with or without a jury, into the cause of sudden or unexpected death.

insanity a legal term for mental illness, roughly equivalent to PSYCHOSIS and implying inability to be responsible for one's acts.

insecticide one of a large group of chemical compounds that kill insect pests.

insemination 1. fertilization of an ovum by a spermatozoon. 2. introduction of semen into the vagina. *Artificial i.* (AI) also known as intrauterine insemination (IUI) insemination by means other than sexual intercourse. The semen can be provided by either the husband (AIH) or partner or some other donor (AID).

insensible 1. unable to perceive with the senses. 2. unconscious. 3. imperceptible to the senses.

insertion 1. the act of implanting. 2. something that is implanted. 3. the attachment of a muscle to the bone that it moves.

insidious approaching by stealth. A term applied to any disease that develops imperceptibly.

insight mental awareness. The capacity of individuals to estimate a situation or their own behaviour or the connection between their present attitudes and past experiences. In psychiatry, a recognition by patients that they are ill. Insight in this connection may be complete, partial or absent, and may alter during the course of the illness.

in situ [L.] *in the original position.*

insoluble not capable of being dissolved in a liquid.

insomnia inability to sleep.

inspiration the act of drawing in the breath.

inspissated thickened, through evaporation, the absorption of fluid (and withdrawal of water) applied to culture medium in the laboratory and sputum.

instillation the act of inserting a liquid into a cavity drop by drop, e.g., into the eye.

instinct a complex of unlearned responses characteristic of a species. *Death i.* in psychoanalysis, the latent instinctive impulse towards death; the drive to reduce tensions by reaching the ultimate tensionless state of death. *Herd i.* the instinct or urge to be one of a group and to conform to its standards of conduct and opinion.

institutionalization a condition of apathy and withdrawal occurring in residents of long-stay institutions, prisons, etc., as a result of rigid routines and lack of independence. The person may resist leaving because the routine has become predictable and familiar, making minimal demands.

insufficiency inadequacy. Used to describe the failure of function of an organ, such as the heart, stomach, liver or muscles.

insufflation the act of blowing air, gas or powder into a cavity of the body.

insulin a peptide hormone formed in the beta cells of the pancreatic islets of Langerhans. The major fuel-regulating hormone, it is secreted into the blood in response to a rise in concentration of blood glucose or amino acids. A deficiency results in diabetes mellitus. Various types of genetically engineered insulin are available. Animal-derived insulin is also available but its use is declining. There are three main groups: rapid-acting, intermediate-acting and long-acting. Diabetic patients react differently in the rate at which they absorb and utilize insulin; therefore, the duration of action varies from patient to patient. Insulin is measured in units. The concentration used is 100 units/ml. This strength allows for accurate measurement of dosage and reduces the possibility of error in calculating an individual dose. *I. pump* a device consisting of a syringe filled with a predetermined amount of short-acting insulin, a plastic cannula and a needle, and a pump that periodically delivers the desired amount of insulin.

insulin dependent diabetes mellitus type 1 diabetes mellitus although insulin is prescribed to people with type 2 diabetes if oral medication is ineffective.

insulinoma a rare benign adenoma of the islet cells of the pancreas, causing hypoglycaemia.

insult any trauma, irritation, poisoning or injury to the body.

integrated care care that is person-centred and coordinated within healthcare settings, across mental and physical health and across health and social care.

integrated therapy a combination of complementary therapies with orthodox medicine to facilitate healing and promote the wellbeing of the patient. A biopsychosocial approach to care.

integument 1. the skin. 2. a layer of tissue covering a part or organ of the body.

intellect the mind, thinking faculty, reasoning or understanding.

intelligence 1. the capacity to understand. 2. general mental ability. *I. quotient* abbreviated IQ. The ratio of the mental age to the chronological age expressed as a percentage. *I. test* a test designed to measure the level of intelligence, usually expressed as an IQ.

Intensive Care Unit abbreviated ICU. A hospital unit in which are concentrated special equipment and specially trained personnel for the care of seriously ill patients requiring immediate and continuous monitoring and treatment. Also called critical care unit (CCU), intensive therapy unit (ITU). *Neonatal ICU* abbreviated NICU. An intensive care unit that is designated solely for small, preterm neonates and those neonates requiring surgery or other specialized care. *Paediatric ICU* abbreviated PICU. A unit providing intensive care solely for seriously ill children.

intention a process of healing.

intercellular between the cells of a structure. May be applied to the connective tissue or to fluid bathing the cells.

intercostal between the ribs. *I. muscles* muscles situated between the ribs and controlling their movements during inspiration and expiration.

intercourse 1. social exchange. 2. sexual intercourse or coitus.

intercurrent occurring at the same time. Describes a disease occurring during the course of another disease in the same person.

interdisciplinary joint working between professional disciplines: nursing, social work, clergy, medical staff, physiotherapy and other allied health professions.

interferon a protein, produced by cells infected by a virus, which has an inhibitory effect on the multiplication of the invading viruses, thus preventing uninfected cells from becoming infected and hastening recovery from viral disease. Human interferon preparations, products of genetic engineering, are used in the treatment of some cancers, multiple sclerosis and hepatitis B and C.

interlobular between lobules. *I. veins* branches of the portal vein in the liver.

intermediate care the purpose of services designed to assist the transition for a patient or client from medical and social dependence to day-to-day independence. A range of services have the potential to fulfil this function as people move from hospital to home, where the objectives of care are not primarily medical, the patient's discharge destination is anticipated, and a clinical outcome of recovery (or restoration of health) is desired. Intermediate care is also used to prevent hospital admission through provision of care at home.

intermenstrual occurring between two menstrual periods.

intermission a temporary interruption, particularly of a feverish condition.

intermittent occurring at intervals. *I. claudication see* CLAUDICATION. *I. fever* one in which the temperature drops to normal or lower, at times. *I. mandatory ventilation* abbreviated IMV. A type of mechanical ventilation in which the VENTILATOR is set to deliver a prescribed tidal volume at specified intervals, and a high-flow gas system permits the patient to breathe spontaneously between cycles. *I. peritoneal dialysis see* DIALYSIS. *I. pneumatic compression hose* a stocking worn to prevent deep vein thrombosis of upper and lower leg. *I. positive pressure ventilation* abbreviated IPPV. A method of assisted ventilation in which oxygen or air is used under pressure to inflate the lungs when the patient is unable to breathe spontaneously.

intermittent self-catheterization (ISC) a procedure carried out by the patient or their carer to drain urine from the bladder. This procedure is recommended for patients who cannot empty their bladder completely but can retain urine for 2 to 4 hours at a time and who have mental cognition, some manual dexterity and the ability to insert a catheter into the urethra. It can be used successfully by women, men and children. This is a clean rather than a sterile procedure.

internal situated on the inside. *I. haemorrhage* one occurring in a cavity or into the tissues. *I. secretion* one in which the hormones pass directly into the bloodstream from the secreting gland.

International Classification of Diseases abbreviated ICD. A publication of the World Health Organization produced approximately every 10 years listing all known disease categories.

International Council of Nurses abbreviated ICN. Founded in 1899 to represent worldwide international nurses' associations as a corporate organization.

internet a global computer network with millions of connected computers. By connecting to this network, it is possible to access a wide range of information including health-related information and provide for the transmission of electronic mail. NHSNet links all NHS Trusts and can securely exchange information with other health care organizations and agencies. *I. addiction syndrome see* PROBLEMATIC INTERNET USE (PIU).

interphase the period between two cell divisions during which the chromosomes are not easily visible.

intersex 1. a congenital abnormality in which anatomical features of both sexes are evident. 2. a person displaying intersexuality.

intersexuality an intermingling of the characters of each sex, including physical form, reproductive tissue and sexual behaviour, in one individual, as a result of some flaw in embryonic development.

interstitial situated within the tissue spaces or between the tissues. *I. cell stimulating hormone* abbreviated ICSH. Luteinizing hormone. *I. fluid* the fluid in which body cells are bathed. It acts as an intermediary between the cells and the blood. Extracellular fluid. *I. keratitis see* KERATITIS. *I. nephritis* chronic nephritis associated with fibrosis and hypertension.

intertrigo an irritating, eczematous skin eruption caused by the chafing of two moist skin surfaces.

intervention in health care, any act carried out to prevent harm to patients or to improve, promote or enhance their physical, mental or spiritual wellbeing.

intervertebral between the vertebrae. *I. disc* the pad of fibrocartilage between the bodies of the vertebrae. Protrusion of the contents of the disc may give rise to sciatica by exerting pressure on the nerve roots.

interviewing process involving a structured, semi-structured or conversational style meeting that allows the interviewer to probe for information and is widely used in research as well as in everyday situations. This technique is also used at the initial stage of patient assessment. Interviews are used as a method of data collection involving face-to-face or telephone questioning by the researcher; most often used in qualitative research.

intestinal referring to the intestine.

intestine that part of the alimentary canal that extends from the stomach to the anus. *Small i.* the first 6 m from the pylorus to the caecum, consisting of the duodenum, the jejunum and the ileum. *Large i.* the final 2 m, consisting of the caecum, the ascending, transverse and descending colon, and the rectum.

intima the innermost coat of an artery or vein.

intolerance lack of power to endure. Applied to the effect of some drugs on individuals, e.g., iodine and quinine. *See* IDIOSYNCRASY.

intoxication 1. poisoning by drugs or harmful substances. 2. the condition produced by excessive use of alcohol.

intra-abdominal within the abdomen.

intra-articular within a joint capsule. *I-a. injection* injection into a joint capsule, applicable to hydrocortisone, for example.

intracapsular within a capsule, usually of a joint. *I. extraction* the removal of the whole lens with its capsule in the treatment of cataract.

intracellular within a cell. *I. fluid* the water and its dissolved salts found within the cells.

intracerebral within the brain substance. *I. haemorrhage* an escape of blood in the cerebrum, most often arising from the middle cerebral artery or from an aneurysm.

intracranial within the skull. *I. abscess* one arising within the brain or meninges. *I. aneurysm* dilatation of one of the cerebral vessels. It may be congenital or acquired. *I. pressure* abbreviated ICP. The pressure exerted by the cerebrospinal fluid within the subarachnoid space and ventricles of the brain.

intractable not able to be relieved, controlled or cured.

intradermal between the layers of the skin.

intradural within the dura mater. *I. haemorrhage see* HAEMORRHAGE.

intragastric within the stomach.

intrahepatic within the liver. Referring to a condition of the liver cells or connective tissue.

intralobular within a lobule. *I. veins* veins that collect blood from within the lobules of the liver or kidney.

intramedullary 1. within the medulla oblongata. 2. within the bone marrow. *I. nail* a metal pin used for the internal fixation of fractures.

intramuscular within muscle tissue.

intranet A computer network designed to meet the internal needs of a single organization, e.g., an NHS Trust. It is not necessarily open to the internet and is not accessible by individuals from outside the organization.

intraocular within the eyeball.

intraorbital within the orbit of the eye.

intraosseous within a bone. *I. infusion* the process of supplying fluid into the narrow cavity of a bone in a life-threatening situation.

intraperitoneal within the peritoneal cavity.

intrathecal within the meninges of the spinal cord, usually in the subarachnoid space.

intratracheal endotracheal; within the trachea. *I. anaesthesia* inhalation anaesthesia. *See* ANAESTHESIA.

intrauterine within the uterus. *I. contraceptive device* abbreviated IUCD. A contraceptive device introduced into the uterine cavity. *I. growth retardation* associated with a poor blood supply to the placenta, or maternal disease. Other factors include infection during pregnancy, maternal smoking or drug addiction. The infant at birth is 'small for dates' and falls below the tenth percentile of appropriate gestational age for infants. *I. insemination* abbreviated IUI. Following the induction of ovulation fresh sperm are introduced into the uterus with ultrasound supervision; allows fertilization to take place naturally in the uterine tubes. *See* IN VITRO FERTILIZATION. *I. life* fetal development in the uterus.

intravenous within a vein. *I. flow rate* the rate at which fluids, medications and blood products flow into the bloodstream during intravenous infusion. The flow rate is usually ordered by the doctor as total volume (ml) per total hours or, in the case of drugs, total dose per total hours. *I. infusion* the therapeutic introduction of a fluid, such as saline, into a vein. The infusion works by gravity, in that the container of fluid is higher than the blood vessel

into which the fluid is being introduced. *I. urography* radiographic examination of the urinary tract after the injection of a radio-opaque contrast medium into a vein.

intraventricular within a ventricle; may apply to a cerebral or a cardiac ventricle.

intrinsic particular to or contained within an organ. *I. factor* a glycoprotein, contained in the gastric juices, which is necessary for the absorption of extrinsic factor (vitamin B_{12}).

introitus [L.] an opening or entrance into a hollow organ or cavity. *I. vaginae* the vulva.

introjection a mental process by which individuals take into themselves the personal characteristics of another person, usually those of someone much loved or admired.

introspection a subjective study of the mind and its processes, in which individuals study their own reactions.

introversion 1. a turning inwards within itself of a hollow organ. 2. preoccupation with oneself, with reduction of interest in the outside world.

introvert a person whose interests are turned inwards upon the self. *See* EXTROVERT.

intubation the introduction of a tube into a part of the body, particularly into the air passages to allow air to enter the lungs.

intussusception prolapse of one part of the intestine into the lumen of an immediately adjacent part (*see* Figure on p. 206), causing OBSTRUCTION (INTESTINAL).

inunction 1. rubbing an oily or fatty preparation containing a medicinal ingredient into the skin, with absorption of the drug. 2. any preparation so applied.

invagination 1. the folding inwards of a part, thus forming a pouch. 2. intussusception. *See* Figure on p. 206.

invasion 1. the entry of bacteria into the body. 2. the entrance of parasites into the body of a host.

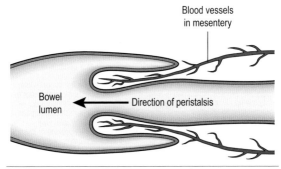

Blood vessels
in mesentery

Bowel
lumen ← Direction of peristalsis

EXAMPLE OF INTUSSUSCEPTION

invasive 1. having the quality of invasiveness. 2. involving puncture or incision of the skin or insertion of an instrument or foreign material into the body; said of diagnostic techniques.

invasiveness 1. the ability of microorganisms to enter the body and spread in the tissues. 2. the ability to infiltrate and actively destroy surrounding tissue, a property of malignant tumours.

inversion a turning upside down or inside out. *Uterine i.* the condition of the uterus after parturition when a part of its upper segment protrudes through the cervix.

investigations procedures performed to establish a diagnosis, to monitor a person's health, disease or the effectiveness of treatment. They are classified as non-invasive where there is no direct entry into the body, e.g., recording body weight, or as invasive, e.g., endoscopy or blood sampling.

in vitro the occurrence of a phenomenon in laboratory experiments (literally 'within a glass', e.g., a test tube) and not necessarily reflecting what happens within the human body. For example, a drug may exhibit certain characteristics in vitro that may or may not occur inside the body. *See* IN VIVO. *I. v.*

fertilization a technique used to treat infertility for women who have blocked uterine tubes. The woman is given hormone therapy which promotes the maturity of more than one egg at the same time. These eggs are harvested by laparoscopy and fertilized with sperm in the laboratory until a blastocyte is formed. Usually two of the fertilized eggs are implanted into the woman's uterus; if these become safely embedded pregnancy continues normally.

in vivo occurrence of a phenomenon or effect within the living body as opposed to in vitro.

involucrum new bone which forms a sheath around necrosed bone, as in chronic osteomyelitis.

involuntary independent of the will. *See* VOLUNTARY. *I. muscle* one that acts without conscious control: for instance, the heart and stomach muscles.

involution 1. turning inwards; describes the contraction of the uterus after labour. The process whereby the uterus returns to its normal size. 2. the progressive degeneration occurring naturally with advancing age, resulting in shrivelling of organs or tissues.

iodine *symbol* I. A non-metallic element with a distinctive odour, obtained from seaweed. Iodine is essential in nutrition, being especially prevalent in the colloid of the THYROID (GLAND). It is used in the treatment of HYPOTHYROIDISM. Iodine is bactericidal and is used as povidone iodine for skin disinfection prior to invasive procedures. Iodine is opaque to X-rays and can be combined with other compounds for use as contrast media in diagnostic radiology.

ion an atom or group of atoms having a positive (cation) or negative (anion) electric charge by virtue of having gained or lost one or more electrons. Substances forming ions are electrolytes (*see* ELECTROLYTE). *See* HYDROGEN.

ionization the breaking up of molecules into electrically charged particles or ions when an electric current is passed through an electrolytic solution.

ionizing radiation *see* RADIATION.

iontophoresis the introduction through the skin of therapeutic ions by ionization.

IPPV intermittent positive pressure ventilation.

ipsilateral occurring on the same side. Applied particularly to paralysis or other symptoms occurring on the same side as the cerebral lesion causing them.

IQ intelligence quotient. *See* INTELLIGENCE.

IRDS infant respiratory distress syndrome. *See* RESPIRATORY.

iridectomy excision of a part of the iris, usually for the treatment of glaucoma.

iridium *symbol* Ir. A radioactive metal, often used in the form of brachytherapy to treat malignancies, e.g., those of the prostate, biliary tract, cervix and some head and neck cancers.

iridocele herniation of a part of the iris through a corneal wound.

iridocyclitis inflammation of the iris and ciliary body.

iridodonesis trembling of the iris due to lack of support from the lens in dislocation of the lens or after a cataract extraction.

iridoptosis prolapse of the iris.

iris the coloured part of the eye, made of two layers of muscle, the contraction of which alters the size of the pupil and so controls the amount of light entering the eye. *I. bombé* a bulging forwards of the iris due to pressure of the aqueous humour when its passage into the anterior chamber is obstructed.

iritis inflammation of the iris, causing pain, photophobia, contraction of the pupil and discoloration of the iris. *See* UVEITIS.

iron *symbol* Fe. A metallic element, present in the body in small quantities and essential to life. A deficiency may produce anaemia.

irradiation the treatment of disease by electromagnetic radiation.

irreducible incapable of being replaced in a normal position. Applied to a fracture or a hernia.

irrigation the washing out of a cavity or wound with a stream of lotion or water.

irritable reacting excessively to a stimulus. *I. bowel syndrome* (IBS) mucous colitis; spastic colon. The patient complains of disordered bowel function with abdominal pain, but no organic disease can be found.

irritant an agent causing stimulation or excitation.

irritation 1. a condition of undue nervous excitement resulting from abnormal sensitiveness. 2. itching of the skin.

ischaemia a deficiency in the blood supply to a part of the body. *Myocardial i.* ischaemia of the heart muscles, which causes angina pectoris.

ischioanal concerning the ischium and the anus. *I. abscess* a collection of pus in the ischiorectal connective tissue. An anal fistula may result.

ischium the lower posterior bone of the pelvic girdle.

Ishihara colour charts *S. Ishihara, Japanese ophthalmologist, 1879–1963.* Patterns of dots of the primary colours on similar backgrounds which make numbers or patterns. The numbers or patterns can be seen by a normal-sighted person, but one who is colour-blind will only be able to identify some of them, depending on the type of colour-blindness.

islet of Langerhans *P. Langerhans, German pathologist, 1847–1888.* One of a group of cells in the pancreas that produce insulin and glucagon; islet of the pancreas.

isograft a tissue graft from one identical twin to another.

isoimmunization the development of antibodies against an antigen derived from an individual of the same species, e.g., a rhesus-negative woman may immunize herself against her fetus, if it is rhesus-positive, by forming specific ANTIBODY.

isolation the separation of a person with an infectious disease from those non-infected. *I. period* quarantine; the length of time during which a patient with an infectious fever is considered capable of infecting others by contact.

isoleucine one of the ten essential amino acids that are vital for health in the adult.

isometric having equal dimensions. *I. exercises* the contraction and relaxation of muscles without producing movement; used to maintain muscle tone after a fracture.

isotonic having uniform tension. *I. solution* a solution of the same osmotic pressure as the fluid with which it is compared. Normal saline (0.9% solution of salt in water) is isotonic with blood plasma.

isotope one of the several forms of an element with the same atomic number but different atomic weights. *Radioactive i.* also known as radioisotope is an unstable isotope which decays and emits alpha, beta or gamma rays. May be used in the diagnosis and treatment of malignant disease.

isovaleric acidaemia a rare hereditary condition where the body cannot process the amino acid leucine. Screening for the condition takes place as part of NEWBORN BLOOD SPOT SCREENING.

isthmus a narrow connection between two larger bodies or parts, e.g., the band of tissue between the two lobes of the thyroid gland.

itch a skin irritation. A skin sensation that makes the person want to scratch the part. Often associated with eczema and skin conditions. Generalized itching may occur as a result of excessive bathing and using irritant detergent soaps and foams. Itching is common in the elderly who often have a dry skin, and also commonly occurs in pregnancy *I. mite* the cause of scabies, *Sarcoptes scabiei.*

ITP idiopathic thrombocytopenic purpura.

ITU intensive therapy unit.

IUCD intrauterine contraceptive device.

IVF in vitro fertilization. *See* FERTILIZATION.

IVP intravenous pyelography (*see* UROGRAPHY).

IVU intravenous urography (*see* UROGRAPHY).

J

J symbol for *joule*.

Jacksonian epilepsy *J.H. Jackson, British neurologist, 1835–1911.* Focal motor EPILEPSY.

Jacquemier's sign *J.M. Jacquemier, French obstetrician, 1806–1879.* Blueness of the lining of the vagina seen from the early weeks of pregnancy.

Japanese encephalitis a severe inflammation of the brain caused by the Japanese B encephalitis virus that is transmitted by the bite of infected mosquitoes. Around 75% of those affected are under the age of 15 years. There is currently no cure and around 1 in 250 people who contract the disease become severely ill. Of those who develop serious complications around one third will die and others will have permanent brain damage. There is a vaccine that gives protection against the disease available privately.

jargon the terminology used and generally understood only by those who have knowledge of that speciality, e.g., medical jargon, legal jargon.

jaundice icterus; a yellow discoloration of the skin and conjunctivae, due to the presence of bile pigment in the blood often associated with pruritus. It may be one of the following types: (a) *Haemolytic j.* due to excessive destruction of red blood cells, causing increase of bilirubin in the blood. The liver is not involved. *Acholuric j.* is of this type. It is characterized by increased fragility of the red blood cells. (b) *Hepatocellular j.* the liver cells are damaged by either infection or drugs. (c) *Obstructive or cholestatic j.* the bile is prevented from reaching the duodenum owing to obstruction by a gallstone, a growth or a stricture of the common bile duct. (d) *Physiological j.* (icterus neonatorum) occurs within the first few days of life, and is caused by the breakdown of the excessive number of red blood cells present in the newborn.

jaw a bone of the face in which the teeth are embedded. *Lower j.* the mandible. *Upper j.* the two maxillae.

jealousy intense concern for the loss of affection or attention of another person; may also be exhibited as being envious of someone else's achievements or advantages. *Morbid j.* also known as Othello syndrome is preoccupation with the potential sexual infidelity of one's partner. Morbid jealousy is usually caused by a personality disorder but may also occur in those suffering from organic brain disease or alcohol dependency.

jejunal biopsy removal of a small piece of the jejunum for histological and enzyme examination. Used to confirm Crohn's disease, coeliac disease and other malabsorption syndromes. The biopsy is taken using a flexible endoscope passed down through the mouth into the jejunum. *See* CROSBY CAPSULE.

jejunoileostomy the making of an anastomosis between the jejunum and the ileum.

jejunostomy the making of an opening into the jejunum through the abdominal wall.

jejunum the portion of the small intestine from the duodenum to the ileum; about 2.4 m in length.

jelly a soft, coherent, resilient substance; generally, a colloidal semisolid mass. *Contraceptive j.* a non-greasy jelly containing spermicide used in the vagina for prevention of conception (*see* CONTRACEPTION). *Petroleum j.* a purified mixture of semisolid hydrocarbons obtained from petroleum (also called petrolatum). *Wharton's j.* the soft, jelly-like intracellular substance of the umbilical cord, which insulates the vein and arteries, preventing occlusion and fetal hypoxia.

jerk a sudden muscular contraction. *Knee j.* also known as the patellar reflex is a kicking movement produced by tapping the tendon below the patella. Used with other jerks, such as the ankle jerk, to test the nervous reflexes.

Jervell and Lange-Nielsen syndrome *see* LONG QT SYNDROME.

jet lag the lack of balance that occurs between local time and the person's biological rhythms that results from air travel over a long distance, especially in an easterly direction and to a lesser extent westwards. Sleep, memory and concentration are disturbed and there is a persistent feeling of tiredness usually lasting 2–3 days as the body adjusts to the time change.

jigger a sand flea, found in the tropics, which burrows into the soles of the feet and causes severe irritation.

jogger's heel a painful condition of the heel caused by repeatedly striking the heel against the ground or road surface when running or jogging. Also known as plantar fasciitis.

jogger's nipple soreness of the nipple(s) caused by friction of clothing against them; occurs in runners and athletes. Prevention is by applying petroleum jelly before running.

jogging running at a slow even pace. A popular form of street exercise.

joint an articulation; the point of junction of two or more bones, particularly one which permits movement of the individual bones relative to each other. *J. hypermobility see* HYPERMOBILITY.

joint strategic needs assessment abbreviated JSNA, involves scrutiny of a wide range of indicators to identify the needs of local populations in order to support the planning of services based on need.

joule symbol J. The SI unit of energy.

judgement the ability of an individual to estimate a situation, to arrive at reasonable conclusions and to decide on a course of action.

judicial review a legal process by which individuals or organizations can challenge government or public body decisions. Any person or organization with sufficient interest and concern regarding a decision that has been made, e.g., by a health sector organization, can apply for a review to the Administrative Court. This relates to the legal process in England and Wales only.

jugular relating to the neck. *J. veins* several veins in the neck which drain the blood from the head.

Jungian theory *C.G. Jung, Swiss psychologist and psychiatrist, 1875–1961.* The concept that certain ideas from past experiences are present in the unconscious and controlled by the way in which the person views the world. Jung called these shared ideas the 'collective unconscious' as an entity common to all human beings. Jung considered that each person also had a 'personal unconscious' containing personal life experiences. Jung separated individuals into personality types: the externally sensitive type who directs energy outwards, and the introvert whose energies are inwardly directed. The goal eof Jungian psychotherapy is to permit the individual to become what they essentially are, i.e., to encourage individual development.

junk food convenience or fast food high in monosodium glutamate.

jurisprudence the science of law. Medical jurisprudence is another name for forensic medicine.

juvenile relating to young people.

juvenile chronic arthritis a rare form of inflammatory arthritis affecting children, most often girls, between the ages of 2 and 4 years or at puberty; usually affects four or more joints. Management is based around the relief of pain, suppression of the inflammatory process and the prevention of deformity. Formerly known as Still's disease.

juxta-articular near a joint.

juxtaglomerular near to a glomerulus of the kidney. *J. cells* specialized cells found in the kidney which appear to play an important part in the control of aldosterone release.

juxtaposition an adjacent, or side by side position.

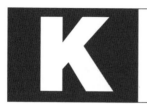

K symbol for *potassium*.

kala-azar visceral leishmaniasis. A tropical disease caused by the protozoan parasite *Leishmania donovani* which is carried by the sandfly. Symptoms include enlargement of the liver and spleen, anaemia and wasting. The disease is often fatal.

kangaroo care the use of skin-to-skin contact between the premature but stable infant and parent or caregiver. The infant in nappy and cap rests on the mother's or father's exposed chest either in a sling or blanket; vital signs can be kept monitored. The skin contact has a soothing effect, calming and warming the infant while promoting bonding between parent and baby.

Kaposi's sarcoma *M.K. Kaposi, Austrian dermatologist, 1837–1902.* A multifocal, metastasizing, malignant reticulosis with angiosarcoma-like features, involving chiefly the skin and mainly seen in people with poorly controlled or severe HIV infection or others with weakened immune systems. It is characterized by the development of bluish-red cutaneous nodules usually on the lower extremities, most often on the toes or feet, increasing in size and number and spreading to more proximal sites especially on the face and nose.

Kaposi's spots a serious complication of atopic eczema occurring on exposure to herpes simplex virus infection. More commonly known as Kaposi's varicelliform eruption.

karyotype 1. the chromosomal constitution and arrangement of a cell of an individual. 2. the pattern that is seen when human chromosomes are photographed during metaphase. The pictures are then enlarged and paired according to the length of their short arm.

Kawasaki disease a rare, acute inflammatory disorder of young children. Cause and mode of transmission not known but may be a sequela of a viral infection. Symptoms include fever, rash, sore throat and cervical lymphadenopathy and in some children cardiac complications. Occurs mainly in Japan and the USA. Also called mucocutaneous lymph node syndrome.

kcal kilocalorie.

Kegel exercises *Dr A.H. Kegel, US gynaecologist, 1894–1981.* Specific exercises to strengthen the pelvic–vaginal muscles as a means of controlling stress incontinence in women.

Keller's operation *W.L. Keller, American surgeon, 1874–1959.* An operation for correcting hallux valgus.

keloid hard, raised scar tissue in the skin, common in people with dark skins. A type occurs in a healed wound due to overgrowth of fibrous tissue, causing the scar to be raised above the skin level.

Kennedy's syndrome *F. Kennedy, American neurologist, 1884–1952.* Ipsilateral optic atrophy caused by a frontal lobe tumour which involves one of the optic nerves.

keratectomy excision of a portion of the cornea.

keratic 1. horny. 2. relating to the cornea. *K. precipitates* inflammatory exudates adhering to the back of the cornea; a sign of iritis and cyclitis.

keratin one of a family of fibrous proteins which forms the main constituent of hair and nails.

keratinize to make or become horny.

keratitis inflammation of the cornea. The causes may be physical (trauma, exposure to dust, vapours or ultraviolet light) or due to infectious conditions such as corneal and dendritic ulcers. *Interstitial k.* deep chronic keratitis, usually arising in congenital syphilis. *Striate k.* inflammation that appears in lines due to the folding over of the cornea after injury or operation, particularly one for cataract.

keratoconjunctivitis inflammation of both the cornea and the conjunctiva of the eye.

keratoconus progressive thinning of the cornea.

keratoiritis inflammation of both the cornea and iris.

keratomalacia ulceration and softening of the cornea due to a deficiency of vitamin A.

keratometer ophthalmometer. An instrument by which the amount of corneal astigmatism can be measured accurately.

keratophakia keratoplasty in which a slice of donor's cornea is shaped to a desired curvature and inserted between layers of the recipient's cornea to change its curvature and to correct hypermetropia.

keratoplasty a plastic operation on the cornea, including corneal grafting.

keratoscope an instrument for examining the eye to detect keratoconus. Also known as Placido's disc.

keratosis a skin disease marked by excessive growth of the epidermis or horny tissue.

keratotomy incision of the cornea.

kerion a complication of ringworm of the scalp, with formation of pustules.

kernicterus a condition in the newborn marked by severe neural symptoms, associated with high levels of bilirubin in the blood; it is commonly a sequela of icterus gravis neonatorum and may result in learning disabilities.

Kernig's sign *V.M. Kernig, Russian physician, 1840–1917.* A sign of meningitis. When the thigh is supported at right angles to the trunk, the patient is unable to straighten the leg at the knee joint.

ketogenic forming or capable of being converted into ketone bodies.

ketone an organic compound containing the carbonyl group (CO) attached to two hydrocarbon groups. Ketones are produced by the metabolization of fats.

ketonuria the presence of ketones in urine; acetonuria.

ketosis the condition in which ketones are formed in excess in the body and accumulate in the blood. Severe acidosis may occur.

ketosteroid a steroid hormone which contains a ketone group attached to a carbon atom. *17-k's* are excreted in the urine and formed from the adrenal corticosteroids, testosterone and, to a lesser extent, oestrogens.

key worker a person (commonly a social worker) designated as coordinator for action where several people are involved in the care of a person or family. The key worker is also responsible for calling a case conference to consider relevant issues for the client.

kick chart a method of fetal assessment carried out by the mother. The number of kicks or movements felt during the day is counted and noted. If fewer than 10 kicks are felt in a 12-hour daytime period on two consecutive occasions, the mother is advised to contact her midwife or doctor immediately. This is a subjective assessment, and is usually combined with other tests of fetal wellbeing. Also known as a fetal movement chart.

kidney one of two organs situated in the lumbar region, which purify the blood and secrete urine. The kidney secretes renin and renal erythropoietic factor. *Artificial k.* the apparatus used to remove retained waste products from the blood when kidney function is impaired. *Granular k.* the small fibrosed kidney of chronic nephritis. *Horseshoe k.* a congenital defect producing a fusion of the two kidneys into a horseshoe shape. *K. failure* the condition in which renal function is severely impaired and the organs are unable to maintain the fluid and electrolyte balance of the body. *K. transplant* the surgical implantation of a kidney taken from a live donor or from one who has recently died. Used in the treatment of renal failure. *Polycystic k.* a congenital bilateral condition of multiple cysts replacing kidney tissue. *See* Figure.

kilocalorie *symbol* kcal. One thousand calories, a unit of food energy.

kilojoule *symbol* kJ. One thousand joules, a unit of food energy (1 kcal = 4.184 kJ).

Kimmelstiel–Wilson syndrome *P. Kimmelstiel, German pathologist, 1900–1970; C. Wilson, British physician, 1906–1997.* A degenerative complication of DIABETES (MELLITUS), with albuminuria, oedema, hypertension, renal insufficiency and retinopathy; may lead to kidney failure. Called also intercapillary glomerulosclerosis.

kinaesthesia the combined sensations by which position, weight and muscular position are perceived.

kinanaesthesia an inability to perceive the sensation of movements of parts of the body.

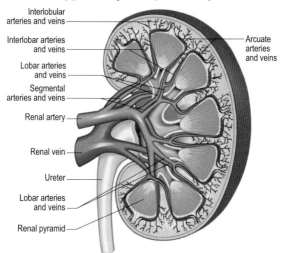

Interlobular arteries and veins

Interlobar arteries and veins

Lobar arteries and veins

Segmental arteries and veins

Renal artery

Renal vein

Ureter

Lobar arteries and veins

Renal pyramid

Arcuate arteries and veins

THE KIDNEY

kinase an enzyme activator; *see* ENTER-OKINASE and THROMBOKINASE.

kineplasty plastic amputation; amputation in which the stump is so formed as to be utilized for producing motion of the prosthesis.

kinetic producing or pertaining to motion.

King's Fund King Edward's Hospital Fund for London was founded in 1897 for the support, by the giving of grants, of voluntary hospitals in London. Since the inception of the National Health Service in 1948, the charitable organisation has been concerned with the shaping of health and social care policy and practice, and leadership development. *K. F. bed* a bed fitted with jointed springs which may be adjusted to various positions, developed as the result of research undertaken on behalf of and funded by the King's Fund.

kinin a polypeptide which occurs naturally and is a powerful vasodilator.

kinship relationship. *K. studies* in anthropology, the study of kin (relatives) and their patterns of marriage, descent, inheritance, habitation, social values, health beliefs and economics.

Kirschner wire M. Kirschner, German surgeon, 1879–1942. A thin wire that may be passed through a bone to apply skeletal traction.

kiss of life the expired air method of artificial respiration, by either mouth-to-nose or mouth-to-mouth breathing. *See* Appendix 2.

kJ symbol for *kilojoule*.

Klebs–Löffler bacillus T.A.E. Klebs, German bacteriologist, 1834–1913; F.A.J. Löffler, German bacteriologist, 1852–1915. Former name for *Corynebacterium diphtheriae*, the causative agent of diphtheria.

Klebsiella a genus of gram-negative bacteria (family Enterobacteriaceae).

Kleihauer test a microscopic test to detect fetal cells in the maternal circulation, usually done immediately after delivery so that, if the mother is rhe-

sus-negative and the fetus rhesus-positive, anti-D immunoglobulin may be given to prevent isoimmunization.

kleptomania an irresistible urge to steal when there is often no need and no particular desire for the objects. Often associated with depression.

Klinefelter's syndrome H.F. Klinefelter, American physician, 1912–1990. A congenital chromosome abnormality in which each cell has three sex chromosomes, XXY, rather than the usual XX or XY, making a total of 47 (normal is 46). Affected men have female breast development and small testes and are infertile.

knee the joint between the femur and the tibia. *K. cap* the patella. *Housemaid's k.* prepatellar bursitis. *K. jerk* an upward jerk of the leg obtained by striking the patellar tendon when the knee is passively flexed. *Knock-k.* a condition in which the knees turn inwards towards each other; genu valgum.

kneecap the patella.

Koch's bacillus R. Koch, German bacteriologist, 1843–1910. Former name for *Mycobacterium tuberculosis*, the causative organism of tuberculosis.

Köhler's disease A. Köhler, German physician and radiologist, 1874–1947. Osteochondritis of the navicular bone of the foot, occurring in children.

koilonychia the development of brittle, spoon-shaped nails which may occur in iron-deficiency anaemia.

Koplik's spots H. Koplik, American paediatrician, 1858–1927. Small white spots that sometimes appear on the mucous membranes inside the mouth in measles on the second day of onset, before the general rash. *See* MEASLES.

Korotkoff's method N.S. Korotkoff, Russian physician, 1874–1920. A method of finding the systolic and diastolic blood pressure by listening to the sounds produced in an artery while the pressure in a previously inflated cuff is gradually reduced.

Korsakoff's syndrome or psychosis *S.S. Korsakoff, Russian neurologist, 1854–1900.* A chronic condition in which there is impaired memory, particularly for recent events, and the patient is disorientated for time and place. It may be present in psychosis of infective, toxic or metabolic origin, or in chronic alcoholism.

kosher food that is prepared and cooked in accordance with Jewish dietary laws; it is eaten by practising Jews.

kraurosis dryness and shrinking of a part of the body. *K. vulvae* a degenerative condition of the vulva. May be treated by giving oestrogen preparations.

Krebs cycle *Sir H.A. Krebs, German–British biochemist, 1900–1981.* A series of reactions during which the aerobic oxidation of pyruvic acid takes place. This is part of carbohydrate metabolism. Also known as the citric acid cycle or tricarboxylic acid cycle. *K. urea c.* the way in which urea is formed in the liver.

Küntscher nail *G. Küntscher, German orthopaedic surgeon, 1902–1972.* An intramedullary nail used in treating fractures of long bones, especially the shaft of the femur.

Kupffer's cells *K.W. von Kupffer, German anatomist, 1829–1902.* Phagocytic reticuloendothelial cells of the liver which form bile from haemoglobin released by disintegrated erythrocytes.

Kveim test *M.A. Kveim, Norwegian physician, 1892–1966.* A test for sarcoidosis in which antigen from the lymph nodes or spleen of a sarcoidosis patient is injected intradermally.

kwashiorkor a condition of protein malnutrition occurring in children in underprivileged populations. Fatty infiltration of the liver arises and may cause cirrhosis.

kymograph an instrument for recording variations or undulations, arterial or other.

kyphoscoliosis an abnormal curvature of the spine in which there is forward and sideways displacement.

kyphosis posterior curvature of the spine; humpback.

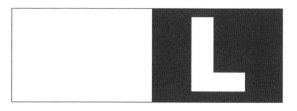

l symbol for *litre*.

label 1. a classifying name given to a person or object. When a label is given to someone there is a tendency for that person to be perceived by others and often by themselves as having the characteristics implied by the label, and being nothing more than that and therefore undervalued. *See* STIGMA. 2. a means of providing data when attached to an item, e.g., drugs, food or surgical dressings.

labial pertaining to the lips or labia.

labile unstable. Applied to those chemicals that are subject to change or readily altered by heat.

lability instability. *L. of mood* the tendency to sudden changes of mood of short duration.

labium a lip. *L. majus pudendi* the large fold of flesh surrounding the vulva. *L. minus pudendi* the lesser fold within the labium majus.

labour parturition or childbirth, which takes place in three stages: (a) dilatation of the cervix uteri; (b) passage of the child through the birth canal; and (c) expulsion of the placenta. *Induced l.* labour brought on by artificial means before term, as in cases of contracted pelvis, or if overdue. *Obstructed l.* labour in which there is a mechanical hindrance, also known as labour dystocia. *Precipitate l.* labour in which the baby is delivered extremely rapidly. *Premature l.* labour which occurs after the 24th week of pregnancy and before fullterm. *Spontaneous l.* that which occurs without being artificially induced or accelerated. *Spurious l.* ineffective labour pains which sometimes precede true labour pains.

labyrinth the structures forming the internal ear, i.e., the cochlea and semicircular canals. *Bony l.* the bony canals of the internal ear. *Membranous l.* the soft structure inside the bony canals.

labyrinthectomy excision of the labyrinth.

labyrinthitis inflammation of the labyrinth, causing vertigo.

laceration a wound with torn and ragged edges.

lacrimal relating to tears. *L. apparatus* the structures secreting the tears and draining the fluid from the conjunctival sac (*see* Figure on p. 218). *L. gland* a gland that secretes tears, which drain through two small openings in the eyelids (*l. puncta*) into a pair of ducts (*l. canaliculi*) into the sac and finally into nasal cavity through the nasolacrimal duct. Situated in the outer and upper corner of the orbit.

lacrimation an excessive secretion of tears.

lacrimator a substance that causes excessive secretion of tears, e.g., tear gas.

lactagogue any agent that promotes the secretion or flow of milk; galactagogue.

lactalbumin an albumin of milk.

lactase an enzyme, produced in the small intestine, which converts lactose into glucose and galactose.

lactate 1. any substance given to promote lactation. 2. any salt of lactic

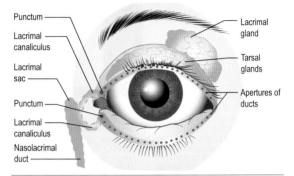

Punctum
Lacrimal canaliculus
Lacrimal sac
Punctum
Lacrimal canaliculus
Nasolacrimal duct

Lacrimal gland
Tarsal glands
Apertures of ducts

LACRIMAL APPARATUS

acid. 3. to secrete milk. *L. dehydrogenase* or lactic acid dehydrogenase abbreviated LD, LDH. An enzyme that catalyses the interconversion of lactate and pyruvate. Widespread in tissues and particularly abundant in kidney, skeletal muscle, liver and myocardium. It has five isoenzymes denoted LD_1 to LD_5. The 'flipped' pattern, in which the serum LD_1 level is greater than the LD_2 level, is indicative of an acute myocardial infarction. This pattern occurs within 12–24 hours after the attack.

lactation 1. the period during which the infant is nourished from the breast. 2. the process of milk secretion by the mammary glands.

lacteal 1. consisting of milk. 2. a lymphatic duct in the small intestine which absorbs chyle.

lactic pertaining to milk. *L. acid* an acid formed by the fermentation of lactose or milk sugar. It is produced naturally in the body as a result of glucose metabolism. An excess of the acid accumulating in the muscles may cause cramp.

lactiferous conveying or secreting milk.

Lactobacillus a genus of gram-positive, rod-shaped bacteria, many of which produce fermentation.

lactoferrin an iron-binding protein found in neutrophils and bodily secretions (milk, tears, saliva, bile, etc.), having bactericidal activity and acting as an inhibitor of colony formation by granulocytes and macrophages.

lactogenic stimulating the production of milk. *See* LUTEOTROPHIN.

lactose milk sugar consisting of glucose and galactose. *L. intolerance* the ingestion of milk containing lactose results in the patient experiencing severe abdominal colic and diarrhoea due to a deficiency of the lactose-splitting enzyme (beta-galactosidase) in the lining of the small intestine.

lactovegetarian 1. a person who subsists on a diet of milk or milk products and vegetables. 2. pertaining to such a diet.

lactulose a synthetic disaccharide which is used as a laxative.

lacuna a small cavity or depression in any part of the body.

Laënnec's cirrhosis *R.T.H. Laënnec, French physician, 1781–1826.* The most common type of cirrhosis of the liver, frequently attributable to high alcohol consumption.

laevulose fruit sugar; fructose.

laking haemolysis of the red blood cells. The cells swell and burst and the haemoglobin is released.

lallation a babbling, infantile form of speech.

Lamaze method *F. Lamaze, French obstetrician, 1890–1957.* A method of preparing for natural childbirth developed by Fernand Lamaze, and based on the technique of training the mind and body for the purpose of modifying perception of pain during labour and delivery. *See* CHILDBIRTH (NATURAL).

lambdoid shaped like the Greek letter lambda, i.e., Λ or λ. *L. suture* the junction of the occipital bone with the parietals.

Lambert-Eaton myasthenic syndrome (LEMS) a rare condition affecting signals sent from nerves to muscles resulting in muscles not being able to contract properly. Some cases are associated with lung cancer.

lambliasis giardiasis.

lamella 1. a thin layer, membrane or plate, as of bone. 2. a thin medicated disc of gelatin used in applying drugs to the eye. The gelatin dissolves and the drugs are absorbed.

lamina a bony plate or layer.

laminectomy excision of the posterior arch of a vertebra, sometimes performed to relieve pressure on the spinal cord or nerves.

Lancefield's groups *R.C. Lancefield, American bacteriologist, 1895–1981.* Divisions of B-haemolytic streptococci, which are classified on the basis of serological action into groups A–R. Most human infections are due to group A.

Landry's paralysis *J.B.G. Landry, French physician, 1826–1865. See* GUILLAIN–BARRÉ SYNDROME; acute ascending polyneuritis.

Landsteiner's classification *K. Landsteiner, Austrian biologist, 1868–1943.* A system of blood groups; the ABO system, consisting of groups A, B, AB and O. *See* BLOOD GROUPS.

Langerhans cell histiocytosis a rare disease of childhood where Langerhans cells proliferate and migrate from the skin to lymph nodes.

language the means of human communication consisting of the use of the spoken or written word in a structured way. Gestures of hands, head and even the body may be involved, although this is reflected differently from one setting to another, e.g., from a formal presentation to the greeting of a friend. Cultural background too plays a part in the use or absence of gestures. *L. disorders* problems affecting the ability to communicate and/or comprehend the spoken and/or written word. *See* SPEECH.

lanugo the fine hair that covers the body of the fetus and newly born infants, especially those who are premature. Also called down.

laparoscopy viewing of the abdominal cavity by passing an endoscope through the abdominal wall.

laparotomy incision of the abdominal wall for exploratory purposes.

laryngeal pertaining to the larynx.

laryngectomy excision of the larynx.

laryngismus a spasmodic contraction of the larynx. *L. stridulus* a crowing sound on inspiration, following a period of apnoea, due to spasmodic closure of the glottis. It occurs in children, particularly those suffering from rickets. *See* CROUP.

laryngitis inflammation of the larynx causing hoarseness or loss of voice due to acute infection or irritation by gases.

laryngopharynx the lower portion of the pharynx connecting with the larynx.

laryngoscope an endoscopic instrument for examining the larynx or for aiding the insertion of endotracheal tubes or the bronchoscope.

laryngospasm a reflex, prolonged contraction of the laryngeal muscles that is liable to occur on insertion or withdrawal of an endotracheal tube.

laryngostenosis contraction or stricture of the larynx.

laryngostomy the making of an opening into the larynx to provide an artificial air passage.

laryngotomy an incision into the larynx to make a temporary opening in an emergency when the larynx is obstructed. Tracheostomy.

laryngotracheal referring to both the larynx and trachea.

laryngotracheitis inflammation of both the larynx and trachea.

laryngotracheobronchitis an acute viral infection of the respiratory tract which occurs particularly in young children. Also known as CROUP.

larynx [Gr.] the muscular and cartilaginous structure, lined with mucous membrane, situated at the top of the trachea and below the root of the tongue and the hyoid bone. The larynx contains the vocal cords and is the source of the sound heard in speech. Also called the voice box.

laser acronym for Light Amplification by Stimulated Emission of Radiation. An apparatus producing an extremely concentrated beam of light that can be used to cut metals. When used in the treatment of neoplasms, detached retina, diabetic retinopathy and macular degeneration, and some skin conditions, eye protection must be worn by the operator.

Lassa fever a West African viral haemorrhagic fever with insidious onset and an incubation period of 6–21 days, and is a significant cause of morbidity and mortality. It is a zoonosis, the reservoir of infection of which is the multimammate rat. Devastating outbreaks of person-to-person transmission have occurred in hospitals in West Africa by direct contact with blood, urine or semen from infected patients. It can also be contracted by the airborne route. In the UK prevention is dependent on the early detection of cases and their isolation, and strict precautions to protect health care staff caring for febrile patients from Africa from inoculation or other accidents.

lassitude a feeling of extreme weakness and apathy.

lasting powers of attorney (LPA) there are two types of LPA—one for financial decisions and one for health and care decisions. These decisions are registered with the Office of the Public Guardian and give the attorney the authority to make treatment decisions in the event that the patient is unable to make such decisions due to incapacity.

latent temporarily concealed; not manifest. *L. heat* the heat absorbed by a substance during a change in state, e.g., from water into steam. When condensation occurs this heat is released. *L. period* 1. the incubation period of an infectious disease. 2. the time between the application of a nerve stimulus and the reaction.

lateral situated at the side; therefore, away from the centre. *L. epicondylitis* tennis elbow. A condition which occurs after strenuous overuse of the muscles and tendons near the elbow joint.

lateroversion a turning to one side, such as may occur of the uterus.

latex a milky fluid derived from tapping the rubber tree *Hevea brasiliensis* found mainly in Thailand, Indonesia and Malaysia. It comprises an aqueous suspension of globules of rubber hydrocarbon coated with proteins. *L. allergy* a reaction to latex proteins, varying in severity. It is a significant occupational health problem for health care workers. Latex is a component of many medical supplies, e.g., various tubes, materials and gloves. Latex gloves have been frequently implicated due either to the latex or to the proteins used in the powders that lubricate the gloves for ease of use.

lavage the washing out of a cavity. *Colonic l.* the washing out of the colon. *Gastric l.* the washing out of the stomach.

laxatives a group of drugs used to treat constipation or to evacuate the bowel before surgery on the large bowel. May be used orally, in suppositories or in enemas. There are different categories of laxative based upon their method of working: (a) bulk forming, e.g., methyl cellulose, that increase volume, encouraging the passage of a softer and bulkier stool; (b) stimulant laxatives that cause the intestinal wall to contract and speed up the elimination of faeces, e.g., senna or bisacodyl; (c) softeners, e.g., liquid paraffin, that lubricate and facilitate the passage of faeces; (d) osmotic laxatives primarily used in enemas that increase the fluid in the bowel by osmosis, e.g., magnesium sulphate or lactulose. Laxatives may also be given in a combined form of softener and stimulant.

LE cell a mature neutrophilic polymorphonuclear leukocyte that has phagocytized a large, spherical inclusion derived from another neutrophil; a characteristic of lupus erythematosus, but also found in analogous connective tissue disorders.

lead *symbol* Pb. A metallic element, many of the compounds of which are highly poisonous. *L. poisoning* a condition that occurs as the result of excessive lead in the atmosphere, or from chewing objects made from lead alloys or covered with paint containing lead. Lead can also be ingested as a result of drinking water contaminated by lead piping or cooking utensils. The symptoms and signs include malaise, diarrhoea and vomiting, and sometimes encephalitis. There is often pallor and a blue line around the gums. The use of lead in paints is now controlled by legislation and safety regulations. The increasing use of 'lead-free petrol' as motor car fuel has reduced previously high levels of lead in the environment.

lean a methodology adopted in health services to minimize waste.

learning knowledge or skills gained, or behaviour modified through being taught or from study. Learning occurs as a result of using intelligence, memory, insight and understanding. *L. curve* a person's rate of progress in gaining experience or new skills which can be represented as a graph. *L. difficulties* problems with learning arising from a result of a range of mental and physical problems. *L. disability* the preferred term to the one formerly used of 'mental handicap'. Essentially disorders are characterized by substantial deficits in scholastic or academic skills.

lecithin one of a group of phospholipids that are found in the cell tissues and are concerned in the metabolism of fat.

leech *Hirudo medicinalis*, an aquatic worm which sucks blood and secretes hirudin (an anticoagulant) in its saliva. Historically used to withdraw blood from patients. May now be used following some forms of surgery, e.g., plastic or microsurgery, to restore the patency of collapsed or blocked blood vessels. Leeches are also occasionally used to drain a haematoma from a wound.

leg the lower limb, from knee to ankle. *Bow-l.* genu varum. *Scissor l.* condition in which the patient is cross-legged, such as occurs in cerebral diplegia. *White l.* phlegmasia alba dolens. Acute oedema in a leg due to lymphatic blockage. Rarely occurs now but was most commonly seen in women after childbirth.

Legionella pneumophila a species of gram-negative, non-acid-fast, rod-shaped bacteria which require both cysteine and iron for growth; the causative agent of LEGIONNAIRES' DISEASE and PONTIAC FEVER.

legionellosis a disease caused by infection with *Legionella* species, such as *L. pneumophila*.

legionnaires' disease pulmonary form of legionellosis, resulting from infection with *Legionella pneumophila*. It is a notifiable disease. It is contagious and may be fatal. Symptoms include fever, confusion, pain in the muscles and across the chest, a dry cough and a partial loss of kidney function. It is associated with an infected water supply in public buildings such as hotels, hospitals and large office blocks, a cause of both community and hospital acquired infection. The infective organism is spread by droplets; there is no person to person spread.

leiomyoma a benign smooth muscle tumour (fibroid) most commonly found in the uterus.

leiomyosarcoma a malignant muscle tumour.

Leishmania a genus of parasitic flagellated protozoa which infect the blood of humans and are the cause of leishmaniasis.

leishmaniasis a group of diseases caused by one of the protozoan *Leishmania* parasites. *See* KALA-AZAR.

lens 1. a piece of glass or other material shaped to transmit light rays in a particular direction. 2. the transparent crystalline body situated behind the pupil of the eye. It serves as a refractive medium for rays of light. *Contact l.* a thin sheet of glass or plastic moulded to fit directly over the cornea. Worn instead of spectacles.

lentigo a brownish or yellowish spot on the skin. A freckle. *L. maligna* Hutchinson's melanotic freckle. *See* FRECKLE.

Lentivirus from Latin *lentus* (slow) + virus. A group of retroviruses that cause disease in animals and humans, including HIV-1 and HIV-2 (*see* HUMAN IMMUNODEFICIENCY VIRUS). These viruses are associated with slowly progressive diseases.

leontiasis an osseous deformity of the face which produces a lion-like appearance. It occurs sometimes in leprosy and rarely in osteitis deformans.

lepidosis any scaly eruption of the skin.

leprosy Hansen's disease. A chronic granulomatous disease of peripheral nerves, mucosa of the upper respiratory tract and the skin. Left untreated, leprosy can be progressive with permanent damage to skin, nerves and eyes. Caused by *Mycobacterium leprae*. It is predominantly a disease of warm climates which is transmitted by prolonged contact, with an incubation period of between 1 and 30 years, the average being between 3 and 5 years. Leprosy is now treated with a combination of drugs including dapsone, rifampicin and clofazimine. None of them is used alone because of the risk of developing resistance.

leptomeningitis inflammation of the pia mater and arachnoid membranes of the brain and spinal cord.

Leptospira a genus of spirochaetes. *L. icterohaemorrhagiae* the cause of spirochaetal jaundice (Weil's disease).

leptospirosis any of a group of rare notifiable infectious diseases due to serotypes of *Leptospira*. The best known is Weil's disease, or leptospiral jaundice; others are mud fever, autumn fever and swineherd's disease. The aetiological agent is a spiral organism that is common in water. Initially the symptoms include fever, rigors, vomiting, headache and often jaundice. Diagnosis may be difficult because the symptoms resemble those of several other diseases. Jaundice is a key symptom. Sanitation measures can reduce the spread of the disease in both humans and animals.

lesbianism sexual and emotional orientation of one woman to another; female homosexuality.

Lesch–Nyhan syndrome *M. Lesch, American physician, 1939–2008; W.L. Nyhan Jr, American physician, b. 1926.* A hereditary disorder of purine metabolism transmitted as an X-linked recessive trait with physical and learning disabilities, compulsive self-mutilation of fingers and lips by biting, spasticity, cerebral palsy and impaired renal function.

lesion any pathological or traumatic discontinuity of tissue or loss of function of a part. Lesion is a broad term, including wounds, sores, ulcers, tumours, cataracts and any other tissue damage. Lesions range from the skin sores associated with eczema to the changes in lung tissue that occur in tuberculosis.

lethargy a condition of drowsiness or stupor that cannot be overcome by the will.

leucine a naturally occurring essential amino acid, vital for growth in infants and for nitrogen equilibrium in adults.

leuco- for words beginning thus, *see* LEUKO-.

leukaemia a progressive, malignant disease of the blood-forming organs, marked by abnormal proliferation and development of leukocytes and their precursors in the blood and bone marrow. It is accompanied by a reduced number of erythrocytes and blood platelets, resulting in anaemia and increased susceptibility to infection and haemorrhage. Other typical symptoms include fever, excessive bruising, breathlessness, pain in the joints and bones and swelling of the lymph nodes, spleen and liver. Leukaemia is classified clinically on the basis of (a) the duration and character of the disease (acute or chronic), and (b) the cell line involved, i.e., myeloid (myelocytic, myeloblastic, granulocytic) or lymphoid (lymphatic, lymphoblastic, lymphocytic). A widely used classification of acute leukaemia based on cell type is the French American British (FAB) classification. The incidence of the disease is growing and the increase is only partially explained by increased efficiency of detection. Treatment options may include a combination of chemotherapy, radiotherapy, steroid therapy, bone marrow or stem cell transplant. Antibiotics are commonly required.

leukaphoresis withdrawal of blood for the selective removal of leukocytes. The remaining blood is retransfused.

leukocyte a white blood corpuscle. There are three types: (a) granular (polymorphonuclear cells) formed in bone marrow, consisting of neutrophils, eosinophils and basophils; (b) lymphocytes (formed in the lymph glands); and (c) monocytes (*see* Figure and Table on p. 224).

leukocytolysis destruction of white blood cells.

leukocytosis an increase in the number of leukocytes in the blood. Often a response to infection.

leukoderma an absence of pigment in patches or bands, producing abnormal whiteness of the skin. Vitiligo.

leukodystrophy a degenerative disorder of the brain which starts during the first few months of life and leads to mental, visual and motor deterioration.

leukonychia white patches on the nails due to air underneath.

leukopenia a decreased number of white cells, usually granulocytes, in the blood.

leukoplakia a chronic inflammation, characterized by white thickened patches on the mucous membranes, particularly on the tongue, gums and inside of the cheeks. *L. vulvae* thickening of the mucous membrane of the labia with the appearance of scattered white patches.

leukopoiesis the formation of white blood cells. Leukocytopoiesis.

leukorrhoea a viscid, whitish discharge from the vagina.

levator a muscle that raises a structure or organ of the body.

Lewy body dementia a type of DEMENTIA where there is a build-up of Lewy bodies, which are clumps of alpha-synuclein protein in neurons.

LH luteinizing hormone.

Li symbol for *lithium*.

liaison communication and contact between groups, units and/or agencies and organizations.

libido 1. the vital force or impulse which brings about purposeful action. 2. sexual drive in Freudian psychoanalysis, the motive force of all human beings.

lichen a group of inflammatory infections of the skin. *L. planus* raised flat patches of dull, reddish-purple colour, with a smooth or scaly surface. *L.*

Basophil

Neutrophil

Eosinophil

Lymphocyte

Monocyte

TYPES OF LEUKOCYTE

Normal leukocyte count	
Cell type	No. cells/litre
Neutrophils	$2.5–7.5 \times 10^9$
Eosinophils	$0.04–0.4 \times 10^9$
Basophils	$0.01–0.1 \times 10^9$
Lymphocytes	$1.5–3.5 \times 10^9$
Monocytes	$0.2–0.8 \times 10^9$

sclerosus a long-term skin disorder with white patches and itching mainly affecting the skins of the genitals.

lichenification the stage of an eruption when it resembles lichen.

lid eyelid. *Granular l.* trachoma. *L. lag* jerky movement of the upper lid when it is being lowered. A sign of exophthalmic goitre (thyrotoxicosis).

lie a position or direction. *L. of fetus* the position of the fetus in the uterus. The normal lie is longitudinal.

life crisis an unpleasant experience which may often be unforeseen and sudden such as being robbed or mugged, redundancy, early retirement, divorce, bereavement and sudden and severe ill health.

life event a sociological term used to describe major events in a person's life, e.g., leaving home for the first time, getting married, moving house, changing a job.

life expectancy the average length of life based upon prevailing mortality trends. It is influenced by health status and illness record, but also by social factors: education, occupation, ethnicity and environmental factors such as sanitation and quality of housing. Currently demographic differences are widening, with life expectancy in the north of England and Scotland being significantly less than in the south.

life long learning a process of personal, social and professional development throughout the life span of the individual.

life support system the equipment and technology used to maintain the life of a patient who is not otherwise able to survive.

lifestyle the pattern of daily living that an individual develops. On the initial assessment of a person entering the health care services this is considered in relation to the delivery of care by health care workers in order that the aims and objectives for care can be individualized.

lift assessment the choice of the most appropriate method to use when moving a patient, as from bed to chair. Factors that need to be taken into account include whether the patient is conscious or unconscious; if there is a visual, hearing or cognitive impairment present; the presence of equipment, e.g., urinary drainage, IV lines or monitors; the body weight of the person. No particular method is suggested as correct or appropriate in all situations; rather, that safe moving and handling practices should be used at all times. Lifting devices are the first option when implementing moving and handling activities. *See also* MOVING AND HANDLING.

ligament 1. a band of fibrous tissue connecting bones forming a joint. 2. a layer or layers of peritoneum connecting one abdominal organ to another or to the abdominal wall. *Annular l.* the ring-like band that fixes the head of the radius to the ulna. *Cruciate l.* crossed ligaments within the knee joint. *Inguinal l.* that between the pubic bone and anterior iliac crest. *Round l.* for example, one of the two anterior ligaments of the uterus, passing through the inguinal canal and ending in the labia majora. There are also round ligaments of the femur and of the liver.

ligation the application of a ligature.

ligature a thread of silk, catgut or other material used for tying round a blood vessel to stop it bleeding.

light electromagnetic waves which stimulate the retina of the eye. *L. adaptation* the changes that take place in the eye when the intensity of the light increases or decreases. *L. coagulation* a method of treating retinal detachment by directing a beam of strong light (including laser) through the pupil to the affected area.

lightening the relief experienced in pregnancy, 2–3 weeks before labour, when the uterus sinks into the pelvis and ceases to press on the diaphragm.

limbus an edge or border. *Corneal l.* the border where the cornea joins the sclera.

liminal pertaining to the threshold of perception.

linctus a thick syrup given to soothe and allay coughing.

linea [L.] *a line. L. alba* the tendinous area in the centre of the abdominal wall into which the transversalis and part of the oblique muscles are inserted. *L. albicantes* white streaks that appear on the abdomen when it is distended by pregnancy or a tumour. *L. aspera* the rough ridge on the back of the femur into which muscles are inserted. *L. nigra* the pigmented line that often appears in pregnancy on the abdomen between the umbilicus and the pubis.

linear pertaining to a line. *L. accelerator* a megavoltage machine for accelerating electrons so that powerful X-rays are given off for use in the treatment of deep-seated tumours.

lingual pertaining to the tongue.

lingula a tongue-like structure, such as the projection of lung tissue from the left upper lobe.

liniment a liquid to be applied externally by rubbing on to the skin.

lip 1. the upper or lower fleshy margin of the mouth. 2. any lip-like part; labium. *Cleft l.* congenital fissure of the upper lip.

lip reading understanding of speech through observation of the speaker's lip movements; called also speech reading.

lipaemia the presence of excess fat in the blood. Sometimes a feature of diabetes. *L. retinalis* condition in which the retinal blood vessels appear to be filled with milk owing to the presence of an excess of fat in the blood.

lipase fat-splitting enzyme; any enzyme that catalyses the splitting of fats into glycerol and fatty acids. Measurement of the serum lipase level is an important diagnostic test for acute and chronic pancreatitis.

lipid one of a group of fatty substances that are insoluble in water but soluble in alcohol or chloroform. They form an important part of the diet and are normally present in the body tissues providing a source of energy and insulation. Lipids are also an important constituent of some cell structures. *L. disorders* metabolic disorders that result in abnormal amounts of lipids in the body leading to hyperlipidaemia; this can cause atherosclerosis and pancreatitis. There are also some rare hereditary disorders. *L. lowering drugs* a group of drugs used in treating hyperlipidaemia to prevent or slow the progression of coronary heart disease and severe atherosclerosis.

lipoedema an abnormal build-up of fat cells in the legs and buttocks and occasionally in the arms.

lipolysis the breakdown of fats by the action of bile salts and enzymes to a fine emulsion and fatty acids.

lipoma a benign tumour composed of fatty tissue, arising in any part of the body, and developing in connective tissue. *Diffuse l.* a tumour of fat in an irregular mass, without a capsule, occurring above the pelvis.

lipoprotein one of a group of fatty proteins present in blood plasma.

liposarcoma a malignant tumour of the fat cells.

liposuction the removal by suction of excess fat in the body through a small skin incision. Most commonly used cosmetically as a means of contour reduction or reshaping. Also called lipectomy.

liquid 1. a substance that flows readily in its natural state. 2. flowing readily, neither solid nor gaseous. *L. diet* a diet limited to the intake of liquids or foods that can be changed to a liquid state. A liquid diet may be restricted to clear liquids or it may be a full liquid diet.

liquor a watery fluid; a solution. *L. amnii* the fluid in which the fetus floats; amniotic fluid.

Listeria Baron J. Lister, British surgeon, 1827–1912. A genus of gram-negative bacteria which produce upper respiratory disease, septicaemia and encephalitic disease in humans. They can be transmitted by the consumption of infected, unpasteurised dairy produce, or by direct contact with infected animals or contaminated soil. Newborn infants, pregnant women, the elderly and the immunosuppressed are more susceptible to infection.

listeriosis infection with organisms of the genus *Listeria*.

lithiasis the formation of calculi. *Conjunctival l.* the formation of small white chalky areas on the inner surface of the eyelids.

lithosis pneumoconiosis resulting from inhalation of particles of silica, etc., into the lungs.

lithotripsy the crushing of calculi in the bladder typically using ultrasound shock waves; lithotrity.

litmus paper a blotting paper impregnated with blue pigment obtained from lichen and used for testing the reaction of fluids. *Blue l.* turned red by an acid. *Red l.* turned blue by an alkali.

litre *symbol* l. The SI unit of capacity. One cubic decimetre.

liver the large gland situated in the right upper area of the abdominal cavity. It is essential to life. Its chief functions are: (a) formation of bile; (b) production of plasma proteins except gamma-globulins; (c) storage of carbohydrates as glycogen, iron and vitamins A, D, E and K; (d) regulation of metabolism of fat, protein and carbohydrate; (e) detoxification of drugs and other substances; (f) the formation and destruction of erythrocytes; (g) production of prothrombin and fibrinogen; (h) heat production; and (i) phagocytic action on bacteria. *Cirrhotic l.* fibrotic changes which occur in the liver as the result of degeneration of the liver cells, often as a result of alcoholism. *L. biopsy* the taking of a small core of liver tissue through a liver biopsy needle under a local anaesthetic. Allows for microscopic examination to aid diagnosis of a wide range of disorders of the liver. *L. function tests* blood tests used to assess liver function including: alanine aminotransferase, alkaline phosphatase, aspartate aminotransferase, coagulation tests, gamma-glutamyltransferase, serum bilirubin and serum proteins. *L. transplant* the transplantation of a liver or a segment of a liver from a suitable donor in the treatment of liver failure. *See* Figure.

livid descriptive of the bluish-grey discoloration of the skin produced by congestion of blood.

living will a statement signed by a person requesting and indicating what should be done in the event of becoming totally incapacitated or terminally ill. It enables the writer, while still alive, to refuse resuscitation or other measures to maintain life. *See* ADVANCE CARE PLAN.

Liverpool Care Pathway for the Dying Patient (LCP) was a UK pathway providing palliative care options for patients in final days or hours of life but no longer in use. *See* END OF LIFE CARE PATHWAYS.

LOA left occipitoanterior. Refers to a possible position of the fetus in the uterus.

loading dose in pharmacotherapeutics, the administration of a drug in larger doses than the body can eliminate in order to bring the concentration

of the drug within the body to an effective level. After this, the daily dose is gradually reduced.

lobar relating to a lobe.

lobe a section of an organ, separated from neighbouring parts by fissures. The liver, lungs and brain are divided into lobes.

lobectomy removal of a lobe, e.g., of the lung.

lobular relating to a lobule.

lobule a small lobe, particularly one making up a larger lobe.

local authority the local government.

local anaesthetic numbing of a part of the body, with no loss of consciousness using medication administered by injection or topically which blocks pain signals from nerves to the brain.

localize 1. to limit the spread, e.g., of disease or infection, to a certain area. 2. to determine the site of a lesion.

lochia the discharge of blood and tissue debris from the uterus after childbirth, lasting for 2–3 weeks. Initially lochia is bright red and gradually becomes paler.

lockjaw tetanus.

locomotor pertaining to movement from one place to another. *L. ataxia* tabes dorsalis. *See* ATAXIA.

loculated divided into small locules or cavities.

loculus a small cystic cavity, one of a number.

locum tenens [L.] *holding the place.* A person, usually a doctor, who substitutes for another over a period of time; usually referred to as a locum.

locus of control the ideas and beliefs that people have about the way in which they can control external events in their lives. Those with an internal locus of control tend to expect that any change or reinforcement is the result of their own efforts or behaviour and will want to be actively involved in any health care measures. Those with an external locus of control see themselves as being dependent upon luck, fate or the actions of 'powerful others' and are

THE LIVER

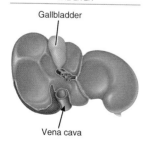

Gallbladder

Vena cava

therefore fatalistic about any health care provision or treatment.

logorrhoea excessive and often unintelligible volubility.

loiasis infestation of the conjunctiva and eyelids with a parasite worm, *Loa loa*. A tropical condition.

loin the area of the back between the thorax and the pelvis.

long QT syndrome irregularity of the electrical activity of the heart as a result of a faulty gene which can cause blackouts, seizures, arrhythmia and cardiac arrest. It is a leading cause of sudden death in young and otherwise healthy people and is thought to be an underlying cause in cases of SUDDEN INFANT DEATH SYNDROME.

long sight hypermetropia.

longitudinal study an investigation that involves making observations of the same group at sequential time intervals. Longitudinal studies are valuable as a means of studying human development or change and may also be used to observe change over time within an institution or organization.

loosening in psychiatry, a disorder of thinking in which associations of ideas become so shortened, fragmented and disturbed as to lack logical relationship.

LOP left occipitoposterior. Refers to a possible position of the fetus in the uterus.

lordosis a form of spinal curvature in which there is an abnormal forward curve of the lumbar spine.

lotion a medicinal solution for external application to the body. Lotions usually have a soothing or antiseptic effect.

louse a general term covering a number of small insects that are parasitic to humans and to other mammals and birds. Three varieties are parasitic to humans: (a) *Pediculus capitis*, the head louse; (b) *Pediculus corporis*, the body louse; and (c) *Phthirus pubis*, which infects the coarse hair on the body and also the eyebrows. Diseases known to be transmitted by

lice are typhus fever, relapsing fever and trench fever.

lozenge a medicated tablet with a sugar basis, used to treat mouth and throat conditions.

LSD *see* LYSERGIC ACID DIETHYLAMIDE.

lubb-dupp representation of the sounds heard through the stethoscope when listening to the normal heart: *lubb* when the atrioventricular valves shut, and *dupp* when the semilunar valves meet each other.

lucid clear, particularly of the mind. *L. interval* period of clear thinking that may occur in cerebral injury between two periods of unconsciousness or as a sane interval in a mental disorder.

lumbago pain in the lower part of the back. It may be caused by muscular strain or by a prolapsed intervertebral disc ('slipped disc').

lumbar pertaining to the loins. *L. puncture* insertion of a trocar and cannula into the spinal canal in the lower back and withdrawal of cerebrospinal fluid for diagnostic and sometimes treatment purposes.

lumbosacral relating to both the lumbar vertebrae and the sacrum. *L. support* a corset aimed at both supporting and restricting movement in that region. *L. vertebra* one of the five vertebrae in the lower back lying between the thoracic vertebrae and the sacrum.

lumen the space inside a tube.

lumpectomy the surgical excision of only the local lesion (benign or malignant) of the breast.

Lund and Browder chart a chart used for the calculation of the surface area of a burn. At birth the size and area of the head is large compared with the adult, and the legs and thighs constitute a much smaller proportion of the total body surface. On admission to a burns unit or ward the area of the body burned is mapped on to the Lund and Browder chart and the area of the burn affecting each portion of the body surface is calculated. *See* Figures on p. 229 and p. 230.

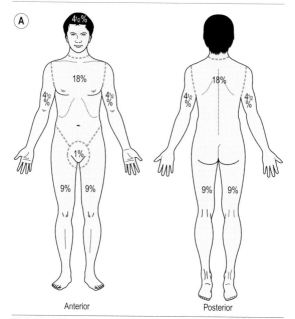

Anterior   Posterior

LUND AND BROWDER CHART FOR ADULTS AND CHILDREN OVER FIVE YEARS

lung one of a pair of conical organs of the respiratory system, consisting of an arrangement of air tubes terminating in air vesicles (alveoli) and filling almost the whole of the thorax. The alveoli are the sites of gaseous exchange in the lungs. Atmospheric oxygen is absorbed and carbon dioxide from the pulmonary capillaries is released and excreted in expiration from the lungs. The right lung has three lobes and the left lung two. They are connected with the air by means of the bronchi and trachea. *See* Figure on p. 231.

lupus a chronic skin disease having many manifestations. *L. erythematosus* a collection of autoimmune diseases in which the immune system becomes hyperactive and attacks normal healthy tissues. Symptoms can affect many different body systems including joints, skin, kidneys, blood cells, heart and lungs. *L. vulgaris* a tuberculous disease of the skin producing brownish nodules, frequently on the nose or cheek, and severe scarring.

luteinizing hormone abbreviated LH. One of three hormones produced by the anterior pituitary gland which control the activity of the gonads.

luteotrophin an anterior pituitary hormone which stimulates the formation

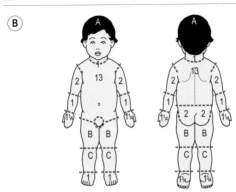

Relative percentages of areas affected by growth

AREA	BIRTH	AGE 1YR	AGE 5YR
A = 1/2 of head	9 1/2	8 1/2	6 1/2
B = 1/2 of one thigh	2 3/4	3 1/4	4
C = 1/2 of one leg	2 1/2	2 1/2	2 3/4

LUND AND BROWDER CHART FOR CHILDREN UP TO FIVE YEARS

of the corpus luteum and the production of milk. Prolactin.

luxation the dislocation of a joint. *L. of the lens* displacement of the lens of the eye into the anterior chamber or posteriorly into the vitreous humour.

Lyme disease a zoonosis transmitted by ticks and characterized by a rash (erythema chronicum migrans), arthritis and aseptic meningitis, caused by the spirochaete *Borrelia burgdorferi*.

lymph the fluid from the blood which has transuded through capillary walls to supply nutriment to tissue cells. It is collected by lymph vessels which ultimately return it to the blood. *L. nodes* or *glands* structures placed along the course of lymph vessels, through which the lymph passes and is filtered of foreign substances, e.g., bacteria. These nodes also make lymphocytes. *Plastic l.* an inflammatory exudate which tends to cause adhesion between structures and so limit the spread of infection.

lymphadenectomy excision of a lymph gland or nodes.

lymphadenitis inflammation of a lymph gland.

lymphadenopathy any disease condition of the lymph nodes.

lymphangiectasis dilatation of the lymph vessels due to some obstruction of the lymph flow.

lymphangiography radiographic examination of lymph vessels after the insertion of a radio-opaque contrast medium.

lymphangioma a swelling composed of dilated lymph vessels.

lymphangitis inflammation of lymph vessels, manifested by red lines on the skin over them. It occurs in cases of severe infection through the skin.

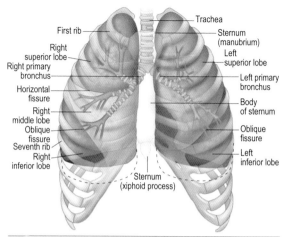

First rib

Right superior lobe

Right primary bronchus

Horizontal fissure

Right middle lobe

Oblique fissure

Seventh rib

Right inferior lobe

Trachea

Sternum (manubrium)

Left superior lobe

Left primary bronchus

Body of sternum

Oblique fissure

Left inferior lobe

Sternum (xiphoid process)

THE LUNGS

lymphatic referring to lymph. *L. system* the system of vessels and glands through which the lymph is returned to the circulation. The vessels end in the thoracic duct and the right lymphatic duct. See Figure on p. 232.

lymphoblast an early developmental cell that will mature into a lymphocyte.

lymphocyte a white blood cell formed in the lymphoid tissue. Lymphocytes produce immune bodies to overcome and protect against infection.

lymphocythaemia an excessive number of lymphocytes in the blood. Lymphocytosis.

lymphocytopenia reduction in the number of lymphocytes in the blood below normal lower limits. Lymphopenia.

lymphoedema a condition in which the intercellular spaces contain an abnormal amount of lymph due to obstruction of the lymph drainage.

lymphogranuloma venereum (LGV) a sexually transmitted disease, caused

by *Chlamydia trachomatis*; primarily a tropical condition although outbreaks have occurred in Europe and the United States.

lymphoma a group of malignant conditions of the lymphoid tissue. Generally, these diseases are classified as either Hodgkin's or non-Hodgkin's lymphomas, although the World Health Organization includes two other categories as types of lymphoma; multiple myeloma and immunoproliferative diseases. *Burkitt's l.* A type of lymphoma found predominantly in East Africa and affecting the jaws of children.

lymphopoiesis the production of lymphocytes. Occurs chiefly in the bone marrow, lymph nodes, thymus, spleen and gut wall.

lymphosarcoma a term formerly used to denote a malignant lymphoma (with the exception of Hodgkin's disease).

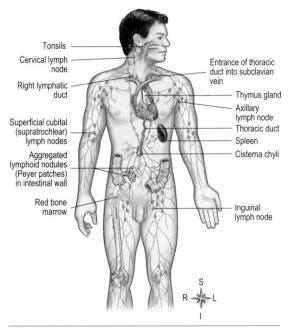

Tonsils

Cervical lymph node

Right lymphatic duct

Superficial cubital (supratrochlear) lymph nodes

Aggregated lymphoid nodules (Peyer patches) in intestinal wall

Red bone marrow

Entrance of thoracic duct into subclavian vein

Thymus gland

Axillary lymph node

Thoracic duct

Spleen

Cisterna chyli

Inguinal lymph node

LYMPHATIC SYSTEM

lyophilization a method of preserving biological substances in a stable state by freeze-drying. It may be used for plasma, sera, bacteria, viruses and tissues.

lysergic acid diethylamide also known as acid and LSD. A powerful hallucinogenic drug, manufactured from lysergic acid which is found in the ergot fungus. LSD is mainly used for recreational purposes and is a Class A drug making it illegal to possess.

lysin a specific antibody present in the blood that can destroy cells. *See* BACTERIOLYSIN.

lysine an essential amino acid formed by the digestion of dietary protein. It is vital for normal health.

lysis 1. the gradual decline of a disease, especially of a fever. The temperature falls gradually, as in typhoid. *See* CRISIS. 2. the destruction of cells.

lysosome a particle, found in the cytoplasm of cells, which causes the breakdown of metabolic substances and foreign particles (e.g., bacteria) within the cell.

lysozyme an enzyme present in tears, nasal mucus and saliva that can kill most bacteria coming into contact with it.

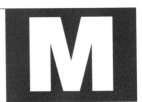

m symbol for *metre*.

McBurney's point *C. McBurney, American surgeon, 1845–1913.* The spot midway between the anterior iliac spine and the umbilicus where pain is felt on pressure if the appendix is inflamed.

maceration softening of a solid by soaking it in liquid. *Neonatal m.* the natural softening of a dead fetus in the uterus.

McKee Farrar prosthesis the first widely used total hip replacement to employ metal on metal articulation.

Mackenrodt's ligaments *A.K. Mackenrodt, German gynaecologist, 1859–1925.* The transverse or cardinal ligaments that support the uterus in the pelvic cavity.

Macmillan nurses qualified nurses who have also received special training in the management of pain relief, palliative care and the provision of emotional support to cancer patients and their families. This nursing service is provided either in the patient's home through the Macmillan home visiting service, in hospital or in a hospice. Supported by the Macmillan Cancer Support charity founded to improve the quality of life for people with cancer and their families.

macrocyte an abnormally large red corpuscle found in the blood in some forms of anaemia.

macrocythaemia the presence of abnormally large red cells in the blood. Macrocytosis.

macronutrient an essential nutrient that has a large minimal daily requirement (greater than 100 mg); calcium, phosphorus, magnesium, potassium, sodium and chloride are macronutrients.

macrophage a large reticuloendothelial cell which has the power to ingest cell debris and bacteria. It is present in connective tissue, especially when there is inflammation.

macroscopic discernible with the naked eye. The opposite of microscopic.

macrostomia an abnormal development of the mouth in which the mandibular and maxillary processes do not fuse and the mouth is excessively wide.

macula a spot or discoloured area of the skin, not raised above the surface; a macule. *M. corneae* a small area of opacity in the cornea, seen through an ophthalmoscope as a deeper red. macular pertaining to the macula. *M. degeneration* the loss of retinal pigment cells and damage to the macula. Occurs with ageing and results in the loss of colour vision and progressive visual impairment. *M.* hole a small gap in the centre of the macula resulting in blurred and distorted vision. *M. lutea* the yellow central area of the retina, where vision is clearest.

maculopapular displaying both maculae and papules. *M. eruption* a rash comprised of both maculae and papules, as in measles.

Madura foot mycetoma of the foot.

maduromycosis a chronic disease caused by *Madurella mycetomatis*. The most common form is Madura foot.

magnesium *symbol* Mg. A bluish-white metallic element. It occurs widely in mineral sources and is present in some of the body tissues. *M. carbonate* and *m. hydroxide* neutralizing antacids used in hyperacidity. *M. sulphate* a saline purgative. Epsom salts. *M. trisilicate* an antacid powder taken after food for dyspepsia and peptic ulceration.

magnetic resonance imaging (MRI) a non-invasive imaging technique based on the NUCLEAR MAGNETIC RESONANCE properties of the hydrogen nucleus. Cross-sectional images in any plane of the body for examination may be obtained.

Makaton one of the sign languages.

mal [Fr.] *disease*. *Grand m., petit m.* former names for forms of EPILEPSY. *M. de mer* seasickness.

malabsorption inability of the small intestine to absorb certain substances. It may be the cause of a deficiency disease due to the lack of an essential factor.

malacia softening of tissues. *See also* OSTEOMALACIA.

maladaptation the inability to make normal adjustments in personal relationships and in society which may result in stress, ill health and abnormal behaviour.

maladjustment in psychiatry, a failure to adjust to the environment.

malaise a feeling of general discomfort and illness.

malalignment displacement, especially of the teeth from their normal relation to the line of the dental arch.

malaria a serious, notifiable infectious illness, is a mosquito-borne infectious disease of humans (and other animals). The symptoms of the disease vary according to the protozoa of the genus *Plasmodium* and begin with a bite from an infected female mosquito of the genus *Anopheles*. This introduces the microorganisms into the circulatory system, and ultimately to the liver where they mature and reproduce. The disease causes symptoms that are typically fever, headache, joint pains, anaemia, jaundice and convulsions. Severe cases may progress to coma or death. The parasite causes haemolysis during its life cycle in the body and relapses are common. The classic symptom of malaria is paroxysm—a cyclical occurrence of sudden coldness followed by rigor with fever and sweating, occurring every two days in *P. vivax and P. ovale* infections, and every 3 days (tertian fever) in *P. malariae*. *P. falciparum* infection can cause recurrent fever every 36–48 hours (quartan fever) or a less pronounced and almost continuous fever. Malaria is widespread in tropical and subtropical regions around the equator, including Sub-Saharan Africa, Asia and Central and South America, and travellers to these regions are at risk of infection. A vaccine RTS,S/AS01 has been developed and trialled and is being further piloted in sub-Saharan Africa. Various anti-malarial drugs are used for treatment and chemoprophylaxis. Prevention of malaria includes the use of medications, vector control with insecticide-treated mosquito nets and indoor residual spray. Health education measures to promote an awareness of malaria and the importance of control measures are important for the populations of and travellers to affected areas. *Airport m.* a term sometimes used to describe malaria occurring at or near an airport, in a country normally free of the disease, and spread by infected mosquitoes brought in on an aeroplane from an endemic area. Control measures include disinsectization of aircraft where appropriate.

male pattern baldness *see* ALOPECIA.

malformation deformity; a structural defect.

malignant tending to become progressively worse and to result in death if untreated; having the properties of anaplasia, invasiveness and metastasis; said of tumours.

malingering wilful, deliberate and fraudulent feigning or exaggeration of the symptoms of illness or injury to attain a consciously desired end.

malleolus one of the two protuberances on either side of the ankle joint. *Lateral m.* that on the outer surface at the lower end of the fibula. *Medial m.* that on the inner surface at the lower end of the tibia.

malleus the hammer-shaped bone in the middle ear.

malnutrition the condition in which nutrition is defective in quantity or quality.

malocclusion an abnormality of dental development which causes overlapping of the bite.

Malpighian body *M. Malpighi, Italian anatomist, physician and physiologist, 1628–1694.* The glomerulus and Bowman's capsule of the kidney.

malposition an abnormal position of any part of the body.

malpractice failure to maintain accepted standards and cause harm. Professional misconduct.

malpresentation any abnormal position of the fetus at birth that renders delivery difficult or impossible.

Malta fever brucellosis; undulant fever.

maltase a sugar-splitting enzyme which converts maltose to glucose. Present in pancreatic and intestinal juice.

maltose the sugar formed by the action of digestive enzymes on starch.

malunion faulty repair of a fracture.

mammary relating to the breasts.

mammography radiographic or infrared examination of the breast to detect abnormalities.

mammoplasty a plastic operation to reduce the size of abnormally large, pendulous breasts or augment the size of very small breasts.

mammothermography an examination of the breast that depends on the

more active cells producing heat that can be shown on a thermograph; it may indicate abnormalities of the breast tissue.

Manchester operation also known as Fothergill operation. A technique used for uterine prolapse.

mandible the lower jawbone.

mania a disordered mental state of extreme excitement, especially the manic type of manic-depressive psychosis. Also used as a word termination to denote obsessive preoccupation with something, as in kleptomania.

manic pertaining to mania. *M.-depressive psychosis* former name for a mental illness characterized by mania or endogenous depression. A bipolar disorder: *see* BIPOLAR.

manipulation use of the hands to produce a desired movement, such as in reducing a fracture or a hernia. Its use is important in orthopaedics, physiotherapy, osteopathy and in chiropractice.

mannitol a sugar alcohol occurring widely in nature; an osmotic diuretic used for forced diuresis.

manometer an instrument for measuring the pressure of liquids or gases.

Mantoux test *C. Mantoux, French physician, 1877–1947.* A tuberculin skin test in which a solution of purified protein derivative (PPD) tuberculin is injected intradermally into either the anterior or posterior surface of the forearm. The test is read 48–72 hours after injection. It is considered positive when the induration at the site of injection is more than 10 mm in diameter.

manual involving the use of the hands. *M. evacuation of the bowel* a nursing technique used to evacuate the bowel following use of faecal softening agents (*see* LAXATIVES) in a severely constipated patient. This procedure is rarely used now due to the possibility of causing rectal trauma and distress to the patient. *M. expression of urine* pressure is placed upon the abdomen by using the hands at regular intervals to encourage the patient to void when the bladder is paralysed.

manubrium the upper part of the sternum to which the clavicle is attached. *M. handling* see MOVING AND HANDLING.

MAOI monoamine oxidase inhibitors.

maple syrup urine disease (MSUD) an inborn error of metabolism in which there is an excess in the urine of certain amino acids; the urine smells like maple syrup. There are learning difficulties, lethargy and convulsions.

marasmus severe and chronic mal-nutrition producing a gradual wasting of the tissues, owing to insufficient or unassimilated food, occurring especially in infants.

Marburg a severe notifiable, often-fatal, haemorrhagic viral disease. Similar to Ebola virus disease, princi-pally seen in central African countries, caused by the Marburg virus, of the family *Filoviridae*. These viruses are among the most virulent pathogens known to infect humans. The incu-bation period ranges from 5 to 10 days and patients present with abrupt onset of high fever, weakness, muscle pain, headache and sore throat. This is quickly followed by more severe symptoms including vomiting, diar-rhoea, rash, decreased kidney and liver functioning, and in some cases, both internal and external bleeding. Case fatality rates vary from 25% in a laboratory-associated outbreak in 1967 to over 80% in Angola in 2004. *See* EBOLA VIRUS DISEASE.

Marfan's syndrome *B.J.A. Marfan, French paediatrician, 1858–1942.* A hereditary disorder in which there is excessive height with very long digits, a high arched palate, hypertonus and dislocation of the lens of the eyes; heart disease commonly occurs.

marijuana *Cannabis indica;* Indian hemp. *See* CANNABIS.

marrow the substance contained in the middle of long bones and in the cancellous tissue of all bones. *M.*

puncture investigatory procedure in which marrow cells are aspirated from the sternum or iliac crest. *Red m.* that found in all cancellous tissue at birth. Blood cells are made in it. *Yellow m.* the fatty substance contained in the centre of long bones in later life.

masculinization the development in a woman of male secondary sexual characteristics.

mask 1. to cover up or to conceal. 2. a covering for the mouth and nose and sometimes the whole face, designed to protect the wearer or patient in pre-venting the inhalation of pathogenic organisms or toxic substances. Masks are also used in the administration of oxygen and other aerosol medications. 3. a facial expression characteristic of a certain disorder or condition. *Aerosol m.* used with a nebulizer that humidifies the inspired air or oxygen. *Parkinson's m.* an unblinking, fixed facial expression characteristic of patients with Parkin-son's disease. *M. of pregnancy.* A brownish patchy discolouration on the face and neck occurring during preg-nancy in some women and disappearing after delivery. Also known as CHLOASMA. *Venturi m.* see VENTURI MASK.

Maslow's hierarchy of needs *A.H. Maslow, American psychologist, 1908– 1970.* A hierarchical ranking, in as-cending order of importance, concern-ing human needs and motivation and the aim of realizing one's full potential. Physiological needs for oxygen, nutri-tion, shelter, sleep, etc., are the most basic and need to be met first before one is able to deal in successive order with the need for safety, security, love and belonging, self-esteem and ulti-mately the need for self-actualization (*see* Figure on p. 237).

masochism a sexual perversion in which pleasure is derived from suffering mental or physical pain.

mass 1. the quantity of material in an object or body. Can be measured in terms of the force that is needed to accelerate it. 2. a lump of undefined

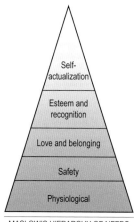

MASLOW'S HIERARCHY OF NEEDS

shape. *M. number* the total mass of protons and neutrons in an atom.

massage the application of diverse manual techniques of touch, stroking, rubbing, kneading and manipulating the body to stimulate circulation and to promote a sense of wellbeing. Used in physio-therapy and as a complementary therapy. *External cardiac m.* the application of rhythmic pressure to the lower sternum to cause expulsion of blood from the ventricles and restart circulation in cases of cardiac arrest.

masseter the muscle of the cheek chiefly concerned in mastication.

mast cell a large connective tissue cell found in many body tissues, including the heart, liver and lungs. Mast cells contain granules which release heparin, serotonin and histamine in response to inflammation or allergy.

mastalgia pain in the breast.

mastectomy amputation of the breast. *Radical m.* removal of the breast, axillary lymph glands and the pectoral muscle.

mastication the act of chewing food.

mastitis inflammation of the breast, usually due to bacterial infection.

mastocytosis a rare condition caused by excessive numbers of mast cells in body tissues.

mastoid breast- or nipple-shaped. *M. antrum* the cavity in the mastoid process which communicates with the middle ear, and contains air. *M. cells* hollow spaces in the mastoid bone. *M. operation* drainage of mastoid cells when infection spreads from the middle ear. *M. process* the breast-shaped prominence on the temporal bone which projects downwards behind the ear and into which the sternocleidomastoid muscle is inserted.

mastoidectomy removal of diseased bone and drainage of the mastoid antrum in severe purulent mastoiditis.

mastoiditis inflammation of the mastoid antrum and cells.

masturbation the production of sexual excitement by friction of the genitals.

materia medica the science of the source and preparation of drugs used in medicine.

maternal pertaining to the mother. *M. mortality rate* the number of deaths in childbirth per 1000 births.

matrix 1. that tissue in which cells are embedded. 2. in research, a matrix is an arrangement of data, which may consist of numbers or text in rows and columns. Matrices are used as part of overall data management, for accessing important data, retaining data for analysis throughout (and after) a research study.

matter substance. *Grey m.* a collection of nerve cells or non-medulled nerve fibres. *White m.* medulled nerve fibres massed together, as in the brain.

maturation ripening or developing.

maxilla one of the pair of bones forming the upper jaw and carrying the upper teeth.

maxillary pertaining to the upper jawbones.

maxillofacial pertaining to the maxilla and the face.

MACE abbreviation for Mothers and babies: Reducing Risk through Audit and Confidential Enquiries in the UK. It is collaboration led by the University of Oxford to undertake surveillance of maternal and deaths in utero or in young infants.

MCADD medium chain acyl-CoA dehydrogenase deficiency. A rare disease screened in the NEWBORN BLOOD SPOT test resulting in an inability to properly break down fat.

MCHC mean corpuscular haemoglobin concentration.

MCV mean corpuscular volume.

ME myalgic encephalomyelitis. *See* CHRONIC FATIGUE SYNDROME.

measles morbilli; rubeola. An acute, infectious, statutorily notifiable disease of childhood caused by a virus spread by droplets. Endemic and worldwide in distribution. Onset is catarrhal before the rash appears on the fourth day. Koplik's spots are diagnostic earlier. Secondary infection may give rise to the serious complication of otitis media or bronchopneumonia. Vaccination provides a high degree of immunity and may be offered with protection against mumps and rubella (MMR). *German m. see* RUBELLA.

measles, mumps and rubella vaccine abbreviated MMR. An injectable vaccine offered to children aged 12 months and 40 months. *See* Appendix 10.

meatus an opening or passage. *Auditory m.* the opening leading into the auditory canal. *Urethral m.* the opening of the urethra to the exterior.

mechanism of labour the sequence of movements whereby the fetus adapts itself to pass through the maternal passages during the process of birth.

Meckel's diverticulum J.F. Meckel, German anatomist and surgeon, 1781–1833. The remains of a passage which, in the embryo, connected the yolk sac and intestine, evident as an enclosed sac or tube in the region of the ileum.

meconium the first intestinal discharges of a newly born child. Dark green and consisting of epithelial cells, mucus and bile. *M. ileus* intestinal obstruction due to blockage of the bowel by a plug of meconium in a neonate with cystic fibrosis.

median 1. placed in the centre. 2. in a series of values, the value middle in position. *M. tibial stress* syndrome pain in the front of the legs caused by exercise. Also known as shin splints.

mediastinum the space in the middle of the thorax, between the two pleurae.

medical pertaining to medicine. *M. audit* also known as clinical audit is an evaluative process applied to the quality of clinical practice, often by peer review of routine or specially collected records of individual cases. Judgements are frequently made on the appropriateness of the processes carried out during the management of the case, in light of the outcome. Deaths are frequently the subject of medical audit, one established example being the Confidential Enquiry into Maternal Deaths (carried out at national level through MBRRACE-UK). *See* AUDIT. *M. certificate* also known as a medical statement *see* FIT NOTE. *M. device* a product used for or by a patient or service user (excluding drugs) for: (a) diagnosis, prevention, monitoring, treatment or alleviation of disease; (b) alleviation of, or compensation for, an injury or impairment; (c) investigation, replacement or modification of the anatomy or of a physiological process. *M. jurisprudence* medical science as applied to aid the law, e.g., in the case of death by poisoning, violence, etc. Forensic medicine. *See* FORENSIC. *M. laboratory scientific officer* abbreviated MLSO also known as Biomedical Scientists. An allied health professional qualified and skilled in the theory and practice of clinical laboratory procedures. *M. model* the traditional approach to the diagnosis and treatment of disease in the Western world. The medical practitioner, using a problem-solving approach, focuses on the disease process and the deficits identified in the body organs and tissues. *M. social worker* a professionally qualified worker who looks after the patients' socioeconomic and welfare needs registered with the Health and Care Professions Council (HCPC). *M. statistics* that branch of statistics concerned with data relating to health and health services. Traditionally these include the use of routine data relating to death, illness and use of hospitals, clinics, etc. The term is also often used to encompass statistics derived from aspects of medical research, such as the conduct of trials of new drugs or procedures.

medicalization 1. the extension of medical authority into areas previously regarded as being non-medical, where the lay or a popular approach prevailed, e.g., pregnancy and childbirth. 2. the tendency to view undesirable conduct as illness and therefore requiring medical intervention.

medically unexplained symptoms also known as functional symptoms. Various symptoms such as pain or dizziness for which no cause can be found.

medicament any medicinal substance used in treatment.

medicated impregnated with a medicinal substance.

medication 1. a substance administered to a patient for therapeutic purposes. 2. the treatment of a patient by means of drugs.

medicinal 1. having therapeutic qualities. 2. pertaining to a medicine.

medicine 1. any drug or remedy. 2. the art and science of the diagnosis and treatment of disease and the maintenance of health. 3. the non-surgical treatment of disease. *Public Health m.* that specialty which deals with all aspects of medical care in the community, including notification and control of infectious diseases, preschool and school health care, and factors affecting the health of the population as a whole. *Emergency m.* that specialty which deals with the acutely ill or injured who require immediate medical treatment. *Forensic m.* the application of medical knowledge to questions of law; medical jurisprudence. Also called legal medicine. *Legal m.* forensic medicine. *Nuclear m.* that branch of medicine concerned with the use of radionuclides in the diagnosis and treatment of disease. *Physical m.* that branch of medicine using physical agents in the diagnosis and treatment of disease. It includes the use of heat, cold, light, water, electricity, manipulation, massage, exercise and mechanical devices. *Preventive m.* the science aimed at preventing disease. *Proprietary m.* any chemical, drug or similar preparation used in the treatment of diseases, if such article is protected against free competition as to name, product, composition or process of manufacture by secrecy, patent, trademark or copyright, or by other means. *Psychosomatic m.* the study of the interrelations between bodily processes and emotional life. *Space m.* that branch of aviation medicine concerned with conditions to be encountered in space. *Sports and Exercise m.* (SEM) the field of medicine concerned with injuries sustained in exercise and athletic endeavours, including their prevention, diagnosis and treatment.

Medicines and Healthcare products Regulatory Agency in the UK abbreviated MHRA. Responsible for the regulation of medicines and health care products. Its primary objective is to promote and protect public health by taking all possible steps to ensure that medicines, health care products and medical equipment meet agreed standards for quality, performance, effectiveness, and are safe for those who use them. MHRA are also responsible for reporting, investigating and monitoring of adverse drug reactions to medicines and incidents with medical devices.

meditation an altered state achieved by concentrating on an object, word or idea. *Transcendental m.* an exercise in contemplative relaxation that promotes a feeling of wellbeing and calmness. It also induces changes in physiological functions, e.g., lowering of the metabolic rate, decreased cardiac output and reduced oxygen consumption, and is used in various complementary therapies.

medium in bacteriology, a preparation for the culture of microorganisms. *Contrast m.* a substance used in radiography to make visible structures that could not otherwise be seen.

MEDLARS *Medical Literature Analysis and Retrieval System* A computerized system of the National Library of Medicine at the National Institutes of Health, Bethesda USA from which the *Index Medicus* is produced. This is available in the UK in the larger academic libraries.

Medline an electronic database providing abstracts of thousands of biomedical studies.

medulla 1. bone marrow. 2. the innermost part of an organ, particularly the kidneys, lymph glands and suprarenal glands. *M. oblongata* that portion of the spinal cord that is contained inside the cranium. In it are the nerve centres that govern respiration, the action of the heart, etc.

medullary pertaining to the marrow or a medulla. *M. cavity* the hollow in the centre of long bones.

medullated having a myelin covering. *M. nerve fibre* one enclosed in a myelin sheath.

medulloblastoma a rapidly growing tumour of neuroepithelial origin occurring in childhood and appearing near the fourth ventricle of the brain. The tumour is highly radiosensitive.

megacolon extreme dilatation and hypertrophy of the large intestine. When the condition is congenital it is known as Hirschsprung's disease.

megakaryocyte a large cell of the bone marrow, responsible for blood platelet formation.

megaloblast an abnormally large nucleated cell from which mature red blood cells are derived.

megalocephaly 1. abnormal largeness of the head. 2. leontiasis ossea.

megalomania delusions of grandeur or self-importance.

megaureter dilatation of the ureter.

meibomian cyst *H. Meibom, German anatomist, 1638–1700.* A small swelling of the meibomian gland caused by obstruction of its duct. If untreated, it may become infected. A chalazion.

meibomian glands Small sebaceous glands situated beneath the conjunctiva of the eyelid; tarsal glands.

meibomianitis a bilateral chronic inflammation of the meibomian glands.

meiosis 1. a stage of reduction in cell division when the chromosomes of a gamete are halved in number ready for union at fertilization. 2. contraction of the pupil of the eye; miosis.

melaena darkening of the faeces by blood pigments.

melancholia a state of extreme DEPRESSION.

melanin a dark pigment found in the hair, the choroid of the eye, the skin and in melanotic tumours.

melanism a condition marked by an abnormal deposit of dark pigment in the skin or other tissue. Melanosis.

melanocyte a cell of the skin pigment melanin. *M.-stimulating hormone* abbreviated MSH. Hormone produced in the pituitary gland which stimulates the formation of melanin.

melanoderma a patchy pigmentation of the skin.

melanoma a malignant tumour arising in any pigment-containing tissues, especially the skin and more rarely the eye. The incidence of melanoma is rising worldwide amongst light skinned people due to increased exposure to sunlight. Preventative measures should be taken such as limiting exposure to sunlight especially between 10 : 00 hours and 16 : 00 hours, avoiding sun burn and tanning. Protective clothing should also be worn with the use of an effective sunscreen of SPF of 15 or higher for children and adults. *Amelanotic m.* an unpigmented malignant melanoma. *Subungual m.* melanoma originating on the big toe or thumb under the nail. Also known as a melanotic whitlow.

melanuria the presence of black pigment in the urine. Occurs in melanotic sarcoma and porphyria.

melisma formation of light to dark brown or greyish pigmentation of the skin, mainly on the face. The cause is not known.

membrane a thin elastic tissue covering the surface of certain organs and lining the cavities of the body. *Basement m.* the interface between epithelial cells and the underlying connective tissue. *Mucous m.* a membrane that secretes mucus and lines all cavities connected directly or indirectly with the skin. *Serous m.* membrane lining the abdominal cavity and thorax and covering most of the organs within.

memory the mental faculty that enables one to register, retain and recall previously experienced sensations, impressions, information and ideas. The ability of the brain to retain and to use knowledge gained from past experience is essential to the process of learning. Short-term memory involves the registration of received information but this is lost quickly unless the information is repeated constantly. Important information that needs to be retained is stored in long-term memory and can be recalled. Memory provides a person with a life history which is central to the concept of the 'individual self'. The exact way in which the brain remembers is not completely understood; it is believed that a portion of the temporal lobe of the brain acts as a memory centre, drawing on memories stored in other parts of the brain. *M. disturbances* any disorder of the memory functions whether of registration, retention, recall or recognition. The disorders are varied in character and in causation. The most common problem is difficulty in recall, i.e., short-term memory, that develops with age. More severe loss of memory may be an early symptom of dementia. *Procedural m.* that part of memory that stores information needed to do routine tasks that involve a sequence of steps, e.g., switching on a computer.

menarche the first appearance of menstruation.

Mendel's theory *G.J. Mendel, Abbot of Brünn, 1822–1884.* The theory that the characters of sexually reproducing organisms are handed on to the offspring in fixed ratios and without blending.

Menière's disease or syndrome *P. Menière, French physician, 1799–1862.* A disease of the inner ear causing attacks of vertigo and tinnitus with progressive deafness.

meninges the membranes covering the brain and spinal cord. There are three: the dura mater (outer), arachnoid mater (middle) and pia mater (inner).

meningioma also known as meningismus, a slow-growing, usually benign tumour developing from the arachnoid and pia mater.

meningism a condition in which there are signs of cerebral irritation similar to meningitis, including photophobia and neck stiffness due to either haemorrhage or infection.

meningitis inflammation of the meninges due to organisms such as bacteria, viruses and fungi. Meningitis causes fever, intense headache, intolerance to light and sound with rigidity of muscles especially those in the neck (*see* KERNIG'S SIGN). Convulsions with severe vomiting and delirium may also occur in the more severely ill patient. A petechial rash that does not disappear when pressure is applied (*see* GLASS TEST) may also occur in patients with meningococcal septicaemia. Therapy involves the use of appropriate antimicrobial drugs, together with intensive care interventions if required, combined with skilled nursing care and support. Meningitis is a notifiable disease, and its causal organism, if known, should also be stated. *Meningococcal m.* cerebrospinal fever. An epidemic form with a rapid onset caused by *Neisseria meningitidis* infection. *Tuberculous m.* inflammation of tuberculous origin.

meningocele a protrusion of the meninges through the skull or spinal column, appearing as a cyst filled with cerebrospinal fluid. *See* SPINA (BIFIDA).

meningococcus *Neisseria meningitidis.* A diplococcus, the microorganism of cerebrospinal meningitis.

meningoencephalitis inflammation of the brain and meninges.

meningomyelocele a protrusion of the spinal cord and meninges through a defect in the vertebral column. Myelomeningocele. *See* SPINA (BIFIDA).

meniscectomy surgical removal of a semilunar cartilage from the knee joint.

meniscus 1. the convex or concave surface of a liquid as observed in its container. 2. a lens having one convex and one concave surface. 3. a semilunar cartilage of the knee joint.

menopause the span of time during which the menstrual cycle wanes and gradually stops; also called change of life and climacteric. It is the period when ovaries stop functioning and therefore menstruation and childbearing cease. Usually occurs between the 48th and 55th years of life. There may be an associated hormonal imbalance which causes symptoms such as night sweats, hot flushes, diminished libido and extreme lethargy. *Artificial m.* an induced cessation of menstruation by surgery or by irradiation.

menorrhagia an excessive flow of the menses; menorrhoea.

menses the discharge from the uterus during menstruation.

menstrual relating to the menses. *M. cycle* the monthly cycle commencing with the first day of menstruation, when the endometrium is shed, proceeding through a process of repair and hypertrophy until the next period. It is governed by the anterior pituitary gland and the ovarian hormones, oestrogen and progesterone (*see* Figure on p. 243). *M. cup* a hygiene product made of re-usable silicon for use during menstruation as an alternative to tampons.

menstruation the monthly discharge of blood and endometrium from the uterus, starting at the age of puberty and lasting until the menopause. *Anovular m., anovulatory m.* periodic uterine bleeding without preceding ovulation. *Vicarious m.* discharge of blood at the time of menstruation from some organ other than the uterus, e.g., epistaxis, which is not uncommon.

mental 1. pertaining to the mind. 2. pertaining to the chin. *M. age* a measurement based on testing a person's intellectual development usually compared to standardized data for a chronological age. For example, a 13-year-old child with learning difficulties may have a mental age of 5. *Mental Capacity Act 2005* governs decision-making by providing a legal framework for acting and making decisions on behalf of adults who lack the capacity to make particular decisions for themselves. *M. disorder* a temporary or permanent change in an individual's mental state which makes the person unable to function in daily life as well as they would normally do. Mental illness or disorder is defined in the English Mental Health Act as 'mental illness, arrested or incomplete development of mind, psychopathic disorder and any other disorder or disability of mind'. *M. handicap* a former term for learning disability. *See* LEARNING DISABILITY. *M. health* a state of wellbeing characterized by the absence of mental or

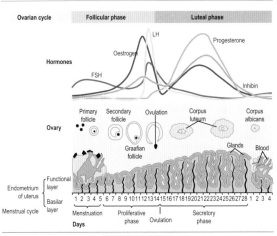

| Ovarian cycle | Follicular phase | Luteal phase |

MENSTRUAL CYCLE

behaviour disorder whereby the person has made a satisfactory adjustment as an individual, and to the community, in relation to emotional, personal, social and spiritual aspects of their life. *M. Health Acts* Laws made by parliament for the care and protection of people with mental illness. The Mental Health Act 1983 details the rights of patients with mental illness and the grounds for detaining mentally ill people against their will. It also outlines the provision of legal guardianship for such patients. The Mental Health Act (Patients in The Community) Act 1995 amended the 1983 Act by providing for supervised discharge of those detained patients requiring a high degree of supervision on discharge from hospital. In Scotland, the Mental Welfare Commission is required to 'exercise protective functions in respect of persons who may by reason of mental disorder be incapable of adequately protecting their persons or interests'. This body also has the power of a court of law, having important functions with regard to detained patients, hospital care, treatment and discharge. It is also required to report annually to the Scottish Assembly. *Mental Health Act managers* NHS Trust non-executive directors who have power under the 1983 Mental Health Act to admit or discharge mentally ill patients. *M. Health Review Tribunal* a committee with the responsibility for hearing applications from or about people detained under the Mental Health Act 1983 (amended by the Mental Health Act 2007). The Tribunal consists of medical members, legal experts and lay members who include people with knowledge of social services. In Scotland, the Mental Health Tribunal was formed as part of The Mental Health Act 2003 to decide issues concerning the compulsory care and treatment of patients with mental health disorders. In England and Wales an Approved Mental Health

Professional (AMHP) acts on behalf of a local social services department and makes application for detention, if required, under the mental Health Act. In Scotland, the Mental Health Officer (MHO) is the equivalent professional to the AMHP in England and Wales and works with people detained under the Mental Health Act. *M. mechanism* an unconscious and indirect manner of gratifying a repressed desire.

mentor 1. a wise or trusted adviser or guide. 2. in nursing, a professional colleague who assists with the career development of a colleague, and facilitates and encourages that person's professional growth and awareness. 3. a nurse and midwife trained to support the learning and assessment of pre-registration students in practice. *Sign-off m.* a specially qualified nurse or midwife who supervises and assesses students in the final placement of the course; mentorship.

mercury *symbol* Hg. Quicksilver; a heavy liquid metallic element. Previously used in the manufacture of various types of thermometer and manometer. If spillage occurs local safety regulations must be followed to prevent contamination.

mercurial poisoning from mercury (mercurialism). Can occur in people in close contact with the metal over a period of time through the skin, by inhalation or ingestion. This may present with a variety of symptoms ranging from gastrointestinal and dental problems, ataxia, visual and auditory disturbances.

meridian a conceptual channel along which qi energy flows in the body. *See* ACUPUNCTURE.

mesentery a fold of the peritoneum which connects the intestine to the posterior abdominal wall.

mesmerism *F.A. Mesmer, Austrian physician, 1734–1815.* Hypnotism.

mesoderm the middle of the three primary layers of cells in the embryo from which the connective tissues develop.

mesometrium the broad ligament connecting the uterus with the abdominal wall.

mesomorph a stocky individual of medium height with well-developed muscles.

mesothelioma a rapidly growing tumour of the pleura, peritoneum or pericardium which may be seen in patients with asbestosis. However, this tumour may also occur in people who have no history of exposure to asbestos.

messenger RNA abbreviated mRNA. The ribonucleic acid which acts as a template for the linking of amino acids during the formation of protein in the cells.

meta-analysis an attempt to improve the findings of research by combining and analysing the results of all discoverable trials on the same subject.

metabolic referring to metabolism. *M. syndrome* term for a combination of diabetes, high blood pressure and obesity.

metabolism the sum of the physical and chemical processes by which living organized substance is built up and maintained (anabolism), and by which large molecules are broken down into smaller molecules to make energy available to the organism (catabolism). Essentially, these processes are concerned with the disposition of the nutrients absorbed into the blood after digestion. *Basal m.* the minimal energy expended for the maintenance of respiration, circulation, peristalsis, muscle tonus, body temperature, glandular activity and the other vegetative functions of the body. *Inborn error of m.* a genetically determined biochemical disorder in which a specific enzyme defect produces a metabolic block that may have pathological consequences at birth, as in phenylketonuria, or in later life.

metabolite any product or substance taking part in metabolism. *Essential m.* a substance that is necessary for normal metabolism, e.g., a vitamin.

metacarpal one of the five bones of the hand which join the fingers to the wrist.

metacarpophalangeal relating to the metacarpal bones and the phalanges.

metacarpus the five bones of the hand uniting the carpus with the phalanges of the fingers.

metamorphosis a structural change or transformation.

metaphase the second stage of mitosis or cell division.

metaphysis the junction of the epiphysis with the diaphysis in a long bone.

metaplasia abnormal change in the structure of a tissue. May be indicative of malignant change.

metastasis the transfer of a disease from one part of the body to another, through the blood vessels, via the lymph channels or across the body cavities. Secondary deposits may occur from a primary malignant growth. Septic infection may arise in other organs from some original focus.

metatarsal one of the five bones of the foot which join the tarsus with the toes.

metatarsalgia pain in the metatarsal bones.

metatarsus the five bones of the foot uniting the tarsus with the phalanges of the toes.

Metazoa the division of the animal kingdom that includes the multicellular animals, i.e., all animals except the PROTOZOA.

methadone a powerful analgesic. Similar in action to morphine, it is used in withdrawal programmes for heroin addicts. Methadone is addictive, but less socially disabling than heroin. Amidone.

methaemalbumin a compound of haem with plasma albumin found in the blood in some types of anaemia.

methaemoglobin an altered form of haemoglobin found in the blood and usually produced by the action of a drug on the red blood corpuscles, causing a reduction in their oxygen-carrying ability. May be associated with the use of phenacetin and other aniline derivatives.

methaemoglobinaemia cyanosis and inability of the red blood cells to transport oxygen owing to the presence of methaemoglobin.

methane marsh gas; an inflammable explosive gas produced by decomposition of organic matter.

methicillin-resistant *Staphylococcus aureus* abbreviated MRSA. A strain of *S. aureus* that is resistant to beta-lactam antibiotics, which include methicillin and flucloxacillin. Treatment depends upon the sensitivity of the particular strain of MRSA to antibacterial drugs and the site of infection. MRSA can affect people in different ways. People can carry the organism in the nose or on the skin without showing any symptoms of illness. This is called MRSA colonization. MRSA can also cause infections, especially in hospitalized patients and particularly in those who are elderly, those with impaired immune systems, for example, those living with HIV/AIDS or transplant recipients, those who are seriously ill or who have an open wound or an indwelling urinary or intravenous catheter. Various types of infections occur, including skin, wound and surgical site infections, bone infections, pneumonia and severe life-threatening bloodstream infections. MRSA is almost always transmitted by direct physical contact, and not through the air. Transmission may also occur through indirect contact by touching objects (fomites) contaminated by the infected skin of a person with MRSA, e.g., towels, sheets, wound dressings, clothes or medical equipment. The most common means by which MRSA is transmitted between patients in hospital is by the contaminated hands of nurses, doctors and other health care workers. Standard infection prevention precautions should be followed, including meticulous attention to hand decontamination, which can effectively reduce the risk of MRSA transmission during health care activities. Environmental prevention measures include:

- Patient screening for nasal/skin carriage of MRSA and isolation while being treated;
- Proper environmental cleaning as MRSA can survive on surfaces or materials, for example, privacy curtains, bed linen;
- Effective, appropriate hand cleansing and the use of alcohol-based hand rubs.

All attendants/visitors/families/ health care professionals should always wash their hands before and after visiting any patient in hospital; use of alcohol hand gel is also effective. Visitors should be advised not to sit on beds (*see* Appendix 11).

methionine 1. a sulphur-containing essential amino acid occurring in proteins that is a vital component of the diet. 2. a drug used orally in the treatment of paracetamol poisoning.

methyl salicylate a compound used externally for rheumatic pains, lumbago, etc. Oil of wintergreen.

methylated spirit a mixture of 95% ethyl alcohol and 5% methyl alcohol. An industrial spirit which, taken as a drink, is poisonous.

methylcellulose a bulk-forming drug used as a laxative.

metra the uterus.

metre *symbol* m. The fundamental SI unit of length.

metritis inflammation of the uterus.

metrocolpocele the protrusion of the uterus into the vagina, the wall of the latter also being pushed forwards.

metrorrhagia irregular uterine bleeding not associated with menstruation.

mg milligram(s).

Mg symbol for *magnesium*.

MHRA Medicines and Healthcare products Regulatory Agency.

microbe a minute living organism, especially one causing disease. A microorganism.

microbiology the study of microorganisms and their effect on living cells.

microcephalic having an abnormally small head.

Micrococcus a genus of bacteria, each of which has a spherical shape. The bacteria occur in pairs or in groups and are gram-positive. Found in soil and water.

microcythaemia the presence of abnormally small red cells in the blood; microcytosis.

micrognathia failure of development of the lower jaw, causing a receding chin.

microgram *symbol* μg. One millionth of a gram.

micrometre *symbol* μm. One millionth of a metre. Formerly called micron.

micron *see* MICROMETRE.

micronutrient a dietary element essential only in small quantities.

microorganism a minute animal or vegetable, particularly a virus, a bacterium, a fungus, a rickettsia or a protozoon.

microphage a minute phagocyte.

microphthalmos a condition in which one or both eyes are smaller than normal. Their function may or may not be impaired.

microscope an instrument which produces a greatly enlarged image of objects that are normally invisible to the human eye. *Electron m.* a microscope in which a beam of electrons is used instead of a light beam, allowing magnification of as much as 500 000 diameters.

microscopic visible only by means of the microscope. The opposite of macroscopic. *M. polyangiitis* a rare but potentially serious form of vasculitis which can affect any organs but which typically affects lungs, kidneys and nerves.

Microsporum a genus of fungi. The cause of some skin diseases, especially ringworm.

microsurgery the carrying out of surgical procedures using a binocular

microscope with magnification and focusing ability. Microsurgery has been developed to enable operating, e.g., on the eye or in the ear, on delicate and previously inaccessible tissues, nerves and blood vessels, in orthopaedics, gynaecology and neurosurgery.

micturition the act of passing urine.

midbrain that portion of the brain that connects the cerebrum with the pons and cerebellum.

midlife crisis experienced by many people usually during the fifth decade of life, resulting in doubt, anxiety and sometimes depression. During this time men and women may reflect on their lives, review the past and be aware of physiological deterioration associated with ageing. Any children are growing up, moving away from home and establishing their own adult relationships: the empty nest syndrome.

midwife the International Confederation of Midwives (ICM) defines a midwife as 'a person who has successfully completed a midwifery education programme that is based on the ICM Essential Competencies for Basic Midwifery Practice and the framework of the ICM Global Standard for Midwifery Education; and is recognised in the country where it is located; who has acquired the requisite qualifications to be registered and/or legally licensed to practice midwifery and use the title 'midwife'; and who demonstrates competency in the practice of midwifery'. Midwives are able to give the necessary support, care and advice to women during pregnancy, labour and the postpartum period, conduct deliveries on her [or his] own responsibility and care for the newborn and the infant. The midwife may practice in hospitals, clinics, health units, domiciliary conditions or in any other service.' The word 'midwife' originates from Middle English meaning 'with woman', thus male practitioners are also called midwives.

midwifery the art and science of caring for women undergoing normal pregnancy, labour and the period following childbirth according to need but usually up to 10–28 days. *Professional M. Advocate* (PMA) experienced practicing midwives trained to support and guide midwives to deliver care.

migraine paroxysmal attacks of severe headache, often with nausea, vomiting and visual disturbance.

milestone one of the norms against which the motor, social and psychological development of a child is measured.

milia small white spots usually occurring in clusters around the nose and cheeks resulting from obstruction of a sebaceous gland. May occur in young adults. *M. neonatorum* milia occurring in the newborn, which are harmless and quickly disappear if left alone.

miliaria prickly heat, an acute itching eruption common among white people in tropical and subtropical areas.

miliary resembling millet seed. *M. tuberculosis see* TUBERCULOSIS.

milieu the environment or setting. *M. interieur* the internal physical and chemical environment experienced by individual cells. *M. therapy* a psychiatric intervention in which the physical surroundings and social setting are used as important elements in the therapeutic process.

milk 1. secretion of the mammary gland. 2. a liquid (emulsion or suspension) resembling the secretion of the mammary gland. *Human breast m.* contains lipids, 98% as triglycerides, which provide more than 50% of the calorific requirements; carbohydrates, mainly lactose, giving 40% of the calorific needs; whey-dominant protein; vitamins; minerals; trace elements; and anti-infective factors, such as leukocytes, immunoglobulins, lysozyme, lactoferrin, bifidus factor, hormones and growth factor. *Pasteurized m.* a process whereby milk is held at 77°C for 15–20 seconds and then rapidly cooled and packed; this method kills non-spore bearing pathogenic organisms without affecting flavour or food properties of the milk. *M. teeth* the first set of a child's teeth.

Miller–Abbott tube *T.G. Miller, American physician, 1886–1981; W.O. Abbott, American physician, 1902–1943.* A double-channel intestinal tube for treating obstruction, especially that due to paralytic ileus of the small intestine. It has an inflatable balloon at its distal end.

milligram *symbol* mg. One thousandth of a gram.

millilitre *symbol* ml. One thousandth of a litre (one cubic centimetre).

millimetre *symbol* mm. One thousandth of a metre.

millimole *symbol* mmol. The amount of a substance that balances or is equivalent in combining power to 1 mg of hydrogen. An SI unit equivalent to $1/1000^{th}$ of a mole. Some medical tests report results in millimoles per litre (mmol/L).

Milwaukee brace a brace consisting of a leather girdle and neck ring connected by metal struts; used to brace the spine in the treatment of SCOLIOSIS.

mineralocorticoid a hormone produced by the adrenal cortex. Its function is to maintain the salt and water balance in the body.

miosis contraction of the pupil of the eye, as in reaction to a bright light; meiosis.

miscarriage abortion; the expulsion of the fetus before the 24th week of pregnancy, i.e., before it is legally viable.

Misuse of Drugs Act 1971 and subsequent regulations controls the manufacture, possession, prescription and sale of certain habit-forming drugs, including narcotic drugs that are liable to misuse with the development of dependence. These are called controlled drugs and are available for treatment only on medical prescription. Heavy penalties invariably follow the illegal sale or supply of these drugs.

mite a minute animal, frequently parasitic on humans and animals, and causing various forms of dermatitis.

mitochondrion a body which is found in the cytoplasm of cells and is concerned with energy production and the oxidation of food.

mitosis a method of multiplication of cells by a specific process of division.

mitral shaped like a mitre. *M. incompetence* the result of a defective mitral valve, when there is a back flow, or regurgitation, after closure of the valve. *M. stenosis* the formation of fibrous tissue, causing a narrowing of the valve; usually due to rheumatic heart disease and endocarditis. *M. valve* the bicuspid valve between the left atrium and left ventricle of the heart. *M. valvotomy* an operation for overcoming stenosis by dividing the fibrous tissue to free the cusps.

mittelschmerz pain occurring between the menses, accompanying ovulation.

ml symbol for *millilitre(s)*.

MLNS mucocutaneous lymph node syndrome.

MLSO medical laboratory scientific officer.

mm symbol for *millimetre(s)*.

mmol symbol for *millimole(s)*.

MMR measles mumps rubella vaccine.

Mn symbol for *manganese*.

mobilization the bringing back into mobility of a limb, joint or person following illness or injury.

model a conceptual paradigm, framework or theory which can be used as an example to illustrate a problem, process or situation.

modelling providing an example that can be imitated, and used as a means of teaching others to learn new behaviour.

modem a device that modulates carrier wave signals to encode digital information for transmission and demodulates signals to decode transmitted information.

MODS multiple organ dysfunction syndrome.

molar a back tooth used for grinding. There are three on either side of each jaw, making 12 in all (only eight in children). See Figure on p. 108. *M. pregnancy see* MOLE. *M. solution* the concentration of a solution expressed in terms of the weight of the dissolved substance in grams per litre divided by its molecular weight.

mole 1. SI unit of amount of substance. The mole is the amount of substance of a system which contains as many elementary entities as there are atoms in 0.012 kilogram of carbon. 2. a pigmented naevus or dark-coloured growth on the skin. Moles are of various sizes, and are sometimes covered with hair. 3. a uterine tumour. *Carneous m.* an organized blood clot surrounding a shrivelled fetus in the uterus. *Hydatidiform m.* (*vesicular m.*) a condition in pregnancy in which the chorionic villi of the placenta degenerate into clusters of cysts like hydatids. Malignant growth may follow if any remnants are left in the uterus. *See* CHORIOCARCINOMA.

molecular pertaining to or composed of molecules. *M. weight* the weight of a molecule of a substance compared with that of an atom of carbon.

molecule the chemical combination of two or more atoms which form a specific chemical substance, e.g., H_2O (water). The smallest amount of a substance that can exist independently.

molluscum a skin disease characterized by the development of soft, round tumours. *M. contagiosum* a benign tumour arising in the epidermis caused by a virus, transmitted by direct contact or fomites.

monarticular referring to one joint only.

Mongolian spots blue-grey births marks present from birth usually appearing on the lower back and buttocks. They will usually disappear by the time the child is 5 years old. They resemble bruises.

Monilia former name for the genus of fungi now known as *Candida*.

monitor 1. to check constantly on a given condition, state or phenomenon, e.g., blood pressure, heart, respiration rate or standards of care. 2. an apparatus by which such conditions or phenomena can be constantly observed and recorded. *Patient m.* the use of electrodes or transducers attached to the patient so that information such as temperature, pulse, respiration and blood pressure can be seen on a screen or automatically recorded.

Monitor formerly had a role in assessing NHS Trusts for foundation trust status, and for ensuring that, once authorized, foundation trusts are financially viable and well led, in terms of both quality and finances. Now part of NHS IMPROVEMENT (NHSI).

monoamine oxidase an enzyme that breaks down noradrenaline and serotonin in the body. *M. o. inhibitor* abbreviated MAOI. A drug that prevents the breakdown of serotonin and leads to an increase in mental and physical activity.

monochromatism colour blindness. The patient sees all colours as black, grey or white.

monoclonal derived from a single cell. *M. antibodies* antibodies derived from a single clone of cells. All the antibody molecules are identical and will react with the same antigenic site.

monocular pertaining to, or affecting, one eye only.

monocyte a white blood cell having one nucleus, derived from the reticular cells, and having a phagocytic action.

mononucleosis an excessive number of monocytes in the blood; monocytosis. *Infectious m.* an infectious disease due to the EPSTEIN–BARR VIRUS; glandular fever.

monoplegia paralysis of one limb or of a single muscle or a group of muscles.

monosaccharide a simple sugar. The end result of carbohydrate digestion. Examples are glucose, fructose and galactose.

monosodium glutamate a chemical food flavour enhancer commonly added to Chinese dishes. May result in nausea, faintness, facial flushing and headache (sometimes called the Chinese restaurant syndrome).

monosomy a congenital defect in the number of human chromosomes. There is one less than the normal 46.

mons a prominence or mound. *M. pubis* or *m. veneris* the eminence, consisting of a pad of fat, that lies over the pubic symphysis in the female.

Montgomery's glands or tubercles *W.F. Montgomery, Irish obstetrician, 1797–1859.* Sebaceous glands around the nipple, which grow larger during pregnancy. Also known as areolar glands.

mood emotional reaction. Variations in mood are natural, but in certain psychiatric conditions there is severe depression in some cases and wild excitement in others, or alternations between both.

moon face (also known as Cushingoid face) one of the features occurring in Cushing's syndrome and as a result of prolonged treatment with steroid drugs.

morbid diseased, or relating to an abnormal or disordered condition.

morbidity the state of being diseased. *M. rate* a figure that shows the susceptibility of a population to a certain disease. Usually shown statistically as the number of cases which occur annually per 1000 or other unit of population.

morbilli measles.

morbilliform resembling measles.

moribund in a dying condition.

morning sickness nausea and vomiting which sometimes occurs in early pregnancy.

Moro reflex *E. Moro, German paediatrician, 1874–1951.* The reaction to loud noise or sudden movement which should be present in the newborn. Startle reflex.

morphine the principal alkaloid obtained from opium and given mainly to relieve severe pain. It is a drug of addiction. Morphia.

mortality the state of being liable to die. *M. rate* the number of deaths, per 1000 or other unit of population, occurring annually from a certain disease or condition.

mortification gangrene or death of tissue; necrosis.

Morton's neuroma a painful foot condition affecting one of the nerves between the toes. Also known as Morton's metatarsalgia.

morula an early stage of development of the ovum when it is a solid mass of cells.

mosaic an individual who has cells of varying genetic composition.

motile capable of movement.

motion 1. the process of moving. 2. evacuation of the bowels; defecation. *M. sickness* sickness occurring as the result of travel by land, sea or air. Appears to be caused by excessive stimulation of the vestibular apparatus within the inner ear.

motivation the reason or reasons, conscious or unconscious, behind a particular attitude or behaviour.

motive the incentive that determines a course of action or its direction.

motor something that causes movement. *M. end-plate* the nuclei and cytoplasm of muscle fibres at the termination of motor nerves. *M. nerve* one of the nerves which convey an impulse from a nerve centre to a muscle or gland to promote activity. *M. neurone disease* a disease in which there is progressive degeneration of the anterior cells in the spinal cord, the motor nuclei of cranial nerves and the corticospinal tracts. The cause is unknown.

mould 1. a species of fungus. 2. the plastic shell used to immobilize a part of the body, usually the head, during radiotherapy.

moulding the alteration in shape of the infant's head as it is forced through the maternal passages during labour.

mountain sickness dyspnoea, headache, rapid pulse and vomiting, which occur on sudden change to the rarefied air of high altitudes.

mourning *see* BEREAVEMENT.

mouth an opening, particularly the external opening (in the face) of the alimentary canal. *M. ulcers* painful, greyish-white sores occurring inside the mouth. Most are of unknown cause and usually disappear after a few days. Aphthous ulcers. *M.-wash* a solution for rinsing the mouth.

movement 1. an act of moving; motion. 2. an act of defecation. *Active m.* movement produced by the person's own muscles. *Associated m.* movement of parts that act together, as the eyes. *Passive m.* a movement of the body or of the extremities of a patient performed by another person without voluntary motion on the part of the patient. *Vermicular m's* the wormlike movements of the intestines in peristalsis.

moving and handling technically the moving, lifting or supporting of a load. In the work environment, this is now subject to statute (Health & Safety at Work Act 1974) to enforce the regulations and guidelines to reduce the risk of back injuries for nurses and health care workers; these regulations are enforced by the Health and Safety Executive and for any infringements, the HSE can prosecute in the criminal courts. *M. and handling equipment* any piece of equipment that facilitates the transfer of persons or objects, e.g., monkey poles, handling belts, transfer boards (Patslides), mechanical lifters or hoists. *M. and handling risk* following an initial assessment, any hazard or risk that has the potential to cause harm or illness to the patient during the manoeuvre.

MRSA methicillin-resistant *Staphylococcus aureus.*

mucinase an enzyme which acts upon mucin used in the treatment of cystic fibrosis.

mucocele a mucous tumour. *Lacrimal m.* a distension of the lacrimal sac caused by a blockage of the nasolacrimal duct. *M. of the gallbladder* occurs if a stone obstructs the cystic duct.

mucocutaneous pertaining to mucous membrane and skin. *M. lymph node syndrome* usually reported in babies and children. *See* KAWASAKI DISEASE.

mucoid resembling mucus.

mucopurulent containing mucus and pus.

mucosa mucous membrane.

mucositis pain and inflammation of the mucous membrane. A common side effect of chemotherapy and radiotherapy.

mucous pertaining to or secreting mucus. *M. membrane* a membrane that secretes mucus and lines many of the body cavities, particularly those of the respiratory and alimentary tracts.

mucoviscidosis *see* CYSTIC FIBROSIS.

mucus the viscous secretion of mucous membrane.

multicellular consisting of many cells.

multidisciplinary involving two or more professional disciplines.

multigravida a pregnant woman who has had two or more pregnancies.

multilocular having many locules. *M. cyst* a cyst, usually in the ovary, containing many compartments.

multinuclear possessing many nuclei.

multipara a woman who has had two or more children.

multiple manifold, occurring in many parts of the body at once. *M. myeloma* malignant disease of the plasma cells which invade the bone marrow and suppress its functioning. *M. sclerosis* *see* SCLEROSIS.

multiple organ dysfunction syndrome abbreviated MODS and also known as multiple organ failure (MOF). A situation usually precipitated by shock or trauma in which the functioning of interdependent body systems is severely affected, e.g., respiration, gastrointestinal tract, kidneys, blood circulation and coagulation. This multiple organ failure causes physiological disturbance requiring vital system support to maintain life. Other systems too may be compromised.

multivariate analysis the analysis of data collected on several different variables but all having a relevance to the study; e.g., in a survey of the provision of community nursing services for a specific population, data may be collected on age, family size and previous use of the services. In analysing the data the effect of each of these variables and their interaction can be examined and considered.

mumps a communicable paramyxovirus disease mainly of childhood, which is statutorily notifiable. Incubation period 2–3 weeks. It attacks one or both of the parotid glands, the largest of the three pairs of salivary glands; also called epidemic parotitis or epidemic parotiditis. Characterized by inflammation and swelling of the parotid glands. The symptoms are fever, and a painful swelling in front of the ears, making mastication difficult.

Münchhausen's syndrome *Baron von Münchhausen, 16th-century German traveller noted for his lying tales.* Habitual seeking of medical treatment for apparent acute illness, the patient giving a plausible and dramatic history, all of which is false. *M. s. by proxy* a situation in which a parent (usually the mother) or both parents fabricate symptoms or signs in a child, who is then presented for hospital treatment; overlaps with other forms of child abuse, and fatal outcomes have been reported.

murmur a sound, heard on auscultation, usually originating in the cardiovascular system. *Aortic m.* one indicating disease of the aortic valve. *Diastolic m.* one heard after the second heart sound. *Friction m.* one present when two inflamed surfaces of serous membrane rub on each other. *Mitral m.* a sign of incompetence of the mitral

valve. *Systolic m.* one heard during systole.

muscae volitantes [L.] *flying flies.* Black spots floating before the eyes. They do not obscure the sight. Floaters.

muscle strong tissue composed of fibres which have the power of contraction, and thus produce movements of the body. *Cardiac m.* muscle composed of partially striped interlocking cells. Not under the control of the will. *M. relaxant* one of a group of drugs used to reduce muscular spasm and also to relax the muscles during surgery. *Smooth* or *non-striated m.* involuntary muscle of spindle-shaped cells, e.g., that of the intestinal wall. Contracts independently of the will. *Striped* or *striated m.* voluntary muscle. Transverse bands across the fibres give the characteristic appearance. It is under the control of the will. *See* Figures on pp. 253–255.

muscular 1. pertaining to muscle. 2. well provided with strong muscles. *M. dystrophy* one of a number of inherited diseases in which there is progressive muscle wasting. *See* DUCHENNE DYSTROPHY.

musculocutaneous referring to the muscles and the skin. *M. nerve* one of the nerves which supply the muscles and the skin of the arms and legs.

musculoskeletal referring to both the osseous and muscular systems.

mutant 1. in genetics, a variation owing to genetic changes. 2. produced by mutation.

mutation a chemical change in the genes of a cell causing it to show a new characteristic. Some produce evolutional changes, others disease.

mute without the power of speech.

mutilation deliberate infliction of bodily injury.

mutism inability or refusal to speak. In almost all cases, individuals are unable to speak because deafness has prevented them from hearing the spoken word. Speech is learned by imitating the speech of others. May also result

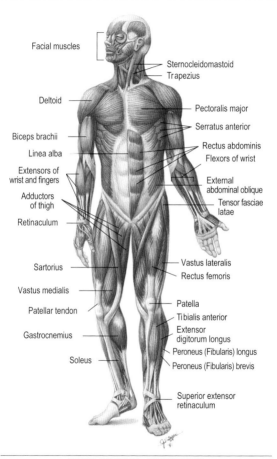

Facial muscles

Sternocleidomastoid
Trapezius

Deltoid

Pectoralis major

Serratus anterior

Biceps brachii

Linea alba

Rectus abdominis
Flexors of wrist

Extensors of
wrist and fingers

External
abdominal oblique

Adductors
of thigh

Tensor fasciae
latae

Retinaculum

Sartorius

Vastus lateralis
Rectus femoris

Vastus medialis

Patellar tendon

Patella
Tibialis anterior

Gastrocnemius

Extensor
digitorum longus

Soleus

Peroneus (Fibularis) longus
Peroneus (Fibularis) brevis

Superior extensor
retinaculum

MUSCULAR SYSTEM – ANTERIOR VIEW

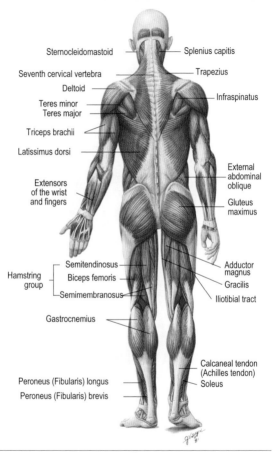

Sternocleidomastoid — Splenius capitis

Seventh cervical vertebra — Trapezius

Deltoid

Teres minor — Infraspinatus
Teres major

Triceps brachii

Latissimus dorsi

External
abdominal
oblique

Extensors
of the wrist
and fingers

Gluteus
maximus

Adductor
magnus

Hamstring group
— Semitendinosus
— Biceps femoris
— Semimembranosus

Gracilis

Iliotibial tract

Gastrocnemius

Calcaneal tendon
(Achilles tendon)

Soleus

Peroneus (Fibularis) longus

Peroneus (Fibularis) brevis

MUSCULAR SYSTEM – POSTERIOR VIEW

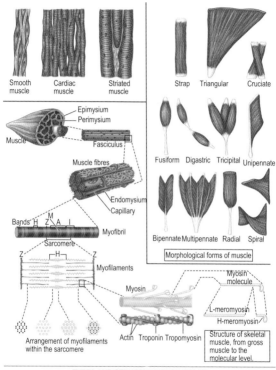

Smooth muscle   Cardiac muscle   Striated muscle

Strap   Triangular   Cruciate

Epimysium
Perimysium
Muscle
Fasciculus
Muscle fibres
Endomysium
Capillary

Fusiform   Digastric   Tricipital   Unipennate

Bands H   M   Z   A   I
Myofibril
Sarcomere

Z   H   Z
Myofilaments

Myosin

Bipennate   Multipennate   Radial   Spiral

Morphological forms of muscle

Myosin molecule

L-meromyosin
H-meromyosin

Actin   Troponin   Tropomyosin

Structure of skeletal muscle, from gross muscle to the molecular level.

Arrangement of myofilaments within the sarcomere

TYPES AND STRUCTURE OF MUSCLES

from disease, the most common being a stroke. *Selective m.* failure to speak in specific situations strongly associated with social anxiety disorder.

myalgia pain in the muscles.

myalgic encephalomyelitis abbreviated ME. *See* CHRONIC FATIGUE SYNDROME.

myasthenia muscle weakness. *M. gravis* an extreme form of muscle weakness which is progressive. There is a rapid onset of fatigue, thought to be due to the too rapid destruction of acetylcholine at the neuromuscular junction. Commonly affected muscles are those of vision, speaking, chewing and swallowing.

mycetoma a chronic fungus infection of the tissues, both external and internal but most commonly affecting the hands and feet. There is swelling and the formation of sinuses. Madura foot.

Mycobacterium a genus of slender, rod-shaped, acid-fast, gram-positive bacteria that cause a variety of diseases. *M. chimaera* a rare complication following open heart surgery or heart or lung transplant linked to a device used to heat and cool blood during surgery. *M. leprae* the causative organism of leprosy. *M. tuberculosis* the cause of tuberculosis.

mycology the study of fungi.

mycosis any disease that is caused by a fungus. *M. fungoides* a rare malignant lymphoreticular neoplasm of the skin which later progresses to the lymph nodes and viscera. Also known as Alibert-Bazin syndrome.

mydriasis abnormal dilatation of the pupil of the eye. Usually caused by injury to the pupil sphincter or by the use of mydriatic drugs.

mydriatic any drug that causes mydriasis. Used in examination of the eye and in the treatment of inflammatory conditions.

myelin the fatty covering of medullated nerve fibres.

myelitis 1. inflammation of the spinal cord, causing pain in the back and sometimes numbness and paralysis of the legs and the lower part of the trunk. 2. inflammation of the bone marrow; osteomyelitis.

myeloblast a primitive cell in the bone marrow, from which develop the granular leukocytes.

myelocyte a cell of the bone marrow, derived from a myeloblast.

myelography radiographic examination of the spinal cord after the introduction of a radio-opaque substance into the subarachnoid space by means of lumbar puncture.

myeloid 1. pertaining to, derived from or resembling bone marrow. 2. pertaining to the spinal cord. 3. having the appearance of myelocytes, but not

necessarily derived from bone marrow. *M. leukaemia* a malignant disease in which there is excessive production of leukocytes in the bone marrow. *M. tissue* red bone marrow.

myeloma a tumour composed of plasma cells. *Multiple m.* a primary malignant tumour of plasma cells, usually arising in bone marrow, and usually associated with anaemia.

myelomatosis a malignant disease of the bone marrow in which multiple myelomas are present.

myelomeningocele meningomyelocele.

myiasis infestation of wounds or body openings by fly larvae (maggots); more commonly seen in the tropics.

myocardial pertaining to the myocardium. *M. infarction* death of part of the heart muscle caused by a blockage in the blood supply. Associated with chest tightness and severe pain that may radiate down, most usually, the left arm. Men are more likely to have a heart attack than women. Risk factors include a family history of the condition, obesity, history of smoking, hypertension, diabetes, raised cholesterol levels together with a sedentary lifestyle. Diagnosis is confirmed by ECG and the measurement of cardiac enzymes. A myocardial infarction is a medical emergency and initial treatment includes aspirin, early thrombolytic therapy, oxygen therapy and analgesia. Increasingly, patients with this condition are treated with an angioplasty, with the insertion of one or more stents to create a passage through the occluded artery for the flow of blood to be re-established. After treatment, preventative lifestyle changes are recommended: take more exercise, reduce weight, stop cigarette smoking and commence a more healthy diet. Statin drugs are usually prescribed to lower blood cholesterol with ACE inhibitors to reduce the risk of further attacks.

myocarditis inflammation of the myocardium.

myocardium the muscle tissue of the heart.

myoclonus spasmodic contraction of the muscles includes HICCUPS.

myofibrosis a degenerative condition in which there is some replacement of muscle tissue by fibrous tissue.

myohaemoglobin a substance, resembling haemoglobin, which is present in muscle cells. It is a pigment and is responsible for the colour of muscle. It acts as an oxygen store. Myoglobin.

myokymia a benign condition in which there is persistent quivering of the muscles.

myoma a benign tumour of muscle tissue. See FIBROMYOMA.

myomectomy removal of a myoma; usually referring to a uterine fibroma.

myometrium the muscular tissue of the uterus.

myoneural relating to both muscle and nerve. *M. junction* the point at which nerve endings terminate in a muscle; neuromuscular junction.

myopathy any disease of the muscles. Muscular dystrophy is one of a group of inherited myopathies in which there is wasting and weakness of the muscles.

myopia shortsightedness. The light rays focus in front of the retina and a biconcave lens is needed to focus them correctly.

myoplasty any operation in which muscle is detached and utilized, as may be done to correct deformities.

myosarcoma a sarcomatous tumour of muscle.

myosin muscle protein.

myositis inflammation of a muscle. *M. ossificans* a condition in which bone cells deposited in muscle continue to grow and cause hard lumps. It may occur after fractures.

myotomy the division or dissection of a muscle.

myotonia lack of muscle tone. *M. congenita* a hereditary disease in which the muscle action has a prolonged contraction phase and slow relaxation.

myringa the eardrum or tympanic membrane.

myringitis inflammation of the tympanic membrane.

myringoplasty a plastic operation to repair the tympanic membrane. See TYMPANOPLASTY.

myringotomy incision of the tympanic membrane to drain fluid from an infected middle ear.

myxoedema a condition, caused by hypothyroidism, which is marked by mucoid infiltration of the skin. There is oedematous swelling of the face, limbs and hands, dry and rough skin, loss of hair, slow pulse, subnormal temperature, slowed metabolism and mental dullness.

myxoma a benign mucous tumour of connective tissue.

myxosarcoma a sarcoma containing mucoid tissue.

myxovirus the group name of a number of related viruses, including the causal viruses of influenza, parainfluenza, mumps and Newcastle disease (of fowl).

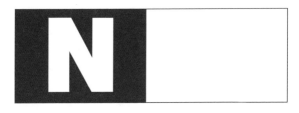

N symbol for *nitrogen* and *newton*.

Na symbol for *sodium*.

nadir the lowest out of a series of measurements, e.g., the lowest level to which the viral load falls after starting antiretroviral treatment. The opposite is ZENITH.

naevus a birthmark; a circumscribed area of pigmentation of the skin due to dilated blood vessels. A haemangioma. *N. flammeus* a flat bluish-red area, usually on the neck or face; popularly known as 'port wine stain'. *N. pilosus* a hairy naevus. *N. araneus* (spider naevus) a small red area surrounded by dilated capillaries. *Strawberry n.* a raised tumour-like structure of connective tissue containing spaces filled with blood.

Nägele's rule rule for calculating the estimated date of labour; add one year, subtract 3 months and add 7 days to the first day of the last menstrual period.

NAI non-accidental injury. *See* CHILD ABUSE.

nail the keratinized portion of epidermis covering the dorsal extremity of the fingers and toes. *Fungal n. infection see* ONYCHOMYCOSIS. *Hang n.* a strip of epidermis hanging at one side or at the root of a nail. *Ingrowing n.* a condition in which the flesh overhangs the edge of the nail, a sharp corner of which may pierce the skin, causing a wound which may become septic. *N. bed* the skin underlying a nail. *N. biting*

a sign of nervousness or tension which occurs in childhood and may persist into adult life. It is a common problem and the most frequent habitual manipulation of the body but is rarely of psychopathological significance. *Spoon n.* a nail with a depression in the centre and raised edges. *See* KOILONYCHIA.

NANDA North American Nursing Diagnosis Association.

nanometre *symbol* nm. A unit of measurement equal to one billionth (10^{-9}) of a metre, or more commonly used to describe a measure equal to one thousandth (10^{-3}) of a micrometre (μm). Nanometres are used to describe the smallest particles in nature, e.g., atoms, small molecules, viruses, electromagnetic radiation). A nanometre is approximately the length of three to six atoms placed side by side, or the width of a single strand of DNA; the thickness of a human hair is between 50 000 and 100 000 nm and represents the smallest feature an unaided human eye can see.

nape the back of the neck.

nappy rash an erythematous rash which may occur in infants in the napkin area. The many causes include the passage of frequent loose stools, thrush and ammoniacal dermatitis.

narcissism the stage of infant development when children are mainly interested in themselves and their own bodily needs. In adults, it may be a symptom of mental disorder. The term is derived from the Greek myth of Narcissus.

narcoanalysis a controversial form of psychotherapy in which an injection of a narcotic drug produces a drowsy, relaxed state during which a patient will talk more freely, and in this way much repressed material may be brought to consciousness. Also known as narcosynthesis.

narcolepsy a rare condition in which there is an uncontrollable desire for sleep.

narcosis a state of unconsciousness produced by a narcotic drug. *Basal n.* a reversible state of unconsciousness produced prior to surgical anaesthesia.

narcotic a drug that produces narcosis or unnatural sleep.

nares the nostrils. *Posterior n.* the opening of the nares into the nasopharynx.

nasal pertaining to the nose. *N. polyp* swelling of the nasal lining inside the nasal passages and sinuses.

nascent 1. at the time of birth. 2. incipient.

nasoduodenal related to the nose and duodenum. *N. tube* a fine-bore tube passed through the nose into the duodenum and used for enteral nutrition.

nasogastric referring to the nose and stomach. *N. tube* one passed into the stomach via the nose.

nasojejunal feeding a method in which a silicone-coated catheter is passed through the nose into the jejunum to provide sufficient nutrition to a sick baby on a ventilator or receiving continuous inflating pressure (CIP) by mask or nasal tube. It is used to prevent the dangers of aspiration with a nasogastric tube feed.

nasolacrimal concerning both the nose and lacrimal apparatus. *N. duct* the duct draining the tears from the inner aspect of the eye to the inferior meatus of the nose.

nasopharynx the upper part of the pharynx; that above the soft palate.

nasosinusitis inflammation of the nose and adjacent sinuses.

National Audit Office (NAO) This is an independent Parliamentary body in the UK, responsible for scrutinizing public spending by auditing the financial statements of all central government departments, agencies and other public bodies. The NAO reports to the Comptroller and Auditor General in Parliament. Audit Scotland performs a similar role in Scotland. The Wales Audit Office is responsible for auditing the Welsh Assembly Government, its public bodies and local government in Wales. The Northern Ireland Audit Office performs similar functions in Northern Ireland.

National Confidential Enquiry into Patient Outcome and Death (NCEPOD) is the system for reviewing the management of patients by undertaking confidential surveys and research. MBRRACE runs the national programme of work conducting investigations into maternal deaths, stillbirths and infant deaths. The national confidential inquiry into suicide and homicide by people with mental illness (NCISH) delivers the mental health outcome review programme. *See* CONFIDENTIAL ENQUIRY.

National Institute for Health and Care Excellence abbreviated NICE. An executive non-departmental public body serving England and Wales, providing formal advice for the NHS and social care through the publication of guidelines in four area: 1. use of new technologies within the NHS e.g., use of new and existing medicines, treatments and procedures. 2. clinical practice focused on care and treatment of people with specific diseases and conditions. 3. guidance for public sectors workers on health promotion. 4. guidance for social care services and users.

natural birth childbirth an approach to birth which advocates avoidance of medical interference, excessive reliance on technology and analgesia in labour, thus encouraging parents to participate in the childbirth experience. Also known as active birth.

natural family planning a method of family planning that uses knowledge of an individual woman's fertility and avoids sexual intercourse during high fertility periods of the menstrual cycle.

natural killer cells abbreviated NK. A type of lymphocyte involved in natural killing (apoptosis) and forming part of the non-specific body defences. NK cells target viral infected cells and tumour cells.

nature–nurture debate the debate surrounding the issue of to what extent human behaviour is the result of hereditary or innate influences (nature) or is determined by the environment and learning (nurture).

naturopathy a drugless system of alternative healing by a combination of diet, fasting, exercise, hydrotherapy and positive thinking.

nausea a sensation of sickness with an inclination to vomit.

navel the umbilicus.

navicular boat-shaped. *N. bone* one of the tarsal bones of the foot.

nebula a slight opacity or cloudiness of the cornea, caused by injury or by corneal ulceration.

nebulizer an apparatus for reducing a liquid to a fine spray. An atomizer.

NEC necrotizing enterocolitis.

neck 1. the narrow part of an organ or bone. 2. the part of the body which connects the head and the trunk. *Wry n.* torticollis.

necrobiosis localized death of a part as a result of degeneration.

necropsy autopsy; a postmortem examination of a body.

necrosis death of a portion of tissue.

necrotizing enterocolitis abbreviated NEC. Inflammatory bowel disease of preterm and low birth weight infants, associated with septicaemia, especially where there is a history of asphyxia,

respiratory distress, hypoglycaemia, hypothermia or cardiovascular disease, possibly due to bacterial proliferation and penetration of the bowel wall in areas of ischaemic damage. May lead to perforation and peritonitis. Treated with parenteral nutrition, antibiotics, and surgery for perforation.

necrotizing fasciitis a bacterial infection of *Streptococcus* type A underneath the skin in the fascia layer; produces necrosis and toxins, resulting in shock and organ failure. Urgent treatment is required with antibiotics and surgical excision of the infected tissues.

needlestick injury an accidental injury with a needle that is contaminated with blood or body fluids. The term is also used sometimes to include other sharps injuries. The injuries have been reported as a means of infecting the nurse or health care professional with hepatitis viruses (hepatitis B or C) or human immunodeficiency virus (HIV). A risk assessment procedure, training policies and clinical guidelines should be in place in all health care situations for staff to follow, should such an injury occur.

need analysis exercise often undertaken by NHS Trusts, service organizations and agencies of a target population to assess a service or situation with a view to change, e.g., alteration in clinic times. Multiple research methods and techniques for data collection and analysis may be used in the process.

needs *see* JOINT STRATEGIC NEEDS ASSESSMENT and MASLOW'S HIERARCHY OF NEEDS.

negative the opposite of positive. The absence of some quality or substance.

negativism a symptom of mental illness in which the patient does the opposite of what is required and so presents an uncooperative attitude. Common in schizophrenia.

negligence in law, the failure to do something that a reasonable person of ordinary prudence would do in certain situations and may provide the basis for a lawsuit when there is a legal duty, as in nursing and midwifery to provide reasonable care to patients/clients, and when negligence results in damage to the patient or client.

Neisseria *A.L.S. Neisser, German bacteriologist, 1855–1916.* A genus of paired, spherical, gram-negative bacteria. *N. gonorrhoeae* the causative organism of gonorrhoea. *N. meningitidis* the cause of meningococcal meningitis.

Nematoda a phylum of worms, including the genus *Ascaris* or roundworm and the genus *Enterobius* or threadworm.

neoadjuvant therapy chemotherapy given prior to radiation treatment or surgery to reduce the size of a tumour.

neoglycogenesis the formation of liver glycogen from non-carbohydrate sources. Glyconeogenesis.

neologism the formation of new words, either completely new ones or ones formed by contraction of two separate words. This is done particularly by patients with schizophrenia.

neonatal referring to the first month of life. *N. mortality rate* the number of deaths of infants up to 4 weeks old per 1000 live births in any one year. *N. herpes* a rare condition in newborn infants where the baby is infected during vaginal delivery to a woman with genital herpes. *N. intensive care unit see* INTENSIVE CARE UNIT. *N. period* the interval from the birth to 28 days of age. *N. respiratory distress syndrome* occurs when newborn babies lungs are not fully developed and there is a lack of surfactant in the lungs. *N. screening see* SCREENING.

neonate newborn; specifically pertaining to a baby under 1 month old.

neonatologist a medically qualified person specializing in the management, assessment, diseases and intensive care of newborn babies, especially those of low birth weight and those with congenital abnormalities.

neonatology the branch of medicine dealing with disorders of the newborn infant.

neoplasm a morbid new growth; a tumour. It may be benign or malignant.

nephrectomy excision of a kidney.

nephritis inflammation of the kidney; a focal or diffuse proliferative or destructive disease that may involve the glomerulus, tubule or interstitial renal tissue. The most usual form is glomerulonephritis.

nephroblastoma a rapidly developing malignant mixed tumour of the kidneys, made up of embryonic cells, and occurring chiefly in children before the fifth year; Wilms' tumour.

nephrocalcinosis a condition in which there is deposition of calcium in the renal tubules, resulting in calculi formation and renal insufficiency.

nephrolith stone in the kidney; renal calculus.

nephrolithiasis the presence of a calculus or of gravel in the kidney.

nephrolithotomy removal of a renal calculus by incising the kidney or by extracorporeal shock wave lithotripsy.

nephroma tumour of the kidney.

nephron the functional unit of the kidney, comprising Bowman's capsule, the proximal and distal tubules, the loop of Henle and the collecting duct, which conveys urine to the renal pelvis. *See* Figure on p. 262.

nephropexy the fixation of a floating (mobile) kidney, usually by sutures, to neighbouring muscle.

nephroptosis downward displacement, or undue mobility, of a kidney.

nephropyeloplasty any plastic operation on the pelvis of the kidney.

nephrosclerosis constriction of the arterioles of the kidney. Seen in benign and malignant hypertension and in arteriosclerosis in old age.

nephrosis any disease of the kidney, especially that characterized by oedema, proteinuria and a low plasma albumin. Caused by non-inflammatory degenerative lesions of the tubules.

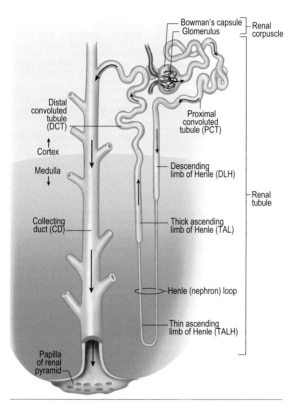

NEPHRON

nephrostomy creation of a permanent opening into the renal pelvis.

nephrotic referring to or caused by nephrosis. *N. syndrome* a clinical syndrome in which there is proteinuria, low plasma protein and gross oedema. The result of increased capillary permeability in the glomeruli. It may occur as a result of acute glomerulonephritis, in subacute nephritis, diabetes mellitus, amyloid disease, systemic lupus erythematosus and renal vein thrombosis.

nephrotomy incision of the kidney.

nephrotoxic poisonous or destructive to the cells of the kidney.

nephroureterectomy surgical removal of the kidney and the ureter.

nerve a bundle of conducting fibres enclosed in a sheath called the epineurium. Its function is to transmit impulses between any part of the body and a nerve centre. *Motor (efferent) n.* one that conveys impulses causing activity from a nerve centre to a muscle or gland. *N. block* a method of producing regional anaesthesia by injecting a local anaesthetic into the nerves supplying the area to be operated on. *N. fibre* the prolongation of the nerve cell, which conveys impulses. Each fibre has a sheath. Medullated nerve fibres have an insulating myelin sheath. *N. gas* also known as nerve agent is a gas that interferes with the functioning of the nerves and muscles. Such gases may cause death from respiratory paralysis; some of them act through the skin and cannot be avoided by the use of gas masks. *Sensory (afferent) n.* one that conveys sensation from an area to a nerve centre. *See* Figure on p. 264.

nervous 1. pertaining to, or composed of, nerves. 2. apprehensive. *N. breakdown* a popular and misleading term for any type of mental illness that interferes with a person's normal activities. A so-called 'nervous breakdown' can include any of the mental disorders, including NEUROSIS, PSYCHOSIS or DEPRESSION, but is usually used to describe neurosis.

nervousness excitability of the nervous system, characterized by a state of mental and physical unrest.

nesting the provision of an enclosed space bounded by a small blanket roll encircling the sick or preterm infant in a cot or incubator. This helps to provide a supportive, calming environment for the infant.

nettle rash an allergic skin condition; urticaria.

network 1. an interconnected group or system of voluntary organizations or of colleagues with similar interests. 2. a system of interconnected computer terminals in which the user has access to others using the system for sharing data, etc. *Academic Health Science n.* (AHSN) these bodies set up as part of NHS reforms in England in 2013 align education, clinical research, informatics, innovation, training and education and healthcare delivery. Their goal is to improve patient and population health by translating research into practice and developing and implementing integrated health care services. *Strategic Clinical n.* a group of health professionals and organizations from primary, secondary and tertiary care working together with commissioners in a managed and coordinated way that is not constrained by existing organizational or professional boundaries. The aim is to deliver a patient-focused service that highlights quality of care and clinical effectiveness. These networks may be grouped by client group (maternity, children and young people), or by disease (cancer; cardiovascular; mental health, dementia and neurological conditions). Regions may develop other networks according to local need.

networking 1. forming and maintaining professional connections and contacts through informal social meetings. 2. the interconnection of two or more computer networks in different places.

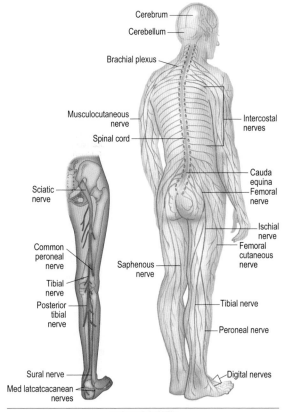

Cerebrum

Cerebellum

Brachial plexus

Musculocutaneous nerve

Spinal cord

Intercostal nerves

Cauda equina

Femoral nerve

Ischial nerve

Femoral cutaneous nerve

Sciatic nerve

Common peroneal nerve

Tibial nerve

Posterior tibial nerve

Saphenous nerve

Tibial nerve

Peroneal nerve

Sural nerve

Med latcatcacanean nerves

Digital nerves

NERVOUS SYSTEM

neural pertaining to the nerves. *N. arch* the bony arch on each vertebra which encloses the spinal cord. *N. tube defect* any of a group of congenital malformations involving the neural tube, including anencephaly, hypocephalus and spina bifida.

neuralgia a sharp stabbing pain, usually along the course of a nerve, owing to neuritis or functional disturbance.

neurapraxia an injury to a nerve resulting in temporary loss of function and paralysis. It is usually caused by compression of the nerve, and there is no lasting damage.

neurilemma the membranous sheath surrounding a nerve fibre.

neurinoma a benign tumour arising in the neurilemma of a nerve fibre.

neuritis inflammation of a nerve, with pain, tenderness and loss of function. *Multiple n.* that involving several nerves; polyneuritis. *Nutritional (alcoholic) n.* that which may be caused by alcoholism or lack of vitamin B complex. *Optic n.* that affecting the optic disc or nerve. *Peripheral n.* that involving the terminations of nerves. *Sciatic n.* sciatica. *Traumatic n.* that which results from an injury to a nerve.

neuroblast an embryonic nerve cell.

neuroblastoma a malignant tumour of immature nerve cells, most often arising in the young.

neurodermatitis a localized prurigo of somatic and psychogenic origin. It irritates, and rubbing causes thickening and pigmentation of the skin.

neurodevelopmental therapy (NDT) a non-invasive approach to the rehabilitation of patients with neurological problems based on current research findings into motor development and neurophysiology.

neuroepithelioma a malignant tumour of the retina of the eye, which may spread into the brain.

neurofibroma a usually benign tumour of nerve and fibrous tissue.

neurofibromatosis von Recklinghausen's disease. A generalized hereditary disease in which there are numerous fibromas of the skin and nervous system.

neurogenic derived from or caused by nerve stimulation. *N. bladder* a disorder of the urinary bladder caused by a lesion of the nervous system.

neuroglia the special form of connective tissue supporting nerve tissues also known as glial cells.

neurolinguistic programming (NLP) an approach to communication based on the notion of a connection between neurological processes, language and behaviour patterns learned through experience.

neurological assessment evaluation of the health status of a patient with a nervous system disorder or dysfunction. Purposes of the assessment include establishing nursing goals to guide the nurse in planning and implementing nursing measures to help the patient cope effectively with daily living activities. Nursing assessment of a patient's neurological status is concerned with identifying functional disabilities that interfere with the person's ability to provide self-care and lead an active life. A functionally oriented nursing assessment includes (a) consciousness; (b) mental functions; (c) motor function; and (d) sensory function. Evaluation of these functions gives the nurse information about the patient's ability to perform everyday activities such as thinking, remembering, seeing, eating, speaking, moving, smelling, feeling and hearing. A patient with an acute and life-threatening alteration in neurological function is evaluated and monitored in four general areas: (a) level of consciousness; (b) sensory and motor function; (c) pupillary changes; and (d) vital signs and pattern of respiration.

neurologist a medical practitioner specializing in neurology.

neurology 1. the scientific study of the nervous system. 2. the branch of medicine concerned with diseases of the nervous system.

neuroma a tumour consisting of nervous tissue.

neuromuscular appertaining to nerves and muscles. *N. junction* the small gap between the end of the motor nerve and the motor end-plate of the muscle fibre supplied. This gap is bridged by the release of acetylcholine whenever a nerve impulse arrives.

neuromyelitis neuritis associated with myelitis. It is a condition akin to multiple sclerosis. *N. optica* a disease in which there is bilateral optic neuritis and paraplegia also known as Devic's disease or syndrome.

neurone a nerve cell. *Lower motor n.* the anterior horn cell and its neurone which convey impulses to the appropriate muscles. *Upper motor n.* that in which the cell is in the cerebral cortex and the fibres conduct impulses to associated cells in the spinal cord. Also called neuron. *See* Figure on p. 267.

neuroparalysis paralysis due to disease of a nerve or nerves.

neuropathy a disease process of nerve degeneration and loss of function. *Alcoholic n.* neuropathy due to thiamine deficiency in chronic alcoholism. *Diabetic n.* that associated with diabetes. *Entrapment n.* any of a group of neuropathies, e.g., carpal tunnel syndrome, due to mechanical pressure on a peripheral nerve also known as nerve compression syndrome. *Ischaemic n.* that caused by a lack of blood supply. *Peripheral n.* occurs when nerves in the body's periphery are damaged.

neuroplasticity the capacity for nerve cells to regenerate and recover function.

neuroplasty the surgical repair of a damaged nerve.

neuropsychiatry the medical specialism concerned with the effects on mind and behaviour of organic disorders of the nervous system, combining both neurology and psychiatry.

neurorrhaphy the operation of suturing a divided nerve.

neurosis now an outdated term for a mental health disorder without loss of touch with reality.

neurosurgery that branch of surgery dealing with the brain, spinal cord and nerves.

neurosyphilis a manifestation of third stage syphilis in which the nervous system is involved. Symptoms of the disease may not occur for 20 years or so after the primary infection.

neurotoxic poisonous or destructive to nervous tissue.

neurotransmitter a substance (e.g., noradrenaline, acetylcholine, dopamine) that is released from the axon terminal to produce activity in other nerves.

neurotripsy the surgical bruising or crushing of a nerve.

neurotropic having an affinity for nerve tissue. *N. viruses* (Japanese encephalitis, measles, rabies, poliomyelitis, etc.) those that particularly attack the nervous system.

neutropenia a decrease in the number of neutrophils in the blood.

neutrophil a polymorphonuclear leukocyte that has a neutral reaction to acid and alkaline dyes.

never events serious events that are entirely preventable and have the potential to cause serious patient harm or death.

newborn blood spot screening a blood test offered to all babies at 5 days old, which screens for a number of diseases which are amenable to healthcare interventions if they are identified early. Blood is taken from the baby's heel.

next of kin technically a person's closest living relative, whose name is often required health care information. Patients should be asked whom they wish to nominate as their 'next-of-kin' or 'significant other' in accordance with their own personal situation.

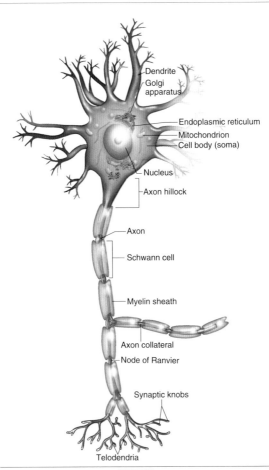

Dendrite
Golgi apparatus
Endoplasmic reticulum
Mitochondrion
Cell body (soma)
Nucleus
Axon hillock
Axon
Schwann cell
Myelin sheath
Axon collateral
Node of Ranvier
Synaptic knobs
Telodendria

NEURONE

NHS Blood and Transplant (NHSBT) Special Health Authority for England and Wales set up for the purpose of providing a reliable and efficient supply of blood, tissues, stem cells and organs for transplantation throughout the NHS. *See also* BLOOD.

NHS 111/NHS 24 (services in Scotland) a telephone health advice service providing 24-hour access to health care assessment and health information. The service (a) is a private, confidential, reliable and consistent source of professional advice; (b) is speedy with simple access to a comprehensive range of the latest health and health-related information; (c) improves quality, increases cost effectiveness and reduces demands on other NHS services; and (d) allows professionals to develop their role in enabling patients to be partners in self-care.

NHS Choices an online service providing a range of resources including an A–Z guide to health information, interactive tools such as a healthy weight calculator and information about local services.

NHS Improvement (NHSI) an organization which aims to support NHS Trusts to provide consistent high quality care through the provision of resources and innovations, and by holding providers to account.

NHS Number ten-digit number used as a unique identifier for every patient.

niacin nicotinic acid.

nicotine a poisonous alkaloid in tobacco. *N. replacement therapy* preparations containing nicotine that are used in place of cigarettes to assist people to stop smoking. Preparations are available in a variety of forms, e.g., as patches, sublingual tablets, chewing gum or nasal sprays; these therapies increase the chances of smokers quitting successfully. Available on NHS prescription. Some side effects may occur, e.g., nausea, headaches, palpitations and flu-like symptoms. *See* E-CIGARETTES.

nicotinic acid niacin. A water-soluble vitamin in the B complex. A deficiency of this vitamin causes pellagra.

nidation implantation of the fertilized ovum in the uterus.

nidus 1. a nest. 2. a place in which an organism finds conditions suitable for its growth and development. 3. the focus of an infection.

Niemann–Pick disease *A. Niemann, German paediatrician, 1880–1921; F. Pick, German physician, 1868–1935.* A group of rare inherited disorders in which there is lipoid storage abnormality and widespread deposition of lecithin in the tissues. Prognosis is poor in type A with most children dying before 18 months. There is an adult form of Neumann–Pick which has a more favourable prognosis.

night blindness nyctalopia; difficulty in seeing in the dark. This may be a congenital defect or be caused by a vitamin A deficiency. Also occurs as a result of retinal degeneration.

nightmare a frightening or unpleasant dream that occurs during REM (rapid eye movement) sleep usually in the middle to later part of the night. The dreamer wakes completely, remembering the dream. Most common in young children; in adults may be a side-effect of certain drugs, e.g., beta-blockers, or associated with a traumatic experience.

night sweat profuse perspiration during sleep, associated with an acute feverish illness or the menopause.

night terror an unpleasant experience in which the subject, usually a young child, screams while asleep and seems terrified. On waking the individual is unable to remember the cause of the fear.

nihilism in psychiatry, a term used to describe feelings of not existing and hopelessness, that all is lost or destroyed.

nipple the small conical projection at the tip of the breast, through which, in the female, milk can be withdrawn. *Accessory n.* a rudimentary nipple anywhere in a line from the breast to the groin. *Depressed n.* one that does not protrude. *N. shield* a shield fitted with a rubber teat which covers the areola of a nursing mother when her nipple is sore or not sufficiently protractile for the baby to suck. *Retracted n.* one that is drawn inwards. It may be a sign of cancer of the breast.

nit the egg of the head louse, attached to the hair near the scalp.

nitrate drugs a group of coronary vasodilator drugs used to treat angina pectoris, e.g., glyceryl trinitrate and isosorbide. These drugs provide rapid relief of symptoms and improve exercise tolerance. They may be given as tablets to be chewed or dissolved sublingually, as skin patches, gel or sublingual sprays.

nitrogen *symbol* N. A gaseous element. Air is largely composed of nitrogen, and it is one of the essential constituents of all protein foods. *N. balance* the state of the body in regard to the rate of protein intake and protein utilization. A negative nitrogen balance occurs when more protein is utilized by the body than is taken in. A positive nitrogen balance implies a net gain of protein in the body. Negative nitrogen balance can be caused by such factors as malnutrition, debilitating disease, blood loss and glucocorticoids. A positive balance can be caused by exercise, growth hormone and testosterone.

nitrous oxide N_2O. An inhalation anaesthetic ensuring a brief spell of unconsciousness.

NK *see* NATURAL KILLER CELLS.

NMC *see* NURSING AND MIDWIFERY COUNCIL.

NNT *see* NUMBERS NEEDED TO TREAT.

noctambulation sleep walking; somnambulism.

nocturia the production of large quantities of urine at night.

nocturnal referring to the night. *N. enuresis* bed-wetting; incontinence of urine during sleep.

node a swelling or protuberance. *Atrioventricular n.* the specialized tissue between the right atrium and the ventricle, at the point where the coronary vein enters the atrium, from which is initiated the impulse of contraction down the atrioventricular bundle. *N. of Ranvier* a constriction occurring at intervals in a nerve fibre to enable the neurilemma with its blood supply to reach and nourish the axon of the nerve. Also known as myelin sheath gaps. *Sinoatrial n.* known as the pacemaker of the heart. A group of specialized cells situated at the opening of the superior vena cava into the right atrium. These cells emit regular electric impulses which initiate and control the heart beat.

nodule a small swelling or protuberance.

noma a gangrenous condition of the mouth; cancrum oris.

nominal the level of measurement that simply assigns data into categories that are mutually exclusive.

nomogram a graph with several scales arranged so that a ruler laid on the graph intersects the scales at related values of the variables; the values of any two variables can be used to find the values of the others.

non compos mentis [L.] *not of sound mind.* Applied to people whose mental state is such that they are unable to manage their own affairs.

non-accidental injury abbreviated NAI. Injuries inflicted upon children or infants by those looking after them, usually the parents. The injuries are usually physical (beating, burnings, biting) but the term includes the giving of poisons and dangerous drugs, sexual abuse, starvation, neglect and any other form of physical assault.

non-allergic rhinitis inflammation of the inside of the nose not caused by allergy leading to a blocked, runny nose and sneezing.

non-compliance describes the decision made by a patient not to comply with a drug regimen, even though fully understanding the rationale for such therapy.

non-experimental research design a research design in which an investigator observes a phenomenon without manipulating the independent variable(s).

non-invasive any medical procedure that does not penetrate the skin or organ of the body, e.g., CT scanning or blood pressure monitoring. The term may also be used to describe non-cancerous tumours that do not metastasize.

non-maleficence the concept in the health care services of the duty to avoid harm to the interests of others.

non-shivering thermogenesis the use of brown adipose tissue by the neonate to produce heat in times of stress. Brown fat is stored in the mediastinum, around the nape of the neck, between the scapulae and around the kidneys and suprarenal glands.

non-specific 1. not due to any single known cause. 2. not directed against a particular agent, but rather having a general effect. *N. urethritis* abbreviated NSU. A common, sexually transmitted disease which may be due to a variety of agents, e.g., *Chlamydia trachomatis* which causes 40% of cases. Also called non-gonococcal urethritis.

non-steroidal anti-inflammatory drugs abbreviated NSAIDs. A group of drugs with analgesic, antipyretic and anti-inflammatory activity due to their ability to inhibit the synthesis of prostaglandins. It includes aspirin, phenylbutazone, indomethacin, tolmetin, ibuprofen and related drugs.

non-union in a fracture, failure of the two pieces of bone to unite.

Noonan syndrome a rare genetic disorder resulting in unusual facial features, short stature and heart defects.

noradrenaline a hormone present in extracts of the suprarenal medulla and at synapses in the peripheral sympathetic nervous system. It causes vasoconstriction and raises both the systolic and the diastolic blood pressure.

norm a fixed standard or value against which values are measured.

normal conforming to a standard; regular or usual. *N. distribution* in statistics, a symmetrical 'bell-shaped' distribution or curve that forms in the plotting of the scores. The most probable scores are concentrated around the mean or average with progressively less probable scores occurring further from the mean. *N. flora* bacteria which normally live on body tissues and have a beneficial effect. *N. saline* isotonic solution of sodium chloride. Physiological solution.

normoblast a nucleated precursor red blood cell in bone marrow. *See* ERYTHROCYTE.

normochromic normal in colour. Applied to the blood when the haemoglobin level is within normal limits.

normocyte a red blood cell that is normal in size, shape and colour.

normoglycaemia normal blood sugar level.

normotension normal tone, tension or pressure. Usually used in relation to blood pressure.

norovirus common cause of vomiting and diarrhoea transmitted through faecal contamination of food and water. Also known as the winter vomiting bug.

North American Nursing Diagnosis Association abbreviated NANDA. Formed as a professional organization of registered nurses in 1982. The purpose of NANDA is 'to promote patient safety by standardizing evidence based nursing diagnoses and to enable nurses to implement interventions with predictable outcomes'.

nose the organ of smell and the airway for respiration. *See* Figure on p. 271.

nosocomial pertaining to, or acquired in hospital. Now most commonly called health care associated infections (HCAI) as many of these acquired infections occur at home or elsewhere in the community. *N. disease* for the patient, a new disorder, not related to the original disease, that is caused or

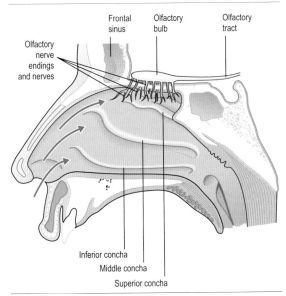

NOSE

precipitated during hospitalization. *N. infection* an infection acquired in hospital at least 72 hours after admission. *Contact transmitted infection* is the most important and frequent mode of transmission of nosocomial infections and may be either direct or indirect. *Direct contact transmitted infections* involve direct body surface-to-body surface contact, such as occurs in patient care activities, e.g., bathing a patient. Direct contact can also occur between two patients, with one serving as the source of infectious microorganisms, the other being a susceptible host. *Indirect contact transmitted infections* involve contact of a susceptible host with a contaminated intermediate object, usually inanimate (*see* FOMITES), e.g., contaminated instruments, needles, dressings or gloves that are not changed between patients. Unwashed, contaminated hands may also be a source of nosocomial infection. *See* Appendix 11.

nosology the classification of disease into groups by criteria, based on (expert) agreement of the boundaries of the groups, e.g., by the DELPHI TECHNIQUE.

nostril one of the anterior orifices of the nose.

notifiable applied to such diseases, incidents or occurrences that must by law be reported. These include measles, scarlet fever, typhus and typhoid fever, cholera, diphtheria, tuberculosis, dysentery and food poisoning.

NPF Nurse Prescribers' Formulary.

NSAIDs non-steroidal anti-inflammatory drugs.

NSU non-specific urethritis.

nuclear pertaining to a nucleus. *N.
medicine* that branch of medicine concerned with the use of radionuclides
in the diagnosis and treatment of
disease. *N. family see* FAMILY.

nuclear magnetic resonance abbreviated NMR. A phenomenon exhibited
by atomic nuclei having a magnetic
moment, i.e., those nuclei that behave
as if they are tiny bar magnets. In the
absence of a magnetic field these
magnets are arranged randomly but
when a strong magnetic field is applied
they align with the field. These signals
can be analysed and used for chemical analysis (NMR spectroscopy) or for
imaging (magnetic resonance imaging).

nuclease an enzyme that breaks down
nucleic acids.

nucleic acids deoxyribonucleic acid
(abbreviated DNA) and ribonucleic acid
(abbreviated RNA), both of which are
found in cell nuclei; RNA is also found
in the cytoplasm. They are composed
of series of nucleotides.

nucleolus a small dense body in the
cell nucleus which contains ribonucleic
acid. It disappears during mitosis.

nucleoprotein a compound of nucleic
acid and protein.

nucleotide a compound formed from
pentose sugar, phosphoric acid and a
nitrogen-containing base (a purine or
a pyrimidine).

nucleotoxic applied to drugs, toxins,
viruses and other agents that are toxic
to cell nuclei.

nucleus 1. the essential part of a cell,
governing nutrition and reproduction,
its division being essential for the formation of new cells. 2. the positively
charged centre portion of an atom. 3.
a group of nerve cells in the central
nervous system. *Caudate n.* and *len-
ticular n.* part of the basal ganglia. *N.
pulposus* the jelly-like centre of an
intervertebral disc. nudge theory a
concept in behavioural science that

proposes behaviour can be modified
by positive reinforcement and indirect
suggestion.

null hypothesis a research concept
indicating that there is no significant
relationship between an independent
variable and a dependent variable, and
that the observed experimental results
can therefore be attributed to chance
alone.

nullipara a woman who has never
given birth to a child.

numbers needed to treat abbreviated NNT. A measure of clinical significance in medicine and pharmacology
used to communicate the effectiveness
of a healthcare intervention. It refers
to the average number of patients who
need to be treated with a specific intervention to prevent one additional bad
outcome. It is used in pharmacology
to make decisions between treatment
options being based upon the number of subjects receiving the medication before one subject has a positive
outcome.

nurse 1. a person who is qualified in
the art and science of nursing and
meets certain prescribed standards
of education and clinical competence.
Is registered with the Nursing and
Midwifery Council (NMC) if practising
in the UK. The person so registered is
entitled legally to use the title of nurse.
2. to provide services that are essential
to or helpful in the promotion, maintenance and restoration of health and
wellbeing. 3. to nourish at the breast
(*see also* BREAST (FEEDING)). *Graduate N.
Apprenticeship* a route to nurse registration funded in England via the
apprenticeship levy. Graduate nurse
apprentices will usually be existing
health care support workers who will
undertake a programme of study at an
approved institution whilst undertaking
practice required for registration. *N.
consultant* an experienced nurse practitioner educated to a Master's level,
with advanced skills in a clinical area,
e.g., mental health, neonatology, critical

care, stroke services, and dermatology; involves considerable patient contact. The nurse consultant will be expected to promote research and evaluation in practice, demonstrate leadership skills, participate in the education and development of staff and the service delivery in the clinical area. *N. practitioner* a nurse with specific preparation and development to function at an advanced level. Nurse practitioners can offer a nurse-led service and patients have a choice of seeing either the doctor or the nurse when they attend. Advanced level nurse practitioners will be educated to masters level and assessed as competent in using their expert knowledge and skills. They have freedom and authority to act making autonomous decisions in the assessment, diagnosis and treatment of patients. *N. prescribing* registered nurses who have undertaken aa additional qualification and demonstrated proficiency in prescribing. There are two types of nurse prescribers; community nurse prescribers and independent and supplementary nurse and midwife prescribers. When deemed competent they may prescribe from the relevant Prescribers' Formulary. *Practice n.* a qualified nurse who works with a general practitioner (GP), or with a group of GPs to assess, screen, treat and educate patients. *Registered n.* in the UK, one whose name is on the register held by the NMC.

Nurse Prescribers' Formulary for Community Practitioners abbreviated NPF. A formulary from which community nurses who are appropriately qualified may prescribe for patients.

nursing the profession of performing the functions of a nurse. *N. assessment* the systematic collection and analysis of patient data pertaining to the individual's health status, abilities and preferences for care and treatment. *See* ASSESSMENT. *N. Associate* a new support role regulated by the Nursing and Midwifery Council. Nursing Associates work alongside registered nurses and healthcare support workers to deliver hands-on nursing care. There is a clear progression route for Nursing Associates to undertake additional training to gain registration as a nurse. *N. audit* a systematic procedure for assessing the quality of nursing care rendered to a specific patient population. *N. auxiliary* an alternative name for health care assistant. *N. care plan* devised by a nurse and based upon a nursing assessment and nursing diagnosis for an individual patient. The plan traditionally had four essential components: (a) identification of the nursing care problems; (b) an outline of the means/methods of solving these; (c) a statement of the anticipated benefit to the patient; and (d) an account of the specific actions used to achieve the goals specified. The nursing diagnosis stage was added later. *N. diagnosis* a statement of a health problem or of a potential health problem in the patient's/client's health status that a nurse is professionally competent to treat. *N. goal* the objective that the nurse hopes to achieve through nursing interventions and activities related to the patient's health status, needs and abilities, e.g., the development of self-care skills. *N. history* a written record providing data for assessing the nursing care needs of a patient. *N. home* a building complex where nursing care is provided by registered nurses for the continuing health needs of the residents, together with their home and social care needs. These homes are provided by independent private sector companies, charitable organizations, social services of the local authority and rarely by the NHS, although the NHS will commission and fund nursing home beds for patients. *N. models* a conceptual framework of nursing practice based on knowledge, ideas and beliefs. Various models were used across the NHS from the 1980 onwards but have now largely fallen out of favour. *N. practice* the performance or compensation of any act in the observation, care and counsel of the ill, injured or infirm, or in the maintenance of health or prevention of illness of others, or in the supervision and teaching of other personnel, or in the administration of medications and treatments as prescribed by a doctor or dentist. This requires substantial specialized judgement and skill and is based on knowledge and application of the principles of biological, physical and social sciences. *N. process* a systematic approach to nursing care derived from many occupational groups. The system itself is not specific to nursing. It has been used as a framework for nursing care by American nurses and subsequently its principles have been adapted to the UK's culture and health care system by British nurses. It is an organized approach to the identification of a patient's nursing care problems and the utilization of nursing actions that effectively alleviate, minimize or prevent the problems being presented from developing. *N. records* accurate record keeping and careful documentation are essential to the delivery of nursing practice to a patient or client, whatever the setting, for example, in general practice premises, the hospital setting, in a nursing home or in the patient's own home. Nursing records whether they are held on paper or electronically provide a record of care planned or given to an individual patient by a registered nurse or other caregivers under the direction of a registered nurse. Records should be made in writing with a black pen or in some other permanent form, for example directly onto a computer. *See* RECORDS. *N. red flags* red flag events are part of the safer staffing initiative and signify to ward managers that they must ensure they have sufficient staff to meet the needs of patients on wards. Guidance has been produced by the National Institute for Health and Care Excellence (NICE).

Nursing and Midwifery Council (NMC) The statutory regulatory body for nursing and midwifery in England, Wales, Scotland and Northern Ireland. Its prime purpose is to protect the public through establishing and monitoring professional standards, setting the standard for education and training, conduct and performance. The council replaced the former UKCC and National Boards. It (a) maintains a register of qualified staff; (b) sets standards for professional education, practice and conduct; (c) provides advice for nurses, midwives and health visitors on professional standards; (d) considers allegations of misconduct or unfitness to practice because of illness; and (e) publishes professional conduct rules and other documents to guide professional practice.

nutation uncontrollable nodding of the head.

nutrient food; any substance that nourishes. The six classes of nutrient are fats, carbohydrates, proteins, vitamins, minerals and water.

nutrition 1. the sum of the processes involved in taking in nutriments and assimilating and utilizing them. 2. nutriment. Nutrition is particularly concerned with those properties of food that build sound bodies and promote health. Good nutrition means a balanced diet containing adequate amounts of the essential nutritional elements that the body must have to function normally. The essential ingredients of a balanced diet are proteins, vitamins, minerals, fats and carbohydrates. The body can manufacture sugars from fats, and fats from sugars and proteins, depending on the need, but it cannot manufacture proteins from sugars and fats. *Enteral n.* the provision of nutrients in fluid form to the alimentary tract by mouth, nasogastric tube or via an opening into the tract such as through a gastrostomy. *N. disease* one that is due to the continued absence of a necessary food factor. *Parenteral n.* a technique for meeting a patient's nutritional needs by means of intravenous feedings; sometimes called hyperalimentation. *See* Appendix 1.

nutritional status the condition of the body as a result of its receiving and using nutrients. Nutritional status may also be affected by biochemical individuality as well as environmental factors.

nyctalopia night blindness. *See* HEMERALOPIA.

nymphomania excessive sexual desire in a woman.

nystagmus an involuntary, rapid movement of the eyeball. It may be hereditary or result from disease of the semicircular canals or of the central nervous system. It can occur from visual defect or be associated with other muscle spasms.

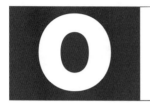

O symbol for *oxygen*.

obese very overweight; corpulent.

obesity corpulence; excessive development of fat throughout the body which impairs health and the most common nutritional disorder worldwide. A body mass index (BMI) of over 30 and up to 39.9. Severe obesity defines someone with greater than 40 BMI. Waist circumference, waist–height ratio and waist–hip ratio are also used as indicators of the amount of fat in the abdomen. Obesity is linked to many conditions—cardiovascular disease, hypertension, sleep apnoea, type 2 diabetes, stroke, arthritis and some cancers. *See* BARIATRICS.

objective 1. in microscopy, the lens nearest the object being looked at. 2. a purpose; a desired end result. 3. concerning matters outside oneself. *O. signs* signs that the observer notes, as distinct from symptoms of which the patient complains (subjective).

oblique slanting. *O. muscles* 1. a pair of muscles, the inferior and the superior, which turn the eye upwards and downwards, and inwards and outwards. 2. muscles found in the wall of the abdomen.

observation the act or faculty of closely noticing and paying attention to someone or something. In nursing this is an active process whereby the nurse uses the senses for the purpose of collecting patient data for developing a nursing diagnosis or care plan.

observational study a research methodology in which the researcher is a non-participant observer and records behaviour without influencing it.

obsession an idea which persistently recurs to an individual, although resisted and regarded as being senseless. A compulsive thought. *See* COMPULSION.

obsessive compulsive disorder (OCD) a mental health condition characterized by obsessional thoughts and/or ideas associated often with compulsive acts which may interfere with daily living.

obstetrician one who is trained and specializes in obstetrics.

obstetrics the branch of medicine and surgery dealing with pregnancy, labour and the puerperium.

obstipation intractable constipation.

obstruction the act of blocking or clogging; the state of being clogged. *Intestinal o.* any hindrance to the passage of faeces.

obstructive sleep apnoea the walls of the throat relax and narrow during sleep, interrupting normal breathing.

obturator that which closes an opening. *O. foramen* the large hole in the hip bone, closed by fascia and muscle.

obtusion weakening or blunting of normal sensations, a condition produced by certain diseases.

occipital relating to the occiput. *O. bone* the bone forming the back and part of the base of the skull.

occipitoanterior referring to the position of the fetal occiput when it is to the front of the maternal pelvis as it comes through the birth canal. The opposite of occipitoposterior.

occipitoposterior referring to the position of the fetal occiput when it is to the back of the maternal pelvis as it comes through the birth canal. The opposite of occipitoanterior.

occiput the back of the head.

occlusion closure, applied particularly to alignment of the teeth in the jaws. *Coronary o.* obstruction of the lumen of a coronary artery. *O. of the pupil* may be congenital or occur in iridocyclitis or after injury. *Retinal artery O.* blockage of one of the small arteries that carry blood to the retina. *Retinal vein O.* blockage of one of the small veins that take blood away from the retina.

occult hidden, concealed. *O. blood* blood excreted in the stools in such a small quantity as to require chemical tests to detect it.

occupational relating to work and working conditions. *O. disease* one likely to occur among workers in certain trades. An industrial disease. *O. health nurse* provides immediate care to ill or injured workers in the workplace and follows up the return to work of the sick and injured. Develops accident prevention programmes and promotes good health amongst the work force. Also has an educational role and a health and safety obligation. *O. health nursing* the branch of nursing that is concerned with the health of people in the workplace. *O. medicine* the branch of medicine concerned with people at work and the effects of work on health. Essentially a branch of preventative or environmental medicine. It is concerned with ensuring that health and safety in the workplace is maintained and legislation complied with. *O. therapy* treatment by provision of support to people whose health problems limit their ability to do activities of daily living. An occupational therapist will identify goals to help patients and service users improve independence by using techniques, changing the environment and equipment.

ocular relating to the eye. *O. myopathy* a rare, gradual bilateral loss of mobility of the eyes. *O. myositis* inflammation of the orbital muscles.

oculogyric causing movements of the eyeballs. *O. crisis* involuntary, violent movements of the eye, usually upwards.

oculomotor relating to movements of the eye. *O. nerves* the third pair of cranial nerves, which control the eye muscles.

odontoid resembling a tooth. *O. process* a tooth-like projection from the axis vertebra upon which the head rotates.

odontoma a tumour of tooth structures.

oedema an excessive amount of fluid in the body tissues. If the finger is pressed upon an affected part, the surface pits and slowly regains its original contour. *Angio o.* characterized by the sudden appearance of urticaria which may involve the skin of the face, hands, feet or genitalia, and with swelling of the mucosal membrane of mouth and throat, oedema of the glottis may be fatal. The swelling may be due to an allergic reaction to food (most common), moulds, pollens, or other allergens, infection or a reaction to an insect bite or sting. In many cases no identifiable cause can be found. *Cardiac o.* a manifestation of congestive heart failure, due to increased venous and capillary pressures and often associated with renal sodium retention. *Dependent o.* oedema affecting most severely the lowermost parts of the body. *Famine o.* that due to protein deficiency. *O. neonatorum* a disease of preterm and feeble infants resembling sclerema, marked by spreading oedema with cold, livid skin. *Pitting o.* oedema in which pressure leaves a persistent depression in the tissues. *Pulmonary o.* diffuse extravascular accumulation of fluid in the tissues and air spaces of the lung due to changes in hydrostatic forces in the capillaries or to increased capillary permeability.

Oedipus complex the suppressed sexual desire of a son for his mother, with hostility towards his father. It is a normal stage in the early development of the child, but may become fixed if the child cannot solve the conflict during his early years or during adolescence. Named after a mythical Greek hero.

oesophageal pertaining to the oesophagus. *O. atresia* a congenital abnormality in which the oesophagus is not continuous between the pharynx and the stomach. May be associated with a fistula into the trachea. *O. varices* varicose veins of the lower oesophagus secondary to portal hypertension.

oesophagitis inflammation of the oesophagus. *Reflux o.* caused by regurgitation of acid stomach contents through the cardiac sphincter.

oesophagojejunostomy an operation to create an anastomosis of the jejunum with the oesophagus after a total gastrectomy.

oesophagus the canal that extends from the pharynx to the stomach. It is about 23 cm long.

oestradiol the chief naturally occurring female sex hormone produced by the ovary. Prepared synthetically, it is used to treat menopausal conditions and amenorrhoea.

oestrogen one of several steroid hormones, including oestradiol, all of which have similar functions. Although they are largely produced in the ovary, they can also be extracted from the placenta, the adrenal cortex and the testis. They control female sexual development.

olecranon the curved process of the ulna which forms the point of the elbow.

oleum [L.] *oil.*

olfactory relating to the sense of smell. *O. nerves* the first pair of cranial nerves; those smell.

oligohydramnios a deficiency in the amount of amniotic fluid.

oligomenorrhoea 1. a diminished flow at the menstrual period. 2. infrequent occurrence of menstruation.

oligospermia also known as oligozoospermia a diminished output of spermatozoa.

oliguria a deficient secretion of urine.

olivary shaped like an olive. *O. body* a mass of grey matter situated behind the anterior pyramid of the medulla oblongata.

ombudsman an official appointed by the government but with a significant degree of independence to receive complaints about unfair administration. The officer for the NHS, appointed as Parliamentary and Health Service Ombudsman or Health Service Commissioner, investigates complaints from the public about actions of the NHS in England, government departments and many public bodies in the UK. *See* HEALTH SERVICE COMMISSIONER.

omentum a fold of peritoneum joining the stomach to other abdominal organs. *Greater o.* the fold reflected from the greater curvature of the stomach and lying in front of the intestines. *Lesser o.* the fold reflected from the lesser curvature and attaching the stomach to the under surface of the liver.

omnivorous eating food of both plant and animal origin.

omphalitis inflammation of the umbilicus.

omphalocele an umbilical hernia.

Onchocerca a genus of filarial worms, found in tropical parts of Africa and America, which may give rise to skin and subcutaneous lesions and attack the eye.

onchocerciasis a tropical skin disease caused by infestation with *Onchocerca.*

oncogenesis the causation and formation of tumours.

oncogenic giving rise to tumour formation.

oncology the scientific and medical study of tumours.

onychia inflammation of the matrix of a nail, with suppuration, which may cause the nail to fall off.

onychogryphosis enlargement of the nails, with excessive ridging and curvature, most commonly affecting the elderly.

onycholysis loosening or separation of a nail from its bed.

onychomycosis a chronic fungal infection of the nail. Can affect toenails and fingernails and, if left untreated, can lead to the destruction of the nail plate.

oöcyte the immature egg cell or ovum in the ovary.

oögenesis the development and production of the ovum.

oöphorectomy excision of an ovary; ovariectomy.

oöphorocystosis the development of one or more ovarian cysts.

oöphoron an ovary.

opacity cloudiness, lack of transparency. Opacities occur in the lens of an eye when a cataract is forming. They also occur in the vitreous humour and appear as floating objects.

open ended items questions that the respondent may answer in their own words.

operant conditioning a form of behaviour therapy in which a reward is given when the subject performs the action required. The reward serves to encourage repetition of the action.

operating framework annually sets out the business and planning arrangements for the NHS in England.

operation a surgical procedure in which instruments or hands are used by the operator upon a part or organ of the body.

operational definition the measurements used to observe or measure a variable; delineates the procedures or operations required to measure a concept.

ophthalmia severe inflammation of the eye or of the conjunctiva or deeper structures of the eye. Also known as ophthalmitis. *O. neonatorum* any

hyperacute purulent conjunctivitis which may be caused by the gonococcus, *Escherichia coli*, staphylococci or *Chlamydia trachomatis*, occurring within the first 28 days of life. *Sympathetic o.* granulomatous inflammation of the uveal tract of the uninjured eye following a wound involving the uveal tract of the other eye, resulting in bilateral granulomatous inflammation of the entire uveal tract. Also called sympathetic uveitis.

ophthalmologist a specialist in diseases of the eye.

ophthalmology the study of the eye and its diseases.

ophthalmoscope an instrument fitted with a light and lenses by which the interior of the eye can be illuminated and examined.

opiate any medicine containing opium.

opisthotonos a muscle spasm causing the back to be arched and the head retracted, with great rigidity of the muscles of the neck and back. This condition may be present in acute cases of meningitis, tetanus and strychnine poisoning.

opium a drug derived from dried poppy juice and used as a narcotic. It is a highly addictive drug. Opium derivatives include codeine, morphine and heroin.

opponens [L.] *opposing.* A term applied to certain muscles controlling the movements of the fingers. *O. pollicis* a muscle that adducts the thumb so that it and the little finger can be brought together.

opportunistic 1. taking advantage of immediate opportunities. 2. denoting a microorganism that does not ordinarily cause disease but becomes pathogenic under certain circumstances. 3. denoting a disease or infection caused by such an opportunistic pathogen.

opsonic index a measurement of the bactericidal power of the phagocytes in the blood of an individual.

opsonin an antibody, present in the blood, which renders bacteria more easily destroyed by the phagocytes.

Each kind of bacterium has its specific opsonin.

optic relating to vision. *O. atrophy* degeneration of the optic nerve. *O. chiasma* the crossing of the fibres of the optic nerves at the base of the brain (*see* Figure on p. 281). *O. disc* the point where the optic nerve enters the eyeball. *O. foramen* the opening in the posterior part of the orbit through which pass the optic nerve and the ophthalmic artery. *O. nerve* a bundle of nerve fibres running from the optic chiasma in the brain to the optic disc on the eyeball.

optical pertaining to sight. *O. density* the refractive power of the transparent tissues through which light rays pass, changing the direction of the ray.

optician a professional trained in the detection of refractive errors and the dispensing of appropriate spectacles or contact lenses.

optimum the best and most favourable.

optometry assessing and measuring visual acuity for the fitting of glasses or contact lenses to correct visual defects.

ora [L.] *a margin. O. serrata* the jagged edge of the retina.

oral 1. pertaining to the mouth; taken through or applied in the mouth, as in oral medication or oral hygiene. 2. denoting that aspect of the teeth which faces the oral cavity or tongue. *O. contraceptive pill* a drug preparation taken orally containing one or more synthetic female hormones taken as part of the monthly cycle to prevent pregnancy. *O. hairy leukoplakia* an unusual form of leukoplakia that is seen only in human immunodeficiency virus (HIV) infected persons. It consists of fuzzy (hairy) patches on the tongue and, less frequently, elsewhere in the mouth. Hairy leukoplakia may be one of the first signs of HIV infection. *See* LEUKO-PLAKIA. *O. rehydration therapy* abbreviated ORT. *See* REHYDRATION. *O. syringe* a calibrated device with a plunger that is used to administer small doses of oral liquid medications to young children. The dose is drawn up into the syringe via the plunger and then squirted onto the inside of the cheek.

orbit 1. the bony cavity containing the eyeball. 2. the path of an object moving around another object.

orchidectomy excision of a testicle. *Bilateral o.* the operation of castration.

orchidopexy an operation to free an undescended testicle and place it in the scrotum.

orchiepididymitis inflammation of a testicle and its epididymis.

orchitis inflammation of a testicle.

ordinal scale a measurement scale in which the data are arranged in order of size or magnitude but where there is no standard measure of difference between the data given.

orf a virus infection transmitted from sheep and goats to humans. It gives rise to boil-like lesions on the hands of meat handlers.

organ a part of the body designed to perform a particular function. *O. of Corti* a spiral structure situated in the inner ear. It contains the basilar membrane that converts sound waves into nerve impulses that are then transmitted to the brain via the cochlear nerve.

organelle a structure within a cell that has specialized functions, e.g., nucleus, endoplasmic reticulum, mitochondrion, etc.

organic 1. pertaining to the organs. 2. pertaining to chemicals containing carbon. *O. disease* disease of an organ, accompanied by structural changes.

organism an individual living being, animal or vegetable.

orgasm the climax of sexual excitement.

orientation a sense of direction. 1. the ability of a person to estimate position in regard to time, place and persons. 2. the imparting of relevant information at the onset of a course or conference so that its content and objects may be understood. *Reality o.* the way in which older people who may be confused or mentally ill are assisted in keeping in

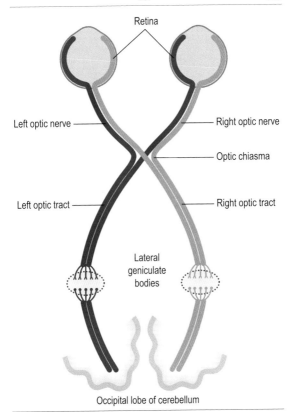

OPTIC CHIASMA

touch with the world around them on a day-to-day basis. This may be achieved in a variety of ways, with large clocks, calendar boards, signs on doors and daily newspapers.

orifice any opening in the body.

origin 1. the point of attachment of a muscle. 2. the point at which a nerve or a blood vessel branches from the main stem.

ornithosis a virus disease of birds, usually pigeons, that may be transmitted to humans in a form resembling bronchopneumonia.

orogenital pertaining to the mouth and external genitalia.

oropharynx the lower portion of the pharynx behind the mouth and above the oesophagus and larynx.

orphan a child whose parents are dead. *O. drugs* those that have been found to be useful in the treatment of rare diseases but which are not commercially produced usually because of high costs involved in manufacture and minimal demand. *O. viruses* those that have been isolated in the laboratory but which do not appear to be associated with any particular disease.

orthodontics dentistry that deals with the prevention and correction of malocclusion and irregularities of the teeth.

orthodox sleep *see* SLEEP.

Orthomyxovirus RNA viruses belonging to the family of *Orthomyxoviridae* which cause influenza in humans and other mammals, e.g., birds and swine. *See* AVIAN FLU and SWINE FLU. These viruses originated in aquatic birds and crossed the species barrier (*see* ZOONOSIS) about 10 000 years ago to infect humans.

orthopaedics the science dealing with deformities, injuries and diseases of the bones and joints.

orthopnoea difficulty in breathing unless in an upright position, e.g., sitting up in bed.

orthoptics the practice of treating by non-surgical methods (usually eye exercises) abnormalities of vision such as strabismus (squint).

orthostatic pertaining to or caused by standing erect. *O. albuminuria see* ALBUMINURIA. *O. hypotension* low blood pressure, occurring when the person stands up. Postural hypotension.

orthotic serving to protect or to restore or improve function.

orthotics the use or application of an orthosis (a supportive appliance that can be applied to or around the body in the care/treatment of physical impairment or disability).

orthotist a person skilled in orthotics and practising its application in individual cases.

Ortolani's sign *M. Ortolani, 20th-century Italian orthopaedic surgeon.* A test performed soon after birth to detect possible congenital dislocation of the hip. A 'click' is felt on reversing the movements of abduction and rotation of the hip while the child is lying with knees flexed.

os [L.] 1. (*pl.* ora) any body orifice. 2. (*pl.* ora) the mouth. 3. (*pl.* ossa) a bone.

oscillation 1. a backwards and forwards motion. 2. vibration.

oscilloscope an apparatus using a cathode-ray tube to depict visibly data fed into it electronically, e.g., the way in which the heart is performing.

Osgood–Schlatter disease pain, swelling and tenderness in the knee in adolescents and young adults due to damage to the bone during growth spurt.

Osler's nodes *Sir W. Osler, Canadian physician, 1849–1919.* Small painful swellings which occur in or beneath the skin, especially of the extremities in subacute bacterial endocarditis, caused by minute emboli. They usually disappear in 1–3 days.

Osler-Weber-Rendu syndrome also known as hereditary haemorrhagic telangiectasia a genetic disorder in which some blood vessels are underdeveloped.

osmoreceptor one of a group of specialized nerve cells which monitor the osmotic pressure of the blood and the extracellular fluid. Impulses from these receptors are relayed to the hypothalamus.

osmosis the passage of fluid from a low concentration solution to one of a higher concentration through a semipermeable membrane.

osmotic pertaining to osmosis. *O. pressure* the pressure exerted by large molecules in the blood, e.g., albumin and globulin proteins, which draws fluid into the bloodstream from the surrounding tissues. *O. diuretics* diuretics, e.g., mannitol, given intravenously to reduce elevated pressure in cerebral oedema or glaucoma, or to produce a diuresis in drug overdose.

osseous bony.

ossicle a small bone. *Auditory o.* one of the three bones in the middle ear: the malleus, incus and stapes.

ossification the process by which bone is developed; osteogenesis.

osteitis inflammation of bone. *O. deformans* Paget's disease. *O. fibrosa cystica* or *parathyroid o.* defects of ossification, with fibrous tissue production, leading to weakening and deformity. It affects children chiefly, and is associated with parathyroid tumour, removal of which checks it.

osteoarthritis often described as degenerative joint disease (DJD). *See* ARTHRITIS.

osteoarthrotomy surgical excision of the jointed end of a bone.

osteoblast a cell that develops into an osteocyte and turns into bone.

osteochondritis inflammation of bone and cartilage, particularly a degenerative disease of an epiphysis, causing pain and deformity. *O. of the tarsal scaphoid bone* Köhler's disease. *O. of the tibial tuberosity* Osgood–Schlatter disease.

osteochondroma a tumour consisting of both bone and cartilage.

osteoclasis 1. the surgical fracture of bones to correct a deformity such as bow-leg. 2. the restructuring of bone by osteoclasts during growth or the repair of damaged bone.

osteoclast 1. a large cell that breaks down and absorbs bone and callus. 2. an instrument designed for surgical fracture of bone.

osteocyte a bone cell.

osteodystrophy a metabolic disease of bone.

osteogenesis the formation of bone. *O. imperfecta* a congenital disorder of the bones, which are very brittle and fracture easily. Fragilitas ossium.

osteoma a benign tumour arising from bone.

osteomalacia a disease characterized by painful softening of bones. Due to vitamin D deficiency.

osteomyelitis inflammation of bone, localized or generalized, due to a pyogenic infection. It may result in bone destruction, stiffening of joints, and, in extreme cases occurring before the end of the growth period, in the shortening of a limb if the growth centre is destroyed. Acute osteomyelitis is caused by bacteria that enter the body through a wound, spread from an infection near the bone, or come from a skin or throat infection. The infection usually affects the long bones of the arms and legs and causes acute pain and fever. It most often occurs in children and adolescents.

osteopath one who practises osteopathy.

osteopathy a system of diagnosis and treatment of disease which involves massage, palpation and manipulation. Osteopathic treatment is aimed at freeing and loosening joints and re-establishing proper relationships of the spinal column, its component bones with the pelvis and limb bones on the basis that many diseases are associated with disorders of the musculoskeletal system.

osteoperiostitis inflammation of bone and periosteum.

osteopetrosis (Albers–Schönberg disease). A rare congenital disease in which the bones become abnormally dense.

osteophyte a small outgrowth of bone, usually in a joint damaged by osteoarthritis.

osteoporosis a loss of bone density which may be idiopathic or secondary to other conditions. The disorder leads to thinning of the skeleton with inadequate calcium absorption into the bone and excessive bone resorption. The principal causes are lack of physical activity, lack of oestrogens or androgens, and nutritional deficiency. Osteoporosis is associated with ageing in both men and women. Symptoms include pathological fractures and collapse of the vertebrae without compression of the spinal cord. Management involves minimizing bone loss with vitamin D, dietary calcium and regular sustained exercise to build and maintain bone strength. Long-term hormone replacement therapy can prevent osteoporosis in postmenopausal women.

osteosarcoma an osteogenic sarcoma; a malignant bone tumour.

osteosclerosis an increase in density and a hardening of bone. *O. congenita* achondroplasia. *O. fragilis* osteopetrosis.

osteotomy the cutting into or through a bone, sometimes performed to correct deformity. *O. of the hip* a method of treating osteoarthritis by cutting the bone and altering the line of weight-bearing.

ostium an opening or entrance. *Abdominal o.* the opening at the end of the uterine tube into the peritoneal cavity.

otoacoustic emission (OAE) a computer linked hearing test used for screening infants in the first few weeks of life to ascertain hearing levels.

OTC drugs *see* OVER-THE-COUNTER DRUGS.

otic relating to the ear.

otitis inflammation of the ear. *Aviation o.* a symptom complex resulting from fluctuations between atmospheric pressure and air pressure in the middle ear; also called barotitis media. *Furuncular o.* the formation of furuncles in the external ear. *O. externa* inflammation of the external ear. *O. interna*, *o. labyrinthica* labyrinthitis. *O. media* inflammation of the middle ear, occurring most often in infants and young children, and classified as serous, secretory and suppurative.

otolith 1. a calculus in the middle ear. 2. one of a number of small calcareous concretions of the inner ear, at the base of the semicircular canals.

otomycosis a fungal infection of the auditory canal.

otorrhoea discharge from the ear, especially of pus.

otosclerosis the formation of spongy bone in the labyrinth of the ear, causing the auditory ossicles to become fixed and less able to pass on vibrations when sound enters the ear. An early symptom is ringing in the ears with a progressive loss of hearing—conductive deafness.

otoscope an auriscope; an instrument for examining the ear.

ototoxic anything that has a deleterious effect on the eighth cranial nerve or on the organs of hearing.

outbreak an epidemic of an infectious disease limited to a localized increase in the incidence of the disease, e.g., in a village, town or institution. *See* EPIDEMIC.

outcome a consequence or objective for a health care intervention, e.g., a patient goal. The implications are that the outcome is (a) measurable and (b) can be expected as a result of the planned intervention. *O. framework* high level indicators which set out the expected priority outcomes the NHS will deliver. *O. indicator* measurement of the success of a clinical treatment/intervention in terms of the impact on the health of the individual.

outlet a means or route of exit or egress. *Pelvic o.* the inferior opening of the pelvis; literally that bounded by the ischial spines, lower border of the symphysis pubis and the sacrococcygeal joint.

out-of-the-body experience a sensation of leaving one's body and travelling through tunnels and lights onto another plane of experience. The condition has been attributed to anoxia of the brain following anaesthesia or severe illness.

outpatient a patient who has a medical consultation or receives treatment at a hospital but who does not require to stay overnight in a hospital bed.

output the yield or total of something produced by a system. *Cardiac o.* the effective volume of blood expelled by either ventricle of the heart per unit of time (usually volume per minute); it is equal to the stroke output multiplied by the number of beats per the time unit used in the computation. *Fluid o.* the amount of urine passed, usually measured in comparison to oral fluid intake.

outreach health care services provided in an alternative setting such as within a community setting, e.g., a specialized clinic held in a general practitioner's surgery, sports centre or other public building enabling patients and/or clients to access care more conveniently and avoid long or difficult journeys. An example of outreach in an acute setting might be staff from ICU providing care for patients and support for staff on general wards.

ovarian relating to an ovary. *O. cyst* a tumour of the ovary containing fluid.

ovariectomy oöphorectomy; excision of an ovary.

ovariotomy 1. surgical removal of an ovary. 2. excision of an ovarian tumour.

ovary one of a pair of glandular organs in the female pelvis. They produce ova, which pass through the uterine tubes into the uterus, and steroid hormones which control the menstrual cycle.

over-the-counter drugs abbreviated OTC drugs. Drugs that can be purchased from a pharmacy without a prescription from a doctor. The list of derestricted drugs available to the public is growing and includes corticosteroid ointments, antihistamines, aciclovir, ibuprofen and nicotine patches.

overbite an overlapping of the lower teeth by the upper teeth.

overcompensation a mental mechanism by which people try to assert themselves by aggressive behaviour or by talking or acting 'big' to compensate for a feeling of inadequacy.

overuse injury injury due to the repetitive movement of a joint or part of the body. *See* REPETITIVE STRAIN INJURY.

oviduct a uterine tube.

ovulation the process of rupture of the mature Graafian follicle when the ovum is shed from the ovary.

ovum [L.] *an egg.* The reproductive cell of the female.

oxidization oxidation. The process by which combustion occurs and breaking up of matter takes place, e.g., oxidization of carbohydrates gives carbon dioxide and water: $C_6H_{12}O_6 + 6\ O_2 = 6\ CO_2 + 6\ H_2O$. The opposite of reduction.

oximeter a photoelectric cell used to determine the oxygen saturation of blood. *Ear o.* one attached to the ear by which the oxygen content of blood flowing through the ear can be measured.

oxygen *symbol* O. A colourless, odourless gas constituting one-fifth of the atmosphere. It is stored in cylinders at high pressure or as liquid oxygen. It is used medicinally to enrich the air when either respiration or circulation is impaired. *O. deficit* a physiological state that exists in cells during episodes of temporary oxygen shortage. *O. saturation* the amount of oxygen bound to haemoglobin in the blood. *O. tent* a large plastic canopy that encloses the patient in a controlled environment; used for oxygen therapy, humidity therapy or aerosol therapy. Not widely used now, but still used for children with severe breathing difficulties. *O. therapy* supplementary oxygen administered for the purpose of relieving hypoxaemia and preventing damage to the tissue cells as a result of oxygen lack.

oxygenation saturation with oxygen; a process which occurs in the lungs to the haemoglobin of blood, which is saturated with oxygen to form oxyhaemoglobin.

oxygenator a machine through which the blood is passed to oxygenate it during open heart surgery.

oxyhaemoglobin haemoglobin that has been oxygenated, as in arterial blood.

oxyntic acid-forming. *O. cell* a parietal cell of the gastric glands which secretes hydrochloric acid.

oxytocic any drug that stimulates uterine contractions and may be used to hasten delivery.

oxytocin a pituitary hormone which stimulates uterine contractions and the ejection of milk. Synthetically prepared, it is used to induce labour and to control postpartum haemorrhage.

oxyuriasis infestation by threadworms of the genus *Enterobius*.

ozena a severe form of rhinitis in which the mucous membrane of the nose atrophies. This is associated with a thick offensive nasal discharge that crusts and often results in severe halitosis.

ozone an intensified form of oxygen containing three O atoms to the molecule (i.e., O_3), and often discharged by electrical machines, such as X-ray apparatus. In medicine it is employed as an antiseptic and oxidizing agent. *O. sickness* sometimes experienced by jet travellers due to the levels of ozone in the aircraft.

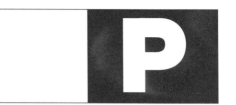

Pa symbol for *pascal*.

pacemaker an object or substance that controls the rate at which a certain phenomenon occurs. The natural pacemaker of the heart is the sinoatrial node. *Electronic cardiac p.* an electrically operated mechanical device which stimulates the myocardium to contract. It consists of an energy source, usually batteries, and electrical circuitry connected to an electrode which is in direct contact with the myocardium. Pacemakers may be temporary or permanent. Temporary ones usually have an external energy source, whereas permanent ones have a subcutaneously implanted one. The rate at which the pacemaker delivers pulses may be either fixed or on demand. *Fixed* pacing means that pulses are delivered to the heart at a predetermined rate irrespective of any cardiac activity. A *demand* pacemaker is programmed to deliver pulses only in the absence of spontaneous cardiac activity.

pachydermia an abnormal thickening of the skin. *P. laryngis* chronic hypertrophy of the vocal cords.

pachyonychia abnormal thickening of the nails.

pacing a series of techniques used by occupational therapists to assist people to perform tasks within their health limitations and to reduce adverse effects such as pain, joint stress and fatigue. Using a contractual arrangement with the patient, the aim is to maximize performance and to meet personal objectives in achieving the desired task.

PACT prescribing analyses and cost.

paediatric advanced life support (PALS) see Appendix 2 and ADVANCED LIFE SUPPORT.

paediatrician a medically qualified person specializing in childhood development and the diseases of children.

paediatrics the branch of medicine dealing with the care and development of children and with the treatment of diseases that affect them.

paedophilia a sexual attraction towards children.

Paget's disease *Sir J. Paget, British surgeon, 1814–1899.* 1. a chronic disease of bone in which overactivity of the osteoblasts and osteoclasts leads to dense bone formation with areas of rarefaction. Osteitis deformans. 2. an inflammation of the nipple caused by cancer of the milk ducts of the breast.

pain a feeling of distress, suffering or agony, caused by stimulation of specialized nerve endings. Its purpose is chiefly protective; it acts as a warning that tissues are being damaged and induces the sufferer to remove or withdraw from the source. Pain is a subjective experience and one person's pain cannot be compared to another's experience. *Bearing-down p.* pain accompanying uterine contractions during the second stage of labour. *False p's* ineffective pains during pregnancy which resemble labour pains, but not accompanied by cervical dilatation; also called false labour. *See also* BRAXTON HICKS CONTRACTIONS. *Gas p's* pains caused by distension of the stomach or intestine by accumulations of air or other gases. *Hunger p.* pain coming on at the time of feeling hunger for a meal; a symptom of gastric disorder. *Intermenstrual p.* pain accompanying ovulation, occurring during the period between the menses, usually about midway. Also called mittelschmerz. *Labour p's* the rhythmic pains of increasing severity and frequency due to contraction of the uterus at childbirth. *See also* LABOUR. *Lancinating p.* sharp, darting pain. *P. assessment* the measurement of a patient's pain and its psychosocial and biological impact upon the individual's personal situation is especially difficult to assess where the patient is unable to articulate their distress, e.g., children, infants and some adults. A number of assessment tools are available for use with children and adults; they are primarily longitudinal scales which list 'no pain' at one end to 'intense pain' at the other. *See* Figure on p. 289. *Phantom p.* pain felt as if it were arising in an absent (amputated) limb. *See also* AMPUTATION. *Referred p.* pain in a part other than that in which the cause that produced it is situated. Referred pain usually originates in one of the visceral organs but is felt in the skin or sometimes in another area deep inside the body. Referred pain probably occurs because pain signals from the viscera travel along the same neural pathways used by pain signals from the skin. The person perceives the pain but interprets it as having originated in the skin rather than in a deep-seated visceral organ. *Rest p.* a continuous burning pain due to ischaemia of the lower leg, which begins or is aggravated after reclining and is relieved by sitting or standing.

painful arc syndrome a condition in which pain occurs when the arm is raised from the side between 45 and 160 degrees. The most usual cause is an inflamed tendon or bursa around the shoulder joint that is being squeezed between the scapula and humerus on movement. *See* FROZEN SHOULDER and SHOULDER IMPINGEMENT SYNDROME.

palate the roof of the mouth. *Artificial p.* a plate made to close a cleft palate. *Cleft p.* a congenital deformity where there is lack of fusion of the two bones forming the palate. *Hard p.* the bony part at the front. *Soft p.* a fold of mucous membrane that continues from the hard palate to the uvula.

palliative treatment that relieves, but does not cure. *P. care* the active total care of patients whose disease no longer responds to curative treatment; should neither hasten nor postpone death. It pays equal attention to the physical, psychological, social and spiritual aspects of care of patients and those close to them.

pallor abnormal paleness of the skin.

palmar relating to the palm of the hand. *Deep p. arches* the deep and superficial palmar arches are the chief arterial blood supply to the hand, formed by the junction of the ulnar and radial arteries. *P. fascia* the arrangement of tendons in the palm of the hand. *Superficial p. arches see earlier, deep p. arches.*

palpation the examination of the organs by touch or pressure of the hand over the part.

palpebral referring to the eyelids. *P. ligaments* a band of ligaments which stretches from the junction of the upper and lower lid to the orbital bones, both medially and laterally.

palpitation rapid and forceful contraction of the heart of which the patient is conscious.

PALS Patient Advice and Liaison Service.

palsy a historical term for paralysis. *Bell's p.* paralysis of the facial muscles

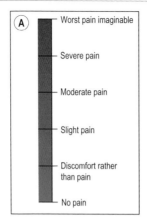

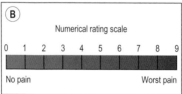

VISUAL ANALOGUE SCALE AND NUMERICAL RATING SCALE
FOR PAIN ASSESSMENT

on one side, supplied by the seventh cranial nerve. *Crutch p.* paralysis due to pressure of a crutch on the radial nerve, and a cause of 'dropped wrist'. *Shaking p.* Parkinsonism; paralysis agitans.

panacea a remedy for all diseases.

panarthritis inflammation of all the joints or of all the structures of a joint.

pancreas an elongated, dual-purpose racemose gland about 15 cm long, lying behind the stomach, with its head in the curve of the duodenum and its tail in contact with the spleen (*see* Figure on p. 290). It secretes a digestive fluid (pancreatic juice) containing ferments which act on all classes of food. The fluid enters the duodenum by the pancreatic duct, which joins the common bile duct. The pancreas also secretes the hormones insulin and glucagon.

pancreatectomy surgical excision of the whole or a part of the pancreas.

pancreatin an extract from the pancreas containing the digestive enzymes. Used to treat deficiency, as in cystic fibrosis, and after pancreatectomy.

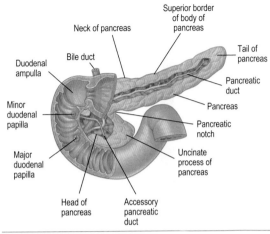

Superior border
of body of
pancreas

Neck of pancreas

Tail of
pancreas

Bile duct

Duodenal
ampulla

Pancreatic
duct

Pancreas

Minor
duodenal
papilla

Pancreatic
notch

Major
duodenal
papilla

Uncinate
process of
pancreas

Head of
pancreas

Accessory
pancreatic
duct

PANCREAS

pancreatitis inflammation of the pancreas. *Acute p.* a severe condition usually associated with alcohol misuse or biliary disease in which the patient experiences sudden pain in the upper abdomen and back. The patient often becomes severely shocked. *Chronic p.* chronic inflammation occurring after acute attacks. Pancreatic failure may lead to diabetes mellitus.

pancreozymin a hormone of the duodenal mucosa that stimulates the external secretory activity of the pancreas, especially its production of amylase.

pancytopenia a reduction in number of all types of blood cell due to failure of bone marrow formation.

pandemic an epidemic spreading over a wide area, sometimes all over the world.

panic an unreasoning and overwhelming fear or terror. It may occur in anxiety states and acute schizophrenia. *P. attack* a brief period of acute anxiety,

distress and fear of dying or of losing one's reason. It may be recognized by the person that this experience is associated with specific situations, e.g., being confined in a small space. Usually associated with other anxiety disorders or mental health problems. *P. disorder* a type of mental health disorder that is characterized by recurrent panic attacks of intense anxiety and distressing physical symptoms.

panniculitis inflammation of the fatty tissue under the skin, usually seen in women on the thighs and lower legs.

pannus increased vascularity of the cornea leading to granulation tissue formation and impaired vision. It occurs in trachoma after inflammation of the cornea.

panophthalmia panophthalmitis; inflammation of all the tissues of the eyeball.

Papanicolaou test *G.N. Papanicolaou, Greek physician, anatomist and* *cytologist, 1883–1962.* A smear test to detect diseases of the uterine cervix and endometrium. Also called Pap test.

papilla a small nipple-shaped protuberance. *Circumvallate p.* one surrounded by a ridge. A number are found at the back of the tongue arranged in a V-shape, and containing taste buds. *Filiform p.* one of the fine, slender filaments on the main part of the tongue which give it its velvety appearance. *Fungiform p.* a mushroom-shaped papilla of the tongue. *Optic p.* the optic disc, where the optic nerve leaves the eyeball. *Tactile p.* a projection on the true skin which contains nerve endings responsible for relaying sensations of pressure to the brain. A touch corpuscle.

papillitis 1. inflammation of the optic disc. 2. inflammation of a papilla.

papilloedema oedema and hyperaemia of the optic disc, usually associated with increased intracranial pressure; also called choked disc.

papilloma a benign growth of epithelial tissue, e.g., a wart.

papillomatosis the occurrence of multiple papillomas.

papovavirus a family of DNA-producing viruses which cause tumours, usually benign, such as warts.

pappataci fever see PHLEBOTOMUS.

papule a pimple, or small solid elevation of the skin.

papulopustular descriptive of skin eruptions of both papules and pustules.

papulosquamous descriptive of skin eruptions that are both papular and scaly. They include such conditions as lichen planus, pityriasis and psoriasis.

paracentesis puncture of the wall of a cavity with a hollow needle in order to draw off excess fluid or to obtain diagnostic material.

paracusis a disorder of hearing. *P. of Willis* an improvement in hearing when surrounded by noise.

paradigm an example or representative instance of a concept or theoretical approach.

paradoxical sleep rapid eye movement (REM) sleep. *See* SLEEP.

paraesthesia an abnormal tingling sensation. 'Pins and needles'.

Paragonimus a genus of trematode parasites. The flukes infest the lungs and are found mainly in tropical countries.

paralysis loss or impairment of motor function in a part owing to a lesion of the neural or muscular mechanism; also, by analogy, impairment of sensory function (sensory paralysis). Paralysis is a symptom of a wide variety of physical and emotional disorders rather than a disease in itself. *P. agitans* Parkinsonism. *Bulbar p. (labioglossopharyngeal p.)* paralysis due to changes in the motor centre of the medulla oblongata. It affects the muscles of the mouth, tongue and pharynx. *Facial p. (Bell's palsy)* paralysis that affects the muscles of the face and is due to injury or to inflammation of the facial nerve. *Flaccid p.* loss of tone and absence of reflexes in the paralysed muscles. *General p. of the insane.* Paralytic dementia occurring in the late stages of syphilis. *Infantile p.* the major form of POLIOMYELITIS. *Spastic p.* paralysis characterized by rigidity of affected muscles.

paralytic affected by or relating to paralysis. *P. ileus* obstruction of the ileum due to absence of peristalsis in a portion of the intestine.

paramedian situated on the side of the median line.

paramedic a person employed in the paramedical services especially ambulance personnel qualified to provide pre-hospital procedures and care.

paramedical associated with the medical profession and the delivery of health care. The paramedical services include trained ambulance personnel, occupational and speech therapy, physiotherapy, radiography and social work.

parametritis inflammation of the parametrium; pelvic cellulitis.

parametrium the connective tissue surrounding the uterus.

paramnesia a defect of memory in which there is a false recollection. The patient may fill in the forgotten period with imaginary events, which are often described in great detail.

paranoia thinking and feeling of being under threat when there is no threat. Paranoid thoughts are delusions and may involve exaggerated suspicions or persecution which may be fully systematized in logical form, with the personality remaining fairly well preserved.

paranoid resembling paranoia. Delusions of persecution are a marked feature. Associated with behaviour that denotes suspicion of others. *P. schizophrenia see* SCHIZOPHRENIA.

paraparesis an incomplete paralysis affecting the lower limbs.

paraphimosis retraction of the prepuce behind the glans penis, with inability to replace it, resulting in a painful constriction.

paraphrenia schizophrenia characterized by delusions (of persecution or grandeur or jealousy) but not accompanied by deterioration of the personality.

paraplegia paralysis of the lower extremities and lower trunk. All parts below the point of lesion in the spinal cord are affected. It may be of sudden onset from injury to the cord or may develop slowly as the result of disease.

parapraxia describes minor aberrations of behaviour such as forgetfulness, the misplacing of things, verbal errors known also as 'Freudian slips' or 'senior moments' commonly associated with ageing.

paraprofessional a person who is specially trained in a particular field or occupation to assist a professional.

parapsychology the branch of psychology dealing with psychical effects and experiences that appear to fall outside the scope of physical laws, e.g., telepathy and clairvoyance.

paraquat a poisonous compound used as a contact herbicide. Contact with concentrated solutions causes irritation of the skin, cracking and shedding of the nails, and delayed healing of cuts and wounds. After ingestion renal and hepatic failure may develop, followed by pulmonary insufficiency and death.

parasite any animal or vegetable organism living upon or within another, from which it derives its nourishment.

parasiticide a drug that kills parasites.

parasuicide a suicidal action such as self-mutilation or the taking of a drug overdose which is motivated by a need to attract attention and seek help rather than commit suicide. Also known as deliberate self-harm (DSH).

parasympathetic nervous system the craniosacral part of the autonomic nervous system.

parasympatholytic anticholinergic; an agent that opposes the effects of the parasympathetic nervous system.

parathormone the endocrine secretion of the parathyroid glands.

parathyroid gland one of four small endocrine glands, two of which are associated with each lobe of the thyroid gland, and sometimes embedded in it. The secretion from these has some control over calcium metabolism, and lack of it is a cause of tetany.

paratyphoid a notifiable infection caused by *Salmonella* of all groups except *S. typhi*. The disease is usually milder and has a shorter incubation period, more abrupt onset and lower mortality rate than does typhoid. Clinically and pathologically, the two diseases cannot be distinguished. Also called paratyphoid fever.

paravertebral near or alongside the vertebral or spinal column. *P. block anaesthesia* induced by the infiltration of a local anaesthetic around the spinal nerve roots emerging from the intervertebral foramina. *P. injection* an injection of local anaesthetic into the sympathetic chain. May be used as a test in ischaemic limbs to ascertain if a sympathectomy would be a useful treatment.

parenchyma the essential active cells of an organ, as distinguished from its vascular and connective tissue.

parent–infant relationship the unique relationship that develops between parents and their infant(s), sometimes referred to as 'bonding', which endures throughout life. Promoted by early touching, fondling, speech, with eye-to-eye contact and breast feeding.

parenteral apart from the alimentary canal. Applied to the introduction into the body of drugs or fluids by routes other than the mouth or rectum, e.g., intravenously or subcutaneously. *P. feeding see* NUTRITION.

paresis partial paralysis.

parietal relating to the walls of any cavity. *P. bones* the two bones forming part of the roof and sides of the skull. *P. cells* the oxyntic cells in the gastric mucosa that secrete hydrochloric acid. *P. pleura* the pleura attached to the chest wall.

parity the classification of a woman with regard to the number of children that have been born live to her.

Parkinson's disease *J. Parkinson, British physician, 1755–1824.* Parkinsonism; paralysis agitans. A slowly progressive disease usually occurring in later life, characterized pathologically by degeneration within the nuclear masses of the extrapyramidal system, and clinically by mask-like facies (*see* FACIES (PARKINSON)), a characteristic tremor of resting muscles, a slowing of voluntary movements, a festinating gait, peculiar posture and muscular weakness. When this symptom complex occurs secondarily to another disorder, the condition is called Parkinsonism.

paronychia an abscess near the fingernail; a whitlow or felon. *P. tendinosa* a pyogenic infection that involves the tendon sheath.

parotid situated near the ear. *P. glands* two salivary glands, one in front of each ear.

parotitis inflammation of a parotid gland. Caused usually by ascending infection via its duct, when hygiene of the mouth is neglected or when the natural secretions are lessened, especially in severe illness or after operation. *Epidemic p.* mumps.

parous having borne one or more children.

paroxysm a sudden attack, worsening or recurrence of symptoms of a disease. A spasm or seizure.

paroxysmal occurring in paroxysms. *P. cardiac dyspnoea* cardiac asthma. Recurrent attacks of dyspnoea associated with pulmonary oedema and left-sided heart failure. *P. tachycardia* recurrent attacks of rapid heartbeats that may occur without heart disease.

parrot disease *see* PSITTACOSIS.

particle a minute piece of substance.

partnership working the relationship between central government, NHS Trusts, NHS Foundation Trusts, Clinical Commissioning Groups, local authorities and patient representatives that has been developed to provide coordinated health care and social services to those in need. One of the core NHS values, this approach aims to achieve improved health for all with the coordinated and collaborative working between all involved agencies.

parturient giving birth; relating to childbirth.

parturition the act of giving birth.

parvovirus B19 *see* FIFTH DISEASE.

pascal *symbol* Pa. The SI unit of pressure.

passive not active. *P. immunity see* IMMUNITY. *P. movements* in massage, manipulation by a physiotherapist without the help of the patient. *P. smoking* inhaling tobacco smoke exhaled by others; associated with a significant risk of increase in lung cancer.

passivity in psychiatry, a delusional feeling that a person is under some outside control and must therefore be inactive.

Pasteurella *L. Pasteur, French chemist and bacteriologist, 1833–1895.* A genus of short gram-negative bacilli.

pasteurization the process of heating foods to destroy disease causing microorganisms, and to reduce the numbers of microorganisms responsible for fermentation and putrefaction. The Pasteurization process using moist heat is also used to disinfect medical instruments and other equipment.

Patau's syndrome a rare and serious genetic disorder caused by having an additional copy of chromosome13. Also known as trisomy 13. Development is severely disrupted and in many cases leads to death in utero or shortly after birth.

patch test a test of skin sensitivity in which a number of possible allergens are applied to the skin under a plaster. The causal agent of the allergy will produce an inflammation.

patella the small, circular, sesamoid bone forming the kneecap.

patellar belonging to the patella. *P. reflex* a knee jerk obtained by tapping the tendon below the patella.

patellectomy excision of the patella.

patent open or unobstructed. *P. ductus arteriosus* failure of the ductus arteriosus to close, causing a shunt of blood from the aorta into the pulmonary artery and producing a continuous heart murmur.

paternity testing the use of blood samples to assist in establishing the paternity of a child. Blood taken from the suspected father, the child and sometimes the mother is tested to ascertain similarities in DNA.

pathogen a microorganism that can cause disease, e.g., *Clostridium tetani* causing tetanus.

pathogenicity the ability of a microorganism to cause disease.

pathognomonic specifically characteristic of a disease. A sign or symptom by which a pathological condition can positively be identified.

pathological 1. pertaining to pathology. 2. causing or arising from disease. *P. fracture* a fracture occurring in diseased bone where there has been little or no external trauma.

pathology the branch of medicine that deals with the essential nature of disease, especially of the structural and functional changes in tissues and organs of the body which cause or are caused by disease.

patient a person who is ill or is undergoing treatment for a health care problem and/or is registered with a general practitioner. *P. advocate, P. representative*, a person who acts on behalf of an incapacitated patient. *P. pathway* the route followed by the patient into, through and out of NHS and social care services. It can involve referral from primary care to hospital, visits to hospital departments and specialties, a pathway through a clinical network, or the experience of joint NHS and social care in the community.

Patient Advice and Liaison Service abbreviated PALS. An advice service for patients in NHS Trusts and Foundation Trusts providing on-the-spot help and information about the health services to patients, their families and carers. PALS also monitors trends, highlighting gaps within the service and provides reports for action to the trust managers. It also represents patients' concerns to the trust management and board.

patients' rights basic rights of patients set out for example in the NHS Constitution for England and the Patients Rights (Scotland) Act 2011.

Paul–Bunnell test *J.R. Paul, American physician, 1893–1971; W.W. Bunnell, American physician, 1902–1966.* An agglutination test which, if positive, confirms the diagnosis of glandular fever.

Pavlov's method *I.P. Pavlov, Russian physiologist, 1849–1936.* A method for the study of the conditioned reflexes. Pavlov noticed that his experimental dogs salivated in anticipation of food when they heard a bell ring.

PDSA *see* PLAN, DO, STUDY, ACT.

peau d'orange [Fr.] a dimpled appearance of the overlying skin. Blockage of the skin lymphatics causes dimpling of the hair follicle openings which resembles orange skin. Particularly associated with breast cancer.

pecten 1. the middle third of the anal canal. 2. a ridge on the pubic crest to which the inguinal ligament is attached.

pectoral relating to the chest. *P. muscles* two pairs of muscles, pectoralis major and pectoralis minor, which control the movements of the shoulder and upper arm.

pectus the chest.

pedicle the stem or neck of a tumour. *P. graft* a tissue graft that is partially detached and inserted in its new position while temporarily still obtaining its blood supply from the original source.

pediculosis the condition of being infested with lice.

Pediculus a genus of lice. *P. humanus* a species that feeds on human blood and is an important vector of relapsing fever, typhus and trench fever. Subspecies are recognized: *P. humanus* var. *capitis* (head louse), found on the scalp hair, *P. humanus* var. *corporis* (body or clothes louse), and *P. pubis* the crab or pubic louse.

peduncle a narrow part of a structure acting as a support. *Cerebellar p.* one of the collections of nerve fibres connecting the cerebellum with the medulla oblongata.

PEEP positive end-expiratory pressure.

peer a colleague usually of equal standing. *P. review* a basic component of a quality assurance (*see* QUALITY) programme in which the results of health and/or nursing care given to a specific patient population are evaluated according to defined criteria established by the peers of the professionals delivering the care. Peer review is focused on the patient and on the results of care given by a group of professionals rather than on individual professional practitioners. Peer review is also a feature of acceptance of journal submissions for publication. *P. support* the social support provided by one's peer group.

Pel–Ebstein syndrome *P.K. Pel, Dutch physician, 1852–1919; W. Ebstein, German physician, 1836–1912.* A recurrent pyrexia, having a cycle of 15–21 days, which is a rare occurrence in people with Hodgkin's lymphoma.

pellagra a syndrome caused by a diet seriously deficient in niacin (or failure to convert tryptophan to niacin). Most persons with pellagra also suffer from deficiencies of vitamin B_2 (riboflavin) and other essential vitamins and minerals. The disease also occurs in persons suffering from alcoholism and drug addiction. Characterized by debility, digestive disorders, peripheral neuritis, ataxia, mental disturbance and erythema with exfoliation of the skin.

pelvic pertaining to the pelvis. *P. exenteration* removal of all the pelvic organs. *P. floor exercises* a programme of exercises to strengthen the muscles and tighten the ligaments at the base of the abdomen which form the pelvic floor. *P. girdle* the ring of bone to which the lower limbs are jointed. It consists of the two hip bones and the sacrum and coccyx. *P. inflammatory disease* (PID) persistent infection of the internal reproductive organs of the female. If not treated can result in infertility.

pelvimetry measurement of the pelvis.

pelvis a basin-shaped cavity. *Bony p.* the pelvic girdle, formed of the hip bones and the sacrum and coccyx. *Contracted p.* narrowing of the diameter of the pelvis. It may be of the true conjugate or the diagonal. Effective antenatal care will recognize this condition, and caesarean section may be necessary. *False p.* the part formed by the concavity of the iliac bones above the iliopectineal line. *Renal p.* the dilatation of the ureter which, by enclosing the hilum, surrounds the pyramids of the kidney substance. *True p.* the basin-like cavity below the false pelvis, its upper limit being the pelvic brim.

pemphigoid 1. resembling pemphigus. 2. a bullous disease of the elderly with the blisters arising beneath the epidermis. The skin and the mucosa are affected, and sometimes the conjunctiva.

pemphigus a distinctive group of rare but serious diseases characterized by successive crops of large bullae ('water blisters'); the name is derived from the Greek word for blister, *pemphix*. Clusters of blisters usually appear first near the nose and mouth (sometimes inside them) and then gradually spread over the skin of the rest of the body. When the blisters burst, they leave round patches of raw and tender skin. Pemphigus is considered to be an auto-immune disorder.

pendulous hanging down. *P. abdomen* the hanging down of the abdomen over the pelvis, due to weakness and laxity of the abdominal muscles.

penicillamine an anti-rheumatic drug used principally to treat active rheumatoid arthritis and Wilson's disease.

penicillin an antibiotic cultured from certain moulds of the genus *Penicillium*. The drug is used in various forms to treat a wide variety of bacterial infections; it was first used therapeutically in 1941.

penicillinase an enzyme that inactivates penicillin. Many bacteria, particularly staphylococci, produce this enzyme.

Penicillium a genus of mould-like fungi, from some of which the penicillins are derived. Some species are pathogenic to humans.

penis the male organ of copulation and urination.

pentose a monosaccharide containing five carbon atoms in a molecule.

pepsin an enzyme found in gastric juice. It partially digests proteins in an acid solution.

pepsinogen the precursor of pepsin, activated by hydrochloric acid.

PEP post-exposure prophylaxis.

peptic relating to pepsin or the action of the gastric juices in promoting digestion. *P. ulcer* an ulcer, usually in the stomach or the duodenum, caused by an erosion of the surface to expose the muscle wall by the stomach acid and digestive enzymes. It is often precipitated by *Helicobacter pylori* organisms.

peptide any of a class of compounds of low molecular weight that yield two or more amino acids on hydrolysis. Peptides form the constituent parts of proteins.

peptone a substance produced by the action of pepsin on protein.

per os [L.] *by the mouth.*

percentile a term used in statistics to show how common some characteristic is. The line represents the percentage of the population who have this characteristic. The 90th percentile (or centile) for height means that 90% of the population will be no taller than the figure. The 50th percentile is the median or average.

percept, perception an awareness and understanding of an impression that has been presented to the senses. The mental process by which we perceive.

percussion a method of diagnosis by tapping with the fingers or with a light hammer upon any part of the body. Information can thus be gained as to the condition of underlying organs.

percutaneous through the skin. *P. endoscopic gastrostomy (PEG)* a gastrostomy tube inserted endoscopically through the abdominal wall to allow feeding and the passage of drugs. *See* Appendix 1.

perforation a hole or break in the containing walls or membranes of an organ or structure of the body. Perforation occurs when erosion, infection or other factors create a weak spot in the organ and internal pressure causes a rupture. It may also result from a deep penetrating wound.

performance indicators abbreviated Pls. A 'package' of measurable statistics against which to benchmark to assess performance usually in relation to quality. Performance indicators are intended to compare services and identify aspects that merit further scrutiny with a view to changes in organization or practice.

perfusion the passage of liquid through a tissue or an organ, particularly the passage of blood through the lung tissue.

perianal surrounding or located around the anus. *P. abscess* a small subcutaneous pocket of pus near the anal margin.

periarteritis inflammation of the outer coat and surrounding tissues of an artery.

periarthritis inflammation of the tissues surrounding a joint.

pericarditis inflammation of the pericardium. *Adhesive p.* the presence of adhesions between the two layers of pericardium owing to a thick fibrinous exudate. *Bacterial p.* inflammation of the pericardium due to bacterial infection. *Chronic constrictive p.* thickening and sometimes calcification of the pericardium, which inhibits the action of the heart. *Rheumatic p.* pericarditis due to rheumatic fever.

pericardium the smooth membranous sac enveloping the heart, consisting of an outer fibrous and an inner serous coat. The sac contains a small amount of serous fluid.

perichondrium the membrane covering cartilaginous surfaces.

pericranium the periosteum of the cranial bones.

perilymph the fluid that separates the bony and the membranous labyrinths of the ear.

perimeter 1. the line marking the boundary of any area or geometrical figure; the circumference. 2. an instrument for measuring the field of vision.

perimetrium the peritoneal covering of the uterus.

perinatal relating to the period shortly before and 7 days after birth. *P. mortality rate* the number of stillbirths plus deaths of babies under 7 days old per 1000 total births in any one year.

perinatologist a medically qualified person specializing in perinatology.

perinatology the branch of medicine (obstetrics and paediatrics) dealing with the fetus and infant during the perinatal period.

perineal relating to the perineum.

perineum the tissues between the anus and external genitals. *Lacerated p.* a torn perineum, which may result from childbirth but is often forestalled by performing an episiotomy. Treatment is by suturing of the laceration.

period *see* MENSTRUATION.

periodic recurring at regular or irregular intervals. *P. apnoea of the newborn* occurring in the normal full-term infant, periodic episodes of rapid breathing followed by a brief period of apnoea which is associated with rapid eye movements. *P. syndrome* recurrent head, limb or abdominal pains in children for which no organic cause can be found. It is often associated with migraine in adult life.

periodontitis inflammation of the periodontium.

periodontium the connective tissue between the teeth and their bony sockets.

perioperative pertaining or relating to the period immediately before or after an operation, as in perioperative care.

periosteal pertaining to or composed of periosteum. *P. elevator* an instrument for separating the periosteum from the bone.

periosteum the fibrous membrane covering the surface of bone. It consists of two layers: the inner or osteogenetic layer, which is closely adherent and forms new cells (by which the bone grows in girth); and, in close contact with it, the fibrous layer richly supplied with blood vessels.

periostitis inflammation of the periosteum, usually as a result of injury.

peripheral relating to the periphery. *P. arterial disease* (PAD) a build up of fatty deposits in the arteries restricting blood supply to leg muscles. *P. iridectomy* excision of a small piece of iris from its peripheral edge. *P. nervous system* those parts of the nervous system lying outside the central nervous system. *P. neuritis* inflammation of terminal nerves. *P. resistance* the resistance in the walls of the arterioles, which is a major factor in the control of blood pressure.

periphery the outer surface or circumference.

peristalsis a wave-like contraction, preceded by a wave of dilatation, that travels along the walls of a tubular organ, tending to press its contents onwards. It occurs in the muscle coat of the alimentary canal. *Reversed p.* a wave of contraction in the alimentary canal which passes *towards* the mouth. *Visible p.* a wave of contraction in the alimentary canal that is visible on the surface of the abdomen.

peritoneal referring to the peritoneum. *P. cavity* the cavity between the parietal and the visceral peritoneum. *P. dialysis* a method of removing waste products from the blood by passing a cannula into the peritoneal cavity, running in a dialysing fluid, and after an interval, draining it off.

peritoneoscopy visual examination of the peritoneum by means of a peritoneoscope.

peritoneum the serous membrane lining the abdominal cavity and forming a covering for the abdominal organs. *Parietal p.* that which lines the abdominal cavity. *Visceral p.* the inner layer which closely covers the abdominal organs and includes the mesenteries.

peritonitis inflammation of the peritoneum. This may be produced by inflammation of abdominal organs, by irritating substances from a perforated gallbladder or gastric ulcer, by rupture of a cyst, or by irritation from blood, as in cases of internal bleeding. Less frequently, it may result from long-standing irritation caused by the presence in the abdomen of a foreign body, such as gunshot, or by chronic peritoneal dialysis.

peritonsillar around the tonsil. *P. abscess* quinsy.

perlèche [Fr.] inflammation with fissuring at the angles of the mouth; often due to vitamin B deficiency, poorly fitting dentures or thrush infection.

permeability the degree to which a fluid can pass from one structure through a wall or membrane to another.

pernicious highly destructive; fatal. *P. anaemia* an anaemia due to lack of absorption of vitamin B_{12} for the formation of red blood cells.

perniosis a condition, resulting from persistent exposure to cold, which produces vascular spasm in the superficial arterioles of the hands and feet, causing thrombosis and necrosis. Perniosis includes chilblains and Raynaud's disease.

peroral by the mouth.

perseveration the constant recurrence of an idea or the tendency to keep repeating the same words or actions.

persistent vegetative state a long-term dependent state that may last for weeks, months or years. Caused by damage to the cerebral cortex of the brain that controls higher mental functions, while the brainstem controlling respiration and circulation remains undamaged. The individual appears awake but is totally dependent on others for all care and remains unresponsive.

persona what one presents of one's self, to be perceived by others.

personal development plan a planned process whereby an individual develops skills and knowledge that are beneficial to themselves and their career. This is part of a life-long learning commitment for nurses and other health professionals.

personality the sum total of heredity and inborn tendencies, with influences from environment and education, which forms the mental make-up of a person and influences attitude to life. *Antisocial p. disorder* (APD) a personality disorder in which repetitive antisocial behaviour is associated with ego eccentricity, lack of guilt or anxiety, and imperviousness to punishment. Also called sociopathic (psychopathic) personality. *Double p., dual p.* multiple personality. *Multiple p.* a dissociative reaction in which an individual adopts two or more personalities alternatively, in none of which is there awareness of the experiences of the other(s). *Psychopathic p.* antisocial personality, sociopathic personality. *Schizoid p.* a personality disorder marked by timidness, self-consciousness, introversion, feelings of isolation and loneliness, and failure to form close interpersonal relationships; the individual is frequently ambitious, meticulous and a perfectionist.

perspiration sweat or the act of sweating. *Insensible p.* water evaporation from the moist surfaces of the body, such as the respiratory tract and skin, that is not due to the activity of the sweat glands. It occurs at a constant rate of about 500 ml/day. When treating dehydration this loss must be taken into account. *Sensible p.* sweat that is visible as droplets on the skin. Part of the mechanism for regulation of body temperature.

Perthes' disease *G.C. Perthes, German surgeon, 1869–1927.* Osteochondritis of the head of the femur. Pseudocoxalgia (Legg–Calvé–Perthes disease).

pertussis See WHOOPING COUGH.

perversion morbid diversion from a normal course. *Sexual p.* abnormal sexual desires and behaviour. A deviation.

pes the foot, or any foot-like structure. *P. cavus* a foot with an abnormally high arch. Claw foot. *P. malleus valgus* hammer toe. *P. planus* flat foot.

pessary 1. a plastic or metal ring-shaped device which is inserted in the vagina to support a prolapsed uterus. 2. a medicated suppository inserted into the vagina for antiseptic or contraceptive purposes.

PET positron emission tomography.

petechia a small spot due to an effusion of blood under the skin, as in purpura.

petit mal former name for a mild form of epilepsy common in children and characterized by a sudden and brief loss of consciousness. *See* EPILEPSY.

pétrissage [Fr.] a kneading action used in massage.

petrositis inflammation of the petrous portion of the temporal bone, usually spread from a middle-ear infection.

Peyer's glands or patches *J. C. Peyer, Swiss anatomist, 1653–1712.* Small lymph nodules situated in the mucous membrane of the lower part of the small intestine.

Peyronie's disease induration of the corpora cavernosa of the penis, producing a fibrous chordee leading to painful erection. Also known as induratio penis plastica (IPP).

pH a measure of the hydrogen ion concentration, and so the acidity or alkalinity of a solution. Expressed numerically 1 to 14; 7 is neutral, below this is acid and above alkaline. *See* HYDROGEN (ION CONCENTRATION).

phaeochromocytoma a rare tumour of the adrenal medulla which gives rise to paroxysmal hypertension.

phage bacteriophage. A virus that lives on bacteria but is confined to a particular strain. *P.-typing* the identification of certain bacterial strains by determining the presence of strain-specific phages. Used in detecting the causative organisms of epidemics, especially food poisoning.

phagocyte a blood cell that has the power of ingesting bacteria, protozoa and foreign bodies in the blood.

phagocytosis the engulfing and destruction of microorganisms and foreign bodies by phagocytes in the blood.

phalanges the bones of the fingers or toes.

phallus the penis.

phantasy *see* FANTASY.

phantom 1. an image or impression not evoked by actual stimuli. 2. a model of the body or of a specific part thereof. 3. a device for simulating the in vivo interaction of radiation with tissues. *P. pain* pain felt as if it were arising in an absent (amputated) limb also known as p. limb pain/experience. *P. pregnancy see* PSEUDOCYESIS. *P. tumour* a tumour-like swelling of the abdomen caused by contraction of the muscles or by localized gas.

pharmacist a person professionally qualified to carry out pharmacy. The traditional role of giving advice, dispensing prescriptions, providing vaccinations and selling over-the-counter medicines from the more than 10 000 community pharmacies in England has been supplemented by the appointment of pharmacy advisers to the NHS at national and local level together with an expanded role associated with community health. *See* Appendix 4.

pharmacogenetics the study of genetically determined variations in drug metabolism and the response of the individual.

pharmacokinetics the study of how drugs are processed within the body, including their absorption, distribution, metabolism and excretion.

pharmacology the science of the nature and preparation of drugs and particularly of their effects on the body.

pharmacopoeia an authoritative publication that gives the standard formulae and preparations of drugs used in a given country. *British P.* that authorized for use in the UK.

pharmacy 1. the activity or study of medicine preparations. 2. the art of preparing, compounding and dispensing medicines. 3. the place where drugs are stored and dispensed. *See* Appendix 4.

pharyngeal relating to the pharynx. *P. pouch* dilatation of the lower part of the pharynx.

pharyngitis inflammation of the pharynx.

pharyngolaryngeal referring to both the pharynx and larynx.

pharyngotympanic tube the tube that joins the middle ear to the pharynx; the eustachian tube.

pharynx the muscular tube, lined with mucous membrane, situated at the back of the mouth. It leads into the oesophagus, and also communicates with the nose through the posterior nares, with the ears through the pharyngotympanic (eustachian) tubes, and with the larynx. *See* LARYNGOPHARYNX, NASOPHARYNX and OROPHARYNX.

phenol carbolic acid. A disinfectant derived from coal tar.

phenomenon 1. an objective sign or symptom. 2. A noteworthy occurrence.

phenomenology an approach in research, as the study of the lived experience of people or a way of thinking about what life experiences are like for people.

phenotype the characteristics of an individual that are due both to the environment and to genetic make-up.

phenylalanine an essential amino acid which cannot be properly metabolized in persons suffering from phenylketonuria.

phenylketonuria abbreviated PKU. A disease due to a defect in the metabolism of the amino acid phenylalanine.

The condition is hereditary. It results from lack of an enzyme, phenylalanine hydroxylase, necessary for the conversion of phenylalanine into tyrosine. Thus, there is accumulation of phenylalanine in the blood, with eventual excretion of phenylpyruvic acid in the urine. If untreated, the condition results in learning difficulties and other abnormalities. The condition can be detected soon after birth, and screening of newborns for PKU is part of the newborn spot blood test at 5 days. Phenylalanine levels are assessed and if necessary treatment is with a diet low in phenylalanine. A special diet is usually recommended throughout life and especially during pregnancy as high phenylalanine levels in the mother's blood can damage the fetus.

phenylpyruvic acid an abnormal constituent of the urine present in phenylketonuria.

pheromone a chemical substance with specific odour secreted externally by an organism and affecting the behaviour or physiology of members of the same species. These substances may be involved in the physiological communication within a species and provide an influence upon sexual behaviour.

phimosis constriction of the prepuce so that it cannot be drawn back over the glans penis. The usual treatment is circumcision.

phlebectomy excision of a vein or a portion of a vein.

phlebitis inflammation of a vein, usually in the leg, which tends to lead to the formation of a thrombus. The symptoms are pain and swelling, and redness along the course of the vein, which is felt later as a hard, tender cord.

phlebography also known as venography. 1. radiographic examination of a vein containing a contrast medium. 2. the graphic representation of the venous pulse.

phlebothrombosis obstruction of a vein by a blood clot, without local inflammation. It is usually in the deep veins of the calf of the leg, causing tenderness and swelling. The clot may break away and cause an embolism.

Phlebotomus a genus of sandflies, the various species of which transmit leishmaniasis in its many forms, and also sandfly fever, which is also known as pappataci fever and three day fever.

phlebotomy the puncture of a vein for the withdrawal of blood. Venesection.

phlegm mucus secreted by the lining of the air passages.

phlegmatic calm and unemotional.

phlycten 1. a small blister caused by a burn. 2. a small vesicle containing lymph occurring in the conjunctiva or cornea of the eye. Often associated with tuberculosis.

phobia an irrational fear produced by a specific situation or object that the patient attempts to avoid.

phocomelia a rare congenital deformity in which the long bones of the limbs are minimal or absent and the individual has stump-like limbs of various lengths. The drug thalidomide, used in the 1960s in early pregnancy, was associated with this deformity.

phonation the art of uttering meaningful vocal sounds.

phonocardiogram a record of the heart sounds made by a phonocardiograph.

phonocardiograph an instrument that graphically records heart sounds and murmurs.

phonology the study of speech sounds, their production and the relationship between sounds as elements of language.

phosphatase one of a group of enzymes involved in the metabolism of phosphate. *Alkaline p.* an enzyme formed by osteoblasts in the bones and by liver cells and excreted in the bile.

phosphate a salt or ester of phosphoric acid.

phospholipid a lipid of glycerol fats found in cells, especially those of the nervous system.

phosphorus *symbol* P. An essential element in the diet. It is a major component of bone, is involved in almost all metabolic processes and also plays an important role in cell metabolism. It is obtained by the body from milk products, cereals, meat and fish. Its use by the body is controlled by vitamin D and calcium. *See* Appendix 1.

phosphorylase an enzyme, found in the liver and kidneys, that catalyses the breakdown of glycogen into glucose 1-phosphate.

photocoagulation the use of a powerful light source to change tissues and blood from a fluid state to a coagulated clotted mass. Used in detachment of the retina and retinopathies.

photophobia intolerance of light. It can occur in many eye conditions, including conjunctivitis, corneal ulceration, iritis and keratitis.

photophthalmia inflammation of the eye due to overexposure to bright light, especially to ultraviolet light.

photopic pertaining to bright light. *P. vision* vision in bright light when the cones of the retina provide the visual appreciation of colour and shape.

photopsia a sensation of flashes of light sometimes occurring in the early stages of retinal detachment.

photosensitivity an abnormal degree of sensitivity of the skin to sunlight.

phototherapy treatment using fluorescent light, containing a high output of blue light, to reduce the amount of unconjugated bilirubin in the skin of a jaundiced neonate.

phrenic 1. relating to the mind. 2. pertaining to the diaphragm. *P. avulsion* the surgical extraction of a part of the phrenic nerve. *P. nerve* one of a pair of nerves controlling the muscles of the diaphragm.

phthisis pulmonary tuberculosis. *P. bulbi* a shrinking of the eyeball following inflammation or injury.

physical in medicine, relating to the body as opposed to the mental processes. *P. abuse*. *See* ABUSE. *P. disability* a term used when a physical disadvantage is due to impairment of physiological or anatomical structure or function. *P. examination* examination of the bodily state of a patient by ordinary physical means, such as inspection, palpation, percussion and auscultation. *P. medicine* the treatment and rehabilitation of patients with physical disabilities. It includes physiotherapy and rehabilitation. *P. signs* those observed by inspection, percussion, etc.

physician a medically qualified person who practises medicine as opposed to surgery. *Community p.* a doctor who practises community medicine (*see* MEDICINE). *Consultant p.* senior doctor in overall charge of patients within a specialist medical field, and responsible for directing junior medical staff working for the same team.

physiological relating to physiology. Normal, as opposed to pathological. *P. jaundice see* JAUNDICE. *P. solutions* those of the same salt composition and same osmotic pressure as blood plasma.

physiology the science of the functioning of living organisms.

physiotherapy a health care profession regulated by the Health and Care Professions Council concerned with function and movement as well as maximizing mobility potential. It provides treatment for physical problems due to accident, illness or disability, promotes normal function and mobility, using skills of manipulation, electrotherapy, with appropriate exercise programmes as necessary. Physiotherapists are also involved in preventative health care and rehabilitation and committed to reviewing evidence that informs its practice and delivery.

physique the structure of the body.

pia mater [L.] the innermost membrane enveloping the brain and spinal cord, consisting of a network of small blood vessels connected by areolar tissue. This dips down into all the folds of the nerve substance.

pica an unnatural craving for strange foods and for things not fit to be eaten. It may occur in pregnancy, and sometimes in children.

Pick's disease a progressive degenerative disease that causes irreversible destruction of brain cells.

picornavirus a family of small RNA-containing viruses including echoviruses and rhinoviruses.

PICU paediatric intensive care unit.

PID abbreviation for prolapse of an intervertebral disc and pelvic inflammatory disease.

pie chart a circular graph divided into sectors proportional to the magnitudes of the quantities represented.

pigeon breast a deformity in which the sternum is unduly prominent. *P. toed* walking with the toes of one foot or of both feet turned inwards.

pigment colouring matter. *Bile p's* bilirubin and biliverdin. *Blood p.* haemoglobin. *Melanotic p.* melanin.

pigmentation the deposition of pigment in the tissues. In some conditions, e.g., jaundice or albinism, there is either an excess or a lack of pigmentation.

pile a haemorrhoid.

pill a rounded mass of one or more drugs. Taken orally.

pilomotor capable of moving the hair. *P. nerves* sympathetic nerves which control muscles in the skin connected with hair follicles. Stimulation causes the hair to be erected, and also the condition of 'goose-flesh' of the skin.

pilonidal having a growth of hair. *P. cyst* a congenital infolding of hair-bearing skin over the coccyx. It may become infected and lead to sinus formation.

pilot study a small-scale version of a planned experiment or observation used initially to test the design of the larger study. A pilot study is helpful to see if any difficulties or problems arise in order that they can be clarified before embarking on the larger study, thus saving time and resources. A pilot study may also indicate possible extensions to the study or suggest restrictions of those aspects likely to be unhelpful.

pimple a small papule or pustule.

pineal shaped like a pine cone. *P. body* a small cone-shaped structure attached by a stalk to the posterior wall of the third ventricle of the brain and composed of glandular substance.

pinguecula [L.] a small, benign, yellowish spot on the bulbar conjunctiva, seen usually in the elderly. Caused by degeneration of the elastic tissue of the conjunctiva.

pinkeye acute contagious conjunctivitis.

pinna the projecting part of the external ear; the auricle.

pinta a non-sexually transmitted skin infection caused by *Treponema carateum* which is similar to the causative agent of syphilis. It is prevalent in the West Indies and Central America.

pinworm a threadworm; *Enterobius vermicularis.*

PIP a type of breast implant withdrawn from the UK in 2010 after discovery that they were prone to splitting.

pituitary an endocrine gland suspended from the base of the brain and protected by the sella turcica in the sphenoid bone. It consists of two lobes: (a) the anterior, which secretes a number of different hormones, including adrenocorticotrophic hormone (ACTH), gonadotrophin, thyroid-stimulating hormone (TSH) and prolactin; (b) the posterior, which secretes oxytocin and vasopressin.

pityriasis a skin disease characterized by fine scaly desquamation. *P. alba* a condition, common in children, in which white scaly patches appear on the face. *P. capitis* dandruff. *P. rosea* an inflammatory form, in which the affected areas are macular and ring-shaped. *P. versicolor* a common condition in which small patches of skin become scaly and discoloured.

PKU phenylketonuria.

place of safety order a court order whereby a child is arbitrarily removed from the care of its parents in the interests of the child's safety.

placebo [L.] a substance given to a patient as medicine or a procedure performed on a patient that has no intrinsic therapeutic value and relieves symptoms or helps the patient in some way only because the patient believes or expects that it will. A placebo may be prescribed to satisfy a patient's psychological need for drug therapy and may also be given during controlled experiments. *P. effect* after the administration of a drug or treatment, a change (usually temporary) in a patient's physical or emotional condition following publicity or media interest in the drug or treatment. The placebo response is due more to the patient's expectations or to the expectations of the person giving the drug or treatment than to the result of any direct physiological or pharmacological substance response.

placenta the afterbirth. A vascular structure inside the pregnant uterus, supplying the fetus with nourishment through the connecting umbilical cord. The placenta develops in about the third month of pregnancy and is expelled after the birth of the child. *Battledore p.* one in which the cord is attached to the margin and not the centre. *P. praevia* one attached to the lower part of the uterine wall. It may cause severe antepartum haemorrhage. *See also* ABRUPTIO PLACENTAE.

plagiocephaly asymmetry of the head resulting from the irregular closing of the sutures.

plague notifiable disease. Acute, febrile, infectious, highly fatal disease caused by the bacillus *Yersinia pestis*. Transmitted to humans by the bites of fleas that have derived the infection from diseased rats. *Bubonic p.* a type in which the lymph glands are infected and buboes form in the groins and armpits. Known in medieval times as 'The Black Death'. *Pneumonic p.* a type in which the infection attacks chiefly the lung tissues. A fatal form. *Septicaemic p.* a very severe and fatal form when the infection enters the bloodstream.

plan a detailed proposal for doing or achieving something.

plan, do, study, act a widely used method used in service improvement methodology to test out small changes.

planes used in the description of location and movement of parts of the body. Three planes are perpendicular to each other passing through the middle of the body. These are defined: *sagittal*, vertical, front-to-back; *frontal*, vertical, side-to-side; *transverse*, horizontal. *See* AXIS.

planned parenthood the practice of measures including contraception that limit the number and the spacing of pregnancies.

planning the stage of the nursing process in which the nurse and the patient together plan how to manage identified needs and problems and consider the measurable goals to achieve and produce an evidence based, patient focused care plan. A forward date is also set for evaluation of whether or not the goals have been achieved.

plantar relating to the sole of the foot. *P. arch* the arch made by anastomosis of the plantar arteries. *P. fasciitis* heel pain usually caused when the plantar fascia becomes damaged and thickens. *P. flexion* bending of the toes downwards and so arching the foot. *P. reflex* contraction of the toes on stroking the sole of the foot. *P. wart* a common wart located on the sole of the foot. Plantar warts are epidermal tumours caused by a virus that may be picked up by going barefoot. Also called verruca plantaris.

plaque 1. a flat patch on the skin. 2. a deposit of food and bacteria on the enamel of teeth which may produce tartar and caries.

plasma the fluid portion of the blood in which corpuscles are suspended. Plasma is to be distinguished from serum, which is plasma from which the fibrinogen has been separated in the process of clotting. *P. proteins* those present in the blood plasma: albumin, globulin and fibrinogen. *P. volume expander* a solution transfused instead of blood to increase the volume of fluid circulating in the blood vessels. Also called artificial plasma extender. *Reconstituted p.* dried plasma when again made liquid by addition of distilled water.

plasmapheresis a method of removing a portion of the plasma from circulation. Venesection is performed, the blood is allowed to settle, the plasma is removed, and the red blood cells are returned to the circulation. Used in the treatment of those diseases caused by antibodies circulating in the patient's plasma.

plasmid deoxyribonucleic acid (DNA) present in the cytoplasm of some bacteria. This genetic material can be transferred during bacterial reproduction thus permitting the genes of antibiotic resistance to be passed on.

plasmin a fibrinolytic, found in blood plasma, which can dissolve fibrin clots.

plasminogen the inactive precursor of plasmin.

Plasmodium a genus of protozoan parasites in the red blood cells of animals and humans. Five species, *P. falciparum, P. knowlesi, P. malariae, P. ovale* and *P. vivax,* cause the four specific types of human malaria.

plaster 1. a mixture of materials that hardens; used for immobilizing or making impressions of body parts. 2. an adhesive substance spread on fabric or other suitable backing material for application to the skin. Lightweight synthetic materials are now used to splint some fractures. Some synthetic materials are less pliable and cannot be moulded as effectively as plaster of Paris (POP) and occasionally cause allergy of the underlying skin. *Bohler's p.* plaster for Pott's fracture. A leg splint of plaster of Paris, in which is embedded an iron stirrup extending below the foot, which enables the patient to walk without putting weight on the joint. *Corn p.* an adhesive strip or patch impregnated with salicyclic acid and applied to corns on the feet. *Frog p.* a plaster of Paris splint used to maintain the position after correction of the deformity due to congenital dislocation of the hip. *P. of Paris* calcium sulphate or gypsum which sets hard when water is added to it; it is used to form a plaster cast to immobilize a part, and in dentistry for making dental impressions.

plastic 1. constructive; tissue-forming. 2. capable of being moulded; pliable. *P. surgery* the branch of surgery that deals with the repair and reconstruction of deformed or injured parts of the body, including their replacement, by tissue grafting or other means to restore function and appearance.

platelet a disc-shaped structure present in the blood and concerned in the process of clotting. A thrombocyte.

play an occupation, for either children or adults, which is voluntary and may be a spontaneous or an organized activity providing enjoyment, entertainment, amusement or a diversion. Play is important in childhood as a necessary part of psychological and physical development. *Normative p.* is by children that is spontaneous and child led, being pleasurable with no intrinsic goals. *P. group* a session of care and activities for preschool children. It can be organized by any interested person at home or in other premises, but it must be registered with Ofsted. *P. specialist* a person who is qualified to use play constructively to help children come to terms with illness and hospitalization. *P. therapist* one trained in the skills of play therapy. *P. therapy* a technique used in child psychotherapy in which play is used to reveal unconscious material. Play is the natural way in which children express and work through unconscious conflicts; thus play therapy is analogous to the technique of free association used in adult psychotherapy.

pleoptics an orthoptic method of improving the sight in cases of strabismus by stimulating the use of the macular part of the retina.

plethora a general term denoting a red, florid complexion or, specifically, an excessive amount of blood.

plethysmography the measurement of changes in the volume of organs or limbs due to alterations in blood pressure.

pleura the serous membrane lining the thorax and enveloping each lung. *Parietal p.* the layer that lines the chest wall. *Visceral p.* the inner layer which is in close contact with the lung.

pleurisy, pleuritis inflammation of the pleura; it may be caused by infection, injury or tumour. It may be a complication of lung diseases, particularly of pneumonia, or sometimes of tuberculosis, lung abscess or influenza. The symptoms are cough, fever, chills, sharp, sticking pain that is worse on inspiration, and rapid shallow breathing. *Dry p., fibrinous p.* pleurisy in which the membrane is inflamed and roughened, but no fluid is formed. *P. with effusion* wet pleurisy. A type that is characterized by inflammation and exudation of serous fluid into the pleural cavity. *Purulent p.* empyema. The formation of pus in the pleural cavity. An operation for drainage is usually necessary. *Wet p.* pleurisy with effusion.

pleurodynia pain in the intercostal muscles, probably rheumatic in origin.

plexus a network of veins or nerves. *Auerbach's p.* the nerve ganglion situated between the longitudinal and circular muscle fibres of the intestine. The nerves are motor nerves. Also known as myenteric plexus. *Brachial p.* the network of nerves of the neck and axilla. *Choroid p.* a capillary network situated in the ventricles of the brain which forms the cerebrospinal fluid. *Coeliac p.* solar plexus. *Meissner's p.* the sensory nerve ganglion situated in the submucous layer of the intestinal wall. Also known as submucous plexus. *Rectal p.* the network of veins that surrounds the rectum and forms a direct communication between the systemic and portal circulations. *Solar p.* coeliac plexus. The network of nerves and ganglia at the back of the stomach, which supply the abdominal viscera.

plication the taking of tucks in a structure to shorten it; a folding to decrease the size of a structure or organ during a surgical procedure.

pneumaturia the passing of flatus with the urine owing to a vesicointestinal fistula and air from the bowel entering the bladder.

pneumococcus the causative agent of a range of illnesses described as pneumococcal disease, e.g., pneumonia, septicaemia and meningitis. A gram-positive, ovoid diplococcus, *Streptococcus pneumoniae*. Immunization with pneumococcal vaccine helps prevent pneumococcal disease, and is recommended for babies, people aged 65 years and over, and those with certain medical conditions, e.g., diabetes, heart and lung conditions.

pneumoconiosis an industrial disease of the lung due to inhalation of dust particles over a period of time. *See* ANTHRACOSIS, ASBESTOSIS and SILICOSIS.

Pneumocystis jirovecii carinii is a yeast-like fungus acquired by the airborne route which frequently causes pneumonia in people with human immunodeficiency virus (HIV) infection and in other immunosuppressed persons. Previously known as *Pneumocystis carinii*.

pneumodynamics the mechanics of respiration.

pneumoencephalography *see* ENCEPHALOGRAPHY.

pneumogastric pertaining to lungs and stomach. *P. nerve* the tenth cranial nerve to the lungs, stomach, etc. The vagus nerve.

pneumomycosis infection of the lung by microfungi, e.g., candidiasis or aspergillosis.

pneumonectomy partial or total removal of a lung.

pneumonia inflammation of the lung with consolidation and exudation. *Aspiration p.* an acute condition caused by the aspiration of infected material into the lungs. *Hypostatic p.* a form that occurs in weak, bedridden patients. *Lobar p.* an acute infectious disease caused by a pneumococcus and affecting whole lobes of either or both lungs. *Viral p.* inflammation of the lung occurring during some virus disease and secondary to it.

pneumonitis an imprecise term denoting any inflammatory condition of the lung.

pneumoperitoneum the presence of air or gas in the peritoneal cavity, occurring pathologically or introduced intentionally for diagnostic or therapeutic purposes.

pneumoradiography radiographic examination of a cavity or part after air or a gas has been injected into it.

pneumotaxic regulating the rate of respiration. *P. centre* the centre in the pons that influences inspiratory effort during respiration.

pneumothorax accumulation of air or gas in the pleural cavity, resulting in collapse of the lung on the affected side. The condition may occur spontaneously, as in the course of a pulmonary disease, or it may follow trauma to, and perforation of, the chest wall. *Spontaneous p.* sometimes occurs when there is an opening on the surface of the lung allowing leakage of air from the bronchi into the pleural cavity. *Tension p.* a particularly dangerous form of pneumothorax that occurs when air escapes into the pleural cavity from a bronchus but cannot regain entry into the bronchus. As a result, continuously increasing air pressure in the pleural cavity causes progressive collapse of the lung tissue.

podalic relating to the feet. *P. version* a method of changing the lie of a fetus so that its feet will present.

podarthritis inflammation of any of the joints of the foot.

podiatry chiropody. The examination, diagnosis, treatment and prevention of diseases and malfunction of the foot, lower limb and related structures. Now a health care profession under regulation by the Health and Care Professions Council (HCPC), the main role of the podiatrist or chiropodist is to assess and treat abnormalities and diseases of the foot, and to give advice on proper care of the foot and the prevention of foot problems.

pointillage [Fr.] a method of massage using the tips of the fingers.

poison any substance that, applied to the body externally or taken internally, can cause injury to any part or cause death.

poisoning the morbid condition produced by a poison. The poison may be swallowed, inhaled (*see* CARBON (MONOXIDE)), injected by a stinging insect as in a bee sting, or spilled or otherwise brought into contact with the skin.

polioencephalitis acute inflammation of the cortex of the brain.

poliomyelitis an acute, notifiable, infectious viral disease that attacks the central nervous system, injuring or destroying the nerve cells that control the muscles and sometimes causing paralysis; also called polio. Paralysis most often affects the limbs but can involve any muscles, including those that control breathing and swallowing. Since the development and the use of vaccines against poliomyelitis, the disease has been virtually eliminated in wealthier countries, where vaccination rates are high, but is still common in many other parts of the world. *See* IMMUNIZATION SCHEDULE.

poliovirus a small RNA-containing virus which causes poliomyelitis.

pollinosis hay fever, allergic rhinitis; an allergy caused by various kinds of pollen. Pollenosis.

pollution 1. the act of destroying the purity of or contaminating something. 2. contamination of the environment by poisons, radioactive substances, accidental chemical spillage, microorganisms or other wastes from industrial activity, vehicle exhausts or untreated sewage. Pollution in the environment has been linked at many levels as being injurious to good health. Air pollution causes respiratory problems while noise pollution has been linked to hearing loss, insomnia and poor concentration.

polyarteritis nodosa (PAN) inflammatory changes in the walls of the small arteries.

polyarthralgia pain in several joints.

polyarthritis inflammation of several joints at the same time, as seen in rheumatoid arthritis.

polycoria a congenital abnormality in which there are one or more holes in the iris in addition to the pupil.

polycystic containing many cysts. *P. kidney disease* a hereditary disease in which there is massive enlargement of the kidney with the formation of many cysts. Severe bleeding into cysts can occur. End-stage renal disease can affect many members of one family. *P. ovary syndrome* abbreviated PCOS, Stein–Leventhal syndrome.

polycythaemia an abnormal increase in the number of red cells in the blood. Erythrocythaemia. *P. vera* a rare disease in which there is a greatly increased production of red blood cells and also of leukocytes and platelets. The skin becomes flushed, with cyanosis, thrombosis and splenomegaly.

polydactylism the condition of having more than the normal number of fingers or toes.

polydipsia abnormal thirst. It may be a symptom of diabetes.

polyhydramnios *see* HYDRAMNIOS. Polymorphic light eruption a common skin condition caused by exposure to sunlight.

polymorphonuclear 1. having nuclei of many different shapes. 2. a polymorphonuclear leukocyte.

polymorphous occurring in several or many different forms.

polymyalgia rheumatica persistent aching pain in the muscles, often involving the shoulder or the pelvic girdle and spine. Associated with morning stiffness. More common in older people.

polymyositis a generalized inflammation of the muscles with weakness and joint stiffness, particularly around the hips and shoulders.

polyneuritis inflammation of many nerves at the same time.

polyneuropathy a number of disease conditions of the nervous system.

polyopia the perception of two or more images of the same object. Multiple vision.

polyp a pedunculated tumour of mucous membrane. A polypus.

polypharmacy 1. the administration of many drugs together. This increases the likelihood of side effects from drug interactions and of non-compliance by the patient. The taking of 'over-the-counter' medications and the use of complementary therapies may enhance the problem. 2. the administration of excessive medication.

polyposis the presence of many polyps in an organ. *Familial adenomatous p.* a hereditary condition in which large numbers of polyps develop in the colon, which may become malignant.

polyuria an abnormally large output of urine due either to an excessive intake of liquid or to disease, often diabetes.

pompholyx an intensely pruritic skin condition in which vesicles appear on the hands and feet, particularly on the palms and soles. Typically occurring in repeated, self-limiting attacks.

pons a bridge of tissue connecting two parts of an organ. *P. varolii* the part of the brain that connects the cerebrum, cerebellum and medulla oblongata.

Pontiac fever an influenza-like illness with little or no pulmonary involvement, caused by *Legionella pneumophila*. It is not life-threatening, as is the pulmonary form known as legionnaires' disease.

popliteal relating to the posterior part of the knee joint. *P. cyst* fluid filled cyst developing at the back of the knee. Also known as Baker's cyst.

poppers a street name for nitrite inhalants generally, or amyl nitrite in particular, taken in substance misuse to achieve 'an elevated mood' or 'high'.

population 1. the total number of persons inhabiting a given geographical area or location. 2. in statistics the aggregate of individuals or items from which a sample for a study is drawn. 3. any group that is distinguished by a particular trait or situation.

pore a minute circular opening on a surface. *Sweat p.* an opening of a sweat gland on the skin surface.

porphyria an inborn error in the metabolism of porphyrins, resulting in porphyrinuria. Several types of porphyria are known depending on the affected gene. The manifestations of porphyria include gastrointestinal, neurological and psychological symptoms, cutaneous photosensitivity, pigmentation of the face (and later of the bones) and anaemia, with enlargement of the spleen.

porphyrin one of a number of pigments used in the production of the haem portion of haemoglobin.

porphyrinuria the presence of an excess of porphyrin in the urine.

porta an opening in an organ through which pass the main vessels.

portacaval pertaining to the portal vein and the inferior vena cava. *P. anastomosis* the joining of the portal vein to the inferior vena cava so that much of the blood bypasses the liver. It is used in the treatment of portal hypertension.

portage system a method of behaviour modification taught to family members to enable them to assist a child with special needs in development and acquiring skills for everyday living.

portfolio a collection of competency evidence assembled by the practitioner/ student which demonstrates the owner's professional development. The portfolio may include such material as journals, marked assessments, evidence of reflective practice or other examples that document the acquisition of new skills, knowledge, understanding and achievements relevant to professional practice. It is a useful tool for REVALIDATION.

port wine stain *see* NAEVUS FLAMMEUS.

position attitude or posture. *Dorsal p.* lying flat on the back. *Genupectoral* or *knee–chest p.* resting on the knees and chest with arms crossed above the head. *Lithotomy p.* lying on the back with thighs raised and knees supported and held widely apart. *Prone p.* face down. *Sims' p.* or *semiprone p.* lying on the left side with the right knee well flexed and the left arm drawn back over the edge of the bed. *Trendelenburg p.* lying down on a tilted plane (usually an operating table at an angle of 30–45 degrees to the floor), with the head lowermost, the shoulders supported and the legs hanging over the raised end of the table.

positive having a value greater than zero; indicating existence or presence, as chromatin positive or Wassermann positive; characterized by affirmation or cooperation. The opposite of negative.

positive end-expiratory pressure abbreviated PEEP. In mechanical ventilation, a positive airway pressure maintained until the end of expiration. A PEEP higher than the critical closing pressure holds alveoli open until the end of expiration and can markedly improve the arterial P_{O_2} in patients with a lowered functional residual capacity (FRC), as in acute respiratory failure.

positron emission tomography abbreviated PET. A diagnostic imaging technique used in nuclear medicine based upon the detection of positively charged particles with a short half-life known as positrons that are emitted by radioactive labelled substances introduced into the body. PET scanning produces three-dimensional images of the metabolic and chemical activity of tissues in the body, e.g., the brain.

posseting regurgitation of a small amount of milk by an infant immediately after a feed.

post-exposure prophylaxis abbreviated PEP. The administration of antibiotics, antiviral agents, or active and/or passive vaccination following exposure to an infectious agent, e.g., antiretroviral drugs after exposure (usually occupationally, but may include sexual exposure) to human immunodeficiency virus (HIV).

post-herpetic neuralgia persistent nerve pain following shingles.

post-traumatic stress disorder (PTSD) following the experience of a major incident—personal, such as injury, rape or drowning, or other serious event, such as a natural disaster, warfare—the person may experience insomnia, acute anxiety, nightmares and 'flashbacks' resulting in depression, loss of concentration, apathy and guilt. This reaction may be immediate or delayed, and may last for a variable time. Support and counselling are needed and many people find antidepressants of the selective serotonin re uptake inhibitor type are beneficial.

postconcussional syndrome constant headaches with mental fatigue, difficulty in concentration and insomnia that may persist after head injury.

posterior behind a part. Dorsal. The opposite of anterior. *P. chamber* that part of the aqueous chamber that lies behind the iris, but in front of the lens.

postgastrectomy syndrome *see* DUMPING.

posthumous occurring after death. *P. birth* one occurring after the death of a biological parent.

postmature a state in which the pregnancy is prolonged after the expected date of delivery. Owing to the many variables it is difficult to estimate, but may exist when a pregnancy has lasted 41–42 weeks from the last menstrual period.

postmenopausal relating to or occurring in the period following the menopause. *See* MENOPAUSE. *P. bleeding* vaginal bleeding that happens at least 12 months after menstruation has ceased.

postmortem after death. *P. examination* autopsy.

postnatal after childbirth. *P. care* includes the care of the mother for at least 6 weeks after delivery. *P. check* an examination of the mother preferably 6 weeks after childbirth (a) regarding the mother's general health; (b) to find out the state of the uterus, pelvic floor and vagina. *P. depression* a common problem affecting more than 1 in 10 women within a year of giving birth. It can also affect fathers. Symptoms include persistent low mood, difficulties in concentration and decision-making occur, loss of interest, lack of energy, feeling tired, disturbances of sleep and appetite and difficulty bonding. May occur shortly after delivery or up to a year later. Treatment includes psychological therapy, self-help, diet, exercise and maybe antidepressant drugs. *See* BABY BLUES. *P. exercises* taught to the mother by the midwife or physiotherapist during the puerperium to strengthen the pelvic floor and abdominal muscles but also includes deep breathing and leg exercises as preventative measures against respiratory tract infection and deep vein thrombosis. *P. period* a period of not less than 10 days (and longer if the midwife considers it necessary), during which the continued attendance of a midwife on the mother and baby is mandatory. This is a rule of the Nursing and Midwifery Council.

postpartum occurring after labour. *P. psychosis* a rare but serious mental health condition occurring shortly after the birth of a baby where the mother has symptoms of hallucinations, delusions, manic mood and depression. Also known as puerperal psychosis.

postprandial occurring after a meal.

postural relating to a position or posture. *P. drainage* drainage of secretions from specific lobes or segments of the lung, aided by careful positioning of the patient *P. orthostatic tachycardia syndrome (POTS)* one of a group of disorders that have orthostatic intolerance (OI) as their primary symptom leading to an abnormal increase in heart rate that occurs after sitting up or standing. It typically caused dizziness and fainting.

potassium *symbol* K. A metallic alkaline element which is a constituent of all plants and animals. Its salts are widely used in medicine.

Pott's disease *P. Pott, British surgeon, 1714–1788.* Tuberculosis of the spine.

Pott's fracture a fracture-dislocation of the ankle, involving fracture of the lower end of the tibia, displacement of the talus and sometimes fracture of the medial malleolus.

pouch a pocket-like space or cavity. *Morison's p.* a fold of peritoneum below the liver also known as the hepatorenal pouch. *P. of Douglas* the lowest fold of the peritoneum between the uterus and rectum.

poultice a soft, moist mass of about the consistency of cooked cereal, spread between layers of muslin, linen, gauze or towels and applied hot to a given area in order to create moist local heat or to counter irritation.

Poupart's ligament *F. Poupart, French anatomist, 1616–1708.* The inguinal ligament. The tendinous lower border of the external oblique muscle of the abdominal wall, which passes from the anterior spine of the ilium to the os pubis.

poverty the lack of sufficient material, economic and cultural resources to sustain an existence compatible with wellbeing. *Absolute p.* the situation of not having sufficient resources to maintain nutrition for good health or to provide shelter and living accommodation. *P. of speech* marked deficit in spontaneous speech; replies to questions are perfunctory, monosyllabic or unforthcoming. *P. trap* a situation whereby an increase in a person's income results in a loss of state benefits leaving them no better off. *Relative p.* where a person's living standards are below those of the community in which the person lives.

power calculation a measure of statistical power used in research. The likelihood of a study to produce statistically significant results.

powerlessness without power or ability, leading to a feeling of being without influence upon their personal situation. People may feel powerless in their dealings with health services and health care professionals.

practice the exercise of a profession. *P. nurse* a member of the primary health care team who is a registered nurse employed by general practitioners to work within the practice setting providing health care services to the population served by the practice. *General p.* the medical specialty concerned with the planning and provision of comprehensive primary health care to a registered practice population on a continuing basis.

practitioner a person who practices a profession.

Prader-Willi syndrome a genetic disorder due to loss of function of specific genes. Symptoms include poor feeding in babies, weak muscles and delayed development. In childhood, there is constant hunger leading to obesity and type 2 diabetes, and mild to moderate learning disability.

pre-eclampsia a condition occurring in late pregnancy. The symptoms include proteinuria, hypertension and oedema.

preceptor 1. a teacher, an instructor. 2. a registered nurse or midwife with experience in the relevant clinical field, who provides newly registered practitioners with support and guidance in making the transition from student to registered practitioner and those returning to practice or joining a new part of the register or overseas registered practitioners making the transition to work in the UK. Preceptors should be provided with specific preparation for their role.

preceptorship a period of support, given by a preceptor, for the first year of registered practice for the newly registered nurse, midwife or health visitor practitioner or for those returning to nursing after a break of more than 5 years.

precipitate labour unusually rapid labour with extremely quick delivery. There is danger to the mother of severe perineal lacerations, and to the child of intracranial trauma as a result of the rapid passage through the birth canal.

precocious developed in advance of the norm, either mentally or physically or both.

precognition a direct perception of a future event which is beyond the reach of inference.

preconception before pregnancy. Ensuring the mother is in optimum health before becoming pregnant.

precursor something that precedes. In biological processes, a substance from which another, usually more active or mature, substance is formed. In clinical medicine, a sign or symptom that heralds another.

prediabetes also known as borderline diabetes is a state which precedes

diabetes mellitus, in which the disease is not yet clinically manifest. In pregnancy, the diabetes may become evident, or the patient may remain well but give birth to an unusually large child. Screening by urine testing can detect the condition.

predisposition susceptibility to a specific disease.

pregnancy being with child; the condition from conception to the expulsion of the fetus. The normal period is 280 days or 40 weeks counted from the first day of the last normal menstrual period. *Ectopic* or *extrauterine p.* pregnancy occurring outside the uterus, in the uterine tube (*tubal p.*) or very rarely in the abdominal cavity. *P. tests* tests used to demonstrate whether conception has occurred. These detect the human chorionic gonadotrophin (HCG) produced by the embryo from the day after the first missed period.

prejudice preconceived opinion, which can be used negatively or positively.

premature occurring before the anticipated time. *P. contraction* a form of cardiac irregularity in which the ventricle contracts before its anticipated time. *See* SYSTOLE. *P. ejaculation* emission of semen before or at the beginning of sexual intercourse. *P. infant* preterm infant. A child born before the 37th completed week of gestation.

premedication drugs given preoperatively in order to reduce fear and anxiety and to facilitate the induction and maintenance of, and recovery from, anaesthesia.

premenstrual preceding menstruation. *P. endometrium* the hypertrophied and vascular mucous lining of the uterus immediately before the menstrual flow starts. *P. syndrome* (PMS) feelings of nervousness, depression, irritability, bloating, breast pain and loss of interest in sex experienced by some women in the days before their menstrual periods. Emotional and physical symptoms usually disappear with the onset of menstruation.

premolar teeth a bicuspid tooth in front of the molars on each side of the upper and lower jaws. *See* DENTITION.

prenatal preceding birth; antenatal. *P. care* care of the pregnant woman before delivery of the infant.

prepuce foreskin; the loose fold of skin covering the glans penis.

presbyopia diminution of accommodation of the lens of the eye, due to a loss of elasticity, occurring normally with ageing and usually resulting in hyperopia, or farsightedness.

prescribed diseases a group of occupational diseases on an annually reviewed official listing, e.g., pneumoconiosis or occupational deafness, that give the sufferers legal entitlement to financial benefits.

prescribing analyses and cost abbreviated PACT. Data on the prescribing of drugs in primary care.

prescription a formula written by a medically qualified doctor, dentist or independent prescriber—a specially qualified nurse, podiatrist/chiropodist, physiotherapist or therapeutic radiographer—directing the pharmacist to supply the medication. Also contains instructions to the patient indicating how the medication is to be taken (*see* prescribing by nurses, midwives and specialist community public health nurses in Appendix 4).

prescription-only medicines drugs and medicines that are not available 'over the counter' and can only be obtained by prescription from the pharmacist.

presenile prematurely aged in mind and body. *See* DEMENTIA.

presentation in obstetrics, that portion of the fetus that appears in the centre of the neck of the uterus (*see* Figure on p. 314).

pressure stress or strain. The force exerted by one object upon another. *P. areas* areas of the body where the tissues may be compressed between the bed or chair and the underlying bone, especially the sacrum, greater trochanters and heels; the tissues become ischaemic (*see* Figure on p. 315). *P. garment* often used in the treatment of burns and scalds to reduce scarring. Made of Lycra (a strong, synthetic, slightly elastic fibre), the garment is worn by the patient to exert firm pressure on the affected area, for example to prevent keloid scarring following burns or scalds. *P. group* an organization or charitable association that seeks to pressurize local and central government to advance the interests of that group. *P. point* the point at which an artery can be compressed against a bone in order to stop bleeding (*see* Figure on p. 316). *P. ulcer* a decubitus ulcer; previously called a bedsore. Ulceration of the skin due to pressure, which causes interference with the blood supply to the area. Causes localized damage to the skin and underlying tissue due to pressure, shear, friction or a combination of these. Pressure ulcers are graded usually using the European Pressure Ulcer Advisory Panel (EPUAP) grading system (*see* Table on pp. 316–318). *P. ulcer assessment scales* regular assessment of the patient's nutrition, general condition especially of the skin and pressure areas, is focal in the prevention of pressure ulcers. Pressure ulcer risk assessment scales are used to monitor and record data for the nursing care plan e.g., *Waterlow scale* which is a comprehensive scale that recognizes there are many factors influencing the development of pressure ulcers. Waterlow's scale includes such factors as build/weight/height, mobility, sex, age, continence, appetite, the state of skin and other influencing factors such as medication, surgery and neurological deficits. Other scales include the *Braden* scale, *Norton* scale.

presystole the period in the cardiac cycle just before systole.

preterm before term, i.e., before the 37th completed week of pregnancy. *P. infant* baby born before 37

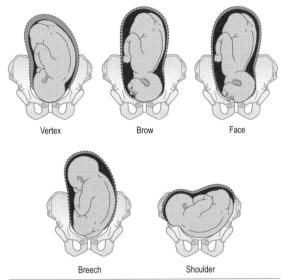

Vertex   Brow   Face

Breech   Shoulder

FETAL PRESENTATIONS

weeks' gestation. The baby will be of low birth weight, but may also be small for gestational age. Gestational age is assessed using the Dubowitz score. Preterm infants are prone to respiratory distress syndrome, feeding problems due to immature sucking, swallowing and coughing reflexes, hypothermia, jaundice and infection. *P. labour* labour that occurs before 37 weeks' gestation. It may occur spontaneously as a result of changing hormone levels, an overstretched uterus or weak cervix or due to infection; the obstetrician may attempt to arrest labour by the administration of tocolytic drugs until conditions are more favourable for the baby to be born. Labour may be induced before term because of poor maternal

or fetal health, and thus the extrauterine environment will be less hazardous for the infant.

prevalence the number of persons who have a specific disease or condition that are present in a defined population at one specific point in time. *See* INCIDENCE.

preventative serving to avert the occurrence of; prophylactic.

priapism persistent erection of the penis, usually without sexual desire. It may be caused by local or spinal cord injury.

prickly heat miliaria; heat rash. A skin eruption characterized by minute red spots with central vesicles.

primary first in order of time or importance. Primary biliary cirrhosis also known as primary biliary cholangitis

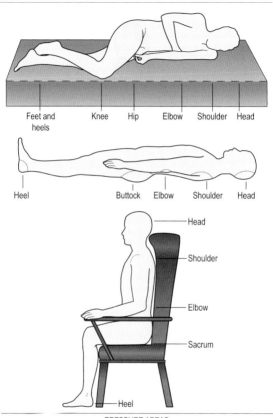

Feet and heels | Knee | Hip | Elbow | Shoulder | Head

Heel | Buttock | Elbow | Shoulder | Head

Head — Shoulder — Elbow — Sacrum — Heel

PRESSURE AREAS

(PBC) is a long-term liver disease in which the bile ducts become damaged, bile builds up and scarring of the liver occurs.

primary care the level of care in the HEALTH CARE SYSTEM that consists of initial care outside institutions. *P. C. Trusts* abbreviated PCTs abolished in 2013 with much of their work taken over by CLINICAL COMMISSIONING GROUPS (CCGS).

primary health care the care given to individuals in the community at the

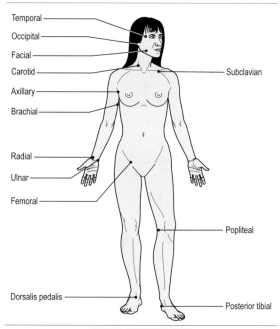

ARTERIAL PRESSURE POINTS

European Pressure Ulcer Grading Scale	
Category/Stage	
Europe **I: Non-blanchable erythema**	Intact skin with non-blanchable redness of a localized area usually over a bony prominence. Darkly pigmented skin may not have visible blanching; its colour may differ from the surrounding area. The area may be painful, firm, soft, warmer or cooler as compared to adjacent tissue. Category I may be difficult to detect in individuals with dark skin tones. May indicate 'at risk' persons.

European Pressure Ulcer Grading Scale—cont'd	
Category/Stage	
II: Partial thickness	Partial thickness loss of dermis presenting as a shallow open ulcer with a red pink wound bed, without slough. May also present as an intact or open/ruptured serum-filled or serosanguinous filled blister. Presents as a shiny or dry shallow ulcer without slough or bruising.[a] This category should not be used to describe skin tears, tape burns, incontinence associated dermatitis, maceration or excoriation.
III: Full thickness skin loss	Full thickness tissue loss. Subcutaneous fat may be visible but bone, tendon or muscle are *not* exposed. Slough may be present but does not obscure the depth of tissue loss. *May* include undermining and tunnelling. The depth of a Category/Stage III pressure ulcer varies by anatomical location. The bridge of the nose, ear, occiput and malleolus do not have (adipose) subcutaneous tissue and Category/Stage III ulcers can be shallow. In contrast, areas of significant adiposity can develop extremely deep Category/Stage III pressure ulcers. Bone/tendon is not visible or directly palpable.
IV: Full thickness tissue loss	Full thickness tissue loss with exposed bone, tendon or muscle. Slough or eschar may be present. Often includes undermining and tunnelling. The depth of a Category/Stage IV pressure ulcer varies by anatomical location. The bridge of the nose, ear, occiput and malleolus do not have (adipose) subcutaneous tissue and these ulcers can be shallow. Category/Stage IV ulcers can extend into muscle and/or supporting structures (e.g., fascia, tendon or joint capsule) making osteomyelitis or osteitis likely to occur. Exposed bone/muscle is visible or directly palpable.

Continued

European Pressure Ulcer Grading Scale—cont'd

Category/Stage

Additional categories/stages for the USA

Unstageable/ unclassified: Full thickness skin or tissue loss, depth unknown	Full thickness tissue loss in which actual depth of the ulcer is completely obscured by slough (yellow, tan, grey, green or brown) and/or eschar (tan, brown or black) in the wound bed. Until enough slough and/or eschar are removed to expose the base of the wound, the true depth cannot be determined; but it will be either a Category/Stage III or IV. Stable (dry, adherent, intact without erythema or fluctuance) eschar on the heels serves as 'the body's natural (biological) cover' and should not be removed.
Suspected deep tissue injury, depth unknown	Purple or maroon localized area of discoloured intact skin or blood-filled blister due to damage of underlying soft tissue from pressure and/or *shear*. The area may be preceded by tissue that is painful, firm, mushy, boggy, warmer or cooler as compared to adjacent tissue. Deep tissue injury may be difficult to detect in individuals with dark skin tones. Evolution may include a thin blister over a dark wound bed. The wound may further evolve and become covered by thin eschar. Evolution may be rapid exposing additional layers of tissue even with optimal treatment.

ᵃBruising indicates deep tissue injury.

first point of contact with the primary health care team. First contact may be the general practitioner, a health visitor, paramedic or a district nurse.

primary source in a research study, the original source of data, e.g., manuscripts, documents or first-hand accounts. Primary sources are preferred over secondary sources because of the reduced potential for bias and distortion beyond the control of the researcher.

primigravida a woman who is pregnant for the first time.

primipara a woman who has given birth to her first child.

prion tiny protein-based infectious agent similar to a virus. Prions transmit diseases, including Creutzfeldt–Jakob disease in humans and bovine spongiform encephalopathy (BSE) in cattle. Prions do not contain nucleic acids and are difficult to destroy.

Private Finance Initiative abbreviated PFI. An agreement between the private and public sector whereby a health care facility, e.g., a hospital, is built using private funding. The facility is then leased to the NHS Trust. The lease agreement may also contain provision for the delivery of on-site services.

probability a statistical term meaning the likelihood of an association between variables being due to chance.

problematic internet use addiction or excessive use of the internet.

problem-oriented record a multi-professional approach to patient care record-keeping that focuses on the patient's specific health problems and the structuring of a health care plan designed to cope with the identified problems.

process in anatomy, a prominence or outgrowth of any part.

procidentia complete prolapse of an organ, particularly the uterus so that the cervix extrudes through the vagina.

proctalgia pain in the rectum and anus; proctodynia.

proctitis inflammation of the rectum.

proctosigmoiditis inflammation of the rectum and sigmoid colon.

prodrome a symptom that appears before the true diagnostic signs of a disease.

prodrug a compound that, on administration, must undergo chemical conversion by metabolic processes before becoming an active pharmacological agent, thus avoiding gastrointestinal side effects.

profession 1. an avowed, public declaration or statement of intention or purpose. 2. a calling or vocation requiring specialized knowledge, methods and skills, as well as preparation, in an institution of higher learning, in the scholarly, scientific and historical principles underlying such methods and skills. Members of a profession are committed to continuing study, to enlarging their body of knowledge, to placing service above personal gain and to providing practical services vital to human and social welfare. A profession functions autonomously and is committed to higher standards of achievement and conduct.

professional 1. pertaining to one's profession or occupation. 2. one who is a specialist in a particular field or occupation. *Allied health p.* a person with special training, and licensed when necessary, who works closely with other health professionals with responsibilities bearing on patient care. *P. disciplinary process* complaints against nurses from members of the public or an employer are reported to the statutory regulatory body. The professional conduct of the nurse is then investigated and judged by peers. The ultimate sanction is that the nurse is removed from the professional register. *P. organization* an organization formed to deal with issues of mutual concern for its members who share common goals and professional status (*see* PRESSURE GROUP). *P. self-regulation* the means whereby a profession monitors its own standards for quality and continuing professional and educational development. Professional regulatory bodies include the General Medical Council for medically qualified practitioners, the Nursing and Midwifery Council for nurses and midwives and the Health and Care Professions Council for dietitians, physiotherapists, etc. *See* Appendix 5.

profile 1. a simple outline, as of the side view of the head or face; by extension, a graph representing quantitatively a set of characteristics determined by tests. 2. a record of achievements developed during a course of study, or subsequently. *See* PORTFOLIO.

progeny issue. Descendants.

progeria premature ageing, the signs of which appear in childhood.

progesterone a hormone of the corpus luteum which plays an important part in the regulation of the menstrual cycle and in pregnancy.

progestogen one of a group of steroid hormones having an action similar to that of progesterone.

prognathism enlargement and protrusion of one or both jaws.

prognosis a forecast of the probable course and outcome of an attack of disease and the prospects of recovery, as indicated by the nature of the disease and the symptoms of the case.

progressive supranuclear palsy a rare and progressive condition caused by damage to brain cells over time due to a build up of the protein tau. Symptoms include problems with balance, movement, speech and swallowing.

projectile vomiting *see* VOMITING.

projection in psychology, an unconscious process by which painful thoughts or impulses are made acceptable by transferring them on to another person or object in the environment.

prolactin a milk-producing hormone of the anterior lobe of the pituitary body which stimulates the mammary gland.

prolapse the downward displacement of an organ or part of one. *P. of the cord* expulsion of the umbilical cord before the fetus presents. *P. of an intervertebral disc* displacement of part of an intervertebral disc; 'slipped disc'; herniated disc. *P. of the iris* protrusion of a part of the iris through a wound in the cornea. *P. of the rectum* protrusion of the mucous membrane through the anal canal to the exterior. *P. of the uterus* descent of the cervix or of the whole uterus into the vagina owing to a weakening of its supporting ligaments.

proliferation rapid multiplication of cells, as may occur in a malignant growth and during wound healing.

prominence in anatomy, a projection, usually on a bone.

prone lying face downwards. *See* SUPINE.

prophylactic 1. relating to prophylaxis. 2. a drug used to prevent a disease developing. *See* PREVENTATIVE.

prophylaxis measures taken to prevent a disease.

proprietary name the name assigned to a drug or device by the manufacturer that first made it.

proprioceptor one of the sensory end-organs that provide information about movements and position of the body. They occur chiefly in the muscles, tendons, joint capsules and labyrinth.

proptosis forward displacement of the eyeball; exophthalmos.

prosopagnosia an inability to recognize faces.

prostaglandin one of several hormone substances produced in many body tissues, including the brain, lungs, uterus and semen. They are active in many ways, having cardiac, gastric and respiratory effects and causing uterine contractions. They are sometimes used for the induction of abortion. Chemically they are fatty acids.

prostate the gland surrounding the male urethra at its junction with the bladder; during ejaculation it produces a fluid which forms part of the semen. It often becomes enlarged after middle age and may require partial removal if it causes obstruction to the outflow of urine. *P. cancer* of unknown cause and one of the most common cancers in men, usually occurring in older men. Treatments include surgery, radiotherapy, chemotherapy and hormone therapy. *P. screening* routine examination and blood testing for prostate-specific antigen (PSA) in older men, as a means to detect cancer of the prostate at an early stage.

prostatectomy surgical removal of the whole or a part of the prostate gland. *Retropubic p.* removal of the gland by incising the capsule of the prostate after making a suprapubic abdominal incision. *Transurethral p.* resection of the gland through the urethra using a resectoscope. *Transvesical p.* removal of the gland by incising the bladder after making a low abdominal incision.

prostatitis inflammation of the prostate gland.

prosthesis 1. the replacement of an absent part by an artificial substitute. 2. an artificial substitute for a missing part.

prostration a condition of extreme exhaustion.

protease a proteolytic enzyme in the digestive juices that causes the breakdown of protein.

protective isolation a type of ISOLATION designed to prevent contact between potentially pathogenic microorganisms and uninfected persons who have seriously impaired resistance. Also called reverse isolation. *See* Appendix 11.

protein one of a group of complex organic nitrogenous compounds formed from amino acids and occurring in every living cell of animal and vegetable tissue. *Bence Jones p.* an abnormal protein found in the urine of patients suffering from multiple myeloma. *First-class p.* one that provides the essential amino acids. Sources are meat, poultry, fish, cheese, eggs and milk. *P.-bound iodine* the iodine in the plasma that is combined with protein. Measurement of this is made when assessing thyroid function. *P.-losing enteropathy* a condition in which protein is lost from the lumen of the intestine. This causes hypoproteinaemia and oedema. *Second-class p.* one that comes from a vegetable source (e.g., peas, beans and whole cereal) that cannot supply all the body's needs.

proteinuria an excess of serum proteins in the urine.

proteolysis the processes by which proteins are reduced to an absorbable form by digestive enzymes in the stomach and intestines.

proteolytic 1. pertaining to, characterized by, or promoting proteolysis. 2. a proteolytic enzyme.

Proteus a genus of gram-negative bacteria common in the intestines of humans and animals and in decaying matter. They are frequently to be found in secondary infections of wounds and in the urinary tract.

prothrombin a constituent of blood plasma, the precursor of thrombin, which is formed in the presence of calcium salts and thrombokinase when blood is shed. *P. time* (PT) a test to measure the activity of clotting factors. Deficiency of any of these factors leads to a prolongation of clotting time. This

test is widely used for the establishment and maintenance of anticoagulant therapy.

protocol a term used by researchers to indicate the method or overall plan for procedures to be carried out in a particular study. Commonly used to indicate a specific programme to be followed or with exclusion criteria for the study.

protoplasm the essential chemical compound of which living cells are made.

prototype the original form from which all other forms are derived.

Protozoa a phylum comprising the unicellular eukaryotic organisms; most are free-living but some lead commensalistic, mutualistic or parasitic existences. Pathogenic protozoa include *Entamoeba histolytica* (cause of amoebic dysentery) and *Plasmodium vivax* (cause of malaria). *See* METAZOA.

protuberance in anatomy, a rounded projecting part.

proud flesh excessive granulation tissue in a wound or ulcer.

provider in the health services, a person, group of people or organization supplying a service.

provitamin a precursor of a vitamin. *P. 'A'* carotene. *P. 'D'* ergosterol.

proxemics the study of how the use of personal space and other spatial aspects affects human behaviour and interactions.

proximal in anatomy, nearest that point which is considered the centre of a system; the opposite to distal.

prurigo a chronic skin disease with an irritating papular eruption.

pruritus great irritation of the skin.

pseudoangina false angina. Precordial pain occurring in anxious individuals without evidence of organic heart disease.

pseudoarthrosis a false joint formed when the two parts of a fractured bone have failed to unite together.

pseudocoxalgia osteochondritis of the head of the femur. Perthes' disease.

pseudocyesis false pregnancy; development of all the signs of pregnancy without the presence of an embryo.

pseudogynaecomastia the deposition of adipose tissue in the male breast which may give the appearance of enlarged mammary glands.

Pseudomonas a genus of gram-negative motile bacilli commonly found in decaying organic matter. *P. aeruginosa* found in pus from wounds ('blue pus') and also in urinary tract infections. Also called *P. pyocyanea*.

pseudomyopia spasm of the ciliary muscle causing the same focusing defect as in myopia.

psittacosis a disease of parrots and budgerigars due to *Chlamydia psittaci*, communicable to humans. The symptoms resemble paratyphoid fever with bronchopneumonia.

psoas a long muscle originating from the lumbar spine and inserting into the lesser trochanter of the femur. It flexes the hip joint. *P. abscess* one that arises in the lumbar region and is due to spinal caries as a result of tuberculous infection.

psoriasis a chronic, recurrent skin disease characterized by reddish marginated patches with profuse silvery scaling on extensor surfaces, such as the knees and elbow, but which may be more widespread and may be associated with arthritis of the joints. It is non-infectious and the cause is unknown. Psoriasis may present in different forms. The most common is discoid or plaque psoriasis in adults. Guttate psoriasis occurs most commonly in children, consisting of small patches that may develop over a wide area of the body. Pustular psoriasis is characterized by small pustules. Treatment includes topical applications, for example emollients containing corticosteroids and vitamin D_3. Other treatments include ultraviolet light, PUVA treatment and systemic drugs such as methotrexate. Psoriasis is a long-term condition.

psyche the mind, both conscious and unconscious.

psychedelic mind-altering; a term applied to hallucinatory or psychotomimetic drugs capable of profound effects upon the nature of the perception and conscious experience. *See also* HALLUCINOGEN.

psychiatrist a medically qualified doctor who specializes in psychiatry.

psychiatry the branch of medicine that deals with the treatment and prevention of mental illness.

psychoanalysis 1. a method of investigating mental processes, developed by Sigmund Freud, which uses the techniques of free association, interpretation and dream analysis. 2. a system of theoretical psychology, formulated by Freud, based on the recognition of unconscious mental processes, such as resistance, repression and transference, and of the importance of infantile experience as a determinant of adult behaviour. 3. a method of psychotherapy based on the psychoanalytical method and psychoanalytical psychology.

psychoanalyst one who specializes in psychoanalysis.

psychodrama group PSYCHOTHERAPY in which patients dramatize their individual conflicting situations of daily life.

psychodynamics the understanding and interpretation of psychiatric symptoms or abnormal behaviour in terms of unconscious mental mechanisms.

psychogenic originating in the mind. *P. illness* a disorder that has a psychological as opposed to an organic origin.

psychologist one who studies normal and abnormal mental processes, development and behaviour.

psychology the study of the mind and mental processes.

psychometrics the measurement of mental characteristics by means of a series of tests.

psychomotor related to the motor effects of mental activity. The term is applied to those mental disorders that affect muscular activity.

psychoneurosis a mental disorder characterized by an abnormal mental response to a normal stimulus. The psychoneuroses include anxiety states, depression, hysteria and obsessive-compulsive neurosis.

psychopathology the study of the causes and processes of mental disorders.

psychopharmacology the study of drugs that have an action on the mind, and how such action is produced.

psychosexual relating to the mental aspects of sex. *P. development* the stages through which an individual passes from birth to full maturity, especially in regard to sexual urges, in the total development of the person. *P. counselling* support for people who fail to achieve emotional and sexual satisfaction within a relationship.

psychosis any major mental disorder of organic or emotional origin, marked by derangement of the personality and loss of contact with reality, often with delusions, hallucinations or illusions. Psychoses are classified into different types including schizophrenia, bipolar disorder and organic brain syndrome.

psychosomatic relating to the mind and the body. *P. disorders* those illnesses in some individuals in which emotional factors (either causative or aggravating) have a profound influence, including anorexia nervosa and asthma respectively.

psychotherapy any of a number of related techniques for treating mental illness by psychological methods. These techniques are similar in that they all rely mainly on establishing communication between the therapist and the patient as a means of understanding and modifying the patient's behaviour. On occasion, drugs may be used, but only in order to make this communication easier.

psychotropic pertaining to drugs that have an effect on the psyche. These include antidepressants, stimulants, sedatives and tranquillizers.

Pthirus pubis the crab louse.

ptosis 1. drooping of the upper eyelid due to paralysis of the third cranial nerve. It may be congenital or acquired. 2. prolapse of an organ.

ptyalin an enzyme (amylase) in saliva which metabolizes starches.

puberty the period during which secondary sexual characteristics develop and the reproductive organs become functional. Generally between the 12th and 17th years.

pubes pubic hair or the area on which it grows.

pubic pertaining to the pubis.

pubis the anterior part of a hip bone. The left and right pubic bones meet at the front of the pelvis at the pubic symphysis.

public domain intellectual property, e.g., published documents, programs or files, usually from government sources and other organizations, that have been released for unconditional access and use by the public.

public health concerned with promoting and protecting health and wellbeing, preventing ill health and prolonging life through organized efforts in the population. To achieve these goals various methods are used including health surveillance, monitoring and analysis of data, assessment of evidence and interventions, the identification of significant trends, the development of policy and strategy, the investigation of outbreaks of disease and of any risks to health, health protection, health improvement and public health intelligence. Public health departments in England are based in Local Authorities. *P. h. England* the body in England with responsibility to protect and improve health and wellbeing and reduce health inequalities. *P. h. laboratory service* a service which aims to protect the public from infection and prevent the spread of infectious disease through a network of laboratories in the UK that provide the necessary resources for investigation, diagnosis and testing in suspected cases or in outbreaks of infectious disease. In Scotland, many of these functions are carried out by Health Protection Scotland; in Wales by Public Health Wales; and in Northern Ireland by the Public Health Agency. *P. h. nurse* one who works within a community service in a variety of settings promoting good health and the prevention of ill health, e.g., a health visitor or school nurse.

pudendal block a form of local analgesia induced by injecting a solution of 0.5% or 1% lignocaine around the pudendal nerve. Used mainly for episiotomy and forceps delivery. *P. neuralgia* chronic pelvic pain due to damage of the pudendal nerve.

pudendum the external genitalia, especially of a woman.

puerperal pertaining to childbirth. *P. fever* or *sepsis* infection of the genital tract following childbirth.

puerperium a period of about 6 weeks following childbirth when the reproductive organs are returning to their normal state.

Pulex a genus of fleas. *P. irritans* those parasitic on humans. The type that infests rats may transmit plague to humans.

pulmonary pertaining to or affecting the lungs. *P. embolism* obstruction of the pulmonary artery or one of its branches by an embolus. *P. hypertension* an increase of blood pressure in the lungs, usually as a result of disease of the lung. *P. oedema* an excess of fluid in the lungs. *P. stenosis* a narrowing of the passage between the right ventricle of the heart and the pulmonary artery. The condition is frequently congenital. *P. tuberculosis see* TUBERCULOSIS. *P. valve* the valve at the point where the pulmonary artery leaves the heart.

pulp any soft, juicy animal or vegetable tissue. *P. cavity* the centre of a tooth containing blood, tissue and nerves.

Splenic p. the reddish-brown tissue of the spleen.

pulsation a beating or throbbing.

pulse the local rhythmic expansion of an artery, which can be felt with the finger, corresponding to each contraction of the left ventricle of the heart. It may be felt in any artery sufficiently near the surface of the body, which passes over a bone, and the normal adult resting rate is 60–100 beats/min. In childhood it is more rapid, varying from 130 in infants to 80 in older children. *Alternating p.* alternate strong and weak beats; pulsus alternans. *Paradoxical p.* pulsus paradoxus; the pulse rate slows on inspiration and quickens on expiration. It may occur in constrictive pericarditis. *P. deficit* a sign of atrial fibrillation; the pulse rate is slower than the apex beat. *P. oximetry* a non-invasive method for measuring haemoglobin oxygen saturation in the body using a sensor from an oximeter that is attached, usually to a finger but may be elsewhere, e.g., nose, finger or ear lobe. *Running p.* there is little distinction between the beats. It occurs in haemorrhage. *Thready p.* thin and almost imperceptible pressure. *Venous p.* that felt in a vein; it is usually taken in the right jugular vein.

pulseless disease progressive obliteration of the vessels arising from the aortic arch, leading to loss of the pulse in both arms and carotids and to symptoms associated with ischaemia of the brain, eyes, face and arms. Also known as Takayasu's disease.

punctate dotted. *P. erythema* a rash of very fine spots.

punctum a point or small spot. *P. lacrimalis* one of the two openings of the lacrimal ducts at the inner canthus of the eye.

puncture 1. the act of piercing with a sharp object. 2. the wound so produced. *Cisternal p.* the withdrawal of fluid from the cisterna magna. *Lumbar p.* the removal of cerebrospinal fluid by puncture between the third and fourth lumbar vertebrae. *Sternal p.* the withdrawal of bone marrow from the manubrium of the sternum. *Ventricular p.* the withdrawal of cerebrospinal fluid from a cerebral ventricle.

pupil the circular aperture in the centre of the iris, through which light passes into the eye. *Argyll Robertson p.* absence of response to light but not to accommodation; characteristic of neuro syphilis of the central nervous system and diabetic retinopathy. *Artificial p.* one made by cutting a piece out of the iris when the centre part of the cornea or the lens is opaque. *Fixed p.* one that fails to respond to light or convergence. *Multiple p.* two or more openings of the iris. *Tonic p.* one that reacts slowly to light or to convergence or both.

pupillary referring to the pupil.

purgative a laxative; an aperient drug. Purgatives may be (a) irritants, like senna, rhubarb and castor oil; (b) lubricants, like liquid paraffin; (c) mechanical agents that increase bulk, like bran and agar preparations.

purine a heterocyclic compound that is the nucleus of the purine bases such as adenine and guanine, which occur in DNA and RNA. *See* PYRIMIDINE.

purpura a condition characterized by extravasation of blood in the skin and mucous membranes, causing purple spots and patches. There are two general types of purpura: primary or idiopathic (usually autoimmune) thrombocytopenic purpura, in which the cause is unknown; and secondary or symptomatic thrombocytopenic purpura, which may be associated with exposure to drugs or other chemical agents, systemic diseases such as systemic lupus erythematosus, diseases affecting the bone marrow, such as leukaemia, and infections such as septicaemia, viral infections and allergic reaction.

purulent containing or resembling pus.

pus a thick, yellow semiliquid substance consisting of dead leukocytes and bacteria, debris of cells, and tissue fluids. It results from inflammation caused by invading bacteria, mainly *Staphylococcus aureus*, which have destroyed the phagocytes and set up local suppuration. *Blue p.* that produced by infection with *Pseudomonas pyocyanea*.

pustule a small pimple or elevation of the skin containing pus. *Malignant p. see* ANTHRAX.

putative supposed, reputed. *P. father* the man believed to be the father of a child born of parents not lawfully married to each other.

putrefaction decomposition of animal or vegetable matter under the influence of microorganisms, usually accompanied by an offensive odour due to gas formation.

***P* value** the symbol used to denote the probability of test results occurring by chance.

pyaemia a condition resulting from the circulation of pyogenic microorganisms from some focus of infection. Multiple abscesses occur, the development of which causes rigor and high fever. *Portal p.* pylephlebitis.

pyarthrosis suppuration in a joint.

pyelography *see* UROGRAPHY.

pyelolithotomy the surgical removal of a stone from the renal pelvis.

pyelonephritis inflammation of the renal pelvis and renal substance, characterized by fever, acute loin pain and increased frequency of micturition, with the presence of pus and albumin in the urine.

pyeloplasty plastic repair of the renal pelvis.

pylephlebitis inflammation of the portal vein which gives rise to severe symptoms of septicaemia or pyaemia.

pyloric relating to the pylorus. *P. stenosis* stricture of the pyloric orifice. It may be (a) hypertrophic, when there is thickening of normal tissue; this is congenital and occurs in infants from 4–7 weeks old, usually males and first babies; (b) cicatricial, when there is ulceration or a malignant growth near the pylorus.

pyloromyotomy Ramstedt's operation; an incision of the pylorus performed to relieve congenital pyloric stenosis.

pyloroplasty plastic operation on the pylorus to enlarge the outlet. A longitudinal incision is made and it is resutured transversely . The procedure is undertaken if conservative treatment with medication is ineffective.

pylorospasm forceful muscle contraction of the pylorus which delays emptying of the stomach and causes vomiting.

pylorus the opening into the duodenum at the lower end of the stomach. It is surrounded by a circular muscle, the *pyloric sphincter*, which contracts to close the opening.

pyoderma any purulent skin disease, e.g., impetigo.

pyogenic producing pus.

pyorrhoea a discharge of pus. *P. alveolaris* pus in the sockets of the teeth; suppurative periodontitis.

pyramidal of pyramid shape. *P. cells* cortical cells shaped like a pyramid from which originate nerve impulses to voluntary muscle. *P. tract* the nerve fibres that transmit impulses from pyramidal cells through the cerebral cortex to the spinal cord.

pyrexia fever; a rise of body temperature to any point between 37 and 40°C; above this is hyperpyrexia.

pyridoxine vitamin B_6. This vitamin is concerned with protein metabolism and blood formation. It is found in many types of food and deficiency is rare.

pyrimidine a nitrogen-containing organic compound. Thymine and cytosine are essential constituents of DNA, and uracil and cytosine of RNA. *See* PURINE.

pyrogen a substance that can produce fever.

pyromania an irresistible desire to set things on fire.

pyrosis heartburn; a symptom of indigestion marked by a burning sensation in the stomach and oesophagus with eructation of acid fluid.

pyuria the presence of pus in the urine; more than three leukocytes per high-power field on microscopic examination.

QALY quality adjusted life year.

Q fever an acute infectious disease of cattle which is transmitted to humans, usually by infected milk. It is caused by a rickettsia, *Coxiella burnetii*, and has symptoms resembling pneumonia.

qi energy in Chinese medicine, the energy believed to be present in all living things. Qi energy is considered to flow through 12 meridian channels in the body mainly connected to the internal organs, and considered essential to good health and wellbeing. This concept is used in a variety of complementary therapies, e.g., reflexology and acupuncture. Complementary therapy practitioners consider that any disturbance or blockage to the flow of qi energy results in illness or bodily and mental disturbance but that with manipulation, e.g., through acupuncture, the qi flow can be increased. Also called chi, prana and aura.

QRS complex a group of waves depicted on an electrocardiogram; also called the QRS wave. It actually consists of three distinct waves created by the passage of the cardiac electrical impulse through the ventricles and occurs at the beginning of each contraction of the ventricles (*see* Figure on p. 328). In a normal ELECTROCARDIOGRAM the R wave is the most prominent of the three; the Q and S waves may be extremely weak and are sometimes absent.

quadriceps four-headed. *Q. femoris muscle* the principal extensor muscle of the thigh.

quadriplegia paralysis in which all four limbs are affected; tetraplegia.

quadruplets four children born at the same labour.

qualitative research a research method widely used in sociology, psychology and anthropology. It is a method that uses a systematic subjective approach to describe life experiences and to give them meaning. In nursing and health care it is used to promote understanding of human experiences of pain, caring and comfort. *See also* QUANTITATIVE RESEARCH.

quality 1. a distinguishing characteristic, property or attribute. 2. a degree or standard of excellence. *Q. account* published by all NHS providers in June each year, setting out performance against measures of quality and safety for the previous year and setting targets for improvement in the coming year. *Q. adjusted life year* abbreviated QALY. A measure which assesses variations in the quality of life for the patient resulting from an intervention, in relation to cost and length of life. Used for measuring the clinical and cost effectiveness of interventions. *Q. assurance* in the health care field, a pledge to the public by those within the various health disciplines that they will work towards the goal of an optimal achievable degree of excellence that is measured

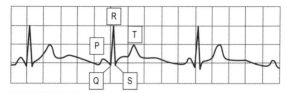

A NORMAL ELECTROCARDIOGRAM SHOWING THE QRS COMPLEX

and evaluated in the services rendered to every patient. *See* COST EFFECTIVENESS and PERFORMANCE INDICATORS. *Q. Assurance Agency* organization which approves higher education institutions offering courses and awards. Monitors delivery of subjects in universities. Has established codes of practice, standards and guidance for programme development. *Q. circle* a group of health care workers from differing levels within an organization who meet regularly to discuss ways in which they can improve their service and raise standards. *Q. indicator* a defined, measurable variable used to monitor the quality or appropriateness of an important aspect of care. Indicators may be activities, events, occurrences or outcomes. *Q. innovation productivity prevention* (abbreviated QIPP) sets out a significant initiative introduced to the NHS by the department of health to support greater efficiencies and encourage services to be transformed. *Q. systems audit* International and British Standards in Quality Systems. An audit programme used to monitor quality in organizations providing health care. The audit programme is an essential management tool, used for verifying objective evidence of processes and to assess how successfully processes have been implemented.

quango a form of government agency used to provide services or to carry out other duties determined by government. Originally an acronym for 'quasi-autonomous non-governmental organization', which initially comprised voluntary and non-profit organizations but became increasingly dependent upon government grants.

quantitative research a formal objective systematic approach to research in which numerical data are utilized to obtain information. It is used to describe variables, examine relationships among variables and to determine cause and effect interactions between variables. Some researchers believe this form of research provides a sounder knowledge base to nursing and midwifery practice than QUALITATIVE RESEARCH.

quarantine the period of isolation of an infectious or suspected case, to prevent the spread of disease. For contacts, this is the longest incubation period known for the specific disease.

quartan 1. recurring in 4-day cycles (every third day). 2. a variety of intermittent fever of which the paroxysms recur on every third day (*see* MALARIA).

quickening the first perceptible fetal movement, felt by the mother usually between the fourth and fifth months of pregnancy.

quiescent inactive or at rest. Descriptive of a time when the symptoms of a disease are not evident.

quinsy a peritonsillar abscess; acute inflammation of the tonsil and surrounding cellular tissue with suppuration.

quintuplets five children born at the same labour.

quotidian recurring every day. *Q. fever* a variety of malaria in which the fever recurs daily.

quotient a number obtained by dividing one number by another. *Intelligence q.* abbreviated IQ. The degree of intelligence estimated by dividing the mental age, reckoned from standard tests, by the age in years. *Respiratory q.* the ratio between the carbon dioxide expired and the oxygen inspired during a specified time.

qwerty the standard typewriter keyboard layout that is also used for computers with some additions.

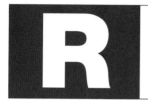

Ra symbol for *radium.*

rabid infected with rabies.

rabies an acute notifiable infectious disease of the central nervous system of animals, especially dogs, foxes, wolves and bats. The virus is found in the saliva of infected animals and is usually transmitted by a bite. Symptoms include fever, muscle spasms and intense excitement, followed by convulsions and paralysis, and death usually occurs. Vaccines are available.

race a term formerly used to describe a group of people sharing the same culture, language, values and beliefs. The preferred terms are now ethnic group or ethnicity. *R. gland* a compound gland composed of a number of small sacs, e.g., the salivary gland.

racism the belief that races are inherently different from one another. A belief that is usually associated with the view that one race has an intrinsic superiority over others, leading to stereotyping, prejudice and discrimination. Also called racialism.

radiant emitting rays.

radiation the emanation of energy in the form of electromagnetic waves, including gamma rays, X-rays, infrared and ultraviolet rays, and visible light rays. Radiation may cause damage to living tissues, e.g., in sunburn. *R. dosimetry* the method used to calculate the amount of radiation received by an individual. Also called radiation monitoring. *Ionizing r.* a form of radiation

that destabilizes an atom to produce highly reactive ions, e.g., X-rays, gamma rays and particle radiation. When used therapeutically ionizing radiation needs careful control and monitoring as it can cause tissue damage. *R. pneumonitis* inflammatory changes in the alveoli and interstitial tissue caused by radiation and which may lead to fibrosis later. *R. sickness* a toxic reaction of the body to radiation. Any or all of the following may be present: anorexia, nausea, vomiting and diarrhoea.

radical dealing with the root or cause of a disease. *R. cure* one which cures by complete removal of the cause.

radioactivity disintegration of certain elements to ones of lower atomic weight, with the emission of alpha and beta particles and gamma rays. *Induced r.* that brought about by bombarding the nuclei of certain elements with neutrons.

radiobiology the branch of medical science that studies the effect of radiation on live animal and human tissues.

radiodermatitis a late skin complication of radiotherapy in which there is atrophy, scarring, pigmentation and telangiectasis of the skin.

radiograph the picture obtained, on specially sensitized film, by passing X-rays through the body.

radiographer a professional health care worker in a diagnostic X-ray department (diagnostic radiographer) or in a radiotherapy department (therapy radiographer).

radiography the making of film records (radiographs) of internal structures of the body by exposure of film specially sensitized to X-rays or gamma rays. *Body-section r.* a special technique to show in detail images and structures lying in a predetermined plane of tissue, while blurring or eliminating detail in images in other planes; various mechanisms and methods for such radiography have been given various names, e.g., laminagraphy, tomography, etc. *Double-contrast r.* largely replaced by other techniques is used for revealing an abnormality of the intestinal mucosa; it involves injection and evacuation of a barium enema, followed by inflation of the intestine with air under light pressure. *Neutron r.* that in which a narrow beam of neutrons from a nuclear reactor is passed through tissues; especially useful in visualizing bony tissue. *Serial r.* the making of several exposures of a particular area at arbitrary intervals.

radioisotope an isotope of an element that emits radioactivity. These isotopes may occur naturally or be produced artificially by bombardment with neutrons.

radiologist a medically qualified doctor who specializes in the science of radiology.

radiology the science of radiation. Using X-rays and other allied imaging techniques in the diagnosis and treatment of disease.

radiomimetic producing effects similar to those of ionizing radiations.

radionuclide a radioactive substance which is inherently unstable. It is used in both radiodiagnosis and in radiotherapy. *R. scanning* a diagnostic technique based on the detection of radiation emitted by radioactive substances introduced into the body. These substances are taken up by different tissues to varying degrees thus allowing specific organs to be studied, e.g., the thyroid gland following the administration of a radionuclide-tagged dose of iodine.

radioscopy the examination of X-ray images on a fluorescent screen.

radiosensitive pertaining to those structures that respond readily to radiotherapy.

radiotherapist a medically qualified doctor specializing in radiotherapy.

radiotherapy a method of treating disease and eradicating tumour cells by aiming to deliver a therapeutic dose of radiation while preserving normal tissue function and structure.

radium *symbol* Ra. A radioactive element, obtained from uranium ores, which gives off emanations of great radioactive power. Used in the treatment of some malignant diseases.

RAI relatives assessment interview.

RAID rapid access interface and discharge team. RAID teams are specialist mental health professionals working in acute settings to ensure that patients with mental health needs are properly managed.

raised intracranial pressure abbreviated ICP. May be associated with a variety of conditions, e.g., haemorrhage, oedema, brain tumour, head injury or disturbance to the flow of cerebrospinal fluid.

râle an abnormal rattling sound, heard on auscultation of the chest during respiration when there is fluid in the bronchi.

Ramsay Hunt syndrome a complication of shingles.

Ramstedt's operation *W.C. Ramstedt, German surgeon, 1867–1963.* A pyloroplasty for congenital stricture of the pylorus in which the fibres of the sphincter muscle are divided, leaving the mucous lining intact.

random sample a sample from a population, obtained by ensuring that each member of that population has an equal chance of being selected. The sample selected should then demonstrate the same profile as the parent population.

randomized controlled trial (RCT) a study in which experimental and control groups are randomly selected for research. There are also a number of other synonyms for this term such as randomized trial, controlled clinical trial and true experiment.

ranula a retention cyst, usually under the tongue when blockage occurs in a submaxillary or sublingual duct, or in a mucous gland.

rape sexual assault or abuse; criminal forcible sexual intercourse (i.e., penetration) without the consent of the adult or child. Many cases are not reported because of feelings of shame, guilt, embarrassment or fear. Rape can occur between men, but it is most usually associated with victims who are female.

raphe a seam or ridge of tissue indicating the junction of two parts.

rapport in psychiatry, a satisfactory relationship based upon respect, understanding and mutuality between two persons, either the doctor and patient or nurse and patient, or the patient with any significant other.

rarefaction the process of becoming less dense, e.g., in bone disease.

rash a superficial eruption on the skin, frequently characteristic of some specific fever.

rate the speed or frequency with which an event or circumstance occurs per unit of time, population, or other standard of comparison. *Basal metabolic r.* abbreviated BMR. An expression of the rate at which oxygen is utilized in a fasting subject at complete rest as a percentage of a value established as normal for such a subject. *Birth r.* the number of live births in a population in a specified period of time (crude birth rate), for the female population (refined birth rate), or for the female population of childbearing age (true birth rate), usually expressed per year per 1000 of the estimated mid-year population. *Death r.* the number of deaths per stated number of persons (1000, 10 000 or 100 000) in a certain

region in a certain time (crude death rate). The death rate calculated with allowances made for age and sex distribution in the population is termed the standardized death rate. Also called *mortality rate. Glomerular filtration r.* an expression of the quantity of glomerular filtrate formed each minute in the nephrons of both kidneys, calculated by measuring the clearance of specific substances, e.g., insulin or creatinine.

ratio an expression of the quantity of one substance or entity in relation to that of another; the relationship between two quantities expressed as the quotient of one divided by the other. *Lecithin–sphingomyelin r.* the ratio of lecithin to sphingomyelin in amniotic fluid.

rationalization in psychiatry, the mental process by which individuals explain their behaviour, giving reasons that are advantageous to themselves or are socially acceptable. It may be a conscious or an unconscious act.

Raynaud's phenomenon or disease M. Raynaud, French physician, 1834–1881. Raynaud's phenomenon is characterized by episodic digital ischaemia producing pallor or cyanosis of the fingers and toes, provoked by stimuli such as emotion, cold, trauma, hormones and drugs. Treatment includes keeping the hands and feet as warm as possible. Vasodilator drugs may be helpful in severe cases.

reaction counteraction; a response to the application of a stimulus. *R. time* the interval between the stimulus and the response. *R. time feedback* ways of gathering feedback from patients about their experiences as near to the point of care as possible. The FRIENDS AND FAMILY TEST was developed and adopted as one way of gaining real time feedback.

reactive in psychiatry, used to describe a mental condition brought about by adverse external circumstances. *R. arthritis* formerly known as Reiter's syndrome. A rare type of arthritis that causes inflammation of the urinary tract, eyes, skins and mucous membrane, and joints usually following an infection. *R. depression* one that arises in this way and is not endogenous.

reagent a substance employed to produce a chemical reaction.

reality agreed as an absolute by members of the same culture as the total of all things related to perception, meaning and behaviour. Not imaginary, fictitious or pretended. *R. orientation see* ORIENTATION.

real-time scanner 1. an ultrasound scanner that gives a moving visual display. 2. Antiviral software which continuously scans files for viruses each time the computer accesses them.

recall to bring back to consciousness.

receptor 1. a sensory nerve ending that receives stimuli for transmission through the sensory nervous system. 2. a molecule on the surface or within a cell that recognizes and binds with specific molecules, producing some effect in the cell.

recessive tending to recede. The opposite to dominant. *R. gene* a gene that will produce its characteristics only when present in a homozygous state; both parents need to possess the particular gene, and there is a 1 in 4 chance of a child inheriting it homozygously.

recipient one who receives, as with a blood transfusion, or a tissue or organ graft. *Universal r.* a person thought to be able to receive blood of any 'type' without agglutination of the donor cells.

recombinant 1. a new cell or individual that results from genetic recombination. 2. pertaining or relating to such cells or individuals. *R. DNA technology* the process of taking a gene from one organism and inserting it into the DNA of another. Also called gene splicing.

recommended daily allowance (RDA) a standard for the daily intake of individual nutrients and calories for groups of people. *See* Appendix 1.

recommended international non-proprietary name a system whereby all drugs have a recommended non-proprietary name that is used internationally.

reconstituted family *see* FAMILY (BLENDED).

record 1. a piece of evidence or information relating to the subject of the record, for example, a change that has occurred or an account of an incident. 2. a document preserving the written account. 3. the state of being set down of information; individual personal details for preservation in writing or some other permanent form. *Summary care R.* (SCR) is an electronic record of important patient information, created from GP records, which can be seen by authorised staff in other areas of the health and care system involved in the direct care of the patient.

recovery position lying a patient who is unconscious on his or her side with a patent airway.

recrudescence renewed aggravation of symptoms after an interval of abatement.

rectal relating to the rectum. *R. examination* inspection by insertion of a glove-covered finger or with the aid of a proctoscope. *R. varices* haemorrhoids.

rectopexy the operation for fixation of a prolapsed rectum.

rectovaginal concerning the rectum and vagina.

rectovesical concerning the rectum and bladder.

rectum the lower end of the large intestine from the sigmoid flexure to the anus.

recumbent lying down in the dorsal position.

recuperation convalescence; recovery of health and strength; rehabilitation.

recurrent liable to recur.

reduction 1. the correction of a fracture, dislocation or hernia. 2. removal of oxygen or the addition of hydrogen to a substance or, more generally, the gain of electrons; the opposite of oxidization. *Closed r.* the manipulative reduction of a fracture without incision. *Open r.* reduction of a fracture after incision into the fracture site.

referred pain that which occurs at a distance from the place of origin due to the sensory nerves entering the cord at the same level, e.g., the phrenic nerve supplying the diaphragm enters the cord in the cervical region, as do the nerves from the shoulder, and so an abscess on the diaphragm may cause pain in the shoulder. *See* SYNALGIA.

reflection 1. a turning or bending back, as in the folds produced when a membrane passes over the surface of an organ and then passes back to the body wall that it lines. 2. in nursing and health care practice, conscious and systematic thinking about one's actions; the review, analysis and evaluation of those situations that have occurred, usually after but maybe during an event. An active process by which the practitioner learns from situations with a view to improving future practice.

reflective practice an active process by which the health care professional is able to review, analyse and evaluate events or situations. This conscious monitoring process can be based on any conceptual model, and may utilize supervision of peers in the process. The aim is to facilitate and enhance professional practice. *See* REVALIDATION.

reflex reflected or thrown back. *Accommodation r.* the alteration in the shape of the lens according to the distance of the image viewed. *Conditioned r.* that which is not natural, but is developed by association and frequent repetition until it appears natural. *Corneal r.* the automatic reaction of closing the eyelids after exertion of light pressure on the cornea. This is a test for unconsciousness which is absolute when there is no response. Also known as the blink reflex. *Deep r.* a muscle reflex elicited by tapping the tendon or bone of attachment. *Light r.* alteration of the size of the pupil in response to exposure to light. *R. action* an involuntary action following immediately upon some stimulus, e.g., the knee jerk, or the withdrawal of a limb from a pin-prick. *R. arc* the sensory and motor neurones, together with the connector neurone, which carry out a reflex action (*see* Figure on p. 335). *R. zone therapy* a system of complementary therapy, similar to reflexology, in which it is believed the body is divided into ten longitudinal and three transverse zones, with corresponding divisions in the feet. Reflex zone therapy can be used to identify areas of disorder or disease in the body and a sophisticated grip technique is used to massage the feet and so treat the problem. The therapy can also be performed on the hands, which correspond closely to the feet, the tongue, the face and the back.

reflexology a technique of deep massage to the soles of the feet, and occasionally the palms of the hands, to relieve somatic symptoms, and promote health and wellbeing. A complementary therapy.

reflux a backward flow; regurgitation.

refraction 1. the bending or deviation of rays of light as they pass obliquely through one transparent medium and penetrate another of different density. 2. in ophthalmology, the testing of the eyes to ascertain the amount and variety of refractive error that may be present in each of them.

refractory not yielding to, or resistant to, treatment. *R. period* the period immediately after some activity during which a nerve or muscle is unable to react to a fresh impulse.

regeneration renewal, as in new growth of tissue in its specific form after injury.

regimen a regulated system, programme or schedule such as diet, therapy or exercise intended to promote health or achieve another beneficial effect for a person's wellbeing. Regimen is used in preference to the

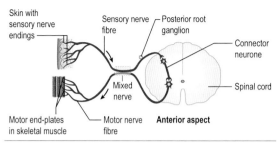

Skin with sensory nerve endings — Sensory nerve fibre — Posterior root ganglion — Connector neurone — Spinal cord — Mixed nerve — Motor end-plates in skeletal muscle — Motor nerve fibre — Anterior aspect

REFLEX ARC

word regime, which usually refers to a political system or structure.

register an epidemiological term meaning an index or file of all cases with a particular disease or condition in a defined population.

Registered Nurse a qualified practitioner whose name appears on the central register of the Nursing and Midwifery Council. The title is protected by law in the UK and other countries too. *See* NURSE.

registrar an official keeper of records. *R. of births, deaths, marriages and civil partnerships* the official recorder of births, marriages, civil partnerships and deaths. Local registry offices are available in most towns. Births should be registered within 42 days in England, Wales and Northern Ireland (21 days in Scotland). Without a death certificate, which indicates that the death has been registered, it is illegal to dispose of a body.

registration the act of recording; in dentistry, the making of a record of the jaw relations, present or desired, in order to transfer them to an articulator to facilitate proper construction of a dental prosthesis.

regression 1. a return to a previous state of health. 2. in psychiatry, a tendency to return to primitive or child-like modes of behaviour. Some degree of regression frequently accompanies physical illness and hospitalization. Patients who are mentally ill may exhibit regression to an extreme degree, reverting all the way back to infantile behaviour (atavistic regression).

regulatory bodies organizations responsible for defining and monitoring preparation and practice of a specific professional group, e.g., Nursing and Midwifery Council, General Medical Council and the Health and Care Professions Council. *See* Appendix 5.

regurgitation backward flow, e.g., of food from the stomach into the mouth. Fluids regurgitate through the nose in paralysis affecting the soft palate. *Aortic r.* backward flow of blood into the left ventricle when the aortic valve is incompetent. *Mitral r.* mitral incompetence. *See* MITRAL.

rehabilitation re-education, particularly where an individual has been ill or injured, to enable them to become capable of useful activity.

rehydration therapy the treatment of dehydration by administering fluid and salts by mouth (oral rehydration) or by intravenous infusion. *See* FLUID BALANCE.

reinforcement the increasing of force or strength. In behavioural science, the process of presenting a reinforcing stimulus to strengthen a response. *See* CONDITIONING. A positive reinforcer is a stimulus that is added to the environment immediately after the desired response. It serves to strengthen the response: that is, to increase the likelihood of its occurring again. Examples of a positive reinforcer are food, money, a special privilege, or some other reward that is satisfying to the subject.

Reiter's syndrome   *H. Reiter, German bacteriologist, 1881–1969.*   former name for REACTIVE ARTHRITIS.

rejection   1. in immunology, the formation of antibodies by the host against transplanted tissue, with eventual destruction of the transplanted tissue. 2. in psychosocial terms, the denial of acceptance or affection, or the exclusion of another person.

relapse   the return of a disease after an interval of convalescence.

relapsing fever   one of a group of similar notifiable infectious diseases transmitted to humans by the bites of ticks. Marked by alternating periods of normal temperature and periods of fever relapse. The diseases in the group are caused by several different species of spirochaetes belonging to the genus *Borrelia*.

relatives   assessment   interview abbreviated RAI. An assessment tool used by mental health nurses and other staff to identify the perceptions and coping skills of relatives of patients with mental health problems. The data obtained forms an important component in the planning and delivery of care to the patient and the family.

relaxant   a drug or other agent that brings about muscle relaxation or relieves tension.

relaxation   a lessening of tension, which may be observed when muscles slacken after they have contracted; it is characterized by feelings of peace and calmness. *R. therapy* classes in which patients are taught breathing and other exercises to use for the relief of pain, stress and tension. Used as part of the preparation for childbirth.

relaxin   a hormone that is produced by the corpus luteum of the ovary; it softens the cervix and loosens the pelvic ligaments to aid the birth of the baby.

releasing hormone   a substance, produced in the hypothalamus, which causes the anterior pituitary gland to release other hormones.

reliability   the quality of being trustworthy or dependable. In research, the consistency of a measure in a study and the likelihood of reproducing the same results, if used again in similar circumstances.

REM   rapid eye movement, a phase of SLEEP associated with dreaming and characterized by rapid movements of the eyes. Paradoxical sleep.

reminiscence therapy   measures to stimulate long-term elderly patients with memorabilia, films and songs meaningful to their generation. Used in conjunction with or as a prelude to reality orientation therapy. *See* ORIENTATION.

remission   subsidence of the symptoms of a disease for a long time.

remittent   decreasing at intervals. *R. fever* one in which a partial fall in the temperature occurs daily.

remotivation   in psychiatry, a group therapy technique administered by the nursing staff in a psychiatric unit, which is used to stimulate the communication skills and an interest in the environment of long-term, withdrawn patients.

renal   relating to the kidney. *R. calculus* stone in the kidney. *R. clearance tests* laboratory tests that determine the ability of the kidney to remove certain substances from the blood. *R. dialysis* the application of the principles of dialysis for treatment of renal failure (*see* later). *See also* HAEMODIALYSIS and peritoneal (dialysis). *R. failure* inability of the kidney to maintain normal function. It may be *acute* or *chronic*. Acute renal failure is a sudden, severe interruption of kidney function. It is normally the complication of another disorder and is reversible.

Chronic renal failure is a progressive loss of kidney function. In its early stage, renal function can remain adequate but the glomerular filtration rate (GFR) is depressed and plasma chemistry begins to show abnormalities as waste products accumulate. In the later stage, known as end-stage renal disease (ESRD), the GFR deteriorates and when uraemia becomes evident and the patient becomes symptomatic, dialysis is started or the patient receives a transplant. *R. threshold* the level of the blood sugar beyond which it is excreted in the urine; normally 10 mmol/litre (180 mg/100 ml). *R. transplant* transfer of a healthy kidney from a donor into the body of someone with serious kidney disease. *R. tubule* the thin tubular part of a nephron. A uriniferous tubule.

renin a proteolytic enzyme released into the bloodstream when the kidneys are ischaemic. It causes vasoconstriction and increases the blood pressure.

reorganization healing by formation of new tissue identical to that which was injured or destroyed.

reovirus any of a group of RNA viruses isolated from healthy children, children with febrile and afebrile upper respiratory disease, or children with diarrhoea.

repetitive strain injury abbreviated RSI. A soft-tissue disorder produced by repetitive use of muscle, especially if the muscle activity involves an awkward or uncomfortable position of the body. Particularly affects keyboard operators, musicians, packers and machine operators.

replication 1. the turning back of a tissue on itself. 2. the process by which DNA duplicates itself when the cell divides.

Replogle tube a double-lumen aspiration catheter attached to low pressure suction apparatus.

repression 1. the act of restraining, inhibiting or suppressing. 2. in psychiatry, a defence mechanism whereby a person unconsciously banishes unacceptable ideas, feelings or impulses from consciousness. A person using repression to obtain relief from mental conflict is unaware that 'forgetting' unpleasant situations is a way of avoiding them (motivated forgetting).

reproductive system all those parts of the male and female body associated with the production of children. (*See* Figures on p. 338.)

Rescue Remedy one of the Bach Flower remedies, based on homeopathic principles, and available in liquid form, which is particularly effective in reducing stress, panic, anxiety and hysteria. Useful for those who have a fear of needles for venepuncture and injections, for the transition stage of labour and at any other time when patients are especially anxious or nervous, e.g., before surgical intervention. Four drops of the remedy are given neat on the tongue or can be added to a small glass of water or applied to the temples or wrists. *See* BACH FLOWER REMEDIES.

research the purposeful, systematic study of sources, data and materials to establish and reach new conclusions. May also be used to find solutions to previously identified problems or to test theories. Nurses and other health care professionals use both qualitative and quantitative research methods, with the ultimate aim being improved practice and better patient care.

resection surgical removal of a part. *Submucous r.* removal of part of a deflected nasal septum, from beneath a flap of mucous membrane, which is then replaced. *Transurethral r.* a method of removing portions of an enlarged prostate gland via the urethra.

reservoir 1. a storage place or cavity. 2. the host or environment in which an organism lives and from which it is able to infect susceptible individuals, e.g., hands, skin, nose and bowel.

residential care the provision of care for frail, elderly people in a variety of

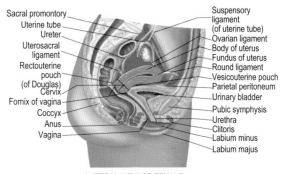

LATERAL VIEW OF FEMALE
REPRODUCTIVE ORGANS AND
ASSOCIATED STRUCTURES

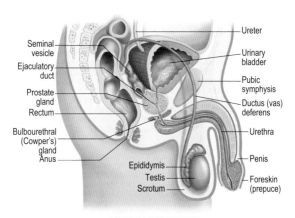

LATERAL VIEW OF MALE
REPRODUCTIVE ORGANS AND
ASSOCIATED STRUCTURES

settings, e.g., local authority residential homes for the elderly or private residential homes.

residual remaining. *R. air* residual volume. The amount of air remaining in the lungs after breathing out fully. *R. urine* urine remaining in the bladder after voiding; seen with bladder outlet obstruction and disorders affecting nerves controlling bladder function. *R. volume* residual air.

resistance the degree of opposition to a force. 1. in electricity, the opposition made by a non-conducting substance to the passage of a current. 2. in psychology, the opposition, stemming from the unconscious, to repressed ideas being brought to consciousness. *Drug r.* the ability of a microorganism to withstand the effects of a drug that are lethal to most members of its species. *Peripheral r.* that offered to the passage of blood through small vessels and capillaries. *R. to infection* the natural power of the body to withstand the toxins of disease.

resolution 1. in medicine, the process of returning to normal. 2. the disappearance of inflammation without the formation of pus. *Conflict R. training* development programme for all front-line NHS staff in the identification, prevention and management of conflict.

resonance the reverberating sound obtained on percussion over a cavity or hollow organ, such as the lung.

respiration the gaseous interchange between the tissue cells and the atmosphere. *Artificial r.* the production of respiratory movements by external effort. *External r.* breathing, which comprises inspiration, when the external intercostal muscles and the diaphragm contract and air is drawn into the lungs, and expiration, when the air is breathed out. *Intermittent positive pressure r.* abbreviated IPPR. Respiration produced by a ventilator. *Internal r.* tissue respiration. The interchange of gases that occurs between tissues and blood through the walls of capillaries.

Laboured r. that which is difficult and distressed. *Stertorous r.* snorting; a noisy breathing. *Tissue r.* internal respiration. *See* CHEYNE–STOKES RESPIRATION.

respirator an apparatus to qualify the air breathed through it, or a device for giving artificial respiration or to assist pulmonary ventilation (*see also* VENTILATOR).

respiratory pertaining to respiration. (*See* Figure on p. 340.) *Acute r. distress syndrome* abbreviated ARDS. A group of signs and symptoms resulting in acute respiratory failure; characterized clinically by tachypnoea, dyspnoea, tachycardia, cyanosis, and low Pa_{O_2} that persists even with oxygen therapy. *R. distress syndrome of newborn* abbreviated NRDS, a condition occurring in preterm infants, full-term infants of diabetic mothers, and infants delivered by caesarean section, and associated with pulmonary immaturity and inability to produce sufficient lung surfactant. Also called hyaline membrane disease, idiopathic respiratory distress syndrome, infant respiratory distress syndrome (abbreviated IRDS). *R. failure* a life-threatening condition in which respiratory function is inadequate to maintain the body's need for oxygen supply and carbon dioxide removal while at rest; also called acute ventilatory failure. *R. insufficiency* a condition in which respiratory function is inadequate to meet the body's needs when increased physical activity places extra demands on it. *R. quotient* the ratio of the volume of expired carbon dioxide to the volume of oxygen absorbed by the lungs per unit of time. *R. shock* circulatory SHOCK due to interference with the flow of blood through the great vessels and chambers of the heart, causing pooling of blood in the veins and the abdominal organs and a resultant vascular collapse. The condition sometimes occurs as a result of increased intrathoracic pressure in patients who are being maintained on a mechanical ventilator. *R. syncytial virus*

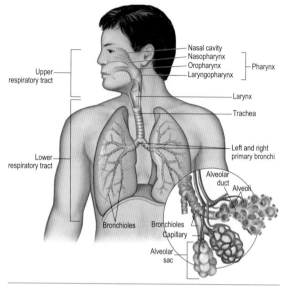

Nasal cavity
Nasopharynx
Oropharynx
Laryngopharynx
} Pharynx

Upper respiratory tract

Larynx

Trachea

Left and right primary bronchi

Lower respiratory tract

Alveolar duct
Alveoli

Bronchioles

Bronchioles
Capillary

Alveolar sac

RESPIRATORY SYSTEM

a virus isolated from children with bronchopneumonia and bronchitis, characteristically causing severe respiratory infection in very young children but less severe infections as the children grow older. *R. therapy* the technical specialty concerned with the treatment, management and care of patients with respiratory problems, including administration of medical gases.

respite care temporary care provided for those with disabilities or serious and terminal conditions to allow relief for the family and other carers. Provision may be on a daily or longer-term basis and in a variety of settings, e.g., in a hospice, nursing or residential home, hostel or in the family home. *See* HOSPICE.

restless legs syndrome characterized by weakness and coldness in the lower limbs with an unpleasant feeling of a creeping tingling sensation, firstly in the lower legs but possibly extending to the thighs, arms and hands. Symptoms most commonly occur in patients in bed at night, or sometimes in those sitting in chairs for prolonged periods during the day. Occurs primarily in the elderly. The cause is unknown but may be due to a vascular disorder. Also known as Willis-Ekbom disease.

resuscitation restoration to life or consciousness of one apparently dead, or whose respirations have ceased. *Cardiopulmonary r.* an emergency technique used in cardiac arrest to re-establish heart and lung function until more advanced life support is available. See Appendix 2.

retching strong, involuntary effort to vomit.

retention holding back. *R. cyst see* CYST. *R. defect* a defect of memory. Inability to retain material in the mind so that it can be recalled when required. *R. of urine* inability to pass urine from the bladder, which may be due to obstruction or be of nervous origin.

reticular resembling a network. *R. formation* areas in the brain stem from which nerve fibres extend to the cerebral cortex.

reticulocyte a red blood cell that is not fully mature; it retains strands of nuclear material.

reticulocytosis the presence of an increased number of immature red cells in the blood, indicating overactivity of the bone marrow.

reticuloendothelial system a collection of endothelial cells in the liver, spleen, bone marrow and lymph glands that produce large mononuclear cells or macrophages. They are phagocytic, destroy red blood cells and have the power of making some antibodies.

retina the innermost coat of the eyeball, formed of nerve cells and fibres, from which the optic nerve leaves the eyeball and passes to the visual area of the cerebrum. The impression of the image is focused upon it.

retinal relating to the retina. *R. detachment* partial detachment of the retina from the underlying choroid layer, resulting in loss of vision. It may result from the presence of a tumour, from trauma or from high myopia. *R. migraine* an eye condition with brief spells of blindness or flashing lights usually in one eye. The episodes are frightening but generally harmless. Also known as ocular migraine.

retinitis inflammation of the retina.

retinoblastoma a rare malignant tumour arising from retinal cells. Occurs in infancy and may be hereditary. Treatment includes cryotherapy, laser treatment, irradiation and chemotherapy, but enucleation may be required.

retinol a light-absorbing molecule obtained from vitamin A. See RHODOPSIN.

retinopathy any non-inflammatory disease of the retina. *R. of prematurity* previously known as retrolental fibroplasia. Scarring and retinal detachment in babies who have received oxygen therapy due to prematurity. *R. pigmentosa* a group of diseases, frequently hereditary, marked by progressive loss of retinal function, especially associated with contraction of the visual field and impairment of vision. The disorder often follows a slow course over a period of many years, but there is considerable variation in the progression of the disease. *Diabetic r.* a complication of diabetes. Retinal haemorrhages occur, resulting in permanent visual damage, and retinal detachment may follow. *Hypertensive r.* retinal change occurring as a result of high blood pressure.

retrobulbar pertaining to the back of the eyeball. *R. neuritis* dimness of vision due to inflammation of the optic nerve.

retroflexion a bending back, particularly of the uterus when it is bent backwards at an acute angle, the cervix being in its normal position. See RETROVERSION.

retrograde going backwards. *R. amnesia* forgetfulness of events occurring immediately before an illness or injury. *R. urography* radiographic examination of the kidney after the introduction of a radio-opaque substance into the renal pelvis through the urethra.

retrolental fibroplasia a fibrous condition of the anterior vitreous body which develops when a premature infant is exposed to high concentrations of oxygen. Both eyes are affected, seriously interfering with vision and leading to retinal detachment. Early treatment with a freezing probe (cryopexy) can prevent retinal detachment.

retroperitoneal behind the peritoneum.

retropharyngeal behind the pharynx.

retrospection a morbid dwelling on memories.

retrospective looking back on or dealing with past events. *R. study* one that examines data from the past, e.g., discharged patients' records, to discover causal factors relevant to outcomes.

retrosternal behind the sternum.

retroversion a lifting backwards, particularly of the uterus when the whole organ is tilted backwards. *See* RETROFLEXION.

retrovirus a group of viruses belonging to the family Retroviridae, principally infecting and frequently causing diseases in animals, but also including viruses that infect and cause disease in humans, e.g., HUMAN IMMUNODEFICIENCY VIRUS (HIV) and human T cell leukaemia/ lymphoma/lymphotropic virus type I (HTLV-I).

Rett syndrome a rare genetic disorder affecting brain development resulting in severe physical and learning disabilities caused by a mutation in the MECP2 gene.

revalidation the requirement of registered nurses and midwives to confirm to the nursing and midwifery council (NMC) that they have met the minimum requirement for practice and continuing professional development hours. They must also provide evidence of reflection and feedback. *See* Appendix 12.

Reverdin's graft *J.L. Reverdin, Swiss surgeon, 1842–1929.* A form of skin graft in which pieces of skin are placed as islands over the area. *See* THIERSCH SKIN GRAFT.

reverse isolation *see* PROTECTIVE ISOLATION; also Appendix 11.

Reye's syndrome *R.D.K. Reye, Australian pathologist, 1912–1977.* An acute, potentially fatal illness that may follow a virus infection occurring in children; there is fatty degeneration of the liver and the brain and raised intracranial pressure, accompanied by vomiting, convulsions and coma. The cause of Reye's syndrome is unknown but administration of salicylates in children under the age of 16 years is not recommended unless advised by a doctor. This follows evidence that aspirin may be a contributory factor in the development of Reye's syndrome.

Rh factor rhesus factor.

rhabdomyosarcoma a rare malignant growth of striated muscle. It grows rapidly and metastasizes early.

rhagades cracks or fissures in the skin, especially those round the mouth.

rhesus factor abbreviated Rh factor. The red blood cells of most humans carry a group of genetically determined antigens and are said to be rhesus positive (Rh^+). Those that do not are said to be rhesus negative (Rh^-). This is of importance as a cause of anaemia and jaundice in the newly born when the infant is Rh^+ and the mother Rh^-. About 83% of Caucasians and 99%–100% of other races are rhesus positive.

rheumatism any of a variety of disorders marked by inflammation, degeneration or metabolic derangement of the connective tissue structures, especially the joints and related structures, and attended by pain, stiffness or limitation of motion. *Acute r.* rheumatic fever. An acute fever associated with previous streptococcal infection and occurring most commonly in children. The onset is usually sudden, with pain, swelling and stiffness in one or more joints. There is fever, sweating and tachycardia, and carditis is present in most cases. Sometimes the symptoms are minor and ignored. This disease is the most common cause of mitral stenosis because scar tissue results from the inflammation.

rheumatoid resembling rheumatism. *R. arthritis see* ARTHRITIS.

rheumatology the branch of medicine dealing with disorders of the joints, muscles, tendons and ligaments.

rhinitis inflammation of the mucous membrane of the nose. *See* ALLERGIC RHINITIS and NON ALLERGIC RHINITIS.

rhinoplasty a plastic operation on the nose; repairing a part of or forming an entirely new nose.

rhinorrhoea an abnormal discharge of mucus from the nose.

rhinoscopy examination of the interior of the nose. *Anterior r.* examination through the nostrils with the aid of a speculum. *Posterior r.* examination through the nasopharynx by means of a rhinoscope.

rhinovirus one of a genus of small RNA-containing viruses that cause respiratory diseases, including the common cold.

Rhipicephalus a genus of ticks that can transmit the *Rickettsia* which cause typhus and relapsing fever.

rhodopsin the visual purple of the retina, the formation of which is dependent upon vitamin A (retinol) in the diet. *See* RETINOL.

rhonchus a wheezing sound, produced in the bronchial tubes, which is caused by partial obstruction and can be heard on auscultation.

rhythm a regular recurring action. *Cardiac r.* the smooth action of the heart when systole is followed by diastole. *R. method* a contraceptive technique in which intercourse is limited to the 'safe period' (avoiding the 2–3 days immediately before and after ovulation).

rhytidectomy commonly known as a face lift, a cosmetic surgical procedure to remove wrinkles and excess skin to improve visible signs of ageing.

rib any one of the 12 pairs of long, flat curved bones of the thorax, joined in front by cartilage to the spinal vertebrae at the back. *Cervical r.* a short extra rib, often bilateral. Pressure on this may cause impairment of nerve or vascular function. *See* SCALENUS (SYNDROME). *False r's* the last five pairs, the upper three of which are attached by cartilage to each other. *Floating r's* the last two pairs, connected only to the vertebrae.

True r's the seven pairs attached directly to the sternum.

riboflavin a chemical factor in the vitamin B complex.

ribonuclease an enzyme from the pancreas which is responsible for the breakdown of nucleic acid.

ribonucleic acid abbreviated RNA. A complex chemical found in the cytoplasm of animal cells and concerned with protein synthesis. Certain viruses contain RNA.

ribosome an RNA- and protein-containing particle which is the site of protein synthesis in the cell.

rickets a condition of infancy and childhood caused by deficiency of vitamin D, which leads to altered calcium and phosphorus metabolism and consequent disturbance of ossification of bone, resulting in deformity, such as bowing of the legs. Since the action of sunlight on the skin produces vitamin D in the human body, rickets often occurs in parts of the world where the winter is especially long, and in children with dark skin who need more sunlight to get enough vitamin D. *Adult r.* OSTEOMALACIA; a rickets-like disease affecting adults. *Fetal r.* achondroplasia. *Late r.* osteomalacia, that occurring in older children. *Vitamin D-resistant r.* an hereditary condition almost indistinguishable from ordinary rickets clinically but resistant to unusually large doses of vitamin D; it is also known as X-linked dominant hypophosphatemic rickets.

Rickettsia a genus of microorganisms which are parasitic in lice and similar insects. The bite of the host is thus the means of transmitting the organisms, some of which are responsible for the typhus group of fevers.

rigidity sustained muscle tension causing the affected part to be stiff and inflexible; may be due to stress, injury or neurological disease.

rigor an attack of intense shivering occurring when the heat regulation is disturbed. The temperature rises rapidly and may either stay elevated or fall rapidly as profuse sweating occurs. *R. mortis* stiffening of the body which occurs soon after death.

Ringer's solution *S. Ringer, British physiologist, 1835–1910.* A physiological solution of saline to which small amounts of calcium and potassium salts have been added. Used to replace fluids and electrolytes intravenously.

ringworm tinea. A contagious skin disease, characterized by circular patches, pinkish in colour with a desquamating surface, and due to a parasitic fungus.

risk hazard, or chance of developing a disease or of complications during or after treatment. This may arise because of inherent problems with the treatment itself (e.g., drug side effects) or because of the frailty of the patient. *Relative r.* the likelihood of developing a disease after a given exposure; in epidemiological terms, calculated as incidence rate of disease in an exposed group divided by incidence rate in the non-exposed group. *R. assessment* 1. a study of a patient by a health care practitioner in which the details of the person's health record are considered together with other relevant factors to assess the likelihood of the development of a particular disease, or, if the disease is already present, the probability of exacerbation or remission. 2. an assessment of a situation or activity for risks with a view to prevention of any damaging effects upon health, e.g., procedures and environment related to moving and handling. *R. factor* a factor which, when added to others, increases the likelihood of a disease or complication (e.g., smoking and obesity are risk factors for the development of coronary artery disease). *R. management* use of a structured approach to reduce identifiable risks in the health services before problems occur in order to protect the interests of the patients and staff by improving the quality of care, reducing costs and potential litigation.

rite of passage the cultural ceremonies and rituals that may accompany the changes in status that occur in the course of a person's life, e.g., 18th birthday parties, or bar mitzvah. These ceremonies serve to draw attention to changes in status and social identity and also to the management of the social tensions that such changes may involve.

RNA ribonucleic acid. *RNA viruses* viruses which contain ribonucleic acid as their genetic material.

Rocky Mountain spotted fever a tick-borne infection caused by a *Rickettsia*, common in the USA, with rash, fever, muscle pain and often an enlarged liver. The disease lasts about 3 weeks.

rod a straight thin structure. *Retinal r.* one of the two types of light-sensitive end-organ of the retina, which contain rhodopsin and are responsible for night vision.

role a pattern of behaviour developed in response to the demands or expectations of others; the pattern of responses to the persons with whom an individual interacts in a particular situation. *R. play* an educational technique used in teaching interpersonal, communication and practice skills. Students are given roles (or parts) and asked to act these roles out. Some members of the group may be given observational tasks related to the exercise. At the end of the session there is an opportunity for the group to evaluate the exercise. This technique may also be used therapeutically, usually in the psychiatric setting. *Sick r.* the role played by people who have defined themselves as ill. Adoption of the sick role changes the behavioural expectations of others towards the sick person, who is exempted from normal social responsibilities and is not held responsible for the condition. The patient is obliged to 'want to get well' and to seek competent medical help.

Romberg's sign *M.H. Romberg, German physician, 1795–1853.* Inability to stand erect without swaying if the eyes are closed. A sign of tabes dorsalis.

Rorschach test *H. Rorschach, Swiss psychiatrist, 1884–1922.* A personality trait test that consists of ten ink-blot designs, some in colours and some in black and white.

rosacea *see* ACNE (ROSACEA).

roseola 1. a rose-coloured rash. 2. roseola infantum. *R. infantum* a common acute viral disease that usually occurs in children under 24 months old; it attacks suddenly but disappears in a few days, leaving no permanent marks. *Syphilitic r.* an eruption of rose-coloured spots in early secondary syphilis.

roughage coarse vegetable fibres and cellulose that give bulk to the diet and stimulate peristalsis.

rouleau a rounded formation found in blood, caused by red cells piling on each other.

roundworm any of various types of parasitic nematode worm, somewhat resembling the common earthworm, which sometimes invade the human intestinal tract and multiply there. Very common among them is the pinworm, or threadworm.

Rovsing's sign *N.T. Rovsing, Danish surgeon, 1868–1927.* A test for acute appendicitis in which pressure in the left iliac fossa causes pain in the right iliac fossa.

RSI repetitive strain injury.

RTS,S/AS01 the first approved malaria vaccine. Approved for use by European regulators in July 2015.

rubefacient an agent causing redness of the skin.

rubella German measles. An acute, notifiable virus infection of short duration, characterized by pyrexia, enlarged cervical lymph glands and a transient rash. The greatest risk from this disease is to the offspring of mothers who contract it during the early weeks of pregnancy. The child may be born with cataract, heart defects, deafness or have other congenital defects including brain damage. When a woman is exposed to rubella during the first 20 weeks of pregnancy, a sample of saliva or blood should be taken to test for immunity to rubella. If this shows immunity and no infection, reassurance can be given to continue the pregnancy. The second serum should be taken 4 weeks later, if the first showed no immunity. If this shows evidence of infection further investigations of the baby will be undertaken to check for any sign of problems in the baby to enable informed choice about termination of the pregnancy be considered. Rubella vaccination is given, in conjunction with immunization against mumps and measles (MMR) when an infant is approximately 1 year old with a second booster before the start of school. *See* Appendix 10.

rumination 1. recurring thoughts. 2. voluntary regurgitation of food, which is then chewed and swallowed again. *Obsessional r.* thoughts which persistently recur against the patient's will.

rupture 1. tearing or bursting of a part, as in rupture of an aneurysm; of the membranes during labour; or of a tubal pregnancy. 2. a term commonly applied to hernia.

Ryle's tube *G.A. Ryle, British physician, 1889–1950.* A thin tube with a weighted end, introduced into the stomach. It may be used for the withdrawal of gastric contents or for the administration of fluids.

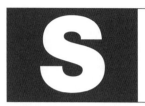

Sabin vaccine *A.B. Sabin, American biologist, 1906–1993.* A live oral attenuated poliovirus vaccine active against poliomyelitis. *See* Appendix 10.

saccharide one of a series of carbohydrates, including the sugars.

saccule a small sac, particularly the smaller of the two sacs within the membranous labyrinth of the ear.

sacral relating to the sacrum.

sacroiliac relating to the sacrum and the ilium.

sacrum a triangular bone composed of five united vertebrae, situated between the lowest lumbar vertebra and the coccyx. It forms the back of the pelvis.

sadism a form of sexual perversion in which the individual takes pleasure in inflicting mental and physical pain on others.

SADS seasonal affective disorder syndrome.

safe motherhood initiative the World Health Organization (WHO) campaign to reduce worldwide maternal mortality and morbidity with the implementation of simple, appropriate and cost effective strategies to enable mothers to have access to high quality, affordable care during pregnancy and childbirth. The campaign also seeks to improve the health, nutrition and the general wellbeing of girls and women of reproductive age and to the reduction of any long-term sequelae of childbirth which often result in lifelong disabilities.

safer sex preventative measures to reduce the risk of sexually transmitted infections; e.g., maintaining a monogamous sexual relationship and using a condom.

safer staffing ensuring that there are the right number of staff with the right skills in the right places—particularly aimed at nursing staff.

sagittal arrow-shaped. *S. suture* the junction of the parietal bones.

salicylate a salt of salicylic acid. *Methyl s.* the active ingredient in ointments and lotions for joint pains and sprains. *Sodium s.* a drug that acts as a non-steroidal anti-inflammatory drug (NSAID) and reduces pyrexia and relieves pain.

saline a solution of sodium chloride and water. *Hypertonic s.* a greater than normal strength. *Hypotonic s.* a lower than normal strength. *Normal* or *physiological s.* a 0.9% solution which is isotonic with blood.

saliva the secretion of the salivary glands. When food is taken, saliva moistens and partially digests carbohydrates by the action of its enzyme, ptyalin (amylase).

salivary relating to saliva. *S. calculus* formation of a calculi in the salivary gland. The calculi can block the flow of saliva causing swelling and pain. *S. fistula* an abnormal opening on the skin of the face, leading into a salivary duct or gland. *S. glands* the parotid, submaxillary and sublingual glands.

salivation 1. the process of salivating. 2. excessive salivation which may lead to soreness of mouth and gums.

Salk vaccine *J.E. Salk, American virologist, 1914–1995.* The first poliomyelitis vaccine of killed viruses, given by injection.

Salmonella any of the genus of gram-negative, non-sporing, rod-like bacteria that are parasites of the intestinal tract of humans and animals. *S. typhi* and *S. paratyphi* are exclusively human pathogens which cause typhoid and paratyphoid fevers.

salmonellosis infection with the genus *Salmonella*, usually caused by the ingestion of food containing salmonellae or their products. The organisms can be found in raw meats, raw poultry, eggs and dairy products; they multiply rapidly at temperatures between 7°C and 46°C. Symptoms of salmonellosis include violent diarrhoea attended by abdominal cramps, nausea and vomiting, and fever. It is rarely fatal and can be prevented by adequate cooking.

salpingectomy excision of one or both of the uterine tubes.

salpingitis 1. inflammation of the uterine tubes. 2. inflammation of the pharyngotympanic (eustachian) tubes. Eustachitis. *Acute s.* most often a bilateral ascending infection due to a streptococcus, a gonococcus or *Chlamydia trachomatis*. *Chronic s.* a less acute form that may be blood-borne.

salpingography radiographic examination of the uterine tubes after injection of a radio-opaque substance to determine their patency.

salpingostomy the making of a surgical opening in a uterine tube near the uterus to restore patency.

salpinx a tube. Applied to the uterine or pharyngotympanic (eustachian) tubes.

salt 1. sodium chloride, common salt, used in solution as a cleansing lotion, a stimulating bath, or for infusion into the blood, etc. 2. any compound of an acid with an alkali or base. 3. a saline purgative such as Epsom salts. *S. depletion* a loss of salt from the body due to sweating or persistent diarrhoea or vomiting. Common in hot climates when it may be prevented by the taking of salt tablets. *Smelling s's* aromatic ammonium carbonate. A restorative in fainting.

sample 1. a selection of individuals made for research purposes from a larger population and intended to reflect that population in all significant aspects. 2. a small part of anything intended as representative of the whole, e.g., blood specimen.

sandfly a very small fly of the genus *Phlebotomus*, common in tropical climates and the vector of most types of leishmaniasis. *S. fever* a fever transmitted by the bites of sandflies, and common in Mediterranean countries. Similar to dengue and sometimes known as three-day fever, pappataci fever or phlebotomus fever.

sanguineous pertaining to or containing blood.

saphenous relating to the venae saphenae (saphenous veins) that carry blood from the foot upwards.

sapphism female homosexuality; lesbianism.

sarcoid 1. tuberculoid; characterized by non-caseating epithelioid cell tubercles. 2. pertaining to or resembling sarcoidosis. 3. sarcoidosis.

sarcoidosis a chronic, progressive, generalized disease resembling tuberculosis which may affect any part of the body but most frequently involves the lymph nodes, liver, spleen, lungs, skin, eyes and small bones of the hands and feet.

sarcoma a malignant tumour developed from connective tissue cells and their stroma. *Ewing s.* a rare type of cancer affecting bones or tissues around bones. Mostly seen in young people and more common in males. *Kaposi's s.* one principally involving the skin, although visceral lesions may be present; it usually begins on the distal parts of the extremities, most often on the toes or feet, as reddish-blue or brownish soft nodules and tumours. It is viral in origin and is frequently associated with AIDS. *Melanotic s.* a highly malignant type, pigmented with melanin. *Round-celled s.* a rare highly malignant growth, composed of a primitive type of cell.

sarcomatosis multiple sarcomatous growths in various parts of the body.

Sarcoptes a genus of mites. *S. scabiei* the cause of scabies.

SARS severe acute respiratory syndrome.

sartorius a long muscle of the thigh, which flexes both the thigh and the lower leg.

satyriasis abnormally excessive sexual appetite in men.

scab the crust on a superficial wound consisting of dried blood, pus, etc.

scabies 'the itch'; a parasitic skin disease caused by the itch mite (*Sarcoptes scabiei*), the female of which burrows beneath the skin and deposits eggs at intervals. It is intensely irritating, and the rash is aggravated by scratching. The sites affected are chiefly between the fingers and toes, the axillae and groins. Acquired by close direct contact and highly contagious. All members of the family should be treated with topical applications containing either permethrin or malathion to the whole body (except for the head). Two applications 1 week apart are required.

scald a burn caused by hot liquid or vapour.

scale 1. a scheme or instrument by which something can be measured. A pair of scales is a balance for measuring weight. 2. compact layers of dead epithelial tissue shed from the skin. 3. to scrape deposits of tartar from the teeth.

scalenus one of four muscles which move the neck to either side and raise the first and second ribs during inspiration. *S. syndrome* symptoms of pain and tenderness in the shoulder, with sensory loss and wasting of the medial aspect of the arm. It may be caused by pressure on the brachial plexus, by spasm of the scalenus anterior muscle or by a cervical rib.

scalp the hairy skin that covers the cranium.

scan an image produced using a moving detector or a sweeping beam of radiation, as in scintiscanning, B-mode ultrasonography, scanography or computed tomography.

scanning 1. visual examination of an area. 2. a speech disorder that may be present in cerebellar disease. The syllables are inappropriately separated from each other and are evenly stressed with rhythmically occurring pauses between them.

scaphoid boat-shaped. *S. bone* a boat-shaped bone of the wrist which articulates with the radius and with the trapezium and the trapezoid bones.

scapula the large flat triangular bone forming the shoulder-blade.

scar the mark left after a wound has healed with the formation of connective tissue.

scarlet fever scarlatina; an acute, notifiable, rare, infectious disease of childhood with an incubation period of 2–4 days. It is caused by a group A beta-haemolytic streptococcus. There is sore throat, high fever and a punctate rash. It is readily treated by antibiotics and the complications of nephritis and middle ear infection are less common.

scattergram used in research and statistics, where two variables are represented by a single plot against an x and y axis.

Schilling test *R.F. Schilling, American haematologist, 1919–2014.* A test used to confirm the diagnosis of pernicious anaemia by estimating the absorption of ingested radioactive vitamin B_{12}.

Schistosoma a genus of minute blood flukes, some of which are parasitic in humans. *S. haematobium* a species that infests the urinary bladder; widely found in Africa and the Middle East, especially in Egypt. *S. japonicum* and *S. mansoni* species that infest the large intestine. They are found respectively in China, Japan and the Philippines, and in Africa, the West Indies and tropical America.

schistosomiasis a parasitic infection of the intestinal or urinary tract by *Schistosoma*. The parasite enters the skin from contaminated water, and causes diarrhoea, haematuria and anaemia. The secondary hosts are freshwater snails. Bilharziasis.

schizoid personality disorder (SPD) a personality disorder that is marked by introspection, self-consciousness, solitariness and a failure in affection towards others. SPD is not the same as schizophrenia or schizotypal disorder.

schizophrenia is a chronic, severe and disabling brain disorder characterized by mental deterioration from a previous level of functioning and characteristic disturbances of multiple psychological processes, including delusions, false beliefs, loosening of associations, poverty of the content of speech, auditory hallucinations, inappropriate affect, disturbed sense of self and withdrawal from the external world. Antipsychotic medication is the mainstay of treatment together with psychotherapy, vocational and social rehabilitation, together with community mental health support to prevent relapse. Family counselling is also supportive. *S. nursing assessment* used by mental health nurses to assess all family members, including the patient, as a means of identifying the main issues for care and treatment.

schizotypal personality disorder a disorder characterized by severe social anxiety, paranoia and often unconventional beliefs. Individuals have great difficulty in establishing and maintaining relationships.

Schlemm's canal *F. Schlemm, German anatomist, 1795–1858.* A

venous channel at the junction of the cornea and sclera for the draining of aqueous humour. Also known as scleral venous sinus.

Schönlein–Henoch purpura or syndrome *J.L. Schönlein, German physician, 1793–1864; E.H. Henoch, German paediatrician, 1820–1910.* See PURPURA.

school health service responsible for delivering the Healthy Child Programme in schools. See HEALTHY CHILD PROGRAMME in schools.

school nurse a registered nurse who has undertaken further education to specialize in the health care of school-age children. Responsibilities include carrying out health assessments, health promotion, advice and education, monitoring growth and development, screening and caring for those with special educational needs and immunisation.

sciatica pain down the back of the leg in the area supplied by the sciatic nerve. It is usually caused by pressure on the nerve roots by a protrusion of an intervertebral disc.

scintillography the visual recording of the distribution of radioactivity in an organ after injection of a small dose of a radioactive substance specifically taken up by that organ.

sclera the fibrous coat of the eyeball, the white of the eye, which covers the posterior part and in front becomes the cornea.

scleroderma a disease marked by progressive hardening of the skin in patches or diffusely, with rigidity of the underlying tissues. It is often a chronic condition. See RAYNAUD'S PHENOMENON.

sclerosis the hardening of any part from an overgrowth of fibrous and connective tissue, often due to chronic inflammation. *Multiple s.* an autoimmune disease of unknown cause affecting the myelin which insulates nerves. It is a long-term condition which results in a wide range of symptoms.

sclerotherapy   treatment of oesoph-ageal varices, varicose veins and hae-morrhoids by the injection of sclerosing solutions to produce fibrosis.

sclerotic   1. hard; indurated; affected by sclerosis. 2. pertaining to the sclera of the eye. *S. coat* the tough membrane forming the outer covering of the eyeball, except in front of the iris, where it becomes the clear horny cornea.

sclerotomy   incision of the sclerotic coat, usually for the removal of a foreign body or for the relief of glaucoma.

scoliosis   lateral curvature of the spine. *See* LORDOSIS and KYPHOSIS.

scotoma   a blind or depressed area in the field of vision, due to some lesion of the retina. It is also found in glaucoma and in detachment of the retina.

SCR   summary care record. An elec-tronic patient record covering patients in England, containing important infor-mation derived from GP records about key medical information including med-ication, allergies and adverse reactions which can be accessed by authorized users involved directly in the patient's care.

screening   the carrying out of a test on a large number of people to identify those that have a particular disease for which treatment may be available. Screening tests include: testing of neo-nates for disorders which benefit from early diagnosis and treatment, for example cystic fibrosis; breast screen-ing with mammography; testing for faecal occult blood; blood pressure measurement, blood tests and ultra-sound examination in pregnancy; testing for prostate specific antigen and abdominal aortic aneurysm in men.

scrotum   the pouch of skin and soft tissues containing the testicles.

scurf   dandruff.

scurvy   hypoascorbaemia a rare defi-ciency disease caused by lack of vitamin C, which is found in raw fruits and vegetables. Clinical features include fatigue, oozing of blood from the gums

and bruising. The condition rapidly improves with adequate diet.

seasonal affective disorder syn-drome   abbreviated SADS. A condi-tion in which the person notices a change in mood or feelings according to the season of the year and hence the amount of exposure to (sun)light.

sebaceous   fatty, or pertaining to the sebum. *S. cyst see* CYST. *S. glands* found in the skin, communicating with the hair follicles and secreting sebum.

seborrhoea   a disease of the seba-ceous glands, marked by an excessive secretion of sebum which collects on the skin in oily scales.

sebum   the fatty secretion of the seba-ceous glands.

secondary   second in order of time or importance. *S. deposits see* METASTASIS. *S. intention* wound healing as the edges of a wound unite after the for-mation of granular tissue. *See* HEALING.

secretin   the hormone originating in the duodenum which, in the presence of bile salts, is absorbed into the blood-stream and stimulates the secretion of pancreatic juice.

secretion   a substance formed or con-centrated in a gland and passed into the alimentary tract, the blood or to the exterior. The secretions of the endo-crine glands include various hormones and are important in the overall regu-lation of body processes.

sedation   the allaying of irritability, the relief of pain or mental distress, and the promotion of sleep, particularly by drugs.

sedative   a drug or agent that lessens excitement and relieves tension. Sed-ative drugs are used to induce sleep.

sedentary   pertaining to sitting; phys-ically inactive.

sedimentation   the deposit of solid particles at the bottom of a liquid. *Erythrocyte s. rate* abbreviated ESR. *See* ERYTHROCYTE.

segregation   1. put or come apart from the rest. 2. the separation during meiosis of allelic genes as the chromosomes migrate towards opposite poles of the cell.

seizure also known as a fit, caused by a disturbance in the electrical activity of the brain. *Absence S.* seizure lasting around 15 seconds is manifested by a brief of staring and lapse in awareness.

selective mutism a severe anxiety disorder where a person is unable to speak in certain situations.

selective serotonin reuptake inhibitors (SSRIs) widely used antidepressive medication.

self 1. a term used to denote an animal's own antigenic constituents, in contrast to 'not-self', denoting foreign antigenic constituents. 2. the complete being of an individual, comprising both physical and psychological characteristics, and including both conscious and unconscious components.

self-actualization a level of psychological development in which innate potential is realized to the full, allowing transcendence of the environment. *See* MASLOW'S HIERARCHY OF NEEDS AND MOTIVATION.

self-care the personal care carried out by the patient, e.g., bathing, personal grooming, eating and toilet hygiene. May be with assistance or instruction from a health care worker. The aim of rehabilitative care is to maximize self-care and personal independence.

self-catheterization men, women and older children can be taught to pass a fine catheter into the urinary bladder to evacuate urine as required.

self-esteem a person's evaluation of their own worth as an individual.

self-examination of breast *see* BREAST.

self-examination of testes *see* TESTICULAR SELF-EXAMINATION.

self-harm deliberate damage to one's own body. Over half of people who die by suicide have a history of self-harm; however, the intention is more often to punish themselves, express their distress or relieve unbearable tension. Self-harm may sometimes be linked to

anxiety and depression. Most often occurs in young adults and is more common in women. Also referred to as self-injury or self-mutilation.

self-image an individual's concept of their own personality and abilities based on their own ideas and perceptions.

self-limited descriptive of a condition affecting health and wellbeing that runs a definite course regardless of external factors or influences, e.g., the common cold.

self-retaining catheter *See* CATHETER.

sella turcica a depression in the sphenoid body which protects the pituitary gland.

semen the secretion of seminal fluid from the prostate gland and spermatozoa from the testicles which is ejaculated from the penis during sexual intercourse.

semicircular formed in a half-circle. *S. canals* part of the labyrinth of the internal ear, consisting of three canals in the form of arches which contain fluid and are connected with the cerebellum by their nerve supply. Impressions of change of position of the body are registered in these canals by oscillation of the fluid, and are conveyed by the nerves to the cerebellum.

semicomatose in a condition of unconsciousness from which the patient can be roused. *See* COMA.

semilunar shaped like a half-moon. *S. cartilages* two crescent-shaped cartilages in the knee joint. *S. valve see* VALVE.

seminoma a malignant tumour of the testis that is highly radiosensitive.

semipermeable of a membrane, permitting the passage of some molecules and hindering that of others.

semiprone partly prone. Applied to a position in which the patient is lying face down but the knees are turned to one side.

senescence the process of growing old.

senile related to the involutional changes associated with old age. *S.*

dementia deterioration of mental activity in the elderly. *See* DEMENTIA.

sensation a feeling resulting from impulses sent to the brain by the sensory nerves.

sense the faculty by which conditions and properties of things are perceived, e.g., hunger or pain. *S. organ* one that receives a sensory stimulus: for instance, the eyes and ears. *Special s.* any one of the faculties of sight, hearing, touch, smell, taste and muscle sense, through which the consciousness receives impressions from the environment.

sensible 1. capable of being perceived. 2. sensitive. *S. perspiration* that which is obvious on the skin as moisture.

sensitization 1. the process of rendering susceptible. 2. an increase in the body's response to a certain stimulus, as in the development of an allergy. *Protein s.* the condition occurring in an individual when a foreign protein is absorbed into the body, e.g., shellfish causing urticaria when eaten. *See* DESENSITIZATION.

sensory relating to sensation. *S. cortex* that part of the cerebral cortex to which information is relayed by the sensory nerves. *S. deprivation* the effecting of a major reduction of sensory information received by the body. This is damaging to the person's ability to function normally, which is dependent upon constant stimulation. *S. nerve* an afferent nerve conveying impressions from the peripheral nerve endings to the brain or spinal cord. *S. overload* exposure to bright lights, constant loud music and noise that may result in distress, confusion and headaches. May occur in intensive care units.

sentiment an emotion directed towards some object or person. Sentiments are acquired and profoundly influence a person's actions.

separation anxiety disorder developmentally, young children experience feelings of distress at separation from home, parents or carers to whom they have formed an attachment. If hospitalized at this time without a 'live-in' parent or carer the child may regress to a former stage of development with food refusal and incontinence. Separation anxiety usually diminishes by the age of 3 or 4 years but occasionally may occur in older children resulting in nightmares, complaints of somatic symptoms (e.g., headaches, nausea or vomiting) and refusal to attend school. May be associated with depression.

sepsis an infection of the body by pus-forming bacteria. *Focal s.* a local focus of infection which produces general symptoms. *Oral s.* infection of the mouth which causes general ill-health by absorption of toxins. *Puerperal s.* infection of the uterus occurring after labour.

septic referring to or produced by sepsis. *S. arthritis* inflammation of a joint due to bacterial infection, most commonly affecting the knees or hips. *S. shock* a life-threatening condition in which there is tissue damage and a severe fall in blood pressure as a result of septicaemia. Toxic shock syndrome is one type of septic shock. *See* TOXIC SHOCK.

septicaemia the presence in the blood of large numbers of bacteria and their toxins. The symptoms are a rapid rise of temperature, which is later intermittent, rigors, sweating, and all the signs of acute fever.

septum a division or partition. *Atrial s., atrioventricular s.* along with ventricular septum, the partitions dividing the various cavities of the heart. *Nasal s.* the structure made of bone and cartilage which separates the nasal cavities. *Ventricular s. see earlier,* atrial septum.

sequela a pathological condition occurring after a disease and resulting from it.

sequestrum a piece of dead bone. Inflammation in bone leads to thrombosis of blood vessels, resulting in necrosis of the affected part, which separates from the living structure.

serious incident abbreviated SI. SIs include acts or omissions in care that result in unexpected or avoidable death, unexpected or avoidable injury resulting in serious harm—including those where the injury required treatment to prevent death or serious harm, abuse, NEVER EVENTS, incidents that prevent (or threaten to prevent) an organisation's ability to continue to deliver an acceptable quality of health care services and incidents that cause widespread public concern resulting in loss of confidence in health care services.

serological relating to serum. *S. tests* those that are dependent on the formation of antibodies in the blood as a response to specific organisms or proteins.

serology the scientific study of serum.

serosa a serous membrane. It consists of two layers: the visceral, in close contact with the organ, and the parietal, lining the cavity.

serotonin an amine present in blood platelets, the intestine and the central nervous system, which acts as a vasoconstrictor. It is derived from the amino acid tryptophan and is inactivated by monoamine oxidase.

serotype the type of organism identified by the kinds of antigens present in the cell. Used to classify microorganisms.

serous related to serum. *S. effusion* an effusion of serous exudate.

serum the clear, fluid residue of blood, from which the corpuscles and fibrin have been removed. *S. hepatitis* jaundice caused by hepatitis B virus, usually after a blood transfusion or an inoculation with contaminated material. *S. sickness* an allergic reaction usually 8–10 days after a serum injection. It may be manifest by an irritating urticaria, pyrexia and painful joints. It readily responds to adrenaline and antihistaminic drugs. *See* ANAPHYLAXIS.

severe acute respiratory syndrome abbreviated SARS. A serious acute respiratory illness caused by the SARS coronavirus known as SARS Co-V. The WHO monitors countries throughout the world for outbreaks; there have been none since 2004. Infected persons develop high fever (>38°C) and cough and/or dyspnoea followed by rapidly progressive respiratory compromise. Infected persons may also experience chills, muscle aches, headache and loss of appetite. The SARS virus is highly contagious and is predominantly transmitted by droplets or by direct and indirect contact. Shedding of the virus in faeces and urine also occurs. Mortality rates vary depending on age and underlying medical conditions. Treatment is symptomatic and intensive respiratory support including mechanical ventilation may be required.

sex 1. either of the two divisions of organic organisms described respectively as male and female. 2. to discover the sex of an organism. *S. chromosome* a chromosome that determines sex. Women have two X chromosomes and men have one X chromosome and one Y chromosome. *S. hormone* a steroid hormone produced by the ovaries or the testes and controlling sexual development. *S.-limited* pertaining to a characteristic found in only one sex. *S.-linked* pertaining to a characteristic that is transmitted by genes that are located on the sex chromosomes, e.g., haemophilia.

sexism a belief in the intrinsic superiority of one sex over the other often accompanied by prejudice, stereotyping and discrimination on the basis of sex.

sexual pertaining to sex. *S. abuse see* ABUSE. *S. development* the biological and psychosocial changes that lead to sexual maturity. *S. deviation* aberrant sexual activity; expression of the sexual instinct in practices which are socially prohibited or unacceptable, or biologically undesirable. *S. intercourse* coitus.

sexuality 1. the characteristic quality of the male and female reproductive elements. 2. the constitution of an individual in relation to sexual attitudes and behaviour.

sexually transmitted infection abbreviated STI. An infection transmitted either by means of sexual intercourse between heterosexual or homosexual individuals, or by intimate contact with the genitals, mouth and rectum. STIs include syphilis, gonorrhoea, human immunodeficiency virus (HIV) infection, acquired immunodeficiency syndrome (AIDS), chlamydial infection, genital herpes, non-specific urethritis, trichomoniasis, genital lice, scabies, genital warts, hepatitis B infection and yaws. 'Sexually transmitted infection' is now the preferred term for what was formerly known as sexually transmitted disease (STD) and venereal disease (VD).

SGA small for gestational age.

SGOT serum glutamic–oxalacetic transaminase, former name for ASPARATE AMINOTRANSFERASE (AST), an enzyme excreted by damaged heart muscle. A raised serum level occurs in myocardial infarction.

SGPT serum glutamic–pyruvic transaminase, former name for ALANINE TRANSAMINASE (ALT).

shaken baby syndrome also known as abusive head trauma. The presence of unexplained subdural haematoma (bleeding under the membrane surrounding the brain), retinal bleed and brain swelling in a baby. These injuries are caused by the violent shaking of the baby resulting in vomiting, convulsions, irritability, coma and death. See ABUSE.

shared care the coordinated care of patients across the primary and secondary health care interface. In obstetrics, a term used to describe antenatal care carried out by a midwife, an obstetrician and/or a general practitioner. *S. c. protocols* consensus protocols for the clinical management of patients across the interface of primary and secondary health care, e.g., for the prescribing of expensive drugs or the use of cytotoxic therapy.

shearing force a strain produced by pressure in the structure of a substance so that each layer slides over the next. In the body this may occur when any part is on a gradient; the deeper tissues slide towards the lower gradient and the skin remains with the supporting contact, e.g., sheets on a bed or on a chair. In the presence of moisture this friction is exacerbated and the deeper tissues become ischaemic. See PRESSURE ULCER.

sheath 1. an enveloping tubular structure or part. 2. a condom, worn on the erect penis during sexual intercourse to trap seminal fluid, preventing the transmission of human immunodeficiency virus (HIV) and other viruses and also reducing the risk of pregnancy.

shiatsu a form of manipulation in which the practitioner uses the thumbs, fingers and palms of the hands, knees, forearms, elbows and feet to apply pressure to the client's body in order to promote and maintain health.

Shigella a genus of gram-negative rod-like bacteria. Some species cause bacillary dysentery. *S. flexneri* and *S. shigae* are common in Asia, *S. dysenteriae* in the USA and *S. sonnei* in Western Europe.

shin the bony front of the leg below the knee. The tibia.

shingles herpes zoster. A severe and debilitating illness that increases with age. Individuals over the age of 70 years are offered a shingles (herpes zoster) vaccination. The aim is to reduce the incidence and severity of shingles in older people. See Appendix 10.

Shirodkar's suture *Shirodkar, Indian obstetrician, 1900–1971.* A cervical cerclage procedure to prevent abortion resulting from cervical incompetence. The internal os is closed by means of a purse-string suture which is removed shortly before term, or earlier if labour should begin.

shock a condition produced by severe illness or trauma in which there is a sudden fall in blood pressure. This leads to lack of oxygen in the tissues and greater permeability of the capillary walls, so increasing the degree of shock by greater loss of fluid. The patient has a cold, moist skin, a feeble pulse and a low blood pressure, and is distressed, thirsty and restless. *Allergic* or *anaphylactic s.* shock produced by the injection of a protein to which the patient is sensitive. *Cardiogenic s.* shock as a result of an acute heart condition such as myocardial infarction. *Hypovolaemic s.* shock resulting from a reduction in the volume of blood in the circulation after haemorrhage or severe burns. *Neurogenic s.* shock due to nervous or emotional factors. *Septic s. see* SEPTIC. *Shell s.* a form of post-traumatic stress disorder, first described in World War I caused by the stresses of warfare (*see* PTSD). *Toxic s. see* TOXIC.

shortsightedness myopia.

shoulder the junction of the clavicle and the scapula where the arm joins the body. *S. impingement syndrome* a common cause of shoulder pain affecting the rotator cuff tendon. *Frozen S.* also known as adhesive capsulitis. Pain and stiffness in the shoulder caused by inflammation and thickening of the capsule.

show the blood-stained discharge that occurs at the onset of labour.

shunt a diversion, particularly of blood, due to a congenital defect, disease or surgery.

sialolith a salivary calculus.

sibling one of a family of children having the same parents. Applied in psychology to one of two or more children of the same parent or substitute parent figure. *S. rivalry* jealousy, compounded of love and hate of one child for its sibling.

sickle-cell disease (SCD) a group of inherited red blood cell disorders. People with SCD have abnormal haemoglobin, called haemoglobin S or sickle haemoglobin, in the red blood cells. (*see* Figure) SCD is particularly common in people with an African or Caribbean family background. *See also* ANAEMIA.

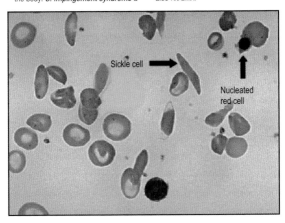

Sickle cell ➤

Nucleated red cell

side effect a result other than the one for which the drug or agent used is being given. Some side effects are predictable, e.g., hair loss with cytotoxic therapy, but others are unpredictable, e.g., skin eruptions or anaphylactic shock.

siderosis 1. chronic inflammation of the lung due to inhalation of particles of iron. 2. excess iron in the blood. 3. the deposit of iron in the tissues.

SIDS sudden infant death syndrome.

sigmoid shaped like the Greek letter sigma, Σ. *S. colon* or *flexure* that part of the colon in the left iliac fossa just above the rectum.

sigmoidoscope an instrument by which the interior of the rectum and sigmoid colon can be seen.

sign 1. any objective evidence of disease or dysfunction. 2. an observable physical phenomenon so frequently associated with a given condition as to be considered indicative of its presence. *S. language* hand and body language used by deaf people to communicate with others. *Vital s's* the signs of life, namely pulse, respiration and temperature.

significant other a person designated by the patient as the person who should be consulted in the event of an emergency or to contact when making arrangements for discharge.

silicosis fibrosis of the lung due to the inhalation of silica dust particles. It occurs in miners, stone masons and quarry workers.

Sims' position *J.M. Sims, American gynaecologist, 1813–1883.* A semiprone position. *See* POSITION.

singultus hiccups.

sinoatrial situated between the sinus venosus and the atrium of the heart. *S. node* the pacemaker of the heart. *See* NODE.

sinus 1. a cavity in a bone. 2. a venous channel, especially within the cranium. 3. an unhealed passage leading from an abscess or internal lesion to the surface. *Cavernous s.* a venous sinus

of the dura mater which lies along the body of the sphenoid bone. *Coronary s.* the vein that returns the blood from the heart muscle into the right atrium. *Ethmoidal s.* air spaces in the ethmoid bone. *Frontal s.* air spaces in the frontal bone. *S. arrhythmia see* ARRHYTHMIA. *S. thrombosis* clotting of blood in a cranial venous channel. In the lateral sinus it is a complication of mastoiditis. *Sphenoidal s.* air spaces in the sphenoid bone.

sinusitis inflammation of the lining of a sinus, especially applied to the bony cavities of the face.

six sigma a set of tools and techniques for improvement of processes.

Sjogren's syndrome a condition affecting parts of the body that produce fluids such as tears and saliva. Symptoms include dry eyes, dry mouth and dry skin.

skeleton the bony framework of the body, supporting and protecting the organs and soft tissues. (*See* Figures on pp. 357–358.)

skewed distribution in statistics, the degree to which the distribution is asymmetric around the mean. The normal distribution is symmetric, thus having a zero skewness.

skill mix the ratio of staff employed in an area of health care activity, whether qualified, trained or untrained, representing the availability of skills possessed by these staff.

skin the outer protective covering of the body. It consists of an outer layer, the epidermis or cuticle, and an inner layer, the dermis or corium, which is known as 'true skin'. (*See* Figure on p. 171.) *S. grafting* transplantation of pieces of healthy skin to an area where loss of surface tissue has occurred. *S. patch* a drug-impregnated adhesive patch which is applied to the skin. The drug is slowly absorbed, allowing its level in the blood to be maintained over a given period of time. *See* TRANSDERMAL PATCH. *S. tags* small, soft, skin-coloured growths that hand from the skin resembling a wart.

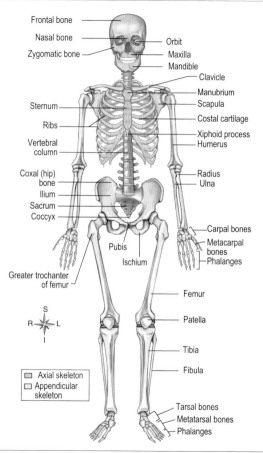

SKELETON – ANTERIOR VIEW

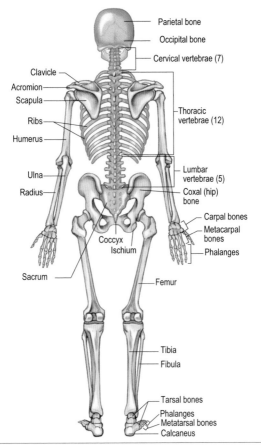

SKELETON – POSTERIOR VIEW

S. test application of a substance to the skin, or intradermal injection of a substance, to permit observation of the body's reaction to it.

skull the bony framework of the head, consisting of the cranium and facial bones. (*See* Figure.)

slapped cheek syndrome also known as fifth disease. A viral infection most commonly seen in children resulting in a bright red rash on the cheeks. It will usually clear up in 1–3 weeks.

sleep a period of rest for the body and mind, during which volition and consciousness are in partial or complete abeyance and the bodily functions partially suspended. It occurs in a 24-hour biological rhythm. Sleep occurs in cycles which have two distinct phases. Each phase lasts approximately 60–90 minutes: orthodox or non-rapid eye movement sleep (NREM), and paradoxical or rapid eye movement sleep (REM). Sleeping requirements vary, with each individual averaging between 4 and 10 hours in a 24-hour period. The purpose of sleep is unknown but sleep deprivation is harmful. *S. apnoea See* OBSTRUCTIVE SLEEP APNOEA. *S. walking see* SOMNAMBULISM.

sleeping sickness trypanosomiasis. A tropical fever occurring in parts of Africa, caused by a protozoal parasite (*Trypanosoma*) which is conveyed by the tsetse fly.

slim disease a term primarily used in Africa and other tropical countries for a progressive wasting disease associated with human immunodeficiency virus infection resulting in a loss of 10% or more of the baseline body weight. *See* AIDS and HUMAN IMMUNODEFICIENCY VIRUS.

slipped disc a prolapsed intervertebral disc which causes pressure on the spinal nerves. It may be very painful.

slough dead tissue caused by injury or inflammation. It separates from the healthy tissue and is ultimately washed away by exuded serum, leaving a granulating surface.

slow taking a long time before acting or showing signs of activity. *S.-acting drugs* those that are absorbed in the small intestine and have a sustained

SKULL

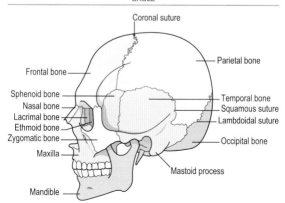

Coronal suture

Parietal bone

Frontal bone

Sphenoid bone

Nasal bone

Lacrimal bone

Ethmoid bone

Zygomatic bone

Maxilla

Mandible

Temporal bone

Squamous suture

Lambdoidal suture

Occipital bone

Mastoid process

release over a period of time. Many of these drugs are now incorporated into skin patches. *S. viruses* those infective agents that produce infection after a latent period in the body which may last weeks to months. *See* PRION.

small for gestational age abbreviated SGA. Term for a baby who is smaller or lighter in weight than expected for its gestational age. There is some variance in definition, from inclusion of babies below the 10th percentile to only those below the 5th percentile.

smallpox once a highly infectious viral disease, associated with high mortality. Eradicated from the world in 1980. Smallpox vaccination is no longer required for travellers to any part of the world.

smear A specimen for microscopic examination that has been prepared by spreading a thin film of the material across a glass slide.

smegma the secretion of sebaceous glands of the clitoris and prepuce.

smell one of the five senses. Air-borne particles are deposited and dissolved in the mucous membrane lining the nose, stimulating the endings of the olfactory nerve. The nose is able to distinguish a wide range of odours.

smoking the act of drawing into the mouth and puffing out the smoke of tobacco contained in a cigarette, cigar or pipe. A close relationship between smoking and lung cancer, heart disease and bronchitis and chronic obstructive airway disease has been established. Smoking is also harmful in pregnancy because the inhaled carbon monoxide reduces oxygen transportation in the body and the nicotine causes vasoconstriction of the arterioles. *Passive s.* the involuntary inhalation of tobacco smoke by people who do not smoke. Passive smoking has been shown to increase the risks of chest infections, coronary disease and tobacco-induced cancers in adults. Smoking in the workplace and other public environments, e.g., restaurants, shops, also planes

and buses, is regarded as an environmental health hazard and is banned throughout the UK. *S. in pregnancy* the infants of mothers who smoke are likely to suffer from fetal growth retardation and development may be delayed. Children exposed to passive smoking are prone to develop ear and chest infections and asthma. *Stop-s. initiatives* a range of programmes to support people to quit. They include the development of the stop smoking programme and nicotine replacement therapy available on the NHS.

snake a limbless reptile; a serpent. The bites of many snakes are poisonous to humans. *S. venom antitoxin* antivenin. A serum made from animals, usually horses, which have been immunized against the venom of a specific type of snake.

Snellen's test types *H. Snellen, Dutch ophthalmologist, 1834–1908.* Square-shaped letters on a chart, used for sight testing.

snow frozen water vapour. *Carbon dioxide s.* solid CO_2, which is used as a refrigerant; 'dry ice'. *S. blindness* photophobia due to the glare of snow also known as photokeratitis.

snuffles a chronic discharge from the nose, occurring in children, as a result of infection of the nasal mucous membrane.

social in health care, the prefix 'social' denotes a state, function or description to do with society, its peoples and its organization. *S. anxiety disorder* fear of social situations. *S. class* a category arising from the division of society into economic or occupational groupings. The most widely used grouping of social class or occupational scale in the UK was the Registrar General's Classification designed originally for use in the 1911 Census but extensively modified for use in later censuses. Occupations are now coded to be comparable with the International Standard Classification of Occupations (*see* Table). *S. drift* the movement of

International Standard Classification of Occupations	
Group	Occupation
1	Managers—such as company directors, senior officials in government, senior executives in large organizations (e.g., NHS Trust Managers)
2	Professionals—such as doctors, lawyers, academics, accountants, pharmacists, nurses, teachers
3	Technicians and associate professionals—such as science technicians, associate nurses, sports and fitness
4	Clerical support workers—such as officers, secretaries, client information workers
5	Service and sales workers—such as cooks, hairdressers, sales workers, teachers' aides
6	Skilled agriculture, forestry and fishery workers
7	Craft and related trade workers
8	Plant and machine operators and assemblers
9	Elementary occupations—such as cleaners and helpers, domestic, hotel and office cleaners, food preparation assistants
0	Armed forces occupations

people from one social class to another usually as a result of socioeconomic circumstances or as a result of morbid processes. Sometimes referred to as social mobility. *S. exclusion* people from groups which for a variety of reasons are not able to participate in community and mainstream activities, e.g., refugees and homeless people. *S. norms* socially accepted patterns of behaviour within a community or population. *S. worker* a professional qualified in the treatment of individual and social problems of patients and their families. *See also* MEDICAL (SOCIAL WORKER).

socialization the process by which society integrates the individual, and the individual learns to behave in socially acceptable ways.

sociology the scientific study of the development of human social relationships and organization, i.e., interpersonal and intergroup behaviour as distinct from the behaviour of an individual.

sociopath a person with an antisocial personality, morally irresponsible and seeking instant gratification; a psychopath.

sodium *symbol* Na. A metallic alkaline element widely distributed in nature, and forming an important constituent of animal tissue. *S. aminosalicylate* an antituberculous drug used in conjunction with other drugs in an established regime of management. *S. bicarbonate* an antacid widely used to treat digestive disorders, especially flatulence. Repeated use can cause alkalosis. *S. chloride* common salt. Its presence in the diet is necessary to health. *S. cromoglycate* a drug used as an inhalant in the treatment of asthma. *S. fluoride* a salt used in the fluoridation of water and also in toothpastes to prevent the formation of caries. *S. hypochlorite* a compound with germicidal properties used in solution to disinfect utensils, and diluted as a topical antibacterial agent in many environmental situations. *S. salicylate* an antipyretic and analgesic drug which acts as a non-steroidal anti-inflammatory (NSAID).

soft tissue mobilization *see* MASSAGE.

software computer data and programs containing instructions that detail how to use a specific computer facility.

solar plexus coeliac plexus. A network of sympathetic nerve ganglia in the abdomen; the nerve supply to abdominal organs below the diaphragm.

solar keratoses rough patches of skins caused by damage from repeated exposure to the sun.

solution a liquid in which one or more substances have been dissolved.

solvent a liquid that dissolves or has power to dissolve. *S. abuse* breathing in fumes from substances such as glue and other volatiles in order to feel high.

soma the body tissue as distinct from the germ cells.

somatic relating to the body wall as distinct from the viscera.

somnambulism walking and carrying out other complex activities during a state of sleep.

Somogyi effect *M. Somogyi, American biochemist, 1883–1971.* A rebound phenomenon occurring in diabetes mellitus; overtreatment with insulin induces hypoglycaemia, resulting in rebound hyperglycaemia and ketosis.

Sonne dysentery *C.O. Sonne, Danish bacteriologist, 1882–1948.* Bacillary dysentery which is common in the UK. The symptoms are diarrhoea, vomiting and abdominal pain. The causative agent is *Shigella sonnei.*

sonogram a record or display obtained by ultrasonic scanning. *See* ULTRASONOGRAPHY.

sonography *see* ULTRASONOGRAPHY.

sorbitol a sweetening agent which is converted into sugar in the body although it is slowly absorbed from the intestine. It is used in some diabetic foods and in intravenous feeding.

sordes brown crusts which form on the teeth and lips of unconscious patients, or those suffering from acute or prolonged fevers.

sore a general term for any ulcer or open skin lesion. *Cold s.* herpes simplex. *Hard s.* a syphilitic chancre. *Pressure s. See* PRESSURE ULCER. *Soft s.* a chancroid ulcer. *S. throat* inflammation of the larynx or pharynx, including tonsillitis.

souffle a blowing sound heard on auscultation. *Uterine s.* a sound due to the blood passing through the uterine arteries of the mother, particularly over the placental site. It is synchronous with the maternal pulse.

soya bean a legume that contains high-quality protein and little starch. *S. milk* historically used as a milk substitute for babies who could not tolerate constituents of breast or cow's milk. Other substitutes are now available and used instead.

spam unsolicited advertising or 'junk' mail sent to an individual address via e-mail.

Spansule trade name for a delayed-release form of capsule.

spasm a sudden involuntary muscle contraction. *Carpopedal s.* spasm of the hands and feet. A sign of tetany. *Clonic s.* alternate muscle rigidity and relaxation. *Habit s.* a tic. *Nictitating s.* spasmodic twitching of the eyelid. *Tetanic s.* violent muscle spasms, including opisthotonos. *Tonic s.* a sustained muscle rigidity.

spastic 1. caused by spasm; convulsive. 2. An offensive term used for one affected by spasticity. *S. colon see* IRRITABLE BOWEL SYNDROME. *S. paralysis* paralysis associated with lesions of the upper motor neurone, as in cerebral vascular accidents, and characterized by increased muscle tone and rigidity.

spasticity marked rigidity of muscles.

spatial pertaining to space.

SPC statistical process control.

special health authorities provide services on behalf of the National Health Service in England. They operate nationally rather than serve a specific geographical area. They are independent but can be subject to ministerial direction. Examples include the NHS

Litigation Authority and NHS Blood and Transplant Authority (NHS BT).

special needs a term generally used to describe the educational or learning needs of a child or adult with a learning disability. The expression may also be used in a wider context to describe the special educational needs of any child, e.g., one who is musically gifted.

specific 1. relating to a species. 2. a remedy that has a distinct curative influence on a particular disease. 3. related to a unit mass of a substance. *S. gravity* the density of fluid compared with that of an equal volume of water.

specimen a sample or part taken to show the nature of the whole, e.g., for chemical testing or microscopic survey.

specular reflection reflecting as from a surface. A term used in ultrasound to describe an interface which gives a strong reflection or echo, e.g., the fetal skull or bony prominence.

speech the act of communicating by sounds by means of a linguistic code. *Clipped s.* speech in which the words are cut short. *Explosive s.* loud, sudden utterances; a sign of brain disorder. *Incoherent s.* disconnected utterances made when the sequence of thought is disturbed, as in delirium. *Oesophageal s.* speech produced after laryngectomy by swallowing air and using it to vibrate within the oesophagus against the closed cricopharyngeal sphincter. *Scanning s.* speech in which the syllables are inappropriately separated from each other and are evenly stressed. Characteristic of cerebellar damage. *S. and language therapist* a professional qualified to identify, assess and rehabilitate persons with speech or language disorders and feeding difficulties. *Staccato s.* speech in which each syllable is separately pronounced. Characteristic of multiple sclerosis.

sperm 1. a spermatozoon. 2. the semen. *S. count* a method of determining the concentration of spermatozoa in a semen sample. *S. donation* seminal fluid provided by donors for

the fertilization of women whose partners are sterile.

spermatocele a cystic swelling in the epididymis, containing semen.

spermatozoon a mature male germ cell consisting of a flat-shaped head, a short middle part and a long tail. There are 300–500 billion spermatozoa in a normal ejaculate.

spermicide any agent that will destroy spermatozoa.

sphenoid wedge-shaped. *S. bone* the central part of the base of the skull.

spherocytosis the presence in the blood of erythrocytes that are more nearly spherical than biconcave. Characteristic of acholuric jaundice, it may also be hereditary.

sphincter a ring-shaped muscle, contraction of which closes a natural orifice.

sphygmomanometer an instrument for non-invasive measuring of the arterial blood pressure. Older versions contain a column of mercury, but are increasingly being replaced by electronic instruments which do not contain mercury.

spica a bandage or plaster cast applied to a joint, e.g., shoulder spica, to hold it in the required position.

spigot a small peg or bung to close the opening of a tube.

spina spine; a slender, thorn-like projection that occurs on many bones. *S. bifida* a congenital defect of non-union of one or more vertebral arches, allowing protrusion of the meninges and possibly their contents. The condition can be detected during pregnancy by ultrasonography, or by testing the blood of the mother or the amniotic fluid for the presence of increased levels of alpha-fetoprotein. Associated with this condition is a folate deficiency in the diet of women of child bearing age who should be encouraged to take sufficient amounts in their diet. See Appendix 1, MENINGOCELE and MENINGOMYELOCELE.

spinal relating to the spine. *S. anaesthesia see* ANAESTHESIA. *S. canal* the hollow in the spine formed by the neural arches of the vertebrae. It contains the spinal cord, meninges and cerebrospinal fluid. *S. caries* disease of the vertebrae, usually tuberculous. *See* POTT'S DISEASE. *S. column* the backbone; the vertebral column. *S. cord see* CORD. *S. cord compression see* CORD. (*See* Figure on p. 365.) *S. curvature* abnormal curving of the spine. If associated with caries, it is known as Pott's disease. *See* KYPHOSIS, LORDOSIS and SCOLIOSIS. *S. jacket* a moulded support for the spine used to provide stabilization to treat a number of spinal conditions including scoliosis. *S. muscular atrophy* a serious progressive genetic disorder causing muscle weakness. *S. nerves* the 31 pairs of nerves which leave the spinal cord at regular intervals throughout its length. They pass out in pairs, one on either side between each of the vertebrae, and are distributed to the periphery. *S. puncture* lumbar or cisternal puncture.

spine 1. the backbone or vertebral column, consisting of 33 vertebrae, separated by fibrocartilaginous discs, and enclosing the spinal cord. 2. a sharp process of bone.

spinnbarkeit [Ger.] a thread of mucus secreted by the cervix uteri. Used to determine ovulation.

spirochaete one of a group of microorganisms in the form of a spiral, some of which are found in impure fresh or salt water. The group includes the species *Treponema, Borrelia* and *Leptospira.*

spirograph an instrument for registering respiratory movements.

spirometer an instrument for measuring the air capacity of the lungs.

Spitz–Holter valve *E.B. Spitz, American paediatric neurosurgeon, 1919–2006; J.W. Holter, American engineer, 1916–2003.* A device used in the treatment of hydrocephalus to drain the cerebrospinal fluid from the ventricles into the superior vena cava or the right atrium.

splanchnic pertaining to the viscera. *S. nerves* sympathetic nerves to the viscera.

spleen a large, vascular, gland-like but ductless organ, coloured a reddish purple and situated in the left hypochondrium under the border of the stomach. It manufactures lymphocytes and breaks down red blood corpuscles.

splenectomy excision of the spleen.

splenomegaly enlargement of the spleen.

splint an appliance used to support or immobilize a part while healing takes place or to correct or prevent deformity.

spondylitis inflammation of the vertebrae. *Ankylosing s.* a rheumatic disease, chiefly of young males, in which there is abnormal ossification with pain and rigidity of the intervertebral, hip and sacroiliac joints.

spondylolisthesis a sliding forwards or displacement of one vertebra over another, usually the fifth lumbar over the sacrum, causing symptoms such as low back pain, as a result of pressure on the nerve roots.

spondylosis ankylosis of the vertebral joints, usually caused by a degenerative disease of the intervertebral discs, such as osteoarthritis.

spontaneous occurring without apparent cause. Applied to certain types of fracture and to recovery from a disease without any specific treatment.

sporadic pertaining to isolated cases of a disease that occurs in various and scattered places (compare ENDEMIC and EPIDEMIC).

spore 1. a reproductive stage of some of the lowest forms of vegetable life, e.g., moulds. 2. a protective state which some bacteria are able to assume in adverse conditions, such as lack of moisture, food or heat. In this form the organism can remain alive, but inert, for years.

sporulation the formation of spores by bacteria, e.g., clostridia or bacilli.

spotted fever a febrile disease characterized by a skin eruption, such as

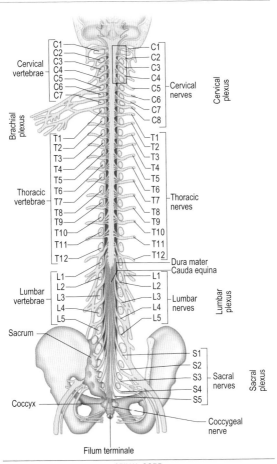

Cervical vertebrae — C1, C2, C3, C4, C5, C6, C7

Brachial plexus

Thoracic vertebrae — T1, T2, T3, T4, T5, T6, T7, T8, T9, T10, T11, T12

Lumbar vertebrae — L1, L2, L3, L4, L5

Sacrum

Coccyx

C1, C2, C3, C4, C5, C6, C7, C8 — Cervical nerves — Cervical plexus

T1, T2, T3, T4, T5, T6, T7, T8, T9, T10, T11, T12 — Thoracic nerves

Dura mater
Cauda equina

L1, L2, L3, L4, L5 — Lumbar nerves — Lumbar plexus

S1, S2, S3, S4, S5 — Sacral nerves — Sacral plexus

Coccygeal nerve

Filum terminale

SPINAL CORD

Rocky Mountain spotted fever, and other infections due to tick-borne rickettsiae.

sprain wrenching of a joint, producing laceration of the capsule or stretching of the ligaments, with consequent swelling, which is due to effusion of fluid into the affected part.

spreadsheet a computer program that aligns data in tables, rows and columns.

sprue a disease of malabsorption in the intestine, which may be tropical or non-tropical in form. There is steatorrhoea, diarrhoea, glossitis and anaemia.

sputum material expelled from the air passages through the mouth. It consists chiefly of mucus and saliva; in diseased conditions of the air passages it may be purulent, blood-stained and frothy and may contain many bacteria. It must always be regarded as highly infectious. *Rusty s.* that in which altered blood permeates the mucus. Characteristic of acute lobar pneumonia.

squamous scaly. *S. bone* the thin part of the temporal bone which articulates with the parietal and frontal bones. *S. cell carcinoma* a malignancy of the squamous cells of the bronchus. *S. epithelium* epithelium composed of flat and scale-like cells.

squint *see* STRABISMUS.

staging 1. the determination of distinct phases or periods in the course of a disease. 2. the classification of neoplasms according to the extent of the tumour. *TNM s.* staging of tumours according to three basic components: primary tumour (T), regional nodes (N) and metastasis (M). Subscripts are used to denote size and degree of involvement; for example, 0 indicates undetectable, and 1, 2, 3 and 4 a progressive increase in size or involvement.

stammering stuttering; a speech disorder in which the utterance is broken by hesitation and repetition or prolongation of words and syllables.

standard deviation in statistics, a measure of the dispersion of a random variable: the square root of the average squared deviation from the mean. For data that have a normal distribution, about 68% of the data points fall within one standard deviation from the mean and about 95% fall within two standard deviations.

standard precautions the current model of best practice in infection control, a synthesis of UNIVERSAL PRECAUTIONS and BODY SUBSTANCE ISOLATION. Standard precautions are designed to reduce the risk of transmission of blood-borne and other pathogens in hospital, from both recognized and unrecognized sources of infection, and apply to all patients all the time. Their implementation requires that nurses and other health care professionals take appropriate measures, e.g., wear gloves, to avoid contact with (a) blood; (b) all body fluids, secretions and excretions except sweat, regardless of whether or not they contain visible blood; (c) non-intact skin; and (4) mucous membranes. Standard precautions are used in association with newer TRANSMISSION-BASED PRECAUTIONS. *See also* INFECTION CONTROL and Appendix 11.

standards statements of the levels of service or care related to specific topics which staff agree to provide. Often accompanied by a description of the structure (staff, equipment, etc.) and process needed to attain specified observable outcomes. *S. of care* a measure by which a professional's conduct is compared, comprises a list of those acts that a prudent professional practitioner would have carried out (or not performed) in similar circumstances within health care.

stapedectomy removal of the stapes and insertion of a vein graft or other device to re-establish conduction of sound waves in otosclerosis.

stapediolysis an operation in which the footpiece of the stapes is mobilized to aid conduction in deafness from otosclerosis.

stapes the stirrup-shaped bone of the middle ear.

Staphylococcus a genus of gram-positive non-mobile bacteria which, under the microscope, appear grouped together in small masses like bunches of grapes. They are normally present on the skin and mucous membranes. *S. pyogenes* (or *S. aureus*) is a common cause of boils, carbuncles and abscesses.

staphyloma a protrusion of the cornea or the scleric coat of the eyeball as the result of inflammation or a wound.

starch carbohydrates are stored as starch in many plants. Starch consists of linked glucose units in two forms, amylose and amylopectin, providing a valuable source of energy and fibre in the diet.

startle reflex SEE MORO REFLEX.

stasis the stagnation or stoppage of the flow of a fluid. *Intestinal s.* sluggish movement of faeces through the bowel, owing to partial obstruction or to impairment of the action of the intestinal muscles also known as gastrointestinal hypomobility or ileus. *Venous s.* congestion of blood in the veins.

statementing the provision by a local authority of a statement following formal assessment of the special educational needs of a child with mental or physical disabilities to attend either a mainstream school with extra help, or a special school.

statistical process control abbreviated SPC. The use of statistical concepts which place the emphasis on the continuous monitoring of a process rather than the reliance on a single outcome as the sole measure for quality assurance in the delivery of a service.

statistical significance in research, a conclusion that the results achieved have little probability of occurring by chance alone.

statistics 1. numerical facts pertaining to a particular subject or body of objects. 2. the science dealing with the collection, tabulation and analysis of numerical facts.

status condition. *S. asthmaticus* a severe and prolonged attack of asthma. *S. epilepticus* a serious condition in which there is rapid succession of epileptic fits. *S. lymphaticus* a condition in which all lymphatic tissues are hypertrophied, also known as lymphatism.

STD sexually transmitted disease now generally called sexually transmitted infections or STI.

steapsin the fat-splitting enzyme (lipase) of the pancreatic juice.

steatoma 1. a sebaceous cyst. 2. a lipoma; a fatty tumour.

steatorrhoea the presence of an excess of fat in the stools owing to malabsorption of fat by the intestines.

Stein–Leventhal syndrome *I.F. Stein, American gynaecologist, 1887–1976; M.L. Leventhal, American gynaecologist, 1901–1971.* Condition affecting females in which obesity, hirsutism and sterility are associated with polycystic ovaries and menstrual irregularities. Polycystic ovary syndrome (PCOS).

Steinmann pin *F. Steinmann, Swiss surgeon, 1872–1932.* A fine metal rod, passed through a bone, by which extension is applied to overcome muscle contraction in certain fractures. *See* KIRSCHNER WIRE.

stellate star-shaped. *S. fracture* a radiating fracture of the patella. *S. ganglion* the inferior cervical ganglion. A star-shaped collection of nerve cells at the base of the neck.

stem cell transplant replacement of damaged blood cells caused by conditions such as leukaemia and lymphoma. An allogeneic transplant involves transplanting cells from a healthy compatible donor. An autologous stem cell transplants involves taking and later replacing cells from the host after any damaged or diseased cells have been removed.

stenosis abnormal narrowing or contraction of a channel or opening. *Aortic* *s.* narrowing of the opening of the aortic valve due to scar tissue formation as the result of inflammation. *Mitral s.* narrowing of the orifice of the mitral valve, usually following rheumatic fever. *Pulmonary s.* a congenital narrowing of the opening from the right ventricle of the heart into the pulmonary artery. *Pyloric s.* narrowing of the pyloric orifice of the stomach due to scar tissue, new growth or congenital hypertrophy.

stent a tube of metal or plastic placed inside a canal, duct or artery to prevent or counteract a disease-induced, localized flow constriction, thus keeping the passageway open.

stercobilin a brown-orange pigment derived from bile and present in faeces.

stereognosis the ability to visualize the shape of an object by touch alone.

stereotype an oversimplified generalization about a group or class of people which is often then applied to an individual. May form a basis for discrimination and prejudice.

stereotypy repetitive actions carried out or maintained for long periods in a monotonous fashion.

sterile 1. aseptic; free from microorganisms. 2. infertile; incapable of producing young.

sterility 1. the state of being free from microorganisms. 2. the inability of a woman to become pregnant, or of a man to produce potent spermatozoa.

sterilization 1. rendering dressings, instruments, etc. aseptic by destroying or removing all microbial life. 2. rendering incapable of reproduction by any means.

sterilizer an apparatus in which objects can be sterilized. *See* AUTOCLAVE.

sternotomy the operation in which the sternum is cut through to enable the heart to be reached.

sternum the breastbone; the flat narrow bone in the centre of the anterior wall of the thorax.

steroid one of a group of hormones chemically related to cholesterol. They include oestrogen and androgen,

progesterone and the corticosteroids. They may be naturally occurring or they may be synthesized.

sterol one of a group of steroid alcohols which includes cholesterol and ergosterol.

stertorous snore-like; applied to a snoring sound produced in breathing during sleep or in coma.

stethoscope the instrument used for listening to internal body sounds, especially from the heart and lung. It consists of a hollow tube, one end of which is placed over the part to be examined and the other at the ear of the examiner.

Stevens–Johnson syndrome *A.M. Stevens, American paediatrician, 1884–1945; F.C. Johnson, American paediatrician, 1894–1934.* A severe form of erythema multiforme in which the lesions may involve the oral and anogenital mucosa, eyes and viscera, associated with such constitutional symptoms as malaise, headache, fever, arthralgia and conjunctivitis.

STI sexually transmitted infection.

stigma any mark characteristic of a condition or defect, or of a disease. May also be applied to any physical or social quality of a person that is perceived by others as a negative attribute.

stillbirth a baby born after the 24th week of pregnancy and who has not, at any time after being completely expelled from its mother, breathed or shown any sign of life. *S. certificate* a certificate issued to the parents by a registered medical practitioner who was present at the birth or examined the body.

Still's disease *Sir G.F. Still, British paediatrician, 1868–1941.* A form of rheumatoid arthritis in children, sometimes associated with enlargement of the lymph glands. Also known as juvenile rheumatoid arthritis.

stimulant an agent that causes increased energy or functional activity of any organ.

stimulus *pl.* stimuli. Any agent, act or influence that produces functional or trophic reaction in a receptor or an irritable tissue. *Conditioned s.* a neutral object or event that is psychologically related to a naturally stimulating object or event and which causes a CONDITIONED RESPONSE (*see also* CONDITIONING). *Discriminative s.* a stimulus, associated with reinforcement, which exerts control over a particular form of behaviour; the subject discriminates between closely related stimuli and responds positively only in the presence of that stimulus. *Eliciting s.* any stimulus, conditioned or unconditioned, that elicits a response. *Structured s.* a well-organized and unambiguous stimulus, the perception of which is influenced to a greater extent by the characteristics of the stimulus than by those of the perceiver. *Threshold s.* a stimulus that is just strong enough to elicit a response. *Unconditioned s.* any stimulus that is capable of eliciting an unconditioned response (*see also* CONDITIONING). *Unstructured s.* an unclear or ambiguous stimulus, the perception of which is influenced to a greater extent by the characteristics of the perceiver than by those of the stimulus.

stitch 1. a popular term used to describe a sudden sharp pain usually due to spasm of the diaphragm. 2. a suture. *S. abscess* pus from a formation where a stitch has been inserted.

Stokes–Adams syndrome *Sir W. Stokes, Irish surgeon, 1804–1878; R. Adams, Irish physician, 1791–1875.* Attacks of syncope or fainting due to cerebral anaemia in some cases of complete heart block. The heart stops temporarily but breathing continues. The syndrome is treated by using an artificial pacemaker.

stoma *pl. stomata* 1. a mouth or mouth-like opening. 2. an artificial opening in the skin surface leading into one of the tubes forming the alimentary canal. *See* COLOSTOMY and ILEOSTOMY.

stomach the dilated portion of the alimentary canal between the oesophagus and the duodenum, just below the diaphragm. *Bilocular* or *hourglass s.* one divided into two parts by a constriction. *S. pH electrode* apparatus used to measure gastric contents in situ. *S. pump* a pump that removes the contents of the stomach by suction. Gastric lavage.

stomatitis inflammation of the mouth, either simple or with ulceration, caused by a vitamin deficiency or by a bacterial or fungal infection. *Angular s.* cracking at the corners of the mouth, usually due to riboflavin deficiency. *Aphthous s.* that characterized by small, white, painful ulcers on the mucous membrane. *Ulcerative s.* painful shallow ulcers on the tongue, cheeks and lips. A severe type that may produce serious constitutional effects.

stone a calculus.

stool a motion or discharge from the bowels.

STP sustainable transformation partnerships. Partnerships between local authorities and all local health providers aimed at improving health and social care in England by ensuring there are inclusive plans to meet the needs of the local population and that there is optimum efficiency across health systems.

strabismus squint; heterotropia. A deviation of the eye from its normal direction. It is called convergent when the eye turns in towards the nose, and divergent when it turns outwards. *Concomitant s.* a squint in which the angle of deviation stays constant.

strabotomy the division of ocular muscles in the treatment of strabismus.

strain 1. overuse or stretching of a part, e.g., a muscle or tendon. 2. a group of microorganisms within a species. 3. to pass a liquid through a filter.

strangulated compressed or constricted so that the circulation of the blood is arrested. *S. hernia see* HERNIA.

strangulation 1. choking caused by compression of the air passages. 2.

arrested circulation to a part, which will result in gangrene.

strangury a painful, frequent desire to micturate, but in which only a few drops of urine are passed with difficulty.

stratified arranged in layers. *S. tissue* a covering tissue in which the cells are arranged in layers. The germinating cells are the lowest, and as surface cells are shed there is continual replacement.

stratum a layer; applied to structures such as the skin and mucous membranes. *S. corneum* the outer, horny layer of the epidermis.

Streptococcus a genus of gram-positive spherical bacteria occurring in chains or pairs. Divided into various groups. The first group includes the beta-haemolytic human and animal pathogens; the second and third include alpha-haemolytic parasitic forms occurring as normal flora in the body; and the fourth is made up of saprophytic forms. *S. mutans* implicated in dental caries. *S. pneumoniae* pneumococcus, the most common cause of lobar pneumonia; also causes serious forms of meningitis, septicaemia, empyema and peritonitis. *S. pyogenes* beta-haemolytic, toxigenic, pyogenic streptococci causing many conditions including pharyngitis, erysipelas and cellulitis, scarlet fever, rheumatic fever, necrotizing fasciitis, glomerulonephritis and toxic shock syndrome.

streptokinase an enzyme derived from a streptococcal culture and used to liquefy clotted blood and pus.

Streptomyces a genus of soil bacteria from which some antibiotics are derived.

stress any factor, mental or physical, the pressure of which can adversely affect the functioning of the body. *S. disorders* those resulting from an individual's inability to withstand stress. *S. fracture* one that occurs as a result of repetitive jarring of a bone, e.g.,

metatarsal bones in the foot associated with long-distance running and walking. *S. incontinence* incontinence, usually of urine, when the intra-abdominal pressure is raised, such as in coughing, sneezing or laughing. *S. ulcer* an acute peptic ulcer, which may be multiple and develop after severe burns, major injuries and occur sometimes during serious illness. The cause is unknown.

stressor any life event or change that causes a person stress and which in some circumstances may precipitate distress or deterioration in mental health. These factors may be physical, physiological or psychosocial, e.g., pain and hunger, loss of job, bereavement, divorce, etc.

stria *pl.* striae. A line or stripe. *Striae gravidarum* the lines that appear on the abdomen of pregnant women. They are red in first pregnancy, but white subsequently, and are due to stretching and rupture of the elastic fibres. Stretch marks.

striated striped. *S. muscle* voluntary muscle. *See* MUSCLE.

stricture a narrowing or local contraction of a canal. It may be caused by muscle spasm, new growth, or scar tissue formation after inflammation.

stridor a harsh, vibrating, shrill sound, produced during respiration when there is partial obstruction of the larynx or trachea.

stroke a term to describe the sudden onset of symptoms that occurs when the blood supply to part of the brain is cut off affecting movement, sensation, speech and vision. There may be paralysis and loss of sensation down one side of the body or one side of the face. Stroke may be ischaemic where the blood supply is stopped due to a blood clot or haemorrhage where a weakened blood vessel supplying the brain bursts. *Heat s.* a hyperpyrexia accompanied by cerebral symptoms. It may occur in someone newly arrived in a very hot climate.

stroma the connective tissue forming the ground substance, framework or matrix of an organ, as opposed to the functioning part or parenchyma.

Strongyloides a genus of nematode worms, one of which, *S. stercoralis*, is common in tropical countries and causes diarrhoea and intestinal ulcers.

strontium *symbol* Sr. A metallic element. Isotopes of strontium are used in bone scanning to detect abnormalities. *S.-90* a radioactive isotope used in radiotherapy in the treatment of bone malignancies.

structuralism in psychology, the view that the important influences on people's lives are the basic content of consciousness including intellect, feelings, memory and behaviour. Structuralist approaches in anthropology and sociology are concerned with the social structures within which people function.

Stryker frame an apparatus specially designed for care of patients with injuries of the spinal cord or paralysis. It is constructed of pipe and canvas and is designed so that one nurse can turn the patient without difficulty.

study skills a set of techniques, strategies and behaviour patterns which form a structured approach to learning.

stupor a state of semi-unconsciousness, occurring in the course of many varieties of mental illness, in which the patient does not move or speak, and usually only responds to noxious stimuli.

Sturge–Weber syndrome *W.A. Sturge, British physician, 1850–1919; Sir H.D. Weber, British physician, 1824–1918.* A rare congenital abnormality in which there is a port wine stain on the face with an angioma of the meninges on the same side. Common symptoms are epilepsy, hemiplegia and associated learning difficulties. Also known as encephalotrigeminal angiomatosis.

stuttering *see* STAMMERING.

stye *see* HORDEOLUM.

stylet a wire or rod for keeping clear the lumen of catheters, cannulae and hollow needles.

styloid like a pen. *S. process* a long pointed spine, particularly one projecting from the temporal bone. Also processes on the ulna and radius.

styptic an astringent which, applied locally, arrests haemorrhage.

subacute moderately acute. Applied to a disease that progresses moderately rapidly, but does not become acute.

subarachnoid below the arachnoid. *S. haemorrhage* bleeding into the subarachnoid space from a vessel in the brain. Commonly, due to a rupture of a cerebral aneurysm or to trauma. Blood is present in the cerebrospinal fluid. *S. space* between the arachnoid and pia mater of the brain and spinal cord, and containing cerebrospinal fluid.

subclavian beneath the clavicle. *S. artery* the main vessel of supply to the neck and arms.

subclinical without clinical manifestations; said of the early stages or a very mild form of a disease.

subconscious 1. not conscious yet able to be recalled to consciousness. 2. in psychoanalysis, the part of the mind that retains memories which cannot without much effort be recalled to mind.

subculture a subgroup that diverges from the dominant culture in a society but may retain some of its customs and values, while rejecting others.

subcutaneous beneath the skin. *S. injection* one given hypodermically.

subdural below the dura mater. *S. haematoma* a blood clot between the arachnoid and dura mater. It may be acute or arise slowly from a minor injury.

subinvolution incomplete or delayed return of the uterus to its pregravid size during the puerperium, usually as the result of retained products of conception and infection.

subjective related to the individual. *S. symptoms* those of which the patient is aware by sensory stimulation, but which cannot easily be seen by others. *See also* OBJECTIVE.

sublimate a substance obtained by sublimation.

sublimation 1. the vaporization of a solid and its condensation into a solid deposit. 2. in psychoanalysis, a redirecting of energy at an unconscious level. The transference into socially acceptable channels of tendencies that cannot be expressed. An important aspect of maturity.

subliminal below the threshold of perception.

sublingual beneath the tongue. *S. glands* two small salivary glands in the floor of the mouth.

subluxation partial dislocation of a joint.

submaxillary beneath the lower jaw. *S. glands* two salivary glands situated under the lower jaw.

submucous beneath mucous membrane. *S. resection* an operation to correct a deflected nasal septum.

subnormal below normal.

subphrenic beneath the diaphragm. *S. abscess* one that develops below the diaphragm, usually after peritonitis or from postoperative infection.

substitution the act of putting one thing in place of another. In psychology, this may be a foster or adoptive mother in the place of the child's own mother.

substrate a substance on which an enzyme acts.

succus a juice. *S. gastricus* gastric juice.

succussion a method of determining when free fluid is present in a cavity in the body. A sound of splashing is heard when the patient moves or is deliberately moved.

sucrose a disaccharide obtained from cane or beet sugar.

suction 1. the process of sucking. 2. the removal of gas or fluid from a cavity or other container by means of reduced pressure. *Post-tussive s.* a sucking noise heard in the lungs just after a cough.

sudamen a small white vesicle formed in the sweat glands after prolonged sweating.

sudden infant death syndrome abbreviated SIDS. The sudden and unexpected death of an apparently healthy infant, typically occurring in the first six months, and not explained by postmortem studies. Called cot death because the infant often is found dead in the cot and dies whilst asleep. The prone position, respiratory illness and infection, tobacco smoke and overheating have been found to be risk factors. Parents and carers are advised to put their babies to sleep on their backs at the foot of the cot to prevent them wriggling under the bed clothes, not to overheat the room, not to smoke in the same room and to seek advice from a health professional if the baby seems unwell. There is also an associated between co-sleeping (sleeping with the baby) and SIDS.

sudor sweat; perspiration.

sudorific diaphoretic; an agent causing sweating.

suffocation asphyxiation; a cessation of breathing caused by occlusion of the air passages, leading to unconsciousness and ultimately to death.

suffusion a process of diffusion or overspreading, as in flushing of the skin; blushing.

sugar a group of sweet carbohydrates classified chemically as monosaccharides or disaccharides. The following are included: *beet s.* obtained from sugar beet; *cane s.* obtained from sugar cane; *fructose* fruit sugar; *grape s.* dextrose, glucose; *milk s.* lactose. *Muscle s.* inositol; a sugar-like compound found in animal tissue, particularly in muscle, and also in many plant tissues.

suggestibility inclination to act on suggestions of others.

suggestion a tool of psychotherapy in which an idea is presented to and accepted by a patient. *Posthypnotic s.* one implanted in a patient under hypnosis, which lasts after return to a normal condition.

SUI serious incident.

suicide the intentional taking of one's own life. Legally, a death suspected of being due to violence that is self-inflicted is not termed a suicide unless the victim leaves positive evidence of the intention to commit suicide, or the method of death is such that a verdict of suicide is inevitable. Attitudes to suicide are culturally determined and vary from one group to another. Depression is the commonest cause of suicide and severely depressed people are always at risk.

sulcus a furrow or fissure; applied especially to those of the brain.

summary care record *see* SCR.

sunburn a dermatitis due to exposure to the sun's rays, causing burning and redness.

sunstroke a profound disturbance of the body's heat-regulating mechanism caused by prolonged exposure to excessive heat from the sun. Persons over 40 and those in poor health are most susceptible to it. *See* STROKE.

superego that part of the personality that is concerned with moral standards and ideals that are derived unconsciously from parents, teachers and environment, and influences the person's whole mental make-up, acting as a control on impulses of the ego.

superfecundation the fertilization of two or more ova, produced during the same menstrual cycle, by spermatozoa from separate coital acts.

superfetation the fertilization of a second ovum when pregnancy has already started, producing two fetuses of different maturity.

supernumerary 1. present in excess of the normal or required number; extra, as in supernumerary digit. 2. students and new staff placed in clinical areas for orientation and/or for supervised practice who are not included in the staffing numbers.

superior above; the upper of two parts.

supine 1. lying on the back, with the face upwards. 2. with the palm of the hand upwards. *See* PRONE.

support in the health care setting, the assistance and aid that is provided to patients and their families. This support may be physical, e.g., in assisting a patient to walk, or psychological, as when listening to the concerns of relatives. *S. worker* fulfilling a supporting role such as a health care assistant, physiotherapy assistant or foot care assistant. In clinical areas all these work under the supervision of a registered practitioner who is responsible for the support worker's practice and activities.

suppository a medicated solid substance, prepared for insertion into the rectum or vagina, which will dissolve at body temperature.

suppression 1. complete cessation of a secretion. 2. in psychology, conscious inhibition as distinct from repression, which is unconscious. *S. of urine* no secretion of urine by the kidneys.

suppuration the formation of pus.

supracondylar above the condyles. *S. fracture* one above the lower end of the humerus or femur.

supraorbital above the orbit of the eye.

suprapubic above the pubic bones. *S. cystotomy* surgical incision of the urinary bladder just above the pubic bones.

suprarenal above the kidney. *S. gland* adrenal gland. One of a pair of triangular endocrine glands situated on the upper surface of the kidneys. *See* ADRENAL.

supraventricular tachycardia (SVT) abnormally fast heartbeat of over 100 beats per minute not connected with exercise.

Sure Start children's centre which gives help and advice on child and family health, parenting, money, training and employment. *See* CHILDREN'S CENTRES.

surfactant a surface-active agent. A mixture of phospholipids that is secreted into the pulmonary alveoli and reduces the surface tension of pulmonary fluids, thus contributing to the elastic properties of pulmonary tissue. Surfactant can be instilled via a tracheal catheter as treatment for respiratory distress syndrome. *See also* RESPIRATORY (DISTRESS SYNDROME OF NEWBORN).

surgeon a medical practitioner who specializes in surgery. By custom the surgeon's title is Mr, Mrs, Miss or Ms, as opposed to physicians who are called Doctor.

surgery the branch of medicine that treats disease by operative measures.

surrogate a real or imaginary substitute for a person or object in someone's life. *S. mother* a woman who carries a child for another (the commissioning parent) with the intention that the child be handed over after birth for adoption.

surveillance the monitoring, recording, analysing and reporting of the occurrence of infectious outbreaks of disease, e.g., hospital-acquired infections, bacterial bloodstream infections and wound infection following orthopaedic surgery. The process can be applied to other incidences, e.g., the cases of notifiable disease in a population.

survey the systematic collection of information, not forming part of a scientific epidemiological study.

susceptibility lack of resistance to infection. The opposite to immunity.

suspensory supporting a part. *S. bandage* one applied to support a part of the body, particularly the scrotum or the lower jaw. *S. ligament* a ligament that supports or suspends an organ, e.g., that of the lens of the eye.

suture 1. a stitch or series of stitches used to close a wound (*see* Figure). 2. the jagged line of junction of the bones of the cranium. *Atraumatic s.* a suture fused to the needle to obtain a single

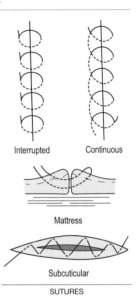

Interrupted   Continuous

Mattress

Subcuticular

SUTURES

thickness through each puncture of the needle. *Cerclage s.* encircling with a ring or loop of non-absorbable suture to keep an incompetent cervix closed to prevent miscarriage. Cervical cerclage. *See* SHIRODKAR'S PROCEDURE. *Continuous s.* a form of oversewing with one length of suture. *Coronal s.* the junction between the frontal and parietal bones. *Everting s.* a type of mattress stitch that turns the edges outwards to give a closer approximation. *Interrupted s.* a series of separate sutures. *Lambdoid s.* the junction between the parietal and occipital bones. *Mattress s.* one in which each suture is taken twice through the wound, giving a loop one side and a knot the other. *Purse-string s.* a circular continuous suture round a small wound or appendix stump. *Sagittal s.* the junction between the two occipital bones. *Subcuticular s.* a continuous suture placed just below the skin. *Tension s.* or *relaxation s.* one taking a large bite and relieving the tension on the true stitch line.

swab 1. a small piece of cotton wool or gauze. 2. in pathology, a dressed sterile stick used in taking bacteriological specimens.

swallowing the taking in of a substance through the mouth and pharynx and into the oesophagus. It is a combination of a voluntary act and a series of reflex actions. Once begun, the process operates automatically. Also called deglutition.

sweat perspiration; a clear watery fluid secreted by the sweat glands. *S. glands* coiled tubular glands situated in the dermis with long ducts to the skin surface.

swine influenza a highly contagious respiratory disease of pigs caused by infection with the swine fever influenza viruses. A/H1N1pdm09 virus (shortened to H1N1). Infected swine can infect and cause symptomatic disease in humans, with fever of sudden onset, cough or shortness of breath associated with headache, tiredness, aching muscles, sneezing and runny nose. The virus was first identified in 2009. The regular flu vaccine protects against H1N1. *See* INFLUENZA, AVIAN INFLUENZA and ORTHOMYXOVIRUS.

sycosis a pustular inflammation of the hair follicles, usually of the beard and moustache.

Sydenham's chorea *T. Sydenham, English physician, 1624–1689.* A disorder of the central nervous system closely linked with rheumatic fever; also called chorea minor or historically St Vitus's dance. The condition, usually self-limited, is characterized by purposeless, irregular movements of the voluntary muscles that cannot be controlled by the patient.

symbiosis in parasitology, an intimate association between two different organisms for the mutual benefit of both.

symblepharon adhesion of an eyelid to the eyeball.

symbolism in psychology, an abnormal mental condition in which events or objects are interpreted as symbols of the patient's own thoughts. In psychiatry, the re-entry into consciousness of repressed material in an acceptable form.

sympathectomy division of autonomic nerve fibres which control specific involuntary muscles. An operation performed for many conditions, among them Raynaud's disease and focal hyperhidrosis.

sympathetic 1. exhibiting sympathy. 2. relating to the autonomic nervous system. *S. nervous system* one of the two divisions of the autonomic nervous system. It supplies involuntary muscle and glands; it stimulates the ductless glands and the circulatory and respiratory systems, but inhibits the digestive system. *S. ophthalmia* inflammation leading to loss of sight in the opposite eye after a perforating injury in the ciliary region.

sympathomimetic pertaining to drugs that produce effects similar to those caused by a stimulation of the sympathetic nervous system.

symphysis a cartilaginous joint along the line of union of two bones. *S. pubis* the cartilaginous junction of the two pubic bones.

symptom any indication of disease perceived by the patient. *Cardinal s's* 1. symptoms of greatest significance to the doctor, establishing the identity of the illness. 2. the symptoms shown in the temperature, pulse and respiration. *Dissociation s.* anaesthesia to pain and to heat and cold, without impairment of tactile sensibility. *Objective s.* one perceptible to others than the patient, such as pallor, rapid pulse or respiration, restlessness, etc. *Presenting s.* the symptom or group of symptoms about which the patient complains or from which relief is sought. *Subjective s.* one perceptible only to the patient, such as pain, pruritus, vertigo, etc. *Withdrawal s's* symptoms that follow sudden abstinence from a drug on which a person is dependent.

symptomatology 1. the study of the symptoms of a disease. 2. the symptoms of a particular disease, taken together.

synalgia pain felt in one part of the body but caused by inflammation of or injury to another part. *See* REFERRED PAIN.

synapse the junction between the termination of an axon and the dendrites of another nerve cell. Chemical transmitters pass the impulse across the space.

syncope a simple faint or temporary loss of consciousness due to cerebral ischaemia, often caused by dilatation of the peripheral blood vessels and a sudden fall in blood pressure.

syndactylism possessing webbed fingers or toes. A condition in which two or more fingers or toes are joined together.

syndrome a group of signs or symptoms typical of a distinctive disease, which frequently occur together and form a distinctive clinical picture.

synergist 1. a muscle that works in conjunction with another muscle. 2. a drug that works in combination with another drug, the two drugs having a greater effect when taken together than when taken separately.

synovectomy excision of a diseased synovial membrane to restore joint movement.

synovial fluid the fluid that surrounds a joint and is secreted by the synovial membrane. It is a thick, colourless, lubricating substance.

synovial membrane a serous membrane lining the articular capsule of a movable joint and terminating at the edge of the articular cartilage.

synovitis inflammation of a synovial membrane, usually with an effusion of fluid within the joint.

synthesis the building up of a more complex structure from simple components. This may apply to drugs or to plant or animal tissues.

syphilis a sexually transmitted infection caused by the spirochaete *Treponema pallidum*. The initial sign is the appearance of a painless sore, appearing either on the genitals, anus, rectum, lips, throat or fingers, which heals within a few weeks. A rash then ensues, which may be transient, recurrent or last for months. Other symptoms include lymphadenopathy, malaise, headaches, fever and fatigue. Following the symptomatic phase, the disease becomes latent for a few years or sometimes indefinitely. For untreated cases, the disease progresses to the development of gummatous lesions involving the cardiovascular and neurological systems. Syphilis can be vertically transmitted from mother to fetus from 9 weeks of gestation, causing miscarriage, stillbirth, neonatal death and long-term morbidity. All pregnant women are offered serological screening. If the results are positive, treatment with penicillin is effective. Practising safer sex can help to prevent syphilis infection. People with syphilis are infectious in the early stages but not in the latent and final stages.

syringe an instrument for injecting fluids or for aspirating or irrigating body cavities. It consists of a hollow tube with a tight-fitting piston. A hollow needle or a thin tube can be fitted to the end. *S. driver* a small battery-operated pump used to give medication continually.

syringomyelia the formation of cavities filled with fluid inside the spinal cord. Impairment of muscle function and sensation result at the level of and below the lesion. Painless injury may be the first symptom. It is a progressive disease.

syringomyelitis inflammation of the spinal cord, as the result of which cavities are formed in it.

syringomyelocele a type of spina bifida in which the protruded sac of fluid communicates with the central canal of the spinal cord.

systematic describing a process that is carried out according to a method or a system. *S. review* a methodical approach to literature reviews that reduces random error and bias. This requires a review of clinical literature in a particular field that has set explicit tests for whether research is valuable enough to be included in an overview of the area. This is often combined with a statistical meta-analysis of clinical trial results. *S. sampling* a type of sampling in which a convenient number is chosen, e.g., every tenth or fourth member of the population is selected into the sample. *S. lupus erythematosus* See LUPUS.

Système International d'Unités [Fr.] *SI units.* The international system for measurement in science, industry and general use. It was agreed in 1960, and it is now illegal in the UK to prescribe or dispense drugs in any other units.

systemic pertaining to or affecting the body as a whole. *S. circulation* circulation of the blood throughout the whole body, other than the pulmonary circulation. *See* SCLEROSIS.

systole the period of contraction of the heart. *See* DIASTOLE. *Atrial s.* the contraction of the heart by which the blood is pumped from the atria into the ventricles. *Extra-s.* a premature contraction of the atrium or ventricle, without alteration of the fundamental rhythm of the pacemaker. *Ventricular s.* the contraction of the heart by which the blood is pumped into the aorta and pulmonary artery.

systolic relating to a systole. *S. murmur* an abnormal sound produced during systole in heart.

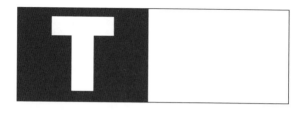

T symbol for *thymine*.

TB tuberculosis.

T cell a lymphocyte which is derived from the thymus and is responsible for cell-mediated immunity. *T. cytotoxic cells* (also known as killer cells) T cells that are activated by circulating T helper cells in the blood and lymphatic systems, and which recognize body cells displaying antigens to which they have become sensitized, targeting those which are viral or bacterially infected, triggering cell-mediated immunity. *T. helper cells* T cells that activate B lymphocytes to release antibodies and T killer cells to destroy cells having a specific antigenic profile. *T. receptor* cells formerly known as suppressor cells T cells keep the immune response at an appropriate level and also stop or slow down the activity of B lymphocytes and other T cells once the immune response has dealt with the antigen.

tabes a wasting away. *T. dorsalis* locomotor ataxia. A slowly progressive disease of the nervous system affecting the posterior nerve roots and spinal cord. It is a late manifestation of syphilis. Also known as syphilitic myelopathy.

taboo any ritual prohibition of certain activities, e.g., incest in many societies, or the open discussion of death and dying.

tachycardia abnormally rapid action of the heart and consequent increase in pulse rate. BRADYCARDIA. *Paroxysmal t.* spasmodic increase in cardiac contractions of sudden onset lasting a variable time, from a few seconds to hours.

tachyphasia, tachyphrasia extreme volubility of speech. It may be a sign of mental disorder.

tachyphrenia hyperactivity of the mental processes.

tachypnoea rapid, shallow respirations; a reflex response to stimulation of the vagus nerve endings in the pulmonary vessels.

tactile relating to the sense of touch.

Taenia a genus of tapeworms. *T. saginata* the beef tapeworm. The most common type of tapeworm found in the human intestine. *T. solium* the pork tapeworm. Can also be parasitic in humans, causing cysticercosis. *See* TAPEWORM.

taeniasis an infestation with tapeworms.

t'ai chi a system of movement, breathing and concentration, Chinese in origin, promoting general health and wellbeing.

Takayasu arteritis a rare type of vasculitis that mainly affects the aorta of young women.

Takotsubo cardiomyopathy also known as acute stress cardiomyopathy. Temporary and reversible symptoms of chest pain and breathlessness after significant emotional or physical stress.

talipes clubfoot. A deformity caused by a congenital or acquired contraction of

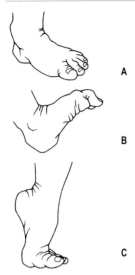

A = talipes valgus,
B = talipes calcaneus with some
cavus deformity,
C = talipes equinus

TALIPES

the muscles or tendons of the foot (*see* Figure). *T. calcaneus* the heel alone touches the ground on standing. *T. equinus* the toes touch the ground but not the heel. *T. valgus* the inner edge of the foot only is in contact with the ground. *T. varus* the person walks on the outer edge of the foot.

talus the astragalus or ankle bone.

tampon a plug of absorbent material inserted in the vagina, the nose or other orifice to restrain haemorrhage or absorb secretion.

tamponade the surgical use of tampons. *Cardiac t.* impairment of heart action by haemorrhage or effusion into the pericardium; may be due to a stab wound or follow surgery.

tantrum an outburst of ill temper. *Temper t.* a behaviour disorder of childhood. A display of bad temper in which the child performs uncontrolled actions in a state of emotional stress.

tapeworm any of a group of cestode flatworms, including the *Taenia* genus, which are parasitic in the intestines of humans and many animals. The adult consists of a round head with suckers or hooklets for attachment (scolex). From this, numerous segments (proglottids) arise, each of which produces ova capable of independent existence for a considerable length of time. Treatment is by anthelmintic drugs.

tapotement [Fr.] a tapping movement used in massage.

tapping *see* PARACENTESIS.

target cells abnormal flat red blood cells seen in liver and spleen disease and in the haemoglobinopathies. The haemoglobin is distributed as a small inner mass with a pale outer ring.

tarsal relating to a tarsus. *T. bones* the seven small bones of the ankle and instep. *T. cyst* meibomian cyst; chalazion. *T. glands* meibomian glands of the eyelids. *T. plates* small cartilages in the upper and lower eyelids.

tarsalgia pain in the foot.

tarsorrhaphy a rarely performed procedure involving partial stitching of the eyelids together to protect the cornea or to allow healing of an abrasion.

tartar a hard incrustation deposited on the teeth and on dentures.

taste the sense by which it is possible to identify what is eaten and drunk. Taste receptors (buds) lie on the tongue and give the sensations of sweet, sour, salt and bitter.

tattoo a permanent discoloration of the skin due to a foreign pigment.

tattooing the deliberate (usually for decorative purposes) or accidental, perhaps as a result of an explosion, insertion of coloured material into the deeper layers of the skin.

taxis manipulation by manual pressure of displaced organs or long bones to restore any part to its normal position.

taxonomy the theory and practice of the classification of animals and plants.

Tay-Sachs disease a rare and usually fatal genetic disorder that causes progressive damage to the nervous system usually within the first six months of life caused by a mutated HEXA gene.

team nursing method of organizing care based on the allocation of each nurse to a team that cares for a group of patients.

tears the watery, slightly alkaline and saline secretion of the lacrimal glands that moistens the conjunctiva. Tears contain lysozyme, a bactericidal enzyme. *Artificial t.* preparations used to supplement tear production in patients with dry eye associated with autoimmune disorder, e.g., rheumatoid arthritis, or to relieve irritation.

teat 1. a nipple of the breast. 2. a manufactured nipple used on infants' feeding bottles.

technetium *symbol* Tc. A metallic element. *Radioactive t.* an isotope ($^{99\,m}$Tc) used in a number of diagnostic tests. As it has a short half-life (6 hours), a high dose may be given for scanning organs, but the patient receives only a low radiation dose.

teeth *see* DENTITION.

tegument the skin.

telangiectasis a group of dilated capillary blood vessels, web-like or radiating in form.

telangioma a tumour of the blood capillaries.

telecare personal alarms that can be used to summons help in the event of falls, unusual movement or hypothermia which can allow people to live independently at home by enabling someone else to remotely monitor their safety.

telemedicine the use of communications systems to provide remote diagnosis, advice, treatment and monitoring. Used in both primary and acute care settings.

telepathy the transmission of thought without any normal means of communication between two persons.

telereceptor a sensory nerve ending which can respond to distant stimuli. Those of the eyes, ears and nose are examples. Teleceptor.

telophase the last stage in the division of cells when the chromosomes have been reconstituted in the nuclei at either end of the cell and the cell cytoplasm divides to form two new cells.

temperament a person's nature; the habitual and emotional attitude, as distinct from mood which is temporary.

temperature the degree of heat of a substance or body as measured by a thermometer. *Normal t.* the normal temperature of the human body is 37°C, with a slight decrease in the early morning and a slight increase at night. It indicates the balance between heat production and heat loss.

template a mould or pattern. In radiotherapy, a map of the area of the patient requiring treatment and of those areas to be protected from radiation.

temple the region on either side of the head above the zygomatic arch.

temporal pertaining to the side of the head. *T. arteritis* giant cell arteritis. A chronic inflammatory condition of the carotid arterial system, occurring usually in elderly people. There is persistent headache and partial or total blindness may result. *T. bone* one of a pair of bones on either side of the skull containing the organ of hearing. *T. lobe* the part of the cerebrum below the lateral sulcus.

temporomandibular relating to the temporal bone and the mandible. *T. joint* the hinge of the lower jaw. *T. joint syndrome* painful dysfunction of the temporomandibular joint, marked by a clicking or grinding sensation in the joint; commonly caused by malocclusion of the teeth. Also known as temporomandibular disorder.

tenacious thick and viscid, as applied to sputum or other body fluids.

tendinitis inflammation of a tendon and its attachments.

tendon a band of fibrous tissue forming the termination of a muscle and attaching it to a bone. *Achilles t.* that inserted into the calcaneum. *T. grafting* an operation which repairs a defect in one tendon by a graft from another. *T. insertion* the point of attachment of a muscle to a bone which it moves. *T. reflex* the muscular contraction produced on percussing a tendon. Tendonitis inflammation of a tendon.

tenesmus a painful, ineffectual straining to empty the bowel or bladder.

tennis elbow a painful disorder which affects the extensor muscles of the forearm at their attachment to the external epicondyle. Also known as lateral epicondylitis.

tenorrhaphy the suturing together of the ends of a divided tendon.

tenosynovitis inflammation of a tendon sheath.

TENS abbreviation for transcutaneous electrical nerve stimulation. A method of treating persistent pain by passing small electrical currents into the spinal cord or sensory nerves by means of electrodes applied to the skin. TENS is non-invasive and non-addictive, with no known side effects. The NMC has approved the use of TENS by midwives and registered nurses on their own responsibility, provided they have been instructed in its use.

tension the act of stretching or the state of being stretched. *Arterial t.* the pressure of blood on the vessel wall during cardiac contraction. *Intraocular t.* the pressure of the contents of the eye on its walls, measured by a tonometer. *Intravenous t.* the pressure of blood within the veins. *Surface t.* tension or resistance which acts to preserve the integrity of a surface, particularly the surface of a liquid.

teratogen an agent or influence that causes physical defects in the developing embryo.

teratoma a solid tumour containing tissues similar to those of a dermoid cyst. Found most often in the ovaries and testes, many of these tumours are malignant.

term the end of pregnancy, normally calculated as 280 days or 40 weeks from the date of the last normal menstrual period but considered to be any time after the 37th week of pregnancy.

termination of pregnancy (TOP) abortion that is induced, legally or illegally.

tertiary third. *T. care* care and treatment that is given in a large regional hospital providing specialist care, e.g., cardiac surgery, intensive, neonatal, oncological services. *T. prevention* prevention of ill health, mitigating the effects of illness and disease that have already occurred.

test 1. an examination or trial. 2. analysis of the composition of a substance by the use of chemical reagents, and/or to determine the presence or absence of a substance.

testicle a testis; one of the two glands in the scrotum which produce spermatozoa. *Undescended t.* a condition in which the organ remains in the pelvis or inguinal canal. testicular feminization syndrome *see* ANDROGEN INSENSITIVITY SYNDROME.

testicular self-examination should be performed regularly once a month for the detection of early tumours of the testis, which are highly curable if detected at an early stage. Self-examination should take place after a warm bath or shower, which relaxes the scrotal skin. It is performed as follows: standing in front of a mirror, look for any swelling. One testicle may appear larger than the other or hang lower; this is usually perfectly normal. Examine each testicle with both hands and gently roll each testicle between the fingers and thumb. A small lump is felt for and, if found, almost always occurs in only one testis and is usually painless. A cord-like structure found on the top and back of each testicle should be found and examined for any swelling.

testicular torsion severe twisting of the spermatic cord.

testis a testicle. (*See* Figure.)

testosterone the hormone produced by the testes which stimulates the development of sex characteristics. It can now be made synthetically, and is used medicinally in cases of failure of sex function and as a palliative treatment in some cases of advanced metastatic breast cancer in females.

tetanus an acute disease of the nervous system caused by the contamination of wounds by the spores of a soil bacterium, *Clostridium tetani*. Muscle stiffness around the site of the wound occurs, followed by rigidity of face and neck muscles; hence 'lockjaw'. All muscles are then affected and opisthotonos may occur. *T. immunoglobulin* also known as tetanus antitoxin and tetanus immune globulin (TIG), a serum that gives a short-term passive immunity and may be used for immediate treatment of a case of tetanus. Also *T. vaccine* or *toxoid* will give an active immunity.

tetany an increased excitability of the nerves due to a lack of available calcium, accompanied by painful muscle spasm of the hands and feet (carpopedal spasm). The cause may be hypoparathyroidism or alkalosis owing to excessive vomiting or hyperventilation.

tetralogy a series of four. *T. of Fallot see* FALLOT'S TETRALOGY.

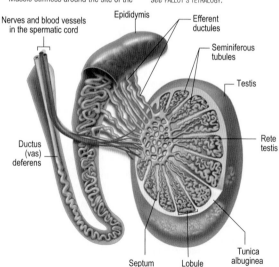

Nerves and blood vessels in the spermatic cord

Epididymis

Efferent ductules

Seminiferous tubules

Testis

Ductus (vas) deferens

Rete testis

Septum

Lobule

Tunica albuginea

TESTIS

tetraplegia quadriplegia. Paralysis of all four limbs.

thalamus a mass of nerve cells at the base of the cerebrum. Most sensory impulses from the body pass to this area and are transmitted to the cortex.

thalassaemia a group of inherited haemolytic anaemias where there is interference with the synthesis of haemoglobin resulting in anaemia. Several types are recognized, according to the symptoms. Thalassaemia is prevalent in the Mediterranean, Middle East and Southeast Asian regions. The only possible cure is a stem cell or bone marrow transplant but this carries significant risks so is not often performed. Genetic counselling is advised for the parents or other close relatives of a child with thalassaemia and also for any person with thalassaemia trait.

thalassotherapy treatment involving sea bathing, sea products or a sea voyage.

thanatology 1. the study of death and dying. 2. the forensic study of the causes of death.

theca a sheath, such as the covering of a tendon. *T. folliculi* the covering of a Graafian follicle. *T. vertebralis* the membranes enclosing the spinal cord; the dura mater.

thenar 1. the palm of the hand. 2. the fleshy part at the base of the thumb.

therapeutic pertaining to therapeutics or treatment of disease; curative. *T. abortion see* ABORTION. *T. community* any treatment setting (usually psychiatric) which provides a living–learning situation through group processes emphasizing social, environmental and personal interactions and which encourages the individual to learn socially from these processes. *T. drug monitoring* abbreviated TDM. Some drugs require that blood levels are maintained within a certain range (often called a therapeutic window) to avoid inefficacy as a result of low blood levels and producing side effects for the patient as a result of levels in the blood being too high. To do this blood levels of the drug concerned need to be measured at appropriate intervals and medication regimens altered as necessary. *T. index* abbreviated TI. The margin of difference between the desired and safe effect that a drug dose achieves, and the dose that is known to produce toxic effects. This measure varies between people, who all process drugs differently, but it does alert the prescriber to the margins of safety in the use of a particular drug. *T. touch* techniques that are used to facilitate healing and wellbeing of a person based on the concept that the body is an energy field and that this field can be influenced from outside itself. Body energies can be transferred to and through the hands of a therapist who has been trained to assume the role of healer. *See* MASSAGE. *T. use of self* the ability of the care giver such as nurse to use therapy and experimental knowledge along with self-awareness and the ability to explore, and use, one's personal impact on others. *T. window* range of blood level in the use of certain drugs. *See earlier* TDM.

therapeutics the science and art of healing and the treatment of disease.

therapy the treatment of disease.

thermal relating to heat.

thermocautery the deliberate destruction of tissue by means of heat. *See* CAUTERY.

thermography a method of measuring the amount of heat produced by different areas of the body, using infrared photography. Used as a diagnostic aid in the detection of breast tumours and the assessment of rheumatic joints; also used in the study of pain.

thermolysis the loss of body heat by radiation, by excretion and by the evaporation of sweat.

thermometer an instrument for measuring temperature. *Clinical t.* one used to measure the body temperature.

thermoreceptor a nerve ending that responds to heat and cold.

thermoregulation the normal regulation of body temperature by the maintenance of the balance between heat production and heat loss.

thermotherapy the treatment of disease by application of heat.

thiamine vitamin B₁, or aneurine. An essential vitamin involved in carbohydrate metabolism. A deficiency causes beriberi. The source is liver and unrefined cereals.

Thiersch skin graft *I. Thiersch, German surgeon, 1822–1895.* The transplantation of areas of partial thickness skin. *See* GRAFT.

thirst an uncomfortable sensation of dryness of the mouth and throat with a desire for oral fluids. *Abnormal t.* polydipsia.

Thomas splint *H.O. Thomas, British orthopaedic surgeon, 1834–1891.* A splint consisting of an oval metal ring that fits over the lower limb. Attached to the ring are two round metal rods which are bent into a W shape at the lower end. It is used to immobilize fractures of the leg during transportation and for use with traction as it supports the limb and moves the weight from the knee joint to the pelvis.

thoracic relating to the thorax. *T. duct* the large lymphatic vessel situated in the thorax along the spine. It opens into the left subclavian vein.

thoracocentesis puncture of the wall of the thorax to allow aspiration of pleural fluid.

thoracoscopy examination of the pleural cavity by means of an endoscopic instrument.

thoracotomy a surgical incision into the thorax.

thorax the chest; a cavity containing the heart, lungs, bronchi and oesophagus. It is bounded by the diaphragm, the sternum, the thoracic vertebrae and the ribs. *Barrel-shaped t.* a development in chronic obstructive pulmonary disease such as emphysema, when the chest is malformed like a barrel.

threadworm a species of roundworm, *Enterobius vermicularis,* parasitic in the large intestine, particularly of children.

threonine one of the essential amino acids.

thrill a tremor discerned by palpation.

throat 1. the anterior surface of the neck. 2. the pharynx. *Sore t.* pharyngitis.

thrombin an enzyme that converts fibrinogen to fibrin during the later stages of blood clotting.

thromboangitis inflammation of blood vessels with clot formation. *T. obliterans* inflammation of the arteries, usually of the legs of young males, causing intermittent claudication and gangrene. Buerger's disease.

thrombocyte a disc-shaped blood platelet; essential for the clotting of shed blood.

thrombocytopenia a reduction in the number of platelets in the blood; bleeding may occur. Destruction of platelets can be caused by infections, certain drugs, transfusion-related purpuras, idiopathic thrombocytopenic purpura and disseminated intravascular coagulation.

thrombocytosis an increase in the number of platelets in the blood.

thromboembolism a clot or embolism, which has become detached from a thrombus formed in another site that is carried in the blood flow to obstruct a blood vessel elsewhere in the body.

thrombokinase thromboplastin. A lipid-containing protein, activated by blood platelets and injured tissues, which is capable of activating prothrombin to form thrombin, which, combined with fibrinogen, forms a clot.

thrombolysis the disintegration or dissolving of a clot by the infusion of an enzyme such as streptokinase into the blood. thrombophilia increased tendency for blood to clot.

thrombophlebitis the formation of a clot, associated with inflammation of the lining of a vein.

thromboplastin   *see* THROMBOKINASE.

thrombosis   the formation of a thrombus. *Cavernous sinus t.* thrombosis of the cavernous sinus, usually the result of infection of the face, when the veins in the sinus are affected via ophthalmic vessels. *Cerebral t.* the occlusion of a cerebral artery, the most common cause of cerebral infarction (a 'stroke'). *Coronary t.* the occlusion of a coronary vessel, by which the heart muscle is deprived of blood, causing myocardial ischaemia and often leading to myocardial infarction (a 'heart attack'). *See* DEEP VEIN THROMBOSIS. *Lateral sinus t.* a rare complication of a middle ear infection when the lateral sinus of the dura mater is infected and there is clot formation.

thrombus   a stationary blood clot caused by coagulation of the blood in the heart or in an artery or a vein.

thrush   an infection of the mucous membranes, most commonly of the skin, mouth and vagina, by a fungus, *Candida albicans*. *See* CANDIDIASIS.

thymectomy   surgical removal of the thymus.

thymine   *symbol* T. One of the pyrimidine bases found in DNA.

thymus   a gland-like structure situated in the upper thorax and neck. Present in early life, it reaches its maximum development during puberty and continues to play an immunological role throughout life, even though its function declines with age.

thyroglossal   relating to the thyroid and the tongue. *T. cyst see* CYST.

thyroid   1. shaped like a shield. 2. pertaining to the thyroid gland. *T. cartilage* the largest cartilage of the larynx. It forms the 'Adam's apple' in the front of the throat. *T. gland* a ductless gland, consisting of two lobes, situated in front and on either side of the trachea. It secretes the hormones thyroxine and tri-iodothyronine which are concerned in regulating the metabolic rate. *Overactive T. see* THYROTOXICOSIS. *T.-stimulating hormone* abbreviated

TSH. *Underactive T.* hypothyroidism. The thyroid gland does not produce sufficient hormones resulting in a range of symptoms including weight gain, tiredness and depression. Thyrotrophin; a hormone, produced by the anterior pituitary gland, which controls the activity of the thyroid gland.

thyroidectomy   partial or complete removal of the thyroid gland.

thyroiditis   inflammation of the thyroid. Acute thyroiditis, usually due to a virus infection, is characterized by sore throat, fever and painful enlargement of the gland. *Hashimoto's t.* also known as chronic lymphocytic thyroiditis is a progressive autoimmune disease of the thyroid gland with degeneration of its epithelial elements and replacement by lymphoid and fibrous tissue.

thyrotoxicosis   hyperthyroidism. The symptoms arise when there is overactivity of the thyroid gland. The metabolism is speeded up and there is enlargement of the gland and exophthalmos.

thyrotrophin   *see* THYROID-(STIMULATING HORMONE).

thyroxine   one of the two hormones secreted by the thyroid gland. It is used in the treatment of hypothyroidism.

TIA   transient ischaemic attack.

tibia   the shin bone; the larger of the two bones of the leg, extending from knee to ankle.

tic   a spasmodic twitching of certain muscles, usually of the face, neck or shoulder. *T. douloureux* paroxysmal trigeminal neuralgia.

tick   a blood-sucking parasite which may transmit the organisms of disease.

tidal volume   the amount of gas passing into and out of the lungs in each respiratory cycle.

tincture   a medical substance dissolved in alcohol.

tinea   a group of skin infections caused by a variety of fungi and named after the area of the body affected, thus *T. barbae*, the beard; *T. capitis*, the head; *T. circinata* or *T. corporis*, the body;

T. cruris, the groin; and *T. pedis*, the feet. *See* RINGWORM.

tinnitus a ringing, buzzing or roaring sound in the ears.

tissue a group or layer of similarly specialized cells that together perform certain special functions.

titration determination of a given component in solution by addition of a liquid reagent of known strength until a given endpoint, e.g., change in colour, is reached, indicating that the component has been consumed by reaction with the reagent.

tobacco the dried leaves of the plant *Nicotiana tabacum*, containing the drug nicotine, which may be smoked, chewed or inhaled. All these activities are potentially dangerous to health. Cigarette smoking in particular is responsible for an increase in cancer of the lungs and mouth and bronchitis. Smoking increases the likelihood of chronic obstructive pulmonary disease, including emphysema and coronary artery disease. It is also harmful during pregnancy, leading to smaller and less healthy babies. *T. withdrawal syndrome* a change in mood or behaviour associated with the stopping of or reduction in cigarette smoking.

tocography the measurement of alterations in the intrauterine pressure during labour.

tocopherol vitamin E, present in wheat germ, green leaves and milk.

token economy programme a behavioural approach to modifying troublesome behaviours and restoring lost self-help behaviours by the systematic rewarding of desired behaviour by giving tokens which may be exchanged for goods or privileges.

tolerance the ability to endure without effect or injury. *Exercise t. test* to determine how much oxygen a patient's myocardium requires during exercise. The results indicate the patient's capacity for exercise and help in the estimation of the extent of coronary disease. *Drug t.* decrease of susceptibility to the effects of a drug due to its continued administration. *Immunological t.* or immune tolerance is a specific non-reactivity of lymphoid tissues to a particular antigen capable, under other conditions, of inducing immunity.

tomography body section radiography in which X-rays or ultrasound waves are used to produce an image of a layer of tissue at any depth.

tone 1. the normal degree of tension, e.g., in a muscle. 2. a particular quality of sound.

tongue a muscular organ attached to the floor of the mouth and concerned in taste, mastication, swallowing and speech. It is covered by a mucous membrane from which project numerous papillae. *T. tie* also known as ankyloglossia is where a strip of skin connecting the tongue and roof of the mouth in a baby is shorter than usual.

tonic 1. a term popularly applied to any drug supposed to brace or tone up the body or any particular part or organ. 2. possessing tone in a state of contraction, e.g., muscles. *T. spasm* a prolonged contraction of one or several muscles, as seen in epilepsy, for example. *See* CLONIC.

tonography the measurement made by an electric tonometer recording the intraocular pressure and so, indirectly, the drainage of aqueous humour from the eye.

tonsil a mass of lymphoid tissue, particularly one of two small, almond-shaped bodies, situated one on each side between the pillars of the fauces. It is covered by mucous membrane, and its surface is pitted with follicles. *Pharyngeal t.* the lymphadenoid tissue of the pharynx between the pharyngotympanic tubes. Adenoids. *T. test* a small sample of tonsil obtained in suspected cases of Creutzfeldt–Jakob Disease (CJD) for the identification of the prion found in new variant CJD, a spongiform encephalopathy. *See* CREUTZFELDT–JAKOB DISEASE.

tonsillectomy excision of one or both tonsils.

tonsillitis inflammation of the tonsils usually due to a viral infection.

tonus the normal state of partial contraction of the muscles.

tooth a structure in the mouth designed for the mastication of food. Each is composed of a crown, neck and root with one or more fangs. The main bulk is of dentine enclosing a central pulp; the crown is covered with a hard white substance called enamel. *See* DENTITION.

tophus a small, hard, chalky deposit of sodium urate in the skin and cartilage, occurring in gout and sometimes appearing on the auricle of the ear.

topical relating to a particular spot; local. *T. lotion* one for local or external application.

topography the study of the surface of the body in relation to the underlying structures.

torpor a sluggish condition in which response to stimuli is absent or very slow.

torsion twisting: (a) of an artery to arrest haemorrhage; (b) of the pedicle of a cyst, which produces venous congestion in the cyst and consequent gangrene (a possible complication of ovarian cyst).

torso the body, excluding the head and the limbs; the trunk.

torticollis wryneck, a contracted state of the cervical muscles, producing torsion of the neck. The deformity may be congenital or secondary to pressure on the accessory nerve, to inflammation of glands in the neck, or to muscle spasm.

total complete, the whole number or amount. *T. body irradiation* abbreviated TBI. The complete exposure of the patient's body to radiotherapy, used in the treatment of some cancers and prior to stem cell or bone marrow transplantation. *T. burn surface area* abbreviated TBSA. A formula for predicting outcomes after a burn injury: (age + TBSA) = percentage chance of surviving. *See* LUND AND BROWDER CHART. *T. lung capacity* abbreviated TLC. The volume of air held in the lungs following deep inspiration. *T. parenteral nutrition* abbreviated TPN. The supplying of all essential nutrients to a patient via the intravenous route. *See* Appendix 1. *T. quality management* (TQM) a largely superseded approach to management based upon the idea that quality of service depends upon the active involvement of all members of staff in achieving and maintaining high standards of care throughout an organization. TQM had great popularity in the 1980s and 1990s but has been replaced by LEAN and SIX SIGMA.

Tourette's syndrome a neurological disorder which starts in childhood. Characterized by repetitive grimaces and tics; involuntary barks, grunts, shouting and other noises may appear as the disease progresses. Some sufferers may also use obscene language (coprolalia). Also known as Gilles de la Tourette's syndrome. Causes are unknown although there may be a genetic cause in some cases.

tourniquet a constrictive band applied to a limb to arrest arterial haemorrhage. Now used to obstruct the venous return from a limb and so facilitate the withdrawal of blood from a vein.

toxaemia of pregnancy a condition affecting pregnant women and characterized by albuminuria, hypertension and oedema, with the possibility of pre-eclampsia and eclampsia developing.

toxic 1. poisonous, relating to a poison. 2. caused by a toxin. *T. shock syndrome* a severe illness characterized by high fever of sudden onset, vomiting, diarrhoea and, in severe cases, death. A sunburn-like rash with peeling of the skin occurs.

toxicity the degree of virulence of a poison.

toxicology the science dealing with poisons.

toxin any poisonous compound, usually referring to that produced by bacteria.

Toxocara a genus of nematode worms, parasitic in the intestines of dogs and cats, which may also infest humans, especially children. The spleen, liver and lungs are most often affected but the parasite may also infest the retina, causing inflammation and granulation.

toxoid a toxin which has been deprived of some of its harmful properties but is still capable of producing immunity and may be used in a vaccine.

Toxoplasma a genus of protozoa which infests birds and animals and may be transmitted from them to humans.

toxoplasmosis a disease due to *Toxoplasma gondii* carried by cats, birds and other animals and in contaminated soil. The congenital form may result in miscarriage or stillbirth of the infant. The disease may also cause enlarged liver and spleen, blindness, brain defects and death. The acquired infection is often asymptomatic but may result in pneumonia, skin rashes and nephritis. Can cause severe multisystem disease in immunocompromised people.

TPN total parenteral nutrition.

trabecula a dividing band or septum, extending from the capsule of an organ into its interior and holding the functioning cells in position.

trabeculectomy an operation to lower the intraocular pressure in glaucoma that cannot be controlled by medication.

trace element an element that is essential in the diet, for the normal functioning of the body, but is required only in minute amounts, e.g., zinc, manganese, fluorine, etc.

tracer a means by which something may be followed, as (a) a mechanical device by which the outline or movements of an object can be graphically recorded, or (b) a material by which the progress of a compound through the body may be observed, e.g., a radioactive isotope tracer.

trachea the windpipe; a cartilaginous tube lined with ciliated mucous membrane, extending from the lower part of the larynx to the commencement of the bronchi.

tracheitis inflammation of the trachea causing pain in the chest, with coughing.

tracheobronchitis acute infection of the trachea and bronchi due to viruses or bacteria.

tracheostomy a surgical opening into the third and fourth cartilage rings of the trachea. *T. tubes* those used to maintain an airway after tracheotomy, either permanently or until the normal use of the air passages is regained.

tracheotomy surgical incision of the trachea. *High t.* superior tracheotomy. *Inferior* or *low t.* that in which the opening is made below the thyroid isthmus. *Superior t.* high tracheotomy. That in which the opening is made above the thyroid isthmus.

trachoma a chronic infectious disease of the conjunctiva and cornea, producing photophobia, pain and lacrimation, caused by an organism once thought to be a virus but now classified as a strain of the bacterium *Chlamydia trachomatis*. Trachoma is more prevalent in Africa and Asia than in other parts of the world.

traction 1. the exertion of a pulling force, such as that applied to a fractured bone or dislocated joint or to relieve muscle spasm, to maintain proper position and facilitate healing. 2. in obstetrics, that along the axis of the pelvis to assist in delivery of a fetal part, or the placenta and membranes. *Hamilton–Russell t.* a form of traction of the leg. *Head t.* traction exerted on the head in the treatment of cervical injury. *Skeletal t.* a method of keeping the fractured ends of bone in position by traction on the bone. A metal pin or wire is passed through the distal fragment or adjacent bone to overcome muscle contraction.

trait an inherited or developed physical or mental characteristic.

trance a condition of semiconsciousness of hysterical, cataleptic or hypnotic origin. It is not due to organic disease.

tranquillizer a drug which allays anxiety, relieves tension and has a calming effect on the patient.

transactional analysis a theory of personality structure and a psychotherapeutic method. The human personality is viewed as consisting of three ego states: the parent, the adult and the child. The aim is to allow the adult ego to take control over the child and parent egos.

transaminase one of a group of enzymes which catalyse the transfer of an amine group from one amino acid into another. Transaminases include *glutamic–oxalacetic t.* (GOT) and *glutamic–pyruvic t.* (GPT).

transcendental meditation a technique for attaining a state of physical relaxation and psychological calm by the regular practice of a relaxation procedure which entails the repetition of a mantra. Has been successfully used by some patients to reduce hypertension.

transcultural nursing being aware of the patient's cultural health beliefs and values and incorporating these into the agreed care plan with the patient.

transcutaneous blood gas monitors the application to the skin of a probe which is heated to a temperature of 44°C and enables measurements of P_{O_2} and P_{CO_2} to be made. Accuracy depends on the quality of the peripheral circulation, thus transcutaneous blood gas monitoring is usually used in conjunction with intermittent arterial sampling.

transcutaneous electrical nerve stimulation *see* TENS.

transdermal through the skin. *T. patch* is a medicated adhesive patch that is placed onto the skin to deliver a specific dose of medication through the skin and into the bloodstream. The main advantage of the transdermal patch is that it provides a controlled release of the medication into the patient. The main disadvantage is that only drugs whose molecules are small enough to penetrate the skin can be delivered by this method.

transference in psychiatry, the unconscious transfer by the patient on to the psychiatrist of feelings that are appropriate to other people significant to the patient.

transferrin a glycoprotein that acts as a carrier for iron in the bloodstream.

transfusion the introduction of whole blood or a blood component into a vein, performed in cases of severe loss of blood, shock, septicaemia, etc. It is used to supply actual volume of blood, or to introduce constituents, such as clotting factors or antibodies, that are deficient in the patient. *Direct t.* the transfer of blood directly from a donor to a recipient. *Exchange t.* replacement transfusion. The removal of most or all of the recipient's blood and its replacement with fresh blood. Used with infants suffering from erythroblastosis. *See* RHESUS FACTOR. *Feto-maternal t.* from fetus to mother via the placenta; transplacental transfusion (TPT). *Replacement t.* exchange transfusion. transgender people who have a gender identity or gender expression that differs from their assigned sex.

transient ischaemic attack abbreviated TIA. A sudden episode of temporary or passing symptoms, caused by diminished blood flow through the carotid or vertebrobasilar blood vessels.

transillumination the illumination of a translucent body structure by a strong light as an aid to diagnosis, particularly of tumours of the retina and of abnormalities in the ethmoidal and frontal sinuses.

translocation in morphology, the transfer of a segment of a chromosome to a different site on the same chromosome or to a different chromosome. It can be a cause of congenital abnormality.

translucent allowing light rays to pass through indistinctly.

transmigration a movement from one place to another, as in the passage of blood cells through the walls of the capillaries. Diapedesis. *External t.* the passage of an ovum from its ovary to the uterine tube on the opposite side. *Internal t.* the movement of an ovum from one uterine tube to the other through the uterus.

transmission-based precautions precautions designed to be applied to patients known or suspected to be infected with pathogens that are highly transmissible or epidemiologically important, and for which additional measures beyond STANDARD PRECAUTIONS are needed to interrupt transmission in hospital. There are three types of transmission-based precaution: airborne, droplet and contact precautions. They may be combined for diseases that have multiple routes of transmission. When employed either singly or in combination, they are used in addition to standard precautions. *See* Appendix 11.

transplacental across the placenta. Movement may be from mother to fetus or vice versa. *T. infection* may affect the unborn child.

transplant 1. an organ or tissue taken from the body and grafted into another area of the same individual or another individual. 2. to transfer tissue from one part to another or from one individual to another.

transplantation the transfer of living organs from one part of the body to another (autotransplant) or from one individual to another (allograft). Transplantation is often called grafting, though the latter is more commonly used to refer to the transfer of skin.

transposition 1. displacement of any of the viscera to the opposite side of the body. 2. the operation which partially removes a piece of tissue from one part of the body to another, complete severance being delayed until it has become established in its new position. *T. of the great vessels* a congenital abnormality of the heart in which the positions of the pulmonary artery and aorta are reversed.

transsexualism experience of gender identity that is inconsistent with a person's assigned sex.

transudate any fluid that passes through a membrane.

transverse cross-wise. *T. presentation* position of the fetus whereby it lies across the pelvis; this position must be corrected before normal birth can take place.

transvestite a person who experiences a habitual and strongly persistent desire to dress and act in a style traditionally associated with a member of the opposite sex. Cross-dressing.. The majority are male and have no desire to physically change sex.

trauma injury. *Birth t.* an injury to the infant sustained during the process of being born. *Psychological t.* an emotional shock that makes a lasting impression.

treatment the mode of dealing with a patient or disease. *Active t.* that in which specific medical or surgical treatment is undertaken. *Conservative t.* that which aims at preserving and restoring injured parts by natural means, e.g., rest, fluid replacement, etc., as opposed to radical or surgical methods. *Empirical t.* treatment based on observation of symptoms and not on science. *Palliative t.* that which relieves distressing symptoms but does not cure the disease. *Prophylactic t.* that which aims at the prevention of disease.

Trematoda a class of fluke worms, some of which are parasitic in humans. Many of them have freshwater snails as secondary hosts.

tremor an involuntary, muscular quivering which may be due to fatigue, emotion or disease. Tremor, first of one hand, and later affecting the other limbs, is the first symptom of Parkinsonism. *Intention t.* one that occurs on attempting a movement, as in disseminated sclerosis.

Trendelenburg's position *F. Trendelenburg, German surgeon, 1844–1924. See* POSITION.

Trendelenburg's sign a test of the stability of the hip. The patient stands on the affected leg and flexes the other knee and hip. If there is dislocation the pelvis is lower on the side of the flexed leg, which is the reverse of normal.

Treponema a genus of spirochaetes. Anaerobic bacteria, they are motile, spiral and parasitic in humans and animals. *T. carateum* the causative agent of pinta. *T. pallidum* the causative agent of syphilis. *T. pallidum pertenue* the causative agent of yaws (framboesia). *T. immobilization test* a serological test for syphilis.

tri-iodothyronine a hormone produced by the thyroid gland together with thyroxine.

triage [Fr.] 1. choosing, classifying or sorting. 2. a process by which a patient is assessed upon arrival to determine the urgency of the problem, and to designate appropriate health care resources to care for the identified problem. *T. nurse* a registered nurse with specialist skills and knowledge who carries out the assessment and classification of casualties according to the type and severity of their injuries in order to assign them for treatment in the accident and emergency department.

triceps having three heads. *T. muscle* that situated on the back of the upper arm, which extends the forearm.

trichiasis 1. a condition of ingrowing hairs about an orifice, or ingrowing eyelashes. 2. the appearance of hair-like filaments in the urine.

trichinosis a disease caused by eating underdone pork containing a parasite, *Trichinella spiralis*. This becomes deposited in muscle and causes stiffness and painful swelling. There may also be nausea, diarrhoea and fever. Trichiniasis.

trichology the study of hair.

Trichomonas a genus of flagellate protozoa that are parasitic to humans. *T. hominis* infests the bowel and may cause dysentery. *T. tenax* infests the mouth and may be present in cases of pyorrhoea. *T. vaginalis* is commonly present in the vagina and may cause leukorrhoea and vaginitis.

trichomoniasis infestation with a parasite of the genus *Trichomonas*.

Trichophyton a genus of fungi that affect the skin, nails and hair.

trichophytosis infection of the skin, nails or hair with one of the genus *Trichophyton. See* TINEA.

trichosis any abnormal growth of hair.

trichuriasis infestation by the whipworm.

Trichuris a genus of nematode worms that may infest the colon and cause diarrhoea. A whipworm.

tricuspid having three flaps or cusps. *T. valve* that at the opening between the right atrium and the right ventricle of the heart.

trifocal pertaining to a spectacle lens that has three foci, one for distant, one for intermediate and one for near vision.

trigeminal divided into three. *T. nerves* the fifth pair of cranial nerves, each of which is divided into three main branches and supplies one side of the face. *T. neuralgia* pain in the face which is confined to branches of the trigeminal nerve. Tic douloureux.

trigger finger a stenosing of the tendon sheath at the metacarpophalangeal joint, allowing flexion of the finger but not extension without assistance, when it 'clicks' into position.

triglyceride 'human fat', an ester of glycerol and three fatty acids.

trigone a triangular area. *T. of the bladder* the triangular space on the floor of the bladder, between the ureteric openings and the urethral orifice.

trimester a period of 3 months. *First t. of pregnancy* the first 3 months, during which rapid development is taking place.

trimethylaminuria a rare genetic disorder that causes a strong body odour due to the inability to process trimethylamine. Also known as fish odour syndrome.

triple vaccine a combined dose of diphtheria, tetanus and pertussis immunization.

triplets three children carried in the uterus at once and born at one labour.

triplopia a condition in which three images of an object are seen at the same time.

trismus lockjaw; a tonic spasm of the muscles of the jaw.

trisomy the presence of an extra chromosome in each cell in addition to the normal paired set of 46. The cause of several chromosome disorders including DOWN'S SYNDROME and KLINEFELTER'S SYNDROME.

trochanter either of two bony prominences below the neck of the femur. *Greater t.* that on the outer side forming the bony prominence of the hip. *Lesser t.* that on the inner side at the neck of the femur.

trochlea any pulley-shaped structure, but particularly the fibrocartilage near the inner angular process of the frontal bone through which passes the tendon of the superior oblique muscle of the eye.

trophoblast the layer of cells surrounding the blastocyst at the time of and responsible for implantation.

tropia a manifest deviation of the eye, one that is present when both eyes are open.

tropical relating to the areas within 23.5 degrees north and south of the equator, termed the tropics. *T. medicine* that concerned with diseases that are more prevalent in hot climates.

tropism an affinity or attraction of one cell to another.

Trousseau's sign A. Trousseau, French physician, 1801–1867. 1. spontaneous peripheral venous thrombosis. 2. a sign for tetany in which carpal spasm can be elicited by compressing the upper arm and causing ischaemia to the nerves distally.

truncus a trunk; the main part of the body, or a part of it, from which other parts spring. *T. arteriosus* the arterial trunk connected to the fetal heart which develops into the aortic and pulmonary arteries.

Trypanosoma a genus of protozoan parasites which pass some of their life cycle in the blood of vertebrates, including humans. *T. gambiense* and *T. rhodesiense* are transmitted by the bite of the tsetse fly, and are the cause of sleeping sickness.

trypanosomiasis a disease caused by infestation with *Trypanosoma*. Sleeping sickness.

trypsin a digestive enzyme that converts protein into amino acids.

trypsinogen the precursor of trypsin. It is secreted in the pancreatic juice and activated by the enterokinase of the intestinal juices into trypsin.

tryptophan one of the essential amino acids.

tsetse fly a fly of the genus *Glossina* which transmits the parasite *Trypanosoma* to humans, causing trypanosomiasis.

TSH thyroid-stimulating hormone.

tsutsugamushi disease scrub typhus, which occurs in Japan and is transmitted by the bite of a mite.

tubal relating to a tube. *T. ligation* tying of the fallopian tubes as a method of female sterilization. *T. pregnancy* extrauterine pregnancy where the embryo develops in the uterine tube. Ectopic pregnancy.

tube feeding administration of liquid and semisolid foods through a nasogastric, gastrostomy or enterostomy tube. Tube feeds are administered to patients who are unable to take foods by mouth.

Tubegauz a proprietary brand of woven circular bandage available in a variety of sizes and applied with a special applicator.

tubercle 1. a small nodule or a rounded prominence on a bone. 2. the specific lesion (a small nodule) produced by the tubercle bacillus.

tubercular pertaining to tubercles.

tuberculin the filtrate from a fluid medium in which *Mycobacterium tuberculosis* has been grown and which contains its toxins. *Old t.* prepared from the human bacillus and used in skin tests in diagnosing tuberculosis. *See* MANTOUX TEST.

tuberculosis abbreviated TB. Chronic, recurrent notifiable infection, most commonly occurring in the lungs, caused by *Mycobacterium tuberculosis* or (rarely in the UK) *M. bovis* or *M. africanum*; transmission is usually by inhalation of bacilli in airborne droplets. *Bovine TB* endemic in cattle and some other animals and transmissible to humans by ingestion of meat or unpasteurized milk; causes extrapulmonary (non-respiratory) TB of the tonsils, abdominal organs, joints and bones and lymph nodes (also lymphadenitis in immunosuppressed patients). *Miliary TB* severe form occurring when tubercle bacilli are spread acutely throughout the bloodstream causing extrapulmonary TB. *Open TB* any type of TB in which infectious patients are excreting bacilli from the body, most often in the sputum. *Pulmonary TB* the most common form of TB, affecting the lungs. *TB of the spine* also known as Pott's disease.

tuberosity an elevation or protuberance on a bone to which tendons are attached.

tuberous covered with tubers. *T. sclerosis* a familial disease with tumours on the surfaces of the lateral ventricles of the brain and sclerotic patches on its surface; marked by mental deterioration and epileptic attacks.

tubule a small tube. *Renal* or *uriniferous t.* the essential secreting tube of the kidney.

tularaemia a plague-like disease of rodents, caused by *Francisella (Pasteurella) tularensis*, which is transmissible to humans. The illness can be contracted by handling diseased animals or their hides, eating infected wild game or being bitten by insects that have fed on infected animals. It causes fever and headache; the lymph glands enlarge and may suppurate.

tumefaction a swelling or the process of becoming swollen. *See* TUMESCENCE.

tumescence 1. a swelling or enlarging of a part. 2. a swollen condition. 3. a penile erection.

tumour an abnormal swelling. The term is usually applied to a morbid growth of tissue which may be benign or malignant. A neoplasm. *Benign* or *innocent t.* one that does not infiltrate or cause metastases, and is unlikely to recur if removed. *Malignant t.* one that invades and destroys tissue, and can spread to neighbouring tissues, and to more distant sites via the blood and the lymphatic systems.

tunica a coat, a covering, or the lining of a vessel. *T. adventitia, t. media, t. intima* the outer, middle and inner coats of an artery, respectively. *T. vaginalis* the membrane covering the front and sides of the testis.

tunnel in anatomy, a canal through a structure. *Carpal t.* the osteofibrous channel in the wrist between the carpal bones and tissue covering the flexor tendons. *C. tunnel syndrome* pain and tingling in the hand and fingers caused by compression of the median nerve in the carpal tunnel. *T. vision* vision that is restricted to the central field. Occurs in chronic glaucoma and in retinitis pigmentosa.

turbinate scroll-shaped. *T. bone* one of the three long thin plates that form the walls of the nasal cavity.

turgid swollen or distended.

Turner syndrome *H.H. Turner, American physician, 1892–1970.* A chromosomal defect in females, causing short stature. Classically, an absence of one X chromosome. Affects 1 in 2000 live female births. The majority have streak ovaries (a form of ovarian dysgenesis) leading to an absence of puberty and infertility. Other features may include webbing of the neck, cubitus valgus, nail abnormalities and coarctation of the aorta. Intelligence is usually normal.

twilight state partial disturbance of consciousness, a state that may follow an epileptic fit and may be associated with alcoholism and some confusional states. The person can still carry out some routine activities but has no awareness or memory of doing so.

twin one of a pair of individuals who have developed in the uterus together. *Binovular (dizygotic) t.* each twin has developed from a separate ovum; fraternal, or non-identical, twins. *Uniovular (monozygotic) t.* both twins have developed from the same cell; identical twins.

tympanectomy excision of the tympanic membrane.

tympanites distension of the abdomen by accumulation of gas in the intestine or the peritoneal cavity.

tympanitis inflammation of the middle ear; otitis media.

tympanoplasty an operation to reconstruct the eardrum and restore conductivity to the middle ear. *See* MYRINGOPLASTY.

tympanosclerosis fibrosis and the formation of calcified deposits in the middle ear which lead to deafness.

tympanum 1. the middle ear. 2. the eardrum or tympanic membrane.

type the general or prevailing character of any particular case of disease, person, substance, etc. *Blood t's see* BLOOD GROUPS. *Phage t.* a subgroup of a bacterial species susceptible to a particular bacteriophage and demonstrated by phage-typing (*see* PHAGE). Also called lysotype and phagotype.

Pyknic t. a type of physical constitution marked by rounded body, large chest, thick shoulders, broad head and short neck.

typhoid fever enteric fever. A notifiable infectious disease caused by *Salmonella typhi*, which is transmitted by water, milk or other foods, especially shellfish, that have been contaminated. There is high fever, a red rash, delirium and sometimes intestinal haemorrhage. Recovery usually begins during the fourth week of the disease. A person who has had typhoid fever gains immunity from it but may become a carrier. Although perfectly well, the person harbours the bacteria and passes them out in the faeces. The typhoid bacillus often lodges in the gallbladder of carriers.

typhus an acute, notifiable, infectious disease caused by species of the parasitic microorganism *Rickettsia*. There is high fever, a widespread red rash and severe headache. Typhus is likely to occur where there is overcrowding, lack of personal cleanliness and bad hygienic conditions, because the infection is spread by bites of infected lice or by rat fleas. *Scrub t.* a form spread by mites and widespread in the Far East. *See* TSUTSUGAMUSHI DISEASE.

tyramine an enzyme present in cheese, game, broad-bean pods, yeast extracts, wine and strong beer, which has a similar effect in the body to that of adrenaline. Foodstuffs containing tyramine should be avoided by patients taking monoamine oxidase inhibitors.

tyrosine an essential amino acid that is the product of phenylalanine metabolism. In some diseases, especially of the liver, it is present as a deposit in the urine. It is a precursor of catecholamines, melanin and thyroid hormones.

tyrosinosis a congenital condition in which there is an error of metabolism and phenylalanine cannot be reduced to tyrosine. Hepatic failure may occur.

U

ulcer an erosion or loss of continuity of the skin or of a mucous membrane, often accompanied by suppuration. *Arterial u.* caused by arterial insufficiency, usually with a deep punched out appearance and is painful at rest with the legs elevated. *Decubitus u.* a pressure ulcer caused by lying immobile for long periods of time. *Duodenal u.* a peptic ulcer in the duodenum. *Gastric u.* one in the lining of the stomach. *Gravitational u.* a varicose ulcer of the leg which heals with difficulty because of its dependent position and the poor venous return. *Indolent u.* one that is painless and heals slowly. *Peptic u.* one that occurs on the mucous membrane of either the stomach or duodenum. *Perforating u.* one that erodes through the thickness of the wall of an organ. *Rodent u.* a slow-growing epithelioma of the face which may cause much local destruction and ulceration, but does not give rise to metastases. *See* BASAL CELL CARCINOMA. *Venous u.* gravitational ulcer. A shallow ulcer usually on the lower leg between the knee and the ankle that is linked with varicose veins resulting in a poor circulation to and from the area. Initially, there is often an area of eczematous skin and the ulcer forms with large amounts of exudate and oozing.

ulcerative characterized by ulceration (the formation of ulcers). *U. colitis* inflammation and ulceration of the colon and rectum thought to be an auto-immune condition.

ultrasonic relating to sound waves having a frequency range beyond the upper limit perceived by the human ear. These waves are widely used instead of X-rays, particularly in the examination of structures not opaque to X-rays.

ultrasonogram an echo picture obtained from using ultrasound.

ultrasonography a radiological technique in which deep structures of the body are visualized by recording the reflections (echoes) of ultrasonic waves directed into the tissues.

ultrasound ultrasonic waves used to examine the interior organs of the body. These waves can also be used in the treatment of soft-tissue pain, and to break up renal calculi or the crystalline lens when cataract is present. *U. screening* a method of body imaging based on the reflectivity of sound. Ultrasound scanning is non-invasive and is widely used in obstetrics to detect the site of the placenta, the presence of fetal abnormalities and the sex of the fetus; it will reveal a multiple pregnancy at an early stage.

ultraviolet rays short wavelength electromagnetic rays. They are present in sunlight and cause tanning and sunburn.

ultra vires a change made beyond powers. An NHS organization must behave reasonably and in accordance with its powers. If an organization acts beyond its powers (ultra vires), it lays itself open to judicial review.

umbilical cord arises from the placenta and enters the fetus at the site of the future navel, providing the nutritional, hormonal and immunological link between mother and fetus during pregnancy. *U. hernia* common in newborn infants where a part of the bowel or a section of fatty tissue protrudes through the abdominal wall near the navel.

umbilicus the navel; the circular depressed scar in the centre of the abdomen where the umbilical cord of the fetus was attached.

unconditioned response an unlearned response, i.e., one that occurs naturally.

unconscious 1. insensible; incapable of responding to sensory stimuli and of having subjective experiences. 2. that part of mental activity which includes primitive or repressed wishes, concealed from consciousness by the psychological censor. *Collective u.* in Jungian psychology, the portion of the unconscious which is theoretically common to human beings.

unconsciousness the state of being unconscious. This may vary in depth from deep unconsciousness, when no response can be obtained, through to lesser degrees of unconsciousness when the patient can be roused by painful stimuli, to a level when the patient can be roused by speech or non-painful stimuli. Deep prolonged unconsciousness is known as coma.

undine a glass flask with a spout used for irrigation of the eye.

undulant rising and falling like a wave. *U. fever see* BRUCELLOSIS.

unguentum an ointment.

uniform resource locator abbreviated URL. Commonly informally referred to as a web address used in the location of a specific website.

unilateral on one side only.

union 1. a joining together. 2. the repair of tissue after separation by incision or fracture. *See* CALLUS and HEALING.

uniovular from one ovum. *U. twins* identical twins, developed from one ovum. Also known as monozygotic twins.

unipara a woman who has given birth to one child.

unit 1. a single thing. 2. a standard of measurement. *Intensive care u.* a hospital department reserved for those with severe medical or surgical disorders. *International insulin u.* a measurement of the pure crystalline insulin arrived at by biological assay. *SI u.* one of the various units of measurement making up the Système International d'Unités (International System of Units).

universal precautions abbreviated UP. A concept developed by nurses during the mid-1980s (largely as a response to human immunodeficiency virus, or HIV, epidemics) that assumes all patients are potentially infected with BLOOD-BORNE VIRUSES; consequently, universal blood and body fluid infection control precautions are used for all patients, all the time. This concept has been further developed and is known as STANDARD PRECAUTIONS. *See also* BODY SUBSTANCE ISOLATION, INFECTION (CONTROL) and Appendix 11.

urachal referring to the urachus. *U. cyst* a congenital abnormality in which a small cyst persists along the course of the urachus. *U. fistula* one that forms when the urachus fails to close. Urine may leak from the umbilicus.

urachus a tubular canal existing in the fetus, connecting the bladder with the umbilicus. In the adult it persists in the form of a solid fibrous cord.

uraemia 1. an excess in the blood of urea, creatinine and other nitrogenous end products of protein and amino acid metabolism; sometimes referred to as azotaemia. 2. in current usage, the entire complex of signs and symptoms of chronic renal failure. Depending upon the cause it may or may not be reversible. Uraemia leads to vomiting and nausea, headache, weakness, metabolic disturbances, convulsions and coma (*see* RENAL (FAILURE)).

urate   a salt of uric acid. *Sodium u.* a compound generally found in concentration around joints in cases of gout.

urea   carbamide. A white crystalline substance which is an end product of protein metabolism and the chief nitrogenous constituent of urine. It is a diuretic. The normal daily output is about 25 g. *Blood u.* that which is present in the blood. Normal value is 6–20 mg of urea nitrogen per 100 ml.

ureter   one of the two long narrow tubes that convey the urine from the kidney to the bladder.

ureterectomy   the surgical removal of a ureter.

ureteric   relating to the ureter. *U. catheter see* CATHETER. *U. transplantation* an operation which changes the way the ureter connects to the bladder by creating a new tunnel into the bladder. Congenital defects may make this necessary.

ureterocele   a cystic enlargement of the wall of the ureter at its entry into the bladder.

ureterolith   a calculus in a ureter.

ureterolithotomy   removal of a calculus from the ureter.

ureterostomy   the surgical creation of a permanent opening through which the ureter discharges urine.

ureterovaginal   relating to the ureter and vagina. *U. fistula* an opening into the ureter by which urine escapes via the vagina.

urethra   the canal through which the urine is discharged from the bladder. The male urethra is about 18 cm long and the female about 3.5 cm.

urethritis   inflammation of the urethra. The condition is frequently a symptom of gonorrhoea but may be caused by other infectious organisms. *Non-gonococcal u.* abbreviated NGU is the term used when the condition is not caused by gonorrhoea. NGU is sometimes referred to as non-specific urethritis abbreviated NSU when no other cause can be found although it is usually a sexually transmitted infection. *See* NON-SPECIFIC (URETHRITIS).

urethrocele   a prolapse of the female urethral wall which may result from damage to the pelvic floor during childbirth.

urethrography   radiographic examination of the urethra. A radio-opaque contrast medium is inserted by catheter.

urethroscope   an instrument for examining the interior of the urethra.

uric acid   lithic acid, the end product of nucleic acid metabolism, a normal constituent of urine. Its accumulation in the blood produces uricacidaemia. Renal calculi are frequently formed of it.

urinalysis   the bacteriological or chemical examination of the urine.

urinary   relating to urine. *U. tract* the system that conducts urine from the kidneys to the exterior, including the ureters, the bladder and the urethra. (*See* Figure on p. 398.)

urination   micturition. The act of passing urine.

urine   the clear fluid of a varying straw colour secreted by the kidneys and excreted through the bladder and urethra. It is composed of 96% water and 4% solid constituents, the most important being urea and uric acid. Specific gravity = 1.003–1.035; slightly acidic. *Residual u.* that which remains in the bladder after micturition. *U. retention* the inability to urinate voluntarily or to empty a full bladder.

urinometer   an instrument used for measuring the specific gravity of urine.

URL   uniform resource locator.

urobilin   the main pigment of urine, derived from urobilinogen.

urobilinogen   a pigment derived from bilirubin which, on oxidation, forms urobilin.

urochrome   the yellow pigment that colours urine.

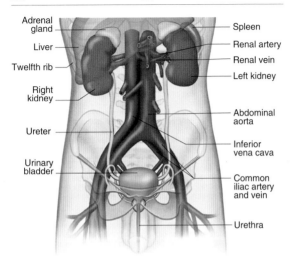

Adrenal gland
Liver
Twelfth rib
Right kidney
Ureter
Urinary bladder

Spleen
Renal artery
Renal vein
Left kidney
Abdominal aorta
Inferior vena cava
Common iliac artery and vein
Urethra

URINARY SYSTEM

urodynamics the dynamics of the propulsion and flow of urine in the urinary tract.

urogenital relating to the urinary and genital organs. Urinogenital.

urography radiographic examination of the urinary tract after the injection of a radio-opaque, water-soluble, iodine-containing medium.

urokinase an enzyme in urine which is secreted by the kidneys and causes fibrinolysis. In certain diseases it may cause bleeding from the kidneys.

urolith a calculus in the urinary tract.

urology the study of diseases of the urinary tract.

urostomy an artificial urinary conduit for deflecting urine from the ureters to the abdominal wall.

urticaria nettle-rash or hives. An acute or chronic skin condition characterized by the recurrent appearance of an eruption of weals, causing great irritation. The cause may be certain foods, infection, drugs or emotional stress. See ALLERGY.

uterine relating to the uterus. *U. tubes* see FALLOPIAN TUBES.

uterosalpingography radiographic examination of the uterus and the uterine tubes.

uterovesical referring to the uterus and bladder. *U. pouch* the fold of peritoneum between the two organs.

uterus the womb; a triangular, hollow, muscular organ situated in the pelvic cavity between the bladder and the rectum. Its function is the nourishment and protection of the fetus during pregnancy and its expulsion at term. (See Figure on p. 338.) *Bicornuate u.* one having two horns. A congenital malformation; see BICORNUATE. *Gravid u.* the pregnant uterus.

utilitarianism a philosophical or ethical view which holds that utility entails the greatest happiness of the greatest number of people and therefore that an action should always produce more benefits than harm.

utricle the delicate membranous sac in the bony vestibule of the ear.

uvea uveal tract. The pigmented layer of the eye, consisting of the iris, ciliary body and choroid.

uveitis inflammation of the uveal tract.

uvula the small fleshy appendage which is the free edge of the soft palate, hanging from the roof of the mouth.

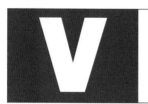

V

vaccination the introduction of vaccine into the body to produce immunity to a specific disease.

vaccine a suspension of killed or attenuated organisms (viruses or bacteria), administered for prevention, amelioration or treatment of infectious diseases. Vaccines are usually given by injection. Some require several doses spaced weeks apart, others require only a single dose. Booster doses may also be required, the interval depending upon the origin vaccine given. *Attenuated v.* one prepared from living organisms which, through long cultivation, have lost their virulence. *Bacille Calmette–Guérin v.* (BCG) an attenuated bovine bacillus vaccine giving immunity from tuberculosis. *Sabin v.* an attenuated poliovirus vaccine that can be administered by mouth, in a syrup or on sugar. *Salk v.* one prepared from an inactivated strain of poliomyelitis virus. *Triple v.* one that protects against diphtheria, tetanus and whooping cough.

vaccinia cowpox; a virus infection of cows, which may be transmitted to humans by contact with the lesions. A local pustular eruption is produced.

vacuum a space from which air or gas has been extracted. *V. bag* a sealed plastic bag containing small expanded polystyrene spheres; the patient is positioned on the bag which has the air pressure inside reduced until it is hardened. This mould is used in radiother-apy to accurately immobilize the patient and to reproduce the position on a daily basis prior to treatment. *V. extractor* an instrument known as a ventouse is used to assist delivery of the fetus. A suction cup is attached to the head and a vacuum created slowly. Gentle traction is applied, which is synchronized with the uterine contractions. *V. wound drainage system* a closed suction drainage system used following surgery for wound exudates.

vagal relating to the vagus nerve.

vagina the canal, lined with mucous membrane, that leads from the cervix of the uterus to the vulva.

vaginismus a painful spasm of the muscles of the vagina, occurring usually when the vulva or vagina is touched, resulting in painful sexual intercourse or dyspareunia.

vaginitis inflammation of the vagina caused by microorganisms. *Atrophic* or *post-menopausal v.* inflammation caused by degenerative changes in the mucous lining of the vagina and insufficient oestrogen secretion. Adhesions may occur, partially closing the vagina. *Trichomonas v.* infection caused by *T. vaginalis,* a protozoon that causes a thin, yellowish discharge, giving rise to local tenderness and pruritus.

vagotomy surgical incision of the vagus nerve or any of its branches. A treatment for gastric or duodenal ulcer when acid production cannot be reduced by other means such as medication or dietary changes. *Highly selective v.* division of only those vagal fibres supplying the acid-secreting glands of the stomach. *Medical v.* interruption of impulses carried by the vagus nerve by administration of suitable drugs.

vagus the tenth cranial nerves (a pair), arising in the medulla and providing the parasympathetic nerve supply to the organs in the thorax and abdomen. *V. resection* vagotomy.

valgus a displacement outwards, particularly of the feet. *See* GENU, HALLUX, TALIPES.

validity the extent to which a measure, indicator or method of data collection possesses the quality of being sound or true, as far as can be judged. *Construct v.* the extent to which an instrument is said to measure a theoretical construct or trait. *Content v.* the degree to which the content of the measure represents the universe of content, or the domain of a given behaviour. *External v.* the degree to which findings of a study can be generalized to other populations or environments. *Face v.* a type of content validity that uses an expert's opinion to judge the accuracy of an instrument. *Internal v.* the degree to which it can be inferred that the experimental treatment, rather than an uncontrolled condition, resulted in the observed effects.

valine an essential amino acid formed by the digestion of dietary protein.

Valsalva's manoeuvre *A.M. Valsalva, Italian anatomist, 1666–1723.* Technique for increasing the intrathoracic pressure by closing the mouth and nostrils and blowing out the cheeks, thereby forcing air back into the nasopharynx. When the breath is released, the intrathoracic pressure drops and the blood is quickly propelled through the heart, producing an increase in the heart rate (tachycardia) and the blood pressure. Immediately after this event a reflex bradycardia ensues. Valsalva's manoeuvre occurs when a person strains to defecate or

urinate, uses the arm and upper trunk muscles to move up in bed, or strains during coughing, gagging or vomiting. The increased pressure, immediate tachycardia and reflex bradycardia can bring about cardiac arrest in vulnerable heart patients.

valve 1. a means of regulating the flow of liquid or gas through a pipe. 2. a fold of membrane in a passage or tube, so placed as to permit passage of fluid in one direction only. Valves are important structures in the heart, in veins and in lymph vessels. *Semilunar v.* either of two valves at the junction of the pulmonary artery and aorta, respectively, with the heart.

valvotomy valvulotomy. A surgical operation to open up a fibrosed valve, e.g., mitral valvotomy to relieve mitral stenosis.

valvulitis inflammation of a valve, particularly of the heart.

vanguard sites across England where new models of care are tested.

vaporizer an apparatus for producing a very fine spray of a liquid.

variable a research term that describes any factor or circumstance that is part of the study. *Confounding v.* one that affects the conditions of the independent variables unequally. *Dependent v.* one that depends upon the experimental conditions. *Independent v.* the variable conditions of an experimental situation, e.g., control or experimental. *Random v's* background factors that may affect any conditions of the independent variables equally.

variance used in statistics. The distribution range of a set of results around a mean. *See* STANDARD DEVIATION.

varicella chickenpox. An infectious disease of childhood with an incubation period of 12–20 days. There is slight fever and an eruption of transparent vesicles on the chest, on the first day of disease; these appear in successive crops all over the body. The vesicles soon dry up, sometimes leaving shallow pits in the skin. The disease is usually mild, but may be severe in neonates, adults and those who are immunocompromised. Anyone who has had chicken pox may develop shingles in later life.

varicella zoster virus abbreviated VZV. A human herpes virus that causes chickenpox during childhood and may reactivate later in life to cause shingles.

varices alternative name for enlarged, distorted varicose veins or lymphatic vessels.

varicose swollen or dilated. *V. ulcer* gravitational ulcer. *See* ULCER. *V. veins* a dilated and twisted condition of the veins (usually those of the leg) caused by structural changes in the walls or valves of the vessels.

varus a displacement inwards. *See* GENU, HALLUX, TALIPES.

vas *pl.* vasa. A vessel or duct. *V. deferens* one of a pair of excretory ducts conveying the semen from the epididymis to the urethra. *V. efferens* one of the many small tubes that convey semen from the testis to the epididymis. *Vasa vasorum* the minute nutrient vessels that supply the walls of the arteries and veins.

vascular relating to, or consisting largely of, blood vessels. *V. dementia* a common type of dementia caused by reduced blood flow to the brain. *See* DEMENTIA. *V. system* the cardiovascular system.

vascularization the development of new blood vessels within a tissue that occurs during healing.

vasculitis angiitis; inflammation of blood vessels. *Allergic v.* a severe allergic response to drugs or to cold. Arising in small arteries or veins, with fibrosis and thrombi formation.

vasectomy excision of a part of the vas deferens. If performed bilaterally, sterility results. Employed as a method of contraception.

vasoconstrictor any agent that causes contraction of a blood vessel wall, and therefore a decrease in the blood flow and a rise in the blood pressure.

vasodilator any agent that causes an increase in the lumen of blood vessels, and therefore an increase in the blood flow and a fall in the blood pressure.

vasomotor controlling the muscles of blood vessels, both dilator and constrictor. *V. centre* nerve cells in the medulla oblongata controlling the vasomotor nerves. *V. nerves* sympathetic nerves regulating the tension of the blood vessels.

vasopressin antidiuretic hormone (ADH). A hormone from the posterior lobe of the pituitary gland which causes constriction of plain muscle fibres and reabsorption of water in the renal tubules. Used in the treatment of diabetes insipidus and bleeding from oesophageal varices.

vasovagal vascular and vagal. *V. attack* fainting or syncope, often evoked by emotional stress associated with fear and pain. There is postural hypotension.

VDU visual display unit.

vector 1. an animal that carries organisms or parasites from one host to another, either to a member of the same species or to one of another species. 2. a quantity with magnitude and direction. *Electrocardiographic v.* the area of the heart that is monitored during electrocardiographic investigation.

vegan a person who does not eat products of animal origin, or use them in general life.

vegetarian a person who does not eat meat or fish. *V. diet* one in which no meat is eaten. A *lacto-vegetarian* diet prohibits the intake of meat, poultry, fish and eggs. An *ovo-lacto-vegetarian* diet allows all foods from plants plus eggs, milk and other dairy products. An *ovo-vegetarian* diet allows eggs and foods of plant origin, but prohibits all meat, fish and dairy products.

vegetation in pathology, a plant-like outgrowth. *Adenoid v.* overgrowth of lymphoid tissue in the nasopharynx.

vegetative 1. the non-sporing stage of a bacterium. 2. profoundly lethargic and passive. *V. state* a type of deep coma that may follow severe head injuries. The patient's eyes may be open with some associated random movements of the head and limbs, but there are no other signs of consciousness or response to stimuli. Only basic functions such as breathing and heart beat are maintained.

vehicle in pharmacy, a substance or medium in which a drug is administered.

vein a vessel carrying blood from the capillaries back to the heart. It has thin walls and a lining endothelium from which the venous valves are formed.

venepuncture the insertion of a needle into a vein for the introduction of a drug or fluid or for the withdrawal of blood.

venereal pertaining to or caused by sexual intercourse. *V. disease* a disease transmitted by sexual intercourse or other genital contact. The term venereal disease (VD) has now been replaced by the term SEXUALLY TRANSMITTED INFECTION.

venereology the study and treatment of venereal diseases.

venesection phlebotomy. Surgical blood-letting by opening a vein or most usually by introducing a wide-bore needle. A procedure used to collect blood from blood donors and occasionally to relieve venous congestion.

venogram 1. a graphic recording of the pulse in a vein. 2. a radiograph taken during venography.

venography radiographic examination of a vein after the instillation of a contrast medium to trace its pathway.

venom a poison secreted by an insect, snake or other animal. *Russell's viper v.* the venom of the Russell viper (*Daboia russelii*), which acts in vitro as an intrinsic thromboplastin and is useful in defining deficiencies of clotting factor X.

venous pertaining to the veins. *See* CENTRAL VENOUS PRESSURE. *V. sinus* one of 14 channels, similar to veins, by

which blood leaves the cerebral circulation. *V. thromboembolism* abbreviated to VTE. The development of a clot. VTE is the collective name for deep vein thrombosis and pulmonary embolism. Most clots are preventable and preventative steps should be taken for patients at risk when in hospital or during periods of ill health. *V. ulcer* *see* ULCER (VARICOSE).

ventilation 1. the process or act of supplying a house or room continuously with fresh air. 2. in respiratory physiology, the process of exchange of air between the lungs and the ambient air. *Pulmonary v.* (usually measured in litres per minute) refers to the total exchange, whereas *alveolar v.* refers to the effective ventilation of the alveoli, where gas exchange with the blood takes place. 3. in psychiatry, the free discussion of one's problems or grievances.

ventilator an apparatus designed to qualify the air that is breathed through it either intermittently or continuously. Ventilators provide an intermittent flow of air and/or oxygen under pressure and are connected to the patient by a tube inserted through the mouth, the nose or an opening in the trachea. *V.-associated pneumonia* (VAP) is a common cause of hospital-acquired pneumonia, diagnosed in a patient more than 48 hours following the insertion of an endotracheal tube and the commencement of mechanical ventilation.

Ventimask an oxygen mask that provides oxygen enrichment of the inspired air while eliminating the need to rebreathe the expired carbon dioxide.

ventouse *see* VACUUM EXTRACTOR.

ventricle a small pouch or cavity; applied especially to the lower chambers of the heart and to the four cavities of the brain.

ventricular pertaining to a ventricle. *V. folds* the outer folds of mucous membrane forming the false vocal cords. *V. septal defect* abbreviated VSD. Congenital abnormality in which there is communication between the two ventricles of the heart as a result of maldevelopment of the intraventricular septum. *V. fibrillation see* FIBRILLATION.

ventriculography 1. radiographic examination of the ventricles of the heart using a radio-opaque contrast medium. 2. radiographic examination of the ventricles of the brain after the injection of air or a contrast medium through a burr hole.

Venturi mask *G.B. Venturi, Italian physicist, 1746–1822.* A type of disposable mask used to deliver a controlled oxygen concentration to a patient. The flow of 100% oxygen through the mask draws in a controlled amount of room air (21% oxygen). Commonly available masks deliver 24%, 28%, 35%, 40% or 60% oxygen. At concentrations above 24%, humidification may be required.

Venturi nebulizer a type of nebulizer used in AEROSOL therapy. The pressure drop of gas flowing through the nebulizer draws liquid from a capillary tube. As the liquid enters the gas stream it breaks up into a spray of small droplets.

venule a minute vein which collects blood from the capillaries.

verbigeration the monotonous repetition of phrases or meaningless words.

vermicide an agent that destroys intestinal worms; an anthelmintic.

vermiform worm-shaped. *V. appendix* the worm-shaped structure attached to the caecum.

vermifuge an agent that expels intestinal worms; an anthelmintic.

verminous infested with worms or other animal parasites, such as lice.

vernix [L.] *varnish. V. caseosa* the fatty covering on the skin of the fetus during the last months of pregnancy. It consists of cells and sebaceous material.

verruca a wart. Condyloma. Hypertrophy of the prickle cell layer of the epidermis and thickening of the horny layer. A virus is the causative organism. *V. acuminata* a venereal wart that appears on the external genitalia. *V.*

plana a small, smooth, usually skin-coloured or light-brown, slightly raised wart, sometimes occurring in great numbers; seen most often in children. Also known as flat warts. *V. plantaris* a viral epidermal tumour on the sole of the foot. *See* CONDYLOMATA.

version the turning of a part; applied particularly to the turning of a fetus in order to facilitate delivery. *External v.* manipulation of the uterus through the abdominal wall in order to change the position of the fetus. *Internal v.* rotation of the fetus by means of manipulation with one hand in the vagina. *Podalic v.* turning of the fetus so that the head is uppermost and the feet presenting. *Spontaneous v.* one that occurs naturally without the application of force.

vertebra one of the 33 irregular bones forming the spinal column: 7 cervical, 12 thoracic, 5 lumbar, 5 sacral (sacrum) and 4 coccygeal (coccyx) vertebrae.

vertebral pertaining to a vertebra. *V. column* the spine or backbone.

vertebrobasilar pertaining to the vertebral and the basilar arteries. *V. insufficiency* abbreviated VBI. A condition affecting the flow of blood through the vertebral and basilar arteries which may cause recurrent attacks of nausea, ataxia, diplopia, vertigo, dysarthria and hemiparesis.

vertex the crown of the head. *V. presentation* position of the fetus such that the crown of the head appears in the vagina first.

vertical transmission transmission of an infection from an infected mother to her newborn child during pregnancy, delivery or in the postpartum period through breast milk. Also called perinatal or mother-to-child transmission.

vertigo a feeling of rotation or of going round, in either oneself or one's surroundings, particularly associated with disease of the cerebellum and the vestibular nerve of the ear. It may occur in diplopia or Menière's syndrome.

vesicle 1. in anatomy, a small bladder, usually containing fluid. 2. a very small blister, usually containing serum. *Seminal v.* one of a pair of sacs which arise from the vas deferens near the bladder and contain semen.

vesicoureteric relating to the urinary bladder and the ureters. *V. reflux* the passing of urine backwards up the ureter during micturition. A cause of pyelonephritis in children.

vesicovaginal relating to the bladder and vagina. *See* FISTULA.

vesicular relating to or containing vesicles. *V. breathing* the soft murmur of normal respiration, as heard on auscultation. *V. mole* hydatidiform mole.

vesiculitis inflammation of a vesicle, particularly the seminal vesicles.

vessel a tube, duct or canal for conveying fluid, usually blood or lymph.

vestibular relating to a vestibule. *V. glands* those in the vestibule of the vagina, including Bartholin's glands. *V. nerve* a branch of the auditory nerve supplying the semicircular canals and concerned with balance and equilibrium. *V. neuronitis* an infection of the vestibular nerve in the inner ear leading to disruption of balance. *V. schwannoma* a benign primary intracranial tumour of the myelin-forming cells of the vestibulocochlear nerve. Also known as acoustic neuroma.

vestibule a space or cavity at the entrance to another structure. *V. of the ear* the cavity at the entrance to the cochlea. *V. of the vagina* the space between the labia minora at the entrance to the vagina.

vestibulocochlear pertaining to the vestibule of the ear and the cochlea. *V. nerve* the eighth cranial nerve. Also known as the auditory nerve.

vestigial rudimentary. Referring to the remains of an anatomical structure which, being of no further use, has atrophied.

viable capable of independent life.

Vibrio a genus of gram-negative bacteria, curved and motile by means of flagella. *V. cholerae* that which causes cholera.

vicarious 1. obtained or undergone at second hand through sympathetic participation in another's experiences. 2. substituted for another; used when one organ functions instead of another. *V. liability* the liability of an employer for the wrongful acts of an employee committed in the course of employment.

villus a small finger-like process projecting from a surface. *Chorionic v. see* CHORIONIC. *Intestinal villi* those of the mucous membrane of the small intestine, each of which contains a blood capillary and a lacteal.

Vincent's angina *J.H. Vincent, French physician, 1862–1950.* Infection of the gingiva or gums. Also known as acute necrotizing ulcerative gingivitis (ANUG) or trench mouth.

viraemia the presence of viruses in the blood.

viral haemorrhagic fevers a group of infectious diseases prevalent in Africa that cause fever, severe malaise and headache, diarrhoea and vomiting with severe bleeding and are commonly fatal. *see* EBOLA, LASSA and MARBURG FEVERS.

virilism masculine traits exhibited by a female owing to the production of excessive amounts of androgenic hormone either in the adrenal cortex or from an ovarian tumour. *See* ARRHENOBLASTOMA.

virion a fully developed complete infectious viral particle consisting of its nucleic acid and a surrounding coat of protein (capsid); the extracellular (cell-free) form of a virus.

virology the scientific study of viruses, their growth and the diseases caused by them.

virtual ward operates like a hospital ward but the patient stays at home and is cared for by a team based in the community.

virulence the power of a microorganism to produce toxins or poisons. This depends on (a) the number and power of the invading organisms, and (b) the power of the microorganism to overcome host resistance.

virulent dangerously infectious or poisonous.

virus any member of a unique class of infectious agents, which were originally distinguished by their smallness and their inability to replicate outside a living host cell; because these properties are shared by certain other microorganisms (rickettsiae, chlamydiae), viruses are now characterized by their simple organization and their unique mode of replication. A virus consists of genetic material, which may be either DNA or RNA, and is surrounded by a protein coat and, in some viruses, by a membranous envelope. They cause many diseases, including chickenpox (varicella), herpes zoster (shingles), herpes infections, measles (rubeola), German measles (rubella), mumps, infectious mononucleosis, hepatitis A and B, yellow fever, the common cold, acquired immune deficiency syndrome (AIDS), influenza, certain types of pneumonia and croup and other respiratory infections, poliomyelitis, and several types of encephalitis. There is evidence that certain viruses can cause cancer, e.g., cancer of the liver and cervix. *See* ORTHOMYXOVIRUS

viscera *pl.* of VISCUS.

viscid sticky and glutinous.

viscosity resistance to flowing. A sticky and glutinous quality.

viscus *pl.* viscera. Any of the organs contained in the body cavities, especially in the abdomen.

vision the faculty of seeing. Sight.

visual relating to sight. *V. acuity* sharpness of vision. It is assessed by reading test types. *V. cells* the rods and cones of the retina. *V. field* the area within which objects can be seen when looking straight ahead. *V. purple* the pigment in the outer layers of the retina. Rhodopsin.

visual display unit abbreviated VDU. The monitor screen attached to a computer.

visualization the technique of using the imagination and relaxation to create any desired changes in an individual's life.

vital relating to life. *V. capacity* the amount of air that can be expelled from the lungs after a full inspiration. *V. signs* the signs of life, namely pulse, respiration and temperature. *V. statistics* the records kept of births and deaths among the population, including the causes of death, and the factors that seem to influence their rise and fall.

vitallium a metal alloy used in dentistry and for prostheses in bone surgery.

vitamin any of a group of accessory food factors which are contained in foodstuffs and are essential to life, growth and reproduction. *See* Appendix 1. *V. B_{12} deficiency* lack of vitamin B_{12} causes the body to produce abnormally large blood cells.

vitiligo a skin disease marked by an absence of pigment, producing white patches on the face and body. Leukoderma.

vitrectomy surgical extraction of the vitreous humour and its replacement by a physiological solution in the treatment of vitreous haemorrhage in diabetic retinopathy. *V. humour* the transparent jelly-like substance filling the posterior of the eye, from lens to retina.

vocal pertaining to the voice, or the organs that produce the voice. *V. cords* the two folds of tissue in the larynx, formed of fibrous tissue covered with squamous epithelium. *V. resonance* the normal sounds of speech heard through the chest wall by means of a stethoscope.

volatile having a tendency to evaporate readily.

volition the conscious adoption by the individual of a line of action.

Volkmann's ischaemic contracture *R. von Volkmann, German surgeon,*

1830–1889. Contraction of the fingers and sometimes of the wrist or of analogous parts of the foot, with loss of power, after severe injury or improper use of a tourniquet or cast.

volume the space occupied by a substance. *Minute v.* the total volume of air breathed in or out in 1 minute. *Packed cell v.* that occupied by the blood cells after centrifuging (about 45% of the blood sample). *Residual v.* the amount of air left in the lungs after breathing out fully.

voluntary under the control of the will. *See* INVOLUNTARY. *V. admission* a patient who voluntarily agrees to enter a psychiatric unit or hospital as an inpatient. *V. muscle* a striated muscle. *See* MUSCLE. *V. organizations* a group of people who join together with a shared common purpose or cause to provide a service to others. Many of these groups are registered charities and may also have grants from local or central government. Some employ professional and managerial staff but most remain dependent upon voluntary help. Many of these organizations provide considerable support to patients, their carers and families.

volvulus twisting of a loop of bowel causing obstruction. Most common in the sigmoid colon.

vomer a thin plate of bone forming the posterior septum of the nose.

vomit 1. matter ejected from the stomach through the mouth (vomitus). 2. to eject material in this way. *Bilious v.* vomit mixed with bile. The vomit is stained yellow or green. *Coffee-ground v.* ejected matter that contains small quantities of altered blood, which has the appearance of coffee grounds. *Faecal* or *stercoraceous v.* vomit mixed with faeces. Occurs in intestinal obstruction when the contents of the upper intestine regurgitate back into the stomach. It is dark brown with an unpleasant odour.

vomiting a reflex act of expulsion of the stomach contents via the oesophagus and mouth. It may be preceded by nausea and excess salivation if the cause is local irritation in the stomach. *Cyclical v.* recurrent attacks of vomiting often occurring in children and associated with acidosis. *Projectile v.* the forcible ejection of the gastric contents, usually without warning. Present in hypertrophic pyloric stenosis and in cerebral diseases. *V. of pregnancy* vomiting occurring in the months of pregnancy. Morning sickness.

von Willebrand's disease *E.A. von Willebrand, Finnish physician, 1870–1949*. A bleeding disorder inherited as an autosomal dominant trait (rarely recessive), characterized by a deficiency of a blood protein called von Willebrand factor (VWF). VWF binds factor VIII which is involved in the clotting process. Symptoms include epistaxis and increased bleeding after trauma or surgery, menorrhagia and postpartum bleeding.

voyeurism sexual deviation, whereby a person gains sexual satisfaction from covertly watching others who are naked or involved in sexual activity.

VSD ventricular septal defect.

vulnerability weakness. Susceptibility to injury or infection.

vulva the external female genital organs.

vulvectomy excision of the vulva.

vulvitis inflammation of the vulva.

vulvovaginitis inflammation of the vulva and vagina.

VZV varicella zoster virus.

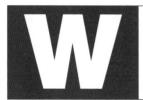

Waldeyer's ring *H.W.G. von Waldeyer-Hartz, German anatomist, 1836–1921.* The circle of lymphoid tissue in the pharynx formed by the lingual, faucial and pharyngeal tonsils.

walk-in centres establishments that deliver accessible health care services on a drop-in basis. They offer NHS consultations and provide treatment for minor injuries and illnesses, general health information, self-treatment advice, information about out-of-hours general practitioner/dental services and local pharmacy services, and are situated in major towns and cities. They generally operate during the day and at weekends, in times and places that people find convenient and are usually nurse-led, though a number of other health professionals and social care staff may be involved. Centres are managed by an NHS body or general practitioner federation and funded by the local health commissioners.

Wangensteen tube *O.H. Wangensteen, American surgeon, 1898–1981.* A gastrointestinal aspiration tube with a tip that is opaque to X-rays.

wart an elevation of the skin, often of a brownish colour, caused by hypertrophy of papillae in the dermis due to a virus infection. *See* VERRUCA and CONDYLOMA.

Wassermann test (reaction) *A.P. von Wassermann, German bacteriologist, 1866–1925.* A complement-fixation test, rarely used today that enables the diagnosis of syphilis.

water a clear, colourless, tasteless liquid composed of hydrogen and oxygen (H_2O). ***W. balance*** fluid balance. That between the fluid taken in by all routes and the fluid lost by all routes. ***W.-borne*** descriptive of certain diseases that are spread by contaminated water. ***W.-brash*** the eructation of dilute acid from the stomach to the pharynx, giving a burning sensation. Pyrosis. Heartburn. ***W. intoxication*** a condition that results from excessive water retention in the brain, resulting in headaches, dizziness and confusion. In severe cases may cause seizures and unconsciousness. Water intoxication can also result from the use of the drug ecstasy, which may be taken by young people in night clubs, leading to excessive quantities of water being drunk. ***W.-seal drainage*** a closed method of drainage from the pleural space allowing the escape of fluid and air but preventing air entering because the drainage tube discharges under water.

Waterhouse–Friderichsen syndrome *R. Waterhouse, British physician, 1873–1958; C. Friderichsen, Danish physician, 1886–1979.* An adrenal gland disease that is characterized by failure of the adrenal gland due to bleeding into the gland marked by sudden onset fever, coma, cyanosis, haemorrhages from the skin and mucous membranes and severe shock. Also known as purpura fulminans.

Waterlow scale *See* PRESSURE ULCER ASSESSMENT SCALES.

waxy flexibility a psychomotor symptom associated with schizophrenia, bipolar disorder or other mental disorders in which a patient's limbs are held indefinitely in any position in which they have been placed. *See* CATATONIA.

weal a raised stripe on the skin or small blister, as is caused by the lash of a whip. Typical of urticaria.

wean 1. to discontinue breast or bottle-feeding and substitute other feeding habits, e.g., solid foods. This should be effected gradually at about the 6th month. 2. in respiratory therapy, to gradually decrease dependence on assisted ventilation until the patient is able to breathe spontaneously.

wear and tear theory the concept of ageing that equates the human body with a machine, and that as parts wear out physiological functions deteriorate affecting the quality of life.

web a network or complex system of interconnected elements. *W. space* the soft tissue between the bases of the fingers and the toes. *W. site* in information technology, one or more pages that can be accessed through the internet to the World Wide Web (WWW) that allows the browser to obtain specific information on the site.

webbing the state of being connected by a membrane or a fold of skin. *W. of the hands* or *feet* congenital abnormality in which the digits are not separated from each other. Syndactyly. *W. of the neck* folds of skin in the neck, giving it a webbed appearance. Occurs in certain congenital conditions, e.g., Turner's syndrome.

Weil's disease *A. Weil, German physician, 1848–1916.* Spirochetal jaundice. The organism, *Leptospira icterohaemorrhagiae*, is harboured and excreted by rats and enters through a bite or skin abrasion, or infected food or water.

Weil–Felix reaction *E. Weil, Austrian physician, 1880–1922; A. Felix, Czech bacteriologist, 1887–1956.* An agglutination test of blood serum used in the diagnosis of typhus.

well-baby clinic parents are encouraged to bring their infants to these clinics for advice and monitoring of the child's health.

wellness the development of a personal lifestyle that promotes feelings of wellbeing, achieves the highest level of health within one's capability, and minimizes chances of becoming ill. It is guided by a developing sense of self-awareness and self-responsibility encompassing emotional, mental, physical, social, spiritual and environmental health.

wen a small sebaceous cyst; a steatoma.

Werdnig–Hoffmann disease *G. Werdnig, Austrian neurologist, 1844–1919; J.E. Hoffmann, German neurologist, 1857–1919.* A genetic condition characterized by progressive spinal muscular atrophy affecting the shoulder, neck, pelvis and eventually the respiratory muscles of infants. Also known as spinal muscular atrophy and autosomal recessive proximal spinal muscular atrophy.

Wernicke–Korsakoff syndrome *K. Wernicke, German neurologist, 1848–1905; S.S. Korsakoff, Russian neurologist, 1854–1900.* A disorder of the central nervous system, usually associated with chronic alcoholism, nutritional deficiency and severe deficiency of vitamin B_1. It can sometimes occur with chronic illness or after weight loss (bariatric) surgery. It is characterized by a combination of motor and sensory disturbances and disordered memory function. One form is Wernicke's encephalopathy, a neurological condition due to vitamin B_1 deficiency. Untreated, it progresses from mental confusion and double vision to lethargy and coma.

Wertheim's operation *E. Wertheim, Austrian gynaecologist, 1864–1920.* *See* HYSTERECTOMY.

West Nile virus a virus spread by mosquitoes occurring across the world.

In around 1 in 100 cases it can be serious with encephalitis developing which can be fatal.

wet nurse an ancient practice common in many cultures where a lactating woman breast feeds another woman's child.

Wharton's jelly *T. Wharton, English physician, 1614–1673.* A gelatinous substance within the umbilical cord, also present in the vitreous humour of the eyeball.

wheezing breathing with a rasp or whistling sound. It results from constriction or obstruction of the throat, pharynx, trachea or bronchi.

whiplash injury injury to the spinal cord, nerve roots, ligaments or vertebrae in the cervical region due to a sudden jerking back of the head and neck. Common in road traffic accidents where there is sudden acceleration or deceleration of the vehicle.

whiplash shake syndrome a constellation of injuries to the brain and eye that may occur when a young child is shaken vigorously with the head unsupported. This causes stretching and tearing of the cerebral vessels and brain substance, commonly leading to subdural haematomas and retinal haemorrhages. It may result in paralysis, blindness and other visual disturbances, convulsions and death. *See* SHAKEN BABY SYNDROME.

Whipple's operation *A.O. Whipple, American surgeon, 1881–1963.* Radical pancreatoduodenectomy performed for carcinoma of the head of the pancreas.

whipworm *see* TRICHURIS.

white leg milk leg.

whitlow a felon; a suppurating inflammation of a finger near the nail. *Melanotic w.* a malignant tumour of the nail bed characterized by formation of melanotic tissue. Also known as subungual melanoma. *Subperiosteal w.* one in which the infection involves the bone covering. *Superficial w.* a pustule between the true skin and cuticle. *See* PARONYCHIA.

WHO *see* WORLD HEALTH ORGANIZATION. An agency of the United Nations.

whole system planning strategic planning and commissioning across a range of services and organizational boundaries. Deals with the impact that changes in one part of the system, whether health and social care or housing, are likely to have on other parts.

whole systems approach the consideration of the interrelatedness of various elements, which come together for a common purpose and continually have impact upon one another. The comprehension of complex systems, e.g., health care and social care, requires understanding of a diverse range of perspectives, and an appreciation that change will often be required across a number of areas to meet needs.

whole time equivalent total weekly contracted hours of full- and part-time staff expressed as a multiple of the standard working week.

whooping cough pertussis a notifiable infectious disease characterized by catarrh of the respiratory tract and paroxysms of coughing, ending in a prolonged whooping respiration; called also pertussis. The causative organism is *Bordetella pertussis*. Whooping cough is a serious disease; most cases occur in children. All babies should be immunized against whooping cough unless there is a sound medical objection.

Widal reaction *G.F.I. Widal, French physician, 1862–1929.* A blood agglutination test for typhoid fever.

Willis-Ekbom syndrome also known as restless leg syndrome results in an uncontrollable urge to move the legs, possibly associated with dopamine. In some people it is temporary and in others permanent and debilitating. The temporary form is very common in pregnancy.

Wilms' tumour *M. Wilms, German surgeon, 1867–1918.* A highly malignant tumour of the kidney occurring in young children. A nephroblastoma.

Wilson's disease *S.A.K. Wilson, British neurologist, 1878–1937.* Hepatolenticular degeneration. A genetic disorder involving the metabolism of copper, leading to neurological degeneration.

wiring the fixing together of a broken or split bone by the use of a wire. Commonly used for the jaw, the patella and the sternum.

wisdom teeth the back molar teeth, the eruption of which is often delayed until maturity.

wish fulfilment a desire, not always acknowledged consciously by the person, which is fulfilled through dreams or by day-dreaming.

withdrawal 1. a pathological retreat from reality. 2. abstention from drugs or activities to which one is habituated or addicted; also denoting the symptoms occasioned by such withdrawal. *W. symptoms* symptoms brought about by abrupt withdrawal of the substance to which a person has become addicted; called also abstinence syndrome. The usual reactions to withdrawal may include anxiety, weakness, gastrointestinal symptoms, nausea and vomiting, tremor, fever, rapid heartbeat, convulsions and delirium.

Wolff–Parkinson–White syndrome *L. Wolff, American cardiologist, 1898–1972; Sir J. Parkinson, British physician, 1885–1976; P. D. White, American cardiologist, 1886–1973.* Abnormal heart rhythm caused by an accessory bundle between the atria and ventricles. A congenital disorder.

womb the uterus.

Wood's light *R.W. Wood, American physicist, 1868–1953.* Ultraviolet light transmitted through a glass filter containing nickel oxide. It produces fluorescence of infected hairs when placed over a scalp affected with ringworm.

woolsorter's disease pulmonary form of anthrax.

word blindness *see* DYSLEXIA.

word salad a colloquial term for rapid speech in which the words are strung together without meaning.

World Health Organization abbreviated WHO. The specialized agency of the United Nations that is concerned with health at an international level. WHO organizes health campaigns against infectious diseases and sponsors research in medical laboratories. It also provides expert advice on all matters directly or indirectly concerned with physical or mental health to all member states.

World Wide Web abbreviated WWW. An information space where documents and other resources are stored and interlinked and accessed via the internet.

worm any one of a number of groups of long soft-bodied invertebrates, some of which are parasitic to humans.

wound a cut or break in continuity of any tissue, caused by injury or operation. It is classified according to its nature. *Abrased w.* the skin is scraped off, but there is no deeper injury. *Contused w.* with bruising of the surrounding tissue. *Incised w.* usually the result of operation, and produced by a knife or similar instrument. The edges of the wound can remain in apposition, and it should heal by first intention. *Lacerated w.* one with torn edges and tissues, usually the result of accident or injury. It is often septic and heals by second intention. *Open w.* a gaping wound on the body surface. *Penetrating w.* often made by gunshot, shrapnel, etc. There may be an inlet and outlet hole and vital organs are often penetrated by the missile. *Punctured w.* made by a pointed or spiked instrument. *Septic w.* any type into which infection has been introduced, causing suppurative inflammation. It heals by second intention. *W. drain. See* DRAIN. *W. dressing* material applied to a surgical or medical wound to provide protection and assist healing. Dressings are made from a variety of materials with or without medication, e.g., hydro-cellular or alginate dressings used in the management of cavities or exuding wounds, and low-adherent absorbent dressings used for clean wounds. The aim is that the dressing should be comfortable, permit the exchange of gases but be impermeable to bacteria, prevent adherence to the wound, and therefore reduce damage to new tissue when it is removed. *W. healing* the restoration of integrity to injured tissues by replacement of dead tissue with viable tissue. In wound healing there are four stages:—haemostasis, inflammation, proliferation (or granulation) and maturation—which may take several months to complete. Wound healing may be delayed by physical stress, inadequate blood supply or by more general factors that include malnutrition, ageing, drugs such as corticosteroids, etc. The process starts immediately after an injury and may continue for months or years. *See* HEALING.

wrist the point of the carpus and bones of the forearm. *W. drop* loss of power in the muscles of the hand. It may be due to nerve or tendon injury, but can result from lack of sufficient support by splint or sling.

writer's cramp a colloquial term for painful spasm of the hand and forearm, caused by excessive writing and poor posture.

wryneck *see* TORTICOLLIS.

Wuchereria a genus of nematode worms which are the principal vectors of filariasis. *W. bancrofti* the most common species in tropical and subtropical areas.

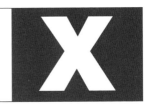

X chromosome the female sex chromosome, being present in all female gametes and only half the male gametes. When union takes place two X chromosomes result in a female child (XX) but one of each results in a male child (XY). *See* Y CHROMOSOME.

X-linked pertaining to the genes, or the effect of these genes, situated on the X chromosome. X-linked disorders are those caused by the genes on the X chromosome.

X-rays electromagnetic waves of short length which are capable of penetrating many substances and of producing chemical changes and reactions in living matter. They are used both to aid diagnosis and to treat disease. Also called Röntgen radiation.

xanthelasma a disease marked by the formation of flat or slightly raised yellow fatty deposits on or around the eyelids.

xanthine a compound found in plant and animal tissues; a rare genetic disorder xanthinuria results from a lack of xanthine oxidase and an inability to convert xanthine to uric acid.

xanthochromia 1. the presence of yellow patches on the skin. 2. the yellow colouring of cerebrospinal fluid seen in patients who have had a subarachnoid haemorrhage.

xanthoma the presence in the skin of flat areas of yellowish pigmentation due to deposits of lipids. There are several varieties.

xanthosis a yellow skin discoloration of degenerating tissue seen in some malignant neoplasms.

Xenopsylla a genus of fleas, some of which are vectors of plague. *X. cheopis* the rat flea, which transmits bubonic plague and murine typhus.

xeroderma also known as xerosis cutis. Dry skin occurring most commonly on the scalp, lower legs, arms, hands, abdomen and thighs. A very common condition especially in winter. *X. pigmentosum* (XP) a rare hereditary disorder of DNA repair where the ability to repair damage caused by ultraviolet light is deficient. It begins in childhood and rapidly progresses. The formation of malignant neoplasms of the skin is common and is a common cause of death in people with XP.

xerophthalmia a condition in which the eye fails to produce tears and the cornea and conjunctiva become dry, thick and wrinkled. It may be caused by a deficiency of vitamin A. Also known as xeroma.

xerostomia dryness of the mouth due to a failure of salivary gland secretion or a change in the composition of saliva.

xylose a pentose sugar, found in connective tissue and sometimes in urine, which is not metabolized in the body. *X. absorption test* an investigation for malabsorption.

XXY a syndrome where boys are born with an additional X chromosome. *See* KLINEFELTER'S SYNDROME.

XYY syndrome an extremely rare condition in males in which there is an extra Y chromosome, making a total of 47 chromosomes in each body cell. Also known as Jacob's syndrome.

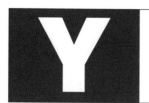

Y chromosome the male sex chromosome, being present in half the male gametes and none of the female. Y is the sex determining chromosome. *See* X CHROMOSOME.

yawning a reflex in which the mouth is opened wide and air is drawn in and exhaled. It may accompany tiredness or boredom.

yaws framboesia. An infection of the skin, bones and joints common in tropical countries. Caused by *Treponema pallidum pertenue*, it is common among people, especially children, who live in poor conditions in at least 13 tropical countries which is disfiguring and debilitating. The World Health Organization (WHO) aims to eradicate yaws by 2020.

yeast any of the fungi of the genus *Saccharomyces*. They produce fermentation in malt and fruit juices, resulting in the formation of alcoholic solutions such as beer and wines.

yellow card scheme a system of reporting side effects from taking or using any prescription medicine, herbal remedy, an over-the-counter (OTC) medicine or medical device; to report a defective or counterfeit medicine; or to report safety concerns about e-cigarettes. A patient, parent, carer or health care professional can report a suspected side effect by telephone or email. This reporting scheme is available in the UK and is monitored and managed by the Medicines and Healthcare Products Agency (MHRA).

yellow fever an acute, notifiable, infectious disease of the tropics caused by a virus and transmitted by the bite of an infected female mosquito (*Aedes aegypti*). The virus attacks the liver and kidneys and the symptoms include rigor, headache, pain in the back and limbs, high fever and nausea. Haemorrhage from the intestinal mucous membrane may occur. There is a high mortality rate. A vaccine is available.

Yersinia a genus of gram-negative bacteria containing the pathogen *Y. pestis* responsible for the bubonic plague. *Yersinia* is also responsible for a variety of other infections, e.g., gastroenteritis in the young and septicaemia in adults.

yin and yang describes how seemingly opposite forces may be complementary —the principles of this Chinese philosophy are incorporated into traditional Chinese medicine. Yin is the black side, dark and negative; yang is the white side, bright and positive. Together, the yin–yang interaction and balance is believed to maintain the harmony of the body and, in a healthy person, maintain a state of dynamic balance (*see* Figure on p. 415).

yoga a Hindu discipline which emphasizes personal physical preparation using meditation, relaxation, breathing control and the attainment of defined

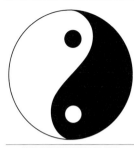

THE CHINESE SYMBOL FOR
YIN–YANG

body positions to achieve relaxation, with physical and emotional harmony and wellbeing.

yolk sac is a membranous sac attached to an embryo and which is important for the blood supply of the early embryo.

yttrium *symbol Y.* A rare chemical element which in its radioactive form is sometimes used in cancer therapy and the treatment of severe arthritis.

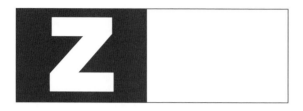

Z-plasty a plastic surgery technique for removing and repairing deformity resulting from a contraction scar (*see* Figure).

Z-track injection an intramuscular injection technique which allows a medication, e.g., an iron preparation, to be given but which prevents the leakage and the staining of tissues surrounding the site. *See* INJECTION.

Zen Zen Buddhism is the teaching that a form of meditation consisting of the contemplation of one's essential nature to the exclusion of everything else is the way to true enlightenment.

zenith the highest point. The opposite is NADIR.

zero nought; *symbol* 0. In the Celsius thermometer 0°C is the melting point of ice; in the Fahrenheit thermometer, 0°F is 32° below the melting point of ice. *See* CELSIUS and FAHRENHEIT.

Ziehl–Neelsen method *F. Ziehl, German bacteriologist, 1857–1926; F.K.A. Neelsen, German pathologist, 1854–1894.* A method of staining tubercle bacilli for microscopic study. Also known as the acid-fast stain.

Zika virus (also known as Zika fever), a viral disease mainly spread by mosquitoes which is serious for pregnant women as it is thought to cause birth defects, particularly microcephaly (small head). There is currently no vaccine.

Zimmer the trade name of a metal, lightweight walking aid, commonly

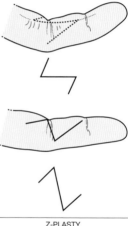

Z-PLASTY

applied to other products of similar design and weight. Predominantly used by the elderly to assist in walking and in rehabilitation.

zinc *symbol* Zn. A trace element which is essential in the body for cell growth and multiplication. The recommended daily intake of zinc is 9.5 mg for an adult man and 7.0 mg for an adult woman. A severe deficiency of zinc can retard growth in children, cause a low sperm count in adult males, and retard wound healing.

Zn symbol for *zinc*.

zona a zone. *Z. pellucida* the membrane surrounding the ovum.

zoonosis a disease of animals that is transmissible to humans, e.g., Ebola, rabies, cat-scratch fever, toxoplasmosis etc.

zoster *see* HERPES.

zygoma the zygomatic bone commonly referred to as the cheek bone or molar bone.

zygote a single fertilized cell formed from the union of a male and a female gamete.

zymosis fermentation.

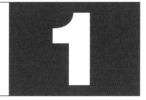
Nutrition

CAROLINE KING and NICOLA BRAMLEY

Nutrition is the study of food in relation to health. It is defined in this dictionary as the sum of the processes involved in taking in nutrients and assimilating and utilizing them.

Nutrients are necessary for growth, maintenance and repair of the human body. The five main groups of nutrients in food are protein, carbohydrate, fat, vitamins and minerals. In this section it should be noted that rich sources of particular nutrients are given as examples, but that foods almost always contain a mixture of many nutrients.

Protein

Protein is required for the body's growth and repair. Any excess protein consumed will be used as energy by the body. Protein provides 4 kcal per gram when used for energy and should provide about 10% of the day's energy needs for healthy adults.

When eaten, protein foods are broken down into amino acids. There are 20 amino acids. The body can make only 12 of the amino acids itself. The remaining 8 are known as the essential amino acids and must come from food.

Protein from animal sources such as meat, fish, eggs and milk usually contains all the essential amino acids; most proteins from vegetable sources are deficient in some essential amino acids. Plant foods need to be combined together if no animal protein is included in the diet, such as baked beans and toast or cereal with nuts.

Most people in the Western world eat more protein than their body requires and deficiency is rare. In times of protein catabolism such as surgery, trauma and burns, the body's requirements for protein may increase.

Foods high in protein: meat, fish, eggs, milk, cheese, nuts, beans.

Carbohydrate

The main function of carbohydrates is to provide energy. Some carbohydrates are also essential components of cells and other parts of the body. Carbohydrate provides approximately 4 kcal per gram. It comes in three forms: sugars, starches and non-starch polysaccharides.

Sugar carbohydrates are either monosaccharides (simple sugars) such as glucose, or disaccharides such as sucrose. They provide quick energy but virtually no nutrients as they are usually refined removing the other nutritious parts of the plant they come from. Only 10% of our total energy requirements should be from this type of carbohydrate.

Starch carbohydrates are made up of large numbers of glucose units joined together, and are found in foods such as rice, bread, pasta, cereals, potatoes and pulses. Starch has to be converted back to glucose during digestion in order for it to be used as energy by the body. Starch carbohydrates provide energy plus vegetable protein and some vitamins and minerals.

There are two types of non-starch polysaccharides (also known as dietary fibre). These are insoluble and soluble. Insoluble fibre is an indigestible carbohydrate that when ingested stimulates peristaltic movement and helps prevent constipation. It is found in cereal grains such as wheat, maize and rice. Soluble fibre such as pectin and guar gum is found in oats, peas, beans and lentils. Evidence shows that soluble fibre can help to reduce levels of cholesterol in the blood and help keep blood sugar levels even (Ho et al., 2017).

For optimal health carbohydrate should be the largest contributor to total energy intake, with the majority from starchy high-fibre varieties.

Foods high in sugar: sweets, cakes, biscuits, soft drinks, honey and jam. Hidden sources in many processed foods and drinks.

Foods high in starchy carbohydrate: breakfast cereals, rice, pasta, potatoes and pulses.

Foods high in non-starch polysaccharides: fruit, vegetables, breakfast cereals, oats.

Fat

Fat is the most concentrated source of energy. It provides 9 kcal per gram. It is a carrier of fat-soluble vitamins, provides a store of concentrated heat and energy, protects vital organs and adds palatability and satiety value to the diet. Essential fatty acids are needed for optimal cell function.

Fat is made up of triglycerides, each of which is made up of three fatty acids and a unit of glycerol. Differences in fat are the result of the different fatty acids found in each. Fats may be saturated, monounsaturated or polyunsaturated. Saturated fatty acids tend to increase the amount of cholesterol in the blood and are usually solid at room temperature. Monounsaturated and polyunsaturated fatty acids have been shown to help reduce cholesterol in the blood. Polyunsaturated fatty acids also play a role in immune function, fat transport and metabolism, and maintenance of the integrity of cell membranes. Essential fatty acids cannot be made by the body, they have to be provided by the diet. Diets containing fatty fish which are high in omega 3 long chain polyunsaturates have been shown to be beneficial for cardiovascular health (Schunck et al., 2017).

Approximately 30% of our total energy should be derived from fat, with approximate ratios of 10% from saturated fat, 5% from polyunsaturated fats and 15% from mono-unsaturated fats. Some schools of thought suggest that energy intake from fat could be higher as long as total energy is kept to a level to avoid overweight or obesity. This is due to the moderating effects of fat on glycaemic control (Tay et al., 2017).

Foods high in saturated fat: butter, cheese, lard, suet.

Foods high in polyunsaturated fat: corn oil, grapeseed oil, sunflower oil, safflower oil, sesame oil, oily fish such as salmon, sardines, mackerel and fresh tuna.

Foods high in monounsaturated fat: olives, olive oil, peanuts, cashew nuts and avocados.

Vitamins

These are found in small amounts in foods and are only required in small amounts by the body for normal biochemical function. Vitamins can be divided into two groups. These are fat-soluble (A, D, E, K) and water-soluble (vitamin B complex and C). In Western countries there are rarely deficiencies in the general population (except vitamin D, see later); however, deficiencies can occur in patients on artificial nutritional support if composition of the feed is not carefully monitored.

There are limited body stores of water-soluble vitamins, but fat-soluble vitamins are stored and if taken in excess over a long period of time can become toxic.

Vitamin A

There are two forms: retinol and carotenes.

Function: needed for growth and normal development of the retina in the eye, healthy skin and mucosal surface tissues.

Retinol

Foods high in retinol: animal foods such as milk, cheese, eggs, fish liver oils, margarine and butter.

Carotene

Can be converted to retinol by the body and is also an important antioxidant (along with other pigments in fruit and vegetables)

Foods high in carotene: cabbage, carrots, peaches and apricots.

Vitamin B Complex

Function of all B vitamins (except vitamin B_{12} and folate): help the body obtain and process energy from food. They enable each cell of the body to metabolize fat and carbohydrate to release energy. Requirements for these B vitamins are calculated in relation to energy need. Pyridoxine (vitamin B_6) plays an important role in protein metabolism.

Foods high in B vitamins are: meat, fish, milk, eggs, cereal grains and fortified cereals.

Deficiencies:

- Vitamin B_1 (thiamine): beri beri.
- Vitamin B_2 (riboflavin): sore mouth.
- Niacin (nicotinic acid): pellagra.
- Biotin: dermatitis, fatigue, nausea and depression.

Vitamin B_{12}

Function: essential for making red blood cells. Required for the correct formation of nerve sheaths. Only absorbed in the presence of intrinsic factor, which is produced in the upper gastrointestinal tract and is reduced as stomach acidity reduces with age, predisposing the elderly to B_{12}-related anaemia.

Deficiency: pernicious anaemia, damage to the nerve sheaths.

Foods high in vitamin B_{12}: found only in animal foods—liver, oily fish, meat and eggs. However, there is some evidence that a healthy gut flora produces B_{12} which can be used by the host (LeBlanc et al., 2013).

Folate (folic acid is the artificial format found in supplements)

Function: involved in production of healthy blood cells. Folate plays a major role in the prevention of neural tube defects such as spina bifida.

Deficiency: megaloblastic anaemia.

Foods high in folate: liver, spinach, brussels sprouts, fortified breakfast cereals, eggs (levels reduced by heat during cooking).

Vitamin C (Ascorbic Acid)

Function: forms a major part of the connective tissue which binds all cells together. Helps tissue to heal and thus is vital for wound healing. Aids absorption of iron from non-animal sources. Antioxidant.

Deficiency: scurvy, wounds not healing, bruising, low resistance to infections.

Foods high in vitamin C: fruit (particularly citrus fruits) and vegetables (if not overcooked as vitamin C is destroyed by heat).

Vitamin D

Function: works to aid the absorption of calcium for the formation and growth of bones and teeth. There is now evidence of its role in immune function and protection against some chronic diseases but this is yet to be proven (Autier ha., 2017). Unlike other nutrients, food is not the main source of this vitamin. It is produced by the action of sunshine on the skin. SACN 2016 recommendations on vitamin D supplementation now recommend routine supplements for the majority of the UK population.

Deficiency: rickets and osteomalacia.

Foods high in vitamin D: margarine (if fortified, which is a statutory obligation in the UK at the moment), some fish such as kippers, mackerel, sardines.

Vitamin E

Function: thought to be necessary for healthy muscles and good blood circulation. It is found in all cell structures and protects polyunsaturated fatty acids both in food and in the body from losing their properties through oxidation (antioxidant).

Foods high in vitamin E: polyunsaturated margarines, wheatgerm, nuts, fish such as tuna and salmon.

Vitamin K

Function: needed for normal blood clotting.

Deficiency: delayed blood clotting, haemorrhagic tendency.

Foods high in vitamin K: green vegetables, cereals and pulses.

Also made by a healthy gut flora.

Minerals

Minerals are an essential part or carrier of enzymes, hormones and proteins such as haemoglobin. They are used by the body's nervous system to transport messages and are essential for strong bones and teeth.

Some minerals (also known as trace elements) are required by the body in very small quantities—zinc, selenium, copper, manganese, chromium, cobalt, fluorine, iodine, molybdenum. They are antioxidants which help to prevent damage to cells from free radicals or cofactors for enzyme systems.

Iron

Function: carries oxygen from the lungs to all cells of the body. Over half of iron is in the form of haemoglobin.

Deficiency: iron-deficiency anaemia.

Foods high in iron: red meat, offal, fortified breakfast cereals, dried fruit, chocolate, nuts.

Calcium

Function: needed for the development and maintenance of the skeleton, good muscle function, nerve functioning and normal clotting of blood.

Deficiency: rickets, osteomalacia.

Foods high in calcium: cheese, yoghurt, milk, dark-green leafy vegetables, white bread, sardines and other tinned fish with edible bones.

Phosphorus

Function: together with calcium it provides the strength of bones and teeth. Required to form adenosine triphosphate and in enzyme systems for energy metabolism. Unlike calcium is not dependent on vitamin D for absorption.

Deficiency: unknown in humans.

Foods high in phosphorus: milk, cheese, wholegrain cereals.

Sodium

Function: regulation of body fluid and transmitting nerve impulses. Also important for energy release, muscle contraction and regulation of blood pressure.

Deficiency: hyponatraemia with symptoms of cramps, weakness, fatigue, nausea and thirst.

Foods high in sodium: salt, bacon, ham, soy sauce.

Potassium

Function: maintenance of acid–base and water balances, osmotic equilibrium, muscle and nerve irritability and normal blood pressure.

Deficiency: rare, secondary deficiency may occur after excessive losses through vomiting, chronic diarrhoea or use of some diuretics, leading to loss of appetite, nausea, muscle weakness, mental disorientation and cardiac arrhythmias.

Foods high in potassium: vegetables including potatoes, fruits and fruit juices, chocolate and instant coffee.

References

Autier, P., Mullie, P., Macacu, A., et al., 2017. Effect of vitamin D supplementation on non-skeletal disorders: a systematic review of meta-analysis and randomised trials. Lancet Diabetes Endocrinol 5 (12), 986–1004. doi:10.1016/S2213-8587(17)30357-1.

Department of Health Standing Advisory Committee on Nutrition (SACN) 2016 Vitamin D and Health. Available on-line https://www.gov.uk/government/groups/scientific-advisory-committee-on-nutrition.

Ho, H.V.T., Jovanovski, E., Zurbau, A., et al., 2017. A systematic review and meta-analysis of randomized controlled trials of the effect of konjac glucomannan, a viscous soluble fiber, on LDL cholesterol and the new lipid targets non-HDL cholesterol and apolipoprotein B. Am. J. Clin. Nutr. 105 (5), 1239–1247.

LeBlanc, J.G., Milani, C., de Giori, G.S., et al., 2013. Bacteria as vitamin suppliers to their host: a gut microbiota perspective. Curr. Opin. Biotechnol. 24 (2), 160–168.

Schunck, W.H., Konkel, A., Fischer, R., et al., 2017. Therapeutic potential of omega-3 fatty acid-derived epoxyeicosanoids in cardiovascular and inflammatory diseases. Pharmacol. Ther. 183, 177–204. doi:10.1016.

Tay, J., Thompson, C.H., Luscombe-Marsh, N.D., et al., 2017. Effects of an energy-restricted low carbohydrate, high unsaturated fat/low saturated fat diet versus a high carbohydrate, low fat diet in type 2 diabetes: a 2 year randomized clinical trial. Diabetes Obes. Metab. 20 (4), 858–871. doi:10.1111/dom.13164.

Artificial Nutritional Support
GERII REILLY

Indications
- An inability to meet nutritional requirements with normal food.
- For prevention or treatment of malnutrition.

Effective nutritional support is capable of treating malnutrition. Nutritional screening tools, such as the Malnutrition Universal Screening Tool (MUST), have been developed by the Malnutrition Advisory Group to help identify patients at risk of malnutrition. For details refer to web address at the end of this section.

Artificial Nutritional Support
There are two types of artificial nutritional support:
- Enteral nutrition, e.g., nutritional supplements (sip feeds) or tube feeding.
- Parenteral nutrition (PN).

Enteral nutrition should be the first-line route for the provision of nutritional support. If the patient is able to absorb food enteral feeding should be used.

Enteral Nutrition
Refer to dictionary entry for definition

Enteral Nutrition Modalities

Oral Diet

Additional snacks or high-protein/energy diets. In addition to normal meals, glucose polymers, protein or milk powder or fat (such as cream or butter) may be added to food to increase its energy and protein content.

Nutritional Supplements

There are a wide variety of sweet supplements (milk shake/yoghurt/mousse/fruit juice style drinks) and savoury supplements (soups) that may be given. If a patient is reliant on the sip feed as the sole source of nutrition, it is important that the supplements are complete in macronutrients (carbohydrates, fat and protein) for energy, and micronutrients (vitamins, minerals and trace elements). A full list of prescribable products can be found in the appendix for borderline substance published in the British National Formulary (BNF).

Tube Feeding

- Prepyloric, e.g., nasogastric, orogastric, gastrostomy (surgical, radiological or endoscopic).
- Postpyloric, e.g., nasoduodenal/jejunal and jejunostomy. Some postpyloric tubes are placed blindly, others rely on endoscopic, radiological or surgical placement. A jejunal extension set can be placed through some gastrostomy tubes to facilitate postpyloric feeding. Nasojejunal feeding tubes are available with a gastric port to facilitate concomitant gastric aspiration with jejunal feeding.

Tube feeding requires a team decision to select the most appropriate route and insertion method. It is important that the date, type of tube, feed exit point (gastric, duodenal, jejunal) and method of tube insertion is documented. This information is vital as it may alter feed and drug administration (refer to drug administration section in the BNF edition 72 on p. 1168), and the daily management of the tube.

Indications for Enteral Tube Feeding

See Table 1.1.

Table 1.1 Indications for enteral tube feeding	
Increased nutritional requirements Inadequate oral intake	• e.g., sepsis, burns, trauma, postoperative stress, head injuries, critically ill • Anorexia • Unable to eat safely due to swallowing difficulties, e.g., cerebral vascular accident (CVA), impaired consciousness, oesophageal carcinoma • Patients not meeting requirements via the oral route alone

Contraindications for Enteral Tube Feeding

Patients with a non-functioning gut (refer to Parenteral Nutrition section).

Composition of Enteral Tube Feeds

All enteral feeds contain protein, carbohydrate, fat, electrolytes, vitamins and minerals.

- Standard feeds: 1 kcal per ml (available with or without fibre).
- High-energy feeds: 1.5 kcal per ml (available with or without fibre).
- High-protein feeds: 8.1g per 100mls (available with or without fibre).

A variety of specialist feeds are also available for the management of a range of acute and chronic medical conditions. These include renal failure, malabsorption, acute respiratory disorders, chronic pulmonary disease, cancer and inflammatory bowel disease. The feed selected will depend on the clinical condition of the patient and their nutritional requirements.

Tube Feeding Regimen

The regimen will depend upon the route of tube feeding, the clinical condition of the patient and the aims of nutritional support. Most prepyloric regimens have a rest period in order to allow the stomach to re-acidify; however, this is not required for feeds administered postpylorically. Feed is either administered using a pump or as a bolus regimen. Bolus regimens should not be used in patients that are deemed at high risk of aspiration.

Check Tube Position Prior to Initiating Feed

The position of the feeding tube should be checked daily prior to feeding as per guidance from the National Patient Safety Agency. Accepted methods for confirming the position of nasogastric tubes include either gastric aspirate checks with Universal pH paper (pH < 5.5) or chest X-ray if aspirates cannot be obtained (please refer to NPSA, MHRA, NNNG websites for further information; the web addresses are provided at the end of this section). Nasal tubes can be easily dislodged; those at high risk are patients who are retching, vomiting or coughing severely or who require frequent nasotracheal suctioning. Gastrostomy and jejunostomy tube sites also need to be checked regularly. These tubes can migrate, leak, kink or become embedded into the lumen wall and result in skin ulceration.

Complications of Enteral Tube Feeding

See Table 1.2

Other Tube Feeding Considerations

Feed Administration Sets

Many plastics are single-use. Scrupulous attention should be paid to hygiene in the handling and administration of feeds. Syringes used to flush tubes should be 50 ml

Table 1.2   Complications of enteral tube feeding

Complication	Recommendation
Diarrhoea (listed below are possible causes)	Monitor bowel frequency; establish a definition, e.g., include frequency and consistency
• Infective diarrhoea	Send stool sample; ensure a cleaning frequency with consistency and the appropriate handling feeds
• Medication, e.g., motility agents, antibiotics, medication	Review medication containing sorbitol
• Bacterial overgrowth	Hydrogen breath test
• Constipation	Review history of bowel function
• Malabsorption	Check for pancreatic, biliary or gastrointestinal disease
• Too rapid infusion of feed	Check rate of feed matches regimen, check for pump malfunction
• Hypoalbuminaemia	Discuss with dietitian
• Hyperosmolar feeds	Discuss with dietitian
N.B. Most feeds are lactose-and gluten-free	
Constipation	
• Inadequate fluid intake	Check fluid intake
• Drug therapy, e.g., opiates	Review medications; consider laxative prescription; consider fibre-based feed
Mucosal erosion and oesophageal strictures	Use fine-bore feeding tubes instead of wide-bore PVC tubes, e.g., Ryle
Regurgitation/aspiration	
• Delayed gastric emptying	Rate of feed must not exceed the patient's absorption. Consider use of prokinetic agents, e.g., metoclopramide or erythromycin
• Tube misplacement:	
– On insertion	Tilt the bed head by 45 degrees when tube feeding supine patients
– During nutritional support	Check tube position prior to commencing feed
Tube occlusion	
• Viscous feeds and drugs	Use liquid drug preparations; dilute viscous drugs; flush tube regularly, before/after the feed/drug is administered; if multiple drugs are given at one time water should be flushed between each drug administered

Table 1.2 Complications of enteral tube feeding—cont'd	
Complication	Recommendation
• Crushed tablets	Flush the tube after aspiration
• Inadequate flushing	Flush regularly, ideally every 4–6 hours
Psychological problems	Where possible involve the patient and carers in the care of the tube feed
• Altered body image	
• Hunger	
• Loss of autonomy	
• Loss of the pleasure of eating	

as the pressure exerted by smaller syringes may rupture the tube lumen. All enteral syringes need to comply with National Patient Safety Agency guidance where they no longer adapt to IV administration sets and are all purple in colour.

Drug Administration
- The route of administration corresponds to absorption site.
- Interactions between drugs and feed must be identified prior to administration. Common interactions between feed and drugs occur with NG administration of phenytoin, warfarin, penicillins, ciprofloxacin, tacrolimus and rifampicin.

N.B. Please discuss with local pharmacist and refer to local policies, drug information departments and BAPEN guidelines (refer to website addresses at the end of this section).

Water
The use of sterile or tap water varies according to local policy, patient's condition and location (home or hospital patient).

Home Tube Feeding
Tube feeding at home needs to be adapted to the home environment and must take into account carer/patient capabilities and social considerations. Feed and its administration set may be delivered by home care companies or collected from a pharmacy.

Monitoring
Effective monitoring can reduce the complications associated with artificial nutritional support. It is very important to:
- Check accurate tube position/inspect tube site prior to commencing feed daily.
- Flush the tube regularly.

- Monitor gastrointestinal function, e.g.:
  - Bowel movements.
  - Vomiting.
  - Bloating.
  - Gastric distension.
- Identify drug–nutrient interactions.

Parenteral Nutrition

Refer to dictionary for definition. Parenteral nutrition (PN) should be used to prevent or treat malnutrition when the gastrointestinal tract is unavailable, or gastrointestinal function is inadequate.

Possible Indications for Parenteral Nutrition

See Table 1.3.

Routes Used for Parenteral Nutrition

The perceived length of feeding will influence the route of nutritional support.

Central Access

- Short-term: multilumen lines.
- Intermediate duration: peripherally inserted central catheter (PICC) >15 cm long (>5 days–4 weeks).
- Long-term: e.g., Hickman line or Portacath.

Table 1.3 Possible indications for parenteral nutrition	
Failure to tolerate enteral nutritional support	e.g., paralytic ileus, vomiting, profuse diarrhoea, radiation enteritis, chronic idiopathic pseudo-obstruction.
Intestinal failure	Intestinal atresia, short bowel syndrome, motility disorders
Severe malabsorption	Cannot be managed by an elemental diet
	Large output enterocutaneous fistula
Inflammatory bowel disease	Crohn's disease, unable to tolerate elemental/semi-elemental diet
Severe mucositis	Unable to pass enteral tube
Bowel rest	Post-gastrointestinal surgery, which cannot be achieved by an elemental diet

Note that full nutritional requirements cannot be met via the enteral route.

Peripheral Access
Peripheral access should not be used for PN due to risk of thrombophlebitis.

Composition of Parenteral Nutrition Feeds
PN is usually administered in an all-in-one preparation (1.5–3 litres) which contains:
- 10%, 20%, 50% glucose.
- 0%, 10%, 20% lipid.
- Amino acids.
- Electrolytes.
- Water.
- Fat- and water-soluble vitamins.
- Trace elements.

A variety of standard preparations are usually available to meet patients' requirements. These may be in a multi-chamber format, in which the separate macronutrient chambers are combined by rolling the bag to break the inner membrane seal prior to administration. The clinical condition of a patient may warrant an individually compounded preparation, such as lipid-free preparations for patients with liver function derangement and cholestasis.

Feeding Regimens
- In all cases the lumen should be dedicated to the use of PN only.
- Strict flow control is essential. This can be done with volumetric pumps fitted with occlusion and air-in-line alarms.
- PN is usually administered continuously over 24 hours; however, this can be reduced in certain cases.

Glutamine
It is now common practice to use intravenous glutamine preparations for critically ill and bone marrow transplant patients who require PN.

Complications
See Table 1.4.

Careful monitoring detects most of the complications associated with nutritional support. Multidisciplinary team management is essential.

Basic Monitoring for Enteral (Tube Feeding) and Parenteral Nutrition
N.B. The frequency of monitoring can be reduced for stable patients; refer to figures in brackets in Table 1.5.

Table 1.4 Complications of parenteral nutrition	
Complication	**Comment**
Catheter-related	Meticulous care of the line and catheter site can prevent sepsis; follow protocols; use a dedicated line for feeding
Catheter-related infection	
Insertion-related	Adhere to policies; experienced staff only to insert; confirm position by X-ray before commencing feed
• Air embolism • Pneumothorax • Catheter malposition	
Catheter occlusion and damage	Discuss with medical team
Central venous thrombosis	Discuss with medical team
Nutritional and metabolic	
Dehydration	Monitor abnormal losses, e.g., fistulae or diarrhoea. N.B. Additional IV fluids may be required
Over-hydration	Monitor all other IV fluids that are administered, e.g., antibiotics, chemotherapy
Hyperglycaemia	Discuss carbohydrate content of PN with dietitian
	Discuss blood sugar management with medical team
Hypoglycaemia	Can occur if PN is stopped immediately. PN infusion rate should be decreased slowly. If this is not possible provide an IV glucose solution and monitor blood glucose 4-hourly for 24 hours.
Lipaemia	At-risk patients include critically ill or septic patients or those with renal failure.
Electrolyte imbalance	Over- or under-administration of electrolytes
Effect on other organ systems	
Hepatobiliary disease	Consider impact of underlying disease and PN composition
Metabolic bone disease	Consider poor nutritional status and exposure to corticosteroid therapy

Parameter	Parameters to assess	Frequency enteral	Parenteral
Clinical	Temperature, pulse, respiration and blood pressure	4-hourly	4-hourly
	Ward urine analysis	Daily	Daily
Fluid balance	Fluid balance	At each bottle change	Hourly
	Serum urea	Daily (2× week once stable)	Daily
Biochemistry	Full serum electrolyte profile	Daily (2× week once stable)	Daily
	Glucose	Daily (2× week once stable)	4-hourly blood (urinalysis)
	Liver function chemistry	2× weekly	2× weekly
	Zinc, copper and selenium	Monthly	Monthly. Assessment is important in patients on long term PN
Nutritional status	Nutrient intake	Daily	Daily
	Body weight	Weekly	Weekly (daily if fluid balance information required)
Haematology	Full blood count	2× weekly	Daily
	Prothrombin time	As indicated	Weekly
Lipaemia	Cholesterol and triacylglycerol	As indicated	On initiation and then weekly

Table 1.5   Monitoring for enteral and parenteral nutrition

Useful Website Addresses

Better Hospital Food: http://www.betterhospitalfood.com

British Association for Parenteral and Enteral Nutrition (BAPEN): http://www.bapen.org.uk (for access to nurse nutrition site, nutrition policies and drug administration)

British National Formulary: http://www.BNF.org

Medicines and Healthcare Products Regulatory Agency: http://www.mhra.gov.uk
National Institute for Health and Care Excellence (NICE): http://www.nice.org.uk
National Nurses Nutrition Group (NNNG): http://www.nnng.org
National Patient Safety Agency: http://www.npsa.nhs.uk
Promoting Excellence in Nutrition Support: http://www.peng.org.uk

Nutritional Management of Coronary Heart Disease

SANDRA ELLIS

In a similar way to obesity and diabetes, coronary heart disease (CHD) is a major cause of morbidity and mortality in the UK. The incidence of CHD is related to modifiable risk factors such as dyslipidaemia and hypertension, which in turn are linked with dietary factors including excess intake of salt and saturated fat, and low intake of fruit and vegetables. Obesity and excess alcohol intake are further diet-related risk factors for CHD. Nutritional advice plays a key role in the prevention and management of CHD.

Cardioprotective Diet

The cardioprotective diet, which originates from the Mediterranean diet, is the first line of dietary advice for the primary and secondary prevention of CHD. It is used in conjunction with specific dietary advice for weight management, diabetes, hypertension and dyslipidaemia. It contains plenty of fruit, vegetables, beans, nuts and wholegrain varieties of starchy foods, with moderate amounts of fish, white meat and low-fat dairy foods and less red and processed meat (Willett et al., 1995). In addition, saturated fat should be replaced by unsaturated fats where possible and alcohol consumed in moderation.

Fats
Saturated Fat
Dietary staturated fat increases total and low-density lipoprotein (LDL) cholesterol. Randomised controlled trials (RCTs) that lowered saturated fats and replaced it with polyunsaturated fats reduced the risk of CHD events by ~30%. Prospective observational studies in many populations showed that lower intake of saturated fat in conjunction with higher intakes of polyunsaturated and monounsaturated fats is associated with lower rates of CHD and all-cause mortality (Sacks et al., 2017). The recommendation is that saturated fat contribute <10% of total energy intake. Foods rich in saturated fat, i.e., hard cheese, butter, whole milk, pastry, coconut oil, fatty meat, processed meat and meat products, should be limited and replaced with unsaturated fats.

Unsaturated Fat

Both monounsaturated and polyunsaturated fats lower total and LDL cholesterol. Avocados; olives; olive and rapeseed oil; nuts (almonds, cashews, hazelnuts, peanuts, pistachios) and spreads made from these nuts are all rich in monounsaturated fats. Oily fish; oils (corn, sesame, and soya) and spreads made from them; seeds (e.g., flaxseeds, sesame and sunflower) and nuts (e.g., walnuts and pine nuts) are rich in polyunsaturated fats.

Trans Fat

Small amounts of naturally occurring trans fats occur in dairy foods and meat. Artificial trans fats, found in pastries, hard margarines, biscuits, cakes, crackers, fried food and takeaways, have been consistently linked to an elevated risk of CHD (de Souza et al., 2015). Trans fats, which increase LDL cholesterol and lower HDL cholesterol, should be reduced. Foods that are labelled as containing 'hydrogenated or partially-hydrogenated fats/oils' are a source of trans fats.

Carbohydrates

High intake of added sugar is associated with a higher risk of cardiovascular disease (CVD) mortality (Yang et al., 2014). A meta-analysis has shown that diets with a high glycaemic index (GI) or glycaemic load (GL) increase the risk of CHD and type 2 diabetes (Barclay et al., 2008). Adults should have no more than 30 g of free sugars per day (roughly equivalent to seven sugar cubes). Sources of free sugars include cakes, biscuits, sweets, chocolate, some fizzy drinks, fruit juices and smoothies.

A meta-analysis of prospective cohort studies showed that an average of 2.5 servings per day of wholegrain foods was associated with lower risks of CV events (Mellen et al., 2008). Wholegrains, such as wheat, barley, oats and rice, are rich in soluble fibre and antioxidants, and tend to have a lower GI.

Fruit and Vegetables

Meta-analyses of prospective cohort studies consistently show that fruit and vegetable consumption is inversely related to the CHD events and mortality (Dauchet et al., 2005, Gan et al., 2015). Fruit and vegetables are a rich source of vitamins, minerals, dietary fibre and a range of healthful plant-based substances including plant sterols and flavonoids. The recommendation is at least 400g (5 × 80 g portions) per day, which includes fresh, frozen or canned fruit and vegetables.

Fish

Meta-analyses of prospective cohort studies show that fish consumption is inversely associated with CHD events and mortality (Whelton et al., 2004, Zheng et al., 2012). Fish and seafood contains several healthful nutrients including protein, unsaturated fats, vitamin D and selenium. Some such as mackerel, pilchards and herring are rich in omega-3 polyunsaturated acids, which lower triglycerides, systolic and diastolic blood pressure and resting heart rate. Individuals should be advised to consume at least two portions of fish per week, including a portion of oily fish. Due to a lack of high quality evidence, people should no longer be advised to consume fish or omega-3 fatty acid capsules for the sole purpose of preventing another myocardial infarction.

Nuts, Seeds and Pulses

Nuts, seeds and pulses are a good source of protein, fibre, vitamins and minerals. Nuts and seeds are also rich in unsaturated fats. The recommendation is to have at least 4–5 portions per day. Regular consumption of unsalted, mixed nuts was shown to reduce CVD mortality in high-risk individuals (Estruch et al., 2013) Meta-analyses of RCTs have shown that a regular intake of pulses significantly reduced cholesterol and blood pressure (Ha et al., 2014, Jayalath et al., 2014).

Salt

Excess dietary salt increases blood pressure, which is a risk factor for CHD. The recommended amount is ≤6 g per day and most of the UK population consumes too much salt. About 75% of this salt is already added to foods we buy e.g., ready meals, soups, crisps, nuts, processed meat and pasta sauces. Salt reduction can be achieved by decreasing the amount of processed food in the diet and choosing foods low in salt. Further reduction can be achieved by using herbs and spices to flavour food when cooking and by reducing the amount added at the table.

Alcohol

Excessive alcohol consumption is associated with hypertension, cardiac arrhythmia and cardiomyopathy, as well as other diseases such as cirrhosis and certain cancers. The recommended safe limit of alcohol is 14 units per week for men and women, with several days alcohol-free each week. 'Binge drinking' (more than 3 alcoholic drinks in 1–2 hours), increases the risk of accidents and injury, and should be avoided. Alcohol is also high in calories and should be limited if weight loss is desired.

Novel Foods

There are a range of foods available containing plant stanols and sterols which can reduce blood cholesterol levels if taken in the correct amounts. Individuals with familial hypercholesterolaemia may benefit for taking these foods if take consistently. However, since there is no evidence that they reduce CHD events or mortality they should not be routinely recommended.

References and Background Reading

Barclay, A.W., Petocz, P., McMillan-Price, J., et al., 2008. Glycemic index, glycemic load, and chronic disease risk–a meta-analysis of observational studies. Am. J. Clin. Nutr. 87 (3), 627–637.

Dauchet, L., Amouyel, P., Dallongeville, J., 2005. Fruit and vegetable consumption and risk of stroke: a meta-analysis of cohort studies. Neurology 65 (8), 1193–1197.

de Souza, R.J., Mente, A., Maroleanu, A., et al., 2015. Intake of saturated and trans unsaturated fatty acids and risk of all-cause mortality, cardiovascular disease, and type 2 diabetes: systematic review and meta-analysis of observational studies. BMJ. 11, 351.

Estruch, R., Ros, E., Salas-Salvadó, J., et al., 2013. Primary prevention of cardiovascular disease with a mediterranean diet. N. Engl. J. Med. 368 (14), 1279–1290.

Gan, Y., Tong, X., Li, L., et al., 2015. Consumption of fruit and vegetable and risk of coronary heart disease: a meta-analysis of prospective cohort studies. Int. J. Cardiol. 183, 129–137.

Ha, V., Sievenpiper, J.L., de Souza, R.J., et al., 2014. Effect of dietary pulse intake on established therapeutic lipid targets for cardiovascular risk reduction: a systematic review and meta-analysis of randomized controlled trials. CMAJ 186 (8), E252–E262.

Jayalath, V.H., de Souza, R.J., Sievenpiper, J.L., et al., 2014. Effect of dietary pulses on blood pressure: a systematic review and meta-analysis of controlled feeding trials. Am. J. Hypertens. 27 (1), 56–64.

Mellen, P.B., Walsh, T.F., Herrington, D.M., 2008. Whole grain intake and cardiovascular disease: a meta-analysis. Nutr. Metab. Cardiovasc. Dis. 18 (4), 283–290.

Sacks, F.M., Lichtenstein, A.H., Wu, J.H.Y., et al., 2017. Dietary fats and cardiovascular disease: a presidential advisory from the American heart association. Circulation 136 (3), e1–e23.

Whelton, S.P., He, J., Whelton, P.K., et al., 2004. Meta-analysis of observational studies on fish intake and coronary heart disease. Am. J. Cardiol. 93 (9), 1119–1123.

Willett, W.C., Sacks, F., Trichopoulou, A., et al., 1995. Mediterranean diet pyramid: a cultural model for healthy eating. Am. J. Clin. Nutr. 61 (6 Suppl.), 1402S–1406S.

Yang, Q., Zhang, Z., Gregg, E.W., et al., 2014. Added sugar intake and cardiovascular diseases mortality among US adults. JAMA Intern. Med. 174 (4), 516–524.

Zheng, J., Huang, T., Yu, Y., et al., 2012. Fish consumption and CHD mortality: an updated meta-analysis of seventeen cohort studies. Public Health Nutr. 15 (4), 725–737.

Nutritional Management of Obesity
CAROLINE KING

Definition

The definition of obesity in adults is usually based on the body mass index (BMI):

$$N.B. \text{ Body Mass Index } (Quetelet\ Index) = \frac{\text{Weight (kg)}}{\text{Height (m}^2)}$$

The international consensus on BMI ranges classifies them as in Table 1.6 (WHO, 2000).

Prevalence

In a government report early in 2017 it was stated that 36% of adults in the UK are overweight and 27% obese (Baker and Bate, 2017).

Our environment has changed drastically over the last 50 years with a reduction in active occupations, a rise in more sedentary occupations, more use of mobile electronic devices and increased car ownership. This has been coupled with changes in food production and an increased availability of high-calorie cheap food. These changes have corresponded with the increasing levels of obesity. Being overweight or obese increases the risk of a number of chronic diseases, including type 2 diabetes, hypertension, heart disease, stroke and certain types of cancers. This is especially true if the weight is carried around the waist (known as apple-shaped or truncal obesity) rather than around the hips (known as pear-shaped obesity).

Waist Circumference

Waist circumference measurements are also important in risk factor assessment, indicating the accumulation of excess intra-abdominal fat. Evidence suggests that an accumulation of fat in the upper body area leading to a high waist to hip circumference

Table 1.6   BMI classification

BMI (kg/m^2)	Classification
<18.5	Underweight
18.5–24.9	Healthy weight
25–29.9	Pre-obese (overweight)
30–34.9	Obese class 1 (moderately obese, commonly referred to as 'fat')
35–39.9	Obese class 2 (severely obese, commonly referred to as 'very fat')
>40	Obese class 3 (morbidly obese)

is associated with an increased risk for developing heart disease and non-insulin dependent diabetes.

Populations differ in the level of risk associated with a particular waist circumference. South Asians have higher levels of abdominal obesity, although they might not be considered obese by conventional BMI criteria (Anoop et al., 2017).

Why Should Individuals Who Are Overweight Lose Weight?

Research shows that losing between 5% and 10% of your current body weight can vastly improve your health (SIGN, 1996). Weight loss has been clearly shown to decrease all causes of mortality (Ma et al., 2017).

What Does Losing Weight Involve?

An individual's body weight represents the balance between all the energy taken in from what they eat and drink and all the energy used up in daily life. To lose weight, energy intake needs to be reduced and energy output or activity increased. The only way to lose weight and keep it off is to change one's eating and physical activity habits permanently. Crash or 'fad' diets may reduce weight in the short term; however, they are unsustainable and usually result in weight regain. This is due to the loss of water and short-term energy storage in the muscles (glycogen) which is easily replaced once the diet is stopped. Some of the fad diets may in fact be dangerous to long-term health. The best approach to weight loss is sensible, healthy eating where weight loss is approximately $\frac{1}{2}$–1 kg (1–2 lbs) each week. This is equivalent to a reduction in energy intake of approximately 500 kilocalories each day or an increase in activity to the equivalent amount. The optimum approach is a little of each as exercise in itself has many health benefits, reducing blood pressure, improving circulation, improving strength and wellbeing.

Practical Guidelines for Weight Loss

- Regular meals.
- Avoidance of high calorie snacks.
- Starchy food at each meal with a focus on wholegrain varieties rather than white.
- 2–3 servings of vegetables and salads each day.
- 2–3 servings of fruit each day.
- At meal times, the vegetables/salad should take up about half the plate.
- Choose low fat foods wherever possible, and eat smaller portions of fat-rich food.
- Avoid sugar and sugary foods.
- Alcohol contains kilocalories—keep to limits of 14 units/week for women and 21 units/week for men.
- Monitor body weight, but not more than once/week.
- Regular activity.

Prevention Is Better Than Cure

All the current reviews of obesity management agree that there should be a greater focus on the prevention of obesity. However, the best way of achieving this is still a topic of current research.

References

Anoop, S., Misra, A., Bhatt, S.P., et al., 2017. High circulating plasma dipeptidyl peptidase-4 levels in non-obese Asian indians with type 2 diabetes correlate with fasting insulin and LDL-c levels, triceps skinfolds, total intra-abdominal adipose tissue volume and presence of diabetes: a case-control study. BMJ Open Diabetes Res Care 5 (1), e000393. doi:10.1136/bmjdrc-2017-000393. eCollection 2017.

Baker, C., Bate, A., 2017. Obesity Statistics House of Commons Briefing paper SNO 3336. Available from http://researchbriefings.files.parliament.uk/documents/SN03336/SN03336.pdf.

Ma, C., Avenell, A., Bollard, M., et al., 2017. Effects of weight loss interventions for adults who are obese on mortality, cardiovascular disease, and cancer: systematic review and meta-analysis. BMJ 359, j4849. doi:10.1136/bmj.j4849.

SIGN, 1996. Obesity in Scotland; Integrating Prevention With Weight Management: A National Clinical Guideline Recommended for Use in Scotland. SIGN, Edinburgh.

World Health Organisation, 2000. Obesity: preventing and managing the global epidemic. Report of a WHO Consultation, WHO Technical Report Series 894.

Nutritional Management of Diabetes

Nutritional Advice for People With Diabetes

There are different types of diabetes and no two people with diabetes are the same. The most common types are type 1, previously called insulin-dependent or juvenile onset diabetes, and type 2, which used to be called non-insulin-dependent diabetes. The main reason for the change is that many people with type 2 diabetes require insulin to treat their diabetes. In both cases, dietary management is an essential part of the treatment and, unless the diet is right, it is impossible to meet the glycaemic control targets. Dietary treatment is not only about controlling blood glucose levels but also about preventing the long-term complications of diabetes, such as heart disease and renal disease.

The recommendations for the nutritional management of diabetes were updated by the Diabetes UK Nutrition Working Group in 2018, and regular updates are available on the Diabetes UK website. These nutritional recommendations are translated into practical advice that will help the person with diabetes to adapt their diet, working towards the following ideal that will help to control their diabetes and reduce the risk of long-term complications.

Nutritional Management

The phrase 'diabetic diet' is no longer promoted. Instead, nutritional management is recommended as part of an integrated package of clinical care and education for people with diabetes and those at high risk of developing type 2 diabetes.

Preventing Type 2 Diabetes

Intensive lifestyle intervention including diet and physical activity has been shown to be effective in delaying the onset of type 2 diabetes. Dietary and lifestyle recommendations for patients at high risk of developing the condition include:

- restricting energy intake to induce weight loss of 5%–7%
- reducing total fat (to less than 35%) and saturated fat (to less than 10%) intake
- increasing fibre intake (to more than 15 g per 1000 calories)
- increasing moderate to vigorous physical activity to at least 30 minutes per day/150 minutes per week.

Dietary patterns associated with reduced risk of diabetes in the population include:

- a Mediterranean diet
- the DASH diet (Dietary Approaches to Stop Hypertension)
- vegetarian and vegan diets
- the Nordic Healthy diet
- moderate carbohydrate restriction.

Diets should include more specific foods such as wholegrains, some fruit, green leafy vegetables, yoghurt and cheese, tea and coffee.

Diets should avoid foods associated with higher risk of diabetes including red and processed meats, potatoes (particularly French fries), sugar-sweetened beverages and refined carbohydrates.

Guidelines emphasise the importance of culturally appropriate dietary advice.

Weight Management for People With Type 2 Diabetes

After diagnosis, obese and overweight people should aim for a weight loss of 15 kg for remission of type 2 diabetes.

For better glycaemic control, it is recommended they aim for a weight loss of at least 5% through a calorie-controlled diet and increased exercise.

The current recommendation regarding very low energy diets is that their use should not extend beyond 12 weeks either continuously or intermittently. Total replacement diets (meal-replacement plans) have been shown to be effective in weight loss but again should be used for no more than 12 weeks.

Glycaemic Control in People With Type 1 Diabetes

There is no convincing evidence for a recommended ideal amount of carbohydrate for maintaining long-term glycaemic control in people with type 1 diabetes. Matching insulin to carbohydrate intake on a meal-by-meal basis has been shown to be effective (carbohydrate counting and insulin adjustment). Diets comprising low-glycaemic-index carbohydrates for glucose control in people with type 1 diabetes are no longer recommended.

The effect of dietary fibre on glycaemic control is also unclear, and the recommendation is to aim for the UK daily recommended amount of fibre for all which is 30 g.

Evidence around fat and protein intake in glycaemic control is poor and more work needs to be undertaken in this area.

Glycaemic Control in People With Type 2 Diabetes

Between 70% and 90% of people with type 2 diabetes are overweight or obese, and weight loss of more than 5% has been shown to be highly effective in glycaemic control. Evidence to support the ideal proportions of micronutrients is inconclusive.

Top Tips From Diabetes UK

Diabetes UK suggests making overall healthier food choices regardless of which type of diabetes people have:

Choose healthier carbohydrates, such as brown rice, buckwheat and whole oats, fruit, vegetables, pulses, e.g. chick peas, beans and lentils, and dairy including unsweetened yoghurt and milk.

Eat less salt aiming to limit intake to a maximum of 6 g per day.

Eat less red and processed meat such as ham, bacon, sausages, beef and lamb.

Eat more whole fruit and vegetables and use these foods for snacks, if required. Fruit juice is not recommended but fresh, frozen, dried or tinned fruit is (avoid tinned fruit in syrup).

Choose healthier fats such as olive oil, rapeseed oil and sunflower oil but cut down where possible by grilling, steaming or baking food. Fats to avoid are those in lard, butter, ghee and fats used in making biscuits, cakes, pies and pastries.

Cut down on added sugar and substitute sugary drinks with low- or zero-calorie options.

Be smart with snacks and, if required, choose unsalted nuts, fruit and vegetables, and healthy yoghurts.

Drink alcohol sensibly and keep to less than 14 units per week, spread throughout the week. Avoid drinking on an empty stomach, particularly if using insulin, as this can increase the risk of hypoglycaemia.

Avoid so-called 'diabetic food'. It is now unlawful to say food is a diabetic food and evidence shows that there is no benefit in eating these foods over other healthy products.

Get your minerals and vitamins from food. There is no evidence that mineral and vitamin supplements help to manage diabetes and a healthy diet should provide these so, unless there is a specific reason for taking them or it is advised by a healthcare professional (such as taking folic acid in pregnancy), then they are not needed.

References

Diabetes UK Nutrition Working Group, 2018. Evidence based nutrition guidelines for the prevention and management of diabetes. Available from https://diabetes-resources-production.s3.eu-west-1.amazonaws.com/resources-s3/2018-03/1373_Nutrition%20guidelines_0.pdf.

www.diabetes.org.uk 10 tips for healthy eating with diabetes

Nutrition in Paediatrics

CAROLINE KING

Nutrient Requirements

Nutrient requirements mirror growth rates, hence children have higher requirements than adults per kg body weight, with the highest being during infancy and adolescence (see Table 1.7).

Infant Feeding

Breast milk is the optimal food for the vast majority of infants whether well or sick, with recent draft government guidelines recommending exclusive breast feeding for 6 months before the introduction of solid food (SACN, 2018).

When breast milk is unavailable proprietary infant formulas are the next choice, as their composition follows agreed nutritional guidelines. Specialized formulas include preterm, nutrient-dense, thickened, soya-based, semi-elemental (hydrolysed and partially hydrolysed), elemental (amino acid based), lactose-free, low-calcium, medium chain triglyceride based and those catering for inborn errors of metabolism. They should only be used with the supervision of an experienced paediatric dietitian.

Nutritional Deficiencies

Preschool children are the most vulnerable group. Those who are socioeconomically disadvantaged and those from some ethnic groups are at highest risk of suboptimal intake of some nutrients. Many are at high risk of iron and vitamin D deficiency. As

Table 1.7	Estimated average requirements/kg body weight in healthy subjects[a]		
Age	Fluid (ml)	Energy (kcal)	Protein (g)
Preterm	150–200	120	3.5
0–3 months	150	115–100	2.1
4–6 months	130	95	1.6
7–9 months	120	95	1.5
10–12 months	110	95	1.5
1–3 years	95	95	1.1
4–6 years	85	90	1.1
7–10 years	75	85	No COMA rec
11–14 years	55	65	No COMA rec
15–18 years	35–50	40	0.6

Note: The higher fluid requirements result in an increased risk of dehydration during illness.
[a]With exception of preterm requirements, source is: Committee on Medical Aspects of Food (COMA) 1991 DOH report on health and social subjects, no. 41. HMSO, London. ISBN 0-11-321397-2.

mentioned in the first part of this appendix, the national recommendations for vitamin D intake for all the population were updated in 2016 and include babies and children.

Obesity

Obesity is increasing in all sectors of industrialized societies but the socially disadvantaged seem to be at highest risk. If the UK continues to follow the childhood obesity trend seen in the USA there will be an increase in short-term morbidity, e.g., diabetes, abnormal liver function tests, weight-bearing-joint problems and psychological issues. In addition, childhood obesity does not bode well for adult health and is likely to lead to increased risk of diabetes and heart disease as these children grow up. Research is ongoing to try and tease out the relative roles of reduced exercise versus increased intake. There are indications that energy intake has not increased sufficiently to explain the rise in obesity; however, there has been a very rapid increase in sedentary behaviour, e.g., computer gaming and television viewing, coupled with less playing outdoors, which could underpin the increased weight of children today. In addition there is evidence that those who are not obese may still be developing an abnormal body composition due to lack of exercise, with an increased proportion of the body's weight being fat compared with several years ago.

Allergies

There is evidence that food allergies are on the increase in industrialized countries, with diagnosis occurring primarily in infancy and early childhood. New research from a group based in the UK suggests that contrary to previous belief, giving some potentially allergenic food early on during weaning may help prevent later development of allergy;

this will be reflected in updated national advice (see SACN publication *Feeding in the first year of life*). However, perceived prevalence is probably much lower than clinically established disease; therefore when exclusion of a nutritionally important food is suggested, this should only be for a trial period after which the food should be added back into the diet if no improvement is seen. Children on cows'-milk-free diets are at risk of poor growth and poor bone mineralization. Any baby or child who is referred for a food exclusion diet should be supervised by an experienced paediatric dietitian with expertise in allergy management.

Chronic Diseases of Childhood

There are many chronic diseases of childhood that require major nutritional or dietetic intervention. For many there is associated poor appetite and supplementation of the diet with tube feeding is necessary; if this is likely to be necessary for an indefinite period a gastrostomy should be considered. For others a fundamental change in the diet is necessary, e.g., coeliac condition, renal and liver disease, cystic fibrosis and many of the inborn errors of metabolism. A lifetime change in diet is often needed which requires monitoring and support of the child and family from a team of medical professionals, including an experienced paediatric dietitian. For many children with chronic diseases faltering growth is common. In 2017 NICE published a document to help identify and manage faltering growth in children.

Useful Resources

NICE guidelines on recognising and managing faltering growth published 2017 can be found at this web address: https://www.ncbi.nlm.nih.gov/pubmedhealth/PMH0097056/pdf/PubMedHealth_PMH0097056.pdf.

SACN Feeding in the first year of life: 2018.

Shaw, V., 2015. Clinical Paediatric Dietetics, fourth ed. Blackwell, Oxford.

WHO guidelines on breast feeding can be found at this web address: http://www.who.int/topics/breastfeeding/en/.

http://www.firststepsnutrition.org/.

Other Useful Websites

British Dietetic Association: http://www.bda.uk.com/.

Cochrane Database of Systematic Review: http://www.nelh.nhs.uk/cochrane.asp.

SACN: https://www.gov.uk/government/groups/scientific-advisory-committee-on-nutrition.

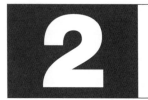

Appendix

2

Resuscitation

ELIZABETH WHITTAKER and LUCY OUGHTON

Introduction

Resuscitation is usually separated into three sections: Basic Life Support (BLS), Immediate Life Support (ILS) and Advanced Life Support (ALS). Basic Life Support is further divided into two sections: in hospital and out of hospital.

This appendix concentrates purely on out-of-hospital basic life support and is based on the 2015 guidelines published by the European Resuscitation Council and the Resuscitation Council (UK). Resuscitation guidelines are currently reviewed and revised every 5 years. Further information on current guidelines can be obtained by visiting the Resuscitation Council (UK) website at www.resus.org.uk.

Although this chapter concentrates on adult and paediatric basic life support it is not intended to replace practical training using resuscitation manikins but is designed as a useful guide for staff working outside of a hospital setting.

As always, the focus of resuscitation is the prevention of cardiac arrest which can be achieved by a knowledge of the early warning signs demonstrated by people who are becoming unwell, and the prompt escalation of these signs to the emergency services who have the advanced skills to manage the situation and thus prevent the person going into full cardiac arrest.

Adult Cardiac Arrest

There are two popular ways to remember the sequence of basic life support and these are SSS ABC and DRS ABC. The second of these seems to be the most memorable, encouraging a quick response.

D = **Danger**
R = **Response**
S = **Shout**
A = **Airway**
B = **Breathing**
C = **Circulation**

Danger

Check for and remove any hazards prior to approaching the person who has collapsed.

Response

Firmly tap the casualty on the shoulders and shout into both their ears, using their name if you know it, to ascertain any signs of consciousness and ensure no further harm is caused with the stimulation.

Shout

It is most likely that you will require assistance with the rescue of this casualty so call for help to anyone nearby. If you are heard, ask them to bring any available rescue equipment as there is a possibility that there might be emergency equipment such as a defibrillator (AED) close by.

Airway

Look in the mouth for any loose objects that may be causing a blockage to the airway. Only remove any objects that you can easily reach with your finger and thumb (dentures can be left in place if they are well fitting). Do not be tempted to push your fingers into the mouth as this could cause damage to the airway by pushing the item further in and the casualty may unintentionally bite your fingers if they begin to regain consciousness.

Then open up the airway by using a head tilt and chin lift (Fig. 2.1). To do this place one of your hands on the patient's forehead and with the other hand place two fingers under the chin, then tilt the head back. This action will lift the tongue from the back of the casualty's throat, thus opening the airway.

Breathing

While keeping the head tilt and chin lift position in placc, check for breathing by bringing your cheek close to the mouth of the casualty (Fig. 2.2). Look down their chest, listen and feel for:

- Movement of the chest
- Breath sounds from the mouth
- Breath on your cheek
- Signs of life such as coughing, swallowing or purposeful movements of limbs.

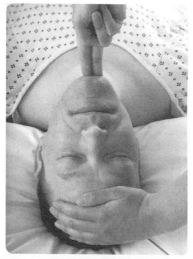

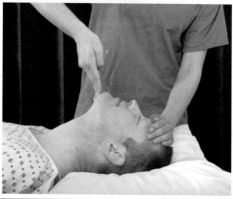

Fig. 2.1 Head tilt and chin lift.

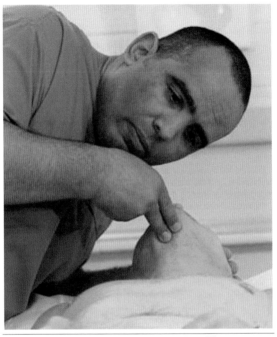

Fig. 2.2   Assessing for breathing and signs of life.

Keep looking for any of these signs for up to 10 seconds. If you should notice the occasional breath or gasp from the casualty, this is not considered a sign of life and must be treated as no breathing present and you should therefore assume cardiac arrest and treat accordingly.

Obtain Help

If the casualty is showing definite signs of life then place them into the recovery position (see Appendix 3 First Aid, page 458).

However, if the person is not showing any signs of life and you obtained no response from your initial call for assistance or you are alone without support, you will need to leave the casualty to summon help yourself without placing the casualty into the recovery position first.

If you have assistance, ensure you focus on one person as you may have several bystanders who have responded. Clearly ask this one person to telephone 999 or 112 to call the emergency services and also to return to you. This will avoid the situation of all the bystanders assuming that someone else has summoned the emergency services and will also ensure that you have help rescuing the casualty with basic life support skills if there are not many people present.

Circulation

This means performing compressions to the casualty's chest. To perform these effectively you must ensure that the person is lying on their back, placed on a firm, flat surface. If necessary, expose the chest to enable you to locate the correct position for your hands.

Place the heel of one of your hands in the centre of the person's chest, place your other hand on top of your first hand and interlock your fingers, attempting to pull your fingers clear of the chest (Fig. 2.3).

Keep your elbows straight and bring your shoulders over the patient's chest. This will mean that you are as close to the casualty as possible. Start pushing down into the chest about 5 to 6 cm and do this 30 times. These compressions should be delivered smoothly with equal attention to gaining the correct depth and relaxation of the chest at a rate of 100 to 120 per minute, two compressions per second.

Attempt Two Ventilations

Ensure the airway is open (with a head tilt and chin lift). The aim is to achieve a rise of the chest only, as over-inflation of the chest can lead to further difficulties in resuscitating the person. With your finger and thumb, pinch the nose of the casualty and place your mouth, which should be open as wide as possible, so it can cover the casualty's mouth completely. Take a breath yourself and deliver this slowly into the patient's mouth. Take your mouth away and repeat the ventilation for a second time.

If you are not prepared to do mouth-to-mouth ventilation or there is failure of the chest to rise and fall when you attempt to do this, then return to achieving good-quality chest compressions. Most health care settings will have airway devices such as pocket masks or a bag valve and mask available. Training in use of these devices should be sought locally.

Research shows that people are more likely to start cardiopulmonary resuscitation (CPR) if they only have to do chest compressions on a casualty. CPR with rescue breaths should remain the gold standard, but if someone is untrained or unsure about how to deliver rescue breaths and compressions, chest

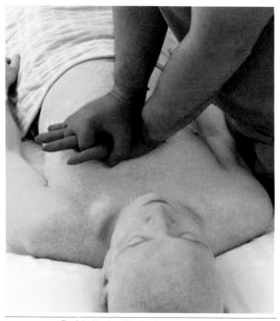

Fig. 2.3 Hand position for chest compressions.

compression-only CPR is still more likely to increase a casualty's chance of survival than no intervention.

Continue Resuscitation

Continue resuscitation with a ratio of 30 compressions to 2 ventilations, until:

- Competent help arrives and takes over
- You are too exhausted to continue
- You notice definite signs of life—in which case stop and reassess the patient.

What else you do will depend on your skill level, training, experience and the local policies on resuscitation in your location.

The stages of adult basic life support are illustrated in Fig. 2.4.

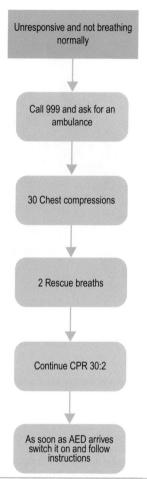

Fig. 2.4   Adult basic life support algorithm. (Reproduced with kind permission of the Resuscitation Council (UK)).

Adult Choking

There are three possible situations as far as choking is concerned:

- Partial or mild
- Complete or severe
- Collapsed.

Partial or Mild Obstruction

Is the person able to speak and cough adequately? If this is not the case then encourage coughing, stay with them and be prepared to intervene should the situation deteriorate.

Complete or Severe Obstruction

If the person is unable to move any air past the obstruction they will be unable to make any noises from the mouth. Often they will clutch at their throat and their face may begin to change colour.

The first action is to confirm that this is indeed a choking episode. If you are in any doubt ask them 'Are you choking?' You may get a nod from them by way of confirmation or a bystander may have witnessed the cause and be able to confirm this.

Support the casualty's chest with one of your hands and lean them forward to ensure that the obstruction comes out of the mouth if it is dislodged. Place the heel of your other hand between the shoulder blades and deliver up to five back slaps, checking between each back slap to see if the obstruction has been removed.

If the obstruction fails to come out and the person is still choking, move on to deliver up to five abdominal thrusts (formerly known as the Heimlich manoeuvre). With the person still leaning forwards, stand yourself behind them and bring your arms underneath theirs. Form a fist with one hand and place this halfway between the belly button (umbilicus) and the V shape where the ribs meet (sternum). Place your second hand over the fist and pull inwards and upwards.

If the abdominal thrusts fail, attempt a further five backslaps and continue alternating between back slaps and abdominal thrusts until the obstruction is removed, help arrives or the person collapses into the third choking situation.

It is advisable that medical help is sought following a choking episode where the back slaps and abdominal thrusts have been used even if the object came out successfully.

Collapsed Choking Casualty

There is no point in reassessing the casualty for breathing, as you will have already ascertained that this is a choking episode. The advice in this situation is to commence BLS immediately, starting with 30 compressions. It is feasible that the pressures created in the chest by doing these compressions will move the obstruction or break it up slightly. Attempt the two rescue breaths as previously described, although they may or may not be successful.

Be aware of your local policies on do not resuscitate (DNACPR) as many of these treat choking as a reversible cause and therefore advise full treatment in this situation.

For treatment of choking in an adult, see the algorithm in Fig. 2.5.

Other Situations
Obstetric Cardiac Arrest

Due to the pressures caused on the inferior vena cava during pregnancy it is preferable for women who are 20 weeks or over in their pregnancy to be placed at a 15-degree angle on their left side during CPR.

However, if a firm device to place between the hip and shoulder is not available to create this tilt, then the casualty should be left flat on their back until specialized help is available. This will ensure that good chest compressions can still be achieved.

Other than the above recommendations all other BLS techniques will still apply.

Tracheostomy

These patients can be ventilated by the stoma in the neck; pocket mask valves can often fit onto these stomas if there are no other more advanced devices available.

Paediatric Cardiac Arrest

Children have a tendency to go into cardiac arrest as a result of respiratory difficulties rather than a primary cardiac cause, so emphasis is placed on rescue breathing first.

The stages of paediatric basic life support for health care professionals with a duty of care to respond are illustrated in Fig. 2.6.

Fig. 2.5   Adult choking treatment algorithm. (Reproduced with kind permission of the Resuscitation Council (UK)).

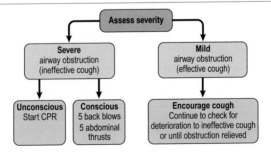

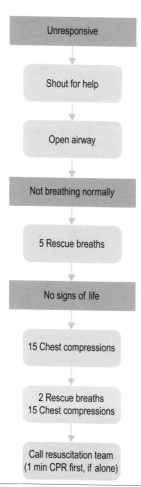

Fig. 2.6 Paediatric basic life support (health care professionals with a duty to respond). (Reproduced with kind permission of the Resuscitation Council (UK)).

Paediatric basic life support is divided into two different age groups; an infant being under 1 year of age and a child above 1 year old.

When opening the airway a head tilt and chin lift technique should still be used, aiming for a neutral position in an infant and a sniffing position in a child.

Rescue breaths should be given to an infant by placing your mouth over the infant's nose and mouth and in a child by using the technique referred to for adults, both techniques aiming to achieve a rise in the chest.

Chest compressions in both age groups should be delivered over the lower half of the sternum. In an infant the tips of two fingers should be used and in a child the heel of one hand. At least one-third of the depth of the chest should be compressed at a rate of 100–120 compressions per minute, two compressions per second.

For staff working in areas that are not specialized in paediatrics or trained in paediatric life support skills, it is recommended that the adult approach is used, if at all possible trying to remember to give five initial rescue breaths. Continue these breaths at a ratio of 30 compressions to two breaths.

Continue in cycles of two breaths and 30 compressions for both the infant and the child until further assistance arrives or you are a lone rescuer and need to leave after a minute of CPR to summon the emergency services.

If you are alone rescuing a child and have no choice other than to leave them to summon help, ensure that you do 1 minute of BLS first before leaving the child to summon further assistance. Should you be expected to be the first responder to a child then it is recommended that you receive targeted training in paediatric life support skills.

Paediatric Choking

The same classifications exist as defined in the adult section, but techniques vary for removing a complete obstruction depending on the age and size of the child. An advantage in smaller children is that gravity can be used very effectively in a choking episode.

Infants (Under 1 Year of Age)

Support the infant's head with one of your hands along the bony part of their jaw, then turn them head down over your lap so their bottom is higher than their head, and they are face down. If the object has not already fallen out at this point deliver up to five back slaps. If these fail to work, continue to support the head and turn the child over, delivering up to five chest thrusts (in the same place as chest compressions but slower and with more force).

Continue in cycles of five back slaps and five chest thrusts until the object comes out or help arrives. If the child loses consciousness, commence basic life support from the initial five rescue breaths.

Child (Above 1 Year Old)

Use the techniques of five back slaps and five abdominal thrusts with less force than for adults. If physically possible, positioning the child over your lap for the back slaps will be helpful for extra gravitational force.

If the child collapses commence BLS, starting at five rescue breaths.

Bibliography

Resuscitation Council (UK), 2015. Immediate Life Support Manual, fourth ed. Resuscitation Council (UK), London.

Resuscitation guidelines are subject to review every five years. Refer to the Resuscitation Council website for the latest guidelines and algorithms http://www.resus.org.uk/.

With thanks to the British Heart Foundation's Heartstart programme for guidance and advice on Basic Life Support in the community setting.

Appendix

First Aid
SUSAN CLEMENTS

First aid is the immediate care given to an injured or ill person before treatment. Effective first aid contributes to reducing the effects of illness and injury. Attention is directed first to the most critical problems: preserving life by securing the airway, looking for bleeding and evaluating the adequacy of cardiac function. Further actions prevent deterioration and promote recovery. This guidance, based on the 2015 guidelines published by the European Resuscitation Council and Resuscitation Council (UK), is aimed at those in medical and social care workplaces where help is available quickly. Following it will enable the reader to respond to a situation, assess the priorities for the casualty and respond. Ensure local procedures are followed, including how to summon appropriate emergency help; 999/112 for an ambulance, or crash team if in a hospital. Remember that a holistic approach is beneficial to the casualty and to those accompanying them.

Action at an Emergency
As you approach the casualty pause to get an overview of the scene (the possible mechanism of the injury, the events leading up to the incident) and evaluate its seriousness. Ensure it is safe before approaching any closer.

Priorities of Treatment: Patient Assessment and Primary Survey
Follow the DRS ABC (Danger, Response, Shout; Airway, Breathing, Circulation) assessment described in Appendix 2 to establish the presence of normal breathing and determine the level of consciousness using AVPU (Alert, Voice, Pain, Unconscious):

- Check it is safe to approach.
- Try to establish a response from the casualty by asking them their name and shaking their shoulders. Use the aide-mémoire AVPU to help remember the steps:
  - Are they **A**lert?
  - Do they respond to your **V**oice?
  - Do they respond to **P**ressure? (squeeze their hand)
  - Are they **U**nresponsive?
  - If they do not respond, or have reduced levels of consciousness, **call for help**.
- Open their airway using the head tilt–chin lift manoeuvre. Check for normal breathing: look for chest movements, listen for breath sounds and feel their breaths on your cheek.

Casualty Breathing Normally: Recovery Position

- If they are breathing normally use the head tilt–chin lift manoeuvre to keep the airway open. If the mechanism of injury suggests a possible neck or spinal injury use the jaw thrust to open the airway. Assess for life-threatening problems: severe bleeding needs to be stopped as soon as possible to prevent the casualty deteriorating. An unconscious casualty breathing normally should be put into the recovery position to maintain an open airway. If the casualty vomits (not uncommon), it will drain from the mouth and not threaten the airway.
- Kneel beside the casualty.
- Remove their spectacles (if worn) and bulky items from their pockets.
- Move the arm nearest you outwards, elbow bent with palm uppermost (Fig. 3.1).
- Bring the furthest arm across their chest, then hold the back of that hand against the cheek nearest you.
- With your other hand, grasp the far leg just above the knee and pull it up, keeping the foot on the ground.
- Keeping the casualty's hand pressed against their cheek, use the knee as a lever to pull the casualty towards you, onto their side (Fig. 3.2).
- Adjust the upper leg so that the hip and knee are bent at right angles. Tilt the head back to keep the airway open (Fig. 3.3).
- Call 999/112 for an ambulance.
- Monitor and record values every 10 minutes for:
  - breathing rate per minute, and listen for any breathing difficulties or unusual noises; and
  - pulse rate per minute, then note the rhythm (regular or irregular) and strength.
- Monitor their level of consciousness.

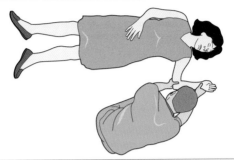

Fig. 3.1 Move the arm nearest you outwards, elbow bent with palm uppermost.

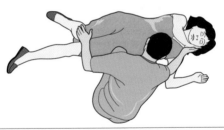

Fig. 3.2 Use the knee as a lever to pull the casualty towards you, onto their side.

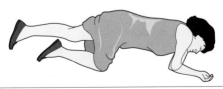

Fig. 3.3 Adjust the upper leg so that the hip and knee are bent at right angles.

- If the person is in the recovery position for 30 minutes, turn them onto the other side to relieve pressure on the lower arm.
- Stay with the casualty until instructed otherwise by the emergency services.

Priorities of Treatment: Patient Assessment and Secondary Survey

After completing the primary survey and dealing with any life-threatening conditions, examine the casualty for other injuries or illnesses in a methodical manner. This can be carried out on a conscious or unconscious casualty. Protect their dignity, and gain their consent if possible.

Protecting the airway always takes priority, so if a casualty is unconscious and breathing but their airway is threatened (e.g., by vomiting), put them into the recovery position immediately. If they are already in the recovery position do the secondary survey with them in that position.

Consider:

History—What happened? Are injuries likely? Is there medical history?

Signs—What you can see, feel, hear and smell (e.g., swelling, bruising, deformity).

Symptoms—What the casualty feels (e.g., pain, nausea). Ask about the site, extent (localized or radiating to other areas) and nature of the pain (e.g., throbbing, stabbing, dull ache), when the pain started and what makes it worse or alleviates it.

Check Them From Head to Toe:

Head and neck—Are breathing and pulse normal? Are pupils dilated, equal, etc. Look for clues such as bruising, swelling, bleeding, discharge from ear or nose.

Shoulders and chest—Compare both sides, look for fractures, wounds, bleeding. Are they able to take a deep breath? If so, does the chest move equally on both sides? Is it painful? Is breathing laboured, wheezy or noisy?

Abdomen and pelvis—Gently feel the abdomen, check for abnormality, bleeding, incontinence and response to pain.

Legs and arms—Look for signs of fracture or deformity. Can they move their limbs and joints without causing pain?

Other Information:

Check for clues such as medical alert bracelets, needle marks, medication, etc. (e.g., injury to a patient taking Warfarin could be life-threatening). If you remove items from pockets have a reliable witness and do so cautiously to reduce the risk of personal injury from sharp objects. Do not put your hand into a pocket; pull the linings out instead.

Disorders of Circulation: External Bleeding

The aims of treatment for severe external bleeding are to stop the bleeding to prevent the casualty going into shock (see later), then to prevent infection.

- Wear disposable gloves if available.
- Sit or lay the casualty down in a position appropriate to wound location and severity of bleeding.
- Examine the wound, note if it is bleeding and how (e.g., spurting, oozing). Look for foreign objects.
- Elevate the wound above the level of the heart. Apply direct pressure over the wound to stem the bleeding.
- Apply a sterile wound dressing. Check the capillary refill by squeezing the tip of a finger or toe on that limb—the skin will become pale—then release the pressure. If the blood flow is not impeded the colour should return within 2 seconds (unless the hands or feet are cold).
- If blood soaks through the dressing put another one on top. If blood seeps through the second dressing, remove both dressings and start again, ensuring sufficient pressure is applied directly over the wound.
- Use a haemostatic dressing when direct pressure cannot control severe external bleeding. Training is required to use haemostatic dressings.

Shock

Shock is a life-threatening condition caused by insufficient fluid circulating around the body, caused by, for example, internal or external bleeding, burns, vomiting, the heart working inefficiently or stopping (e.g., heart attack or acute heart failure). This results in insufficient oxygen reaching the tissues and vital organs, notably the brain and heart.

Recognition

Look for fluid loss (e.g., severe external bleeding). Be aware that the cause may not be obvious (e.g., internal bleeding), so look for signs of shock. The first signs are cold, clammy skin, rapid pulse, sweating and pale, grey skin. As shock develops the pulse become weak and breathing rapid and shallow. The casualty will feel weak, giddy, thirsty, may complain of nausea and possibly vomit. If shock develops further they may become restless, anxious, aggressive, yawn or gasp for air, become unconscious and their heart may eventually stop.

Treatment

- Treat the cause of shock (e.g., external bleeding).
- Lay casualty on their back. Where there is no evidence of trauma raise their legs. A heavily pregnant casualty should have her right hip elevated to prevent the baby restricting the mother's blood flow.

- Keep them warm. Place a coat or blanket under them for insulation. Loosen any tight clothing. They must not eat, drink or smoke.
- Reassure the casualty and stay with them.
- Dial 999/112 for ambulance.
- Monitor their ABC, level of response, and be prepared to resuscitate.

Respiratory Conditions

Many people have conditions that may affect breathing, e.g., emphysema, chronic bronchitis, congestive heart failure, other cardiovascular diseases, lung cancer, asthma, allergies, sleep apnoea, pneumonia or upper respiratory infections. Breathing that is too fast or too slow might indicate a situation requiring first aid so it is important to know what is normal breathing for a particular patient. A change in breathing is the first indication of a change in condition. Some breathing problems warrant immediate emergency attention and are life-threatening.

Asthma

A condition caused by an allergic reaction in the lungs causing the bronchioles to spasm and constrict. Breathing, especially breathing out, becomes difficult.

Recognition

There may be wheezing, difficulty speaking or cyanosed skin, lips, earlobes and nail beds. In severe attacks, there may be exhaustion and possible loss of consciousness.

Treatment

- Calm and reassure the casualty—tell them to breathe slowly and deeply.
- Encourage them to sit with their arms resting on something, e.g., a table in front of them.
- Help them to use their reliever inhaler, with a spacer if possible. Symptoms should improve within minutes. If not, another dose may be taken.
- If their condition fails to improve or talking becomes more difficult call 999/112 for an ambulance.
- Monitor the casualty's ABC and level of response until help arrives.

Heart Conditions: Angina and Myocardial Infarction

Coronary heart disease may cause angina, chest pain or discomfort caused by a temporary deficiency of oxygen to the heart. It may result from stress-induced spasms of the coronary arteries or increased physical demands on the heart. The heart cells are weakened by the temporary lack of oxygen but they do not die.

Far more serious is a prolonged coronary blockage. This prevents oxygen reaching the tissues and can lead to a myocardial infarction (heart attack). Areas of cell death are repaired with scar tissue, so surviving a myocardial infarction depends on the extent and location of the damage.

The signs and symptoms of a heart attack and angina are similar.

Angina

Angina pain is usually caused by exercise or excitement. The casualty experiences central chest pain ('vice-like'), shortness of breath, anxiety, pain or tingling. The pain tends to ease when the patient has rested. This is in contrast to a heart attack in which rest does not ease the pain.

Treatment

- Help the casualty into a comfortable position such as a half-sitting position with the back supported and their knees bent.
- If they have a glyceryl trinitrate (GTN) spray help them to take it.
- Reassure them.
- If the pain persists or returns, call 999/112 for an ambulance.
- Monitor ABC.

Heart Attack

Signs and symptoms are profuse sweating, gasping for air, persistent vice-like central chest pain, sudden fainting or dizziness and cyanosed lips.

Treatment

- Help casualty into a comfortable position, e.g., half sitting with back supported and knees bent.
- Call 999/112 for ambulance.
- For the conscious casualty give them one 300 mg Aspirin to chew (unless they are allergic to Aspirin).
- Monitor ABC.

Cerebrovascular Accidents (Strokes)

Strokes occur when blood circulation to a brain area is disrupted. This causes deficient oxygen and nutrient delivery to cells and results in brain-tissue death. There are two types of stroke. The most common is caused by a clot in a blood vessel blocking the blood flow to the brain. Some are the result of a ruptured blood vessel that causes bleeding into the brain.

Transient Ischaemic Attack (TIA)

A TIA is caused when a small clot blocks a blood vessel temporarily. A TIA lasts from 5 to 50 minutes and is characterized by temporary numbness, paralysis and impaired speech. The patient may recover fully within 24 hours. A TIA may precede a later stroke.

A stroke is a time-critical medical emergency. Strokes due to a blood clot benefit from thrombolytic treatment within 4 hours of the event to be successful, so rapid transfer to specialist care is essential.

Assessment
Carry out the 'FAST' test:

Facial weakness—can the casualty smile? Has their mouth or eye dropped?
Arm weakness—can the casualty raise both arms?
Speech problems—can the casualty speak clearly and understand what you say?
Time to call 999/112—if any tests are failed.

Also look for:
- Sudden numbness of the face or one side of the body.
- Loss of balance; lack of coordination.
- Sudden, severe headache.
- Sudden onset of confusion.
- Sight problems in one or both eyes; unequal pupils.

Treatment
- Maintain airway and breathing; monitor for problems with swallowing.
- Call for emergency help.
- Position casualty with head and shoulders raised.
- Reassure the casualty.

Burns and Scalds

Burns and scalds are caused by intense heat, electricity, radiation or some chemicals. They are painful, may scar and disfigure and be life-threatening, so they need rapid and careful management. The cause may still be present at the scene and present a hazard to everyone present.

The immediate threat from severe burns is a catastrophic loss of body fluids leading to inadequate blood circulation and shock. The lost fluids must be replaced immediately. Burnt or scalded skin may not function effectively as a natural barrier so there is also an increased risk of infection.

Assessment
Consider:
- Whether or not the airway is likely to have been affected.
- The extent, location and depth of the burn. If burns or scalds cover a large area there will be significant fluid loss and a high risk of shock.

Assess the Severity:

- Size—the larger the area of the burn, the more severe. The size is given as a percentage of the body's surface area. An area equal to the size of one side of the casualty's opened hand (including fingers) is equal to 1% of their body area.
- Age—the age of the casualty can affect the severity and recovery rate. The skin of babies and young children may burn more easily. An elderly person may be more susceptible to infection and take longer to heal.
- Location—the location of the burn can affect severity:
  - Inhaling hot gases or smoke can burn the airway.
  - Burns to the eye may result in blindness.
  - Burns extending around the chest may impede breathing; those extending around a limb may impede blood flow.
- Depth—the deeper the burn, the more severe:
  - Superficial burns affect only the outer epidermis of the skin. The burn looks red, sore and swollen. These are most commonly caused by scalds.
  - Partial thickness burns affect the epidermis and the dermis layers of the skin. The burn looks raw and the skin blisters.
  - Full thickness burns burn down to the subcutaneous fat layer and deeper. The area may look pale, charred and waxy. The nerve endings may be destroyed so there may not be any pain. This may be misleading when assessing the severity of the burn.

Treatment

- Actively cool thermal burns as soon as possible using running water for a minimum of 10 minutes using running water or until the pain reduces. Do not touch the burn or burst blisters.
- Cover the injury using a clean non-fluffy pad.
- Do not apply adhesive tape or dressings or remove clothing stuck to the burn.
- Call emergency help if the burn or scald is severe:
  - if superficial burns are larger than 5%;
  - if partial thickness burns are larger than 1%;
  - if the burns are full thickness, mixed pattern or varying depth, to the hands, feet, genitals, face or extending around a limb;
  - or if the casualty is a child.

See the Lund and Browder burn charts on p. 229.

Anaphylaxis

Anaphylaxis is a potentially fatal, rapid allergic response to a previously encountered allergen (e.g., insect stings, peanuts, penicillin). The response releases mediators that may cause a localized wheal and flare reaction or widespread symptoms so fast recognition is essential. The symptoms are:

- Sudden swelling of the face, lips, neck and eyes.
- Swelling of tongue and throat, developing into loud noisy breathing.
- Difficult breathing ranging from tight chest to severe difficulty causing wheezing and gasping for air.
- Red, blotchy skin, itchy rash, red, itchy, watery eyes.
- Rapid, weak pulse.
- Stomach cramps, nausea, vomiting, diarrhoea.
- Anxiety, confusion and agitation.

The outcome may be fatal if no action is taken.

Treatment

- Call urgent emergency help.
- Position the casualty in a comfortable position:
  - If the casualty has airway or breathing problems they may prefer to sit up.
  - If they feel faint, lay them down immediately. Raise their legs if they still feel faint.
- If the casualty has an epinephrine (adrenaline) auto-injector encourage them to use it and assist them if necessary. Repeat the dose at 5-minute intervals if no improvement or if symptoms return.
- Monitor casualty's ABC and level of response until help arrives.

Poisoning

These notes are guidelines. Ensure you are familiar with the procedures of the host establishment.

A poison is any substance (solid, liquid or gas) that causes damage when it enters the body in sufficient quantity. Poisons may be ingested (e.g., foods, alcohol), injected (e.g., drugs), inhaled (e.g., fumes from cleaning) or absorbed (e.g., industrial poisons).

General Advice

- There may be a range of signs and symptoms, depending on the substance.
- Take a history from the casualty (if conscious) and from bystanders. Try to identify what has been taken.
- Look for clues, such as bottles, containers, syringes, smell on the breath.
- Look for signs, such as vomiting or retching, abdominal pains, breathing problems, burns around the entry area (or a burning sensation), breath odour, cyanosis, confusion or hallucination, headache, unconsciousness or fitting.
- Note the:
  - poison(s) involved or suspected;
  - amount or concentration;

- mode of exposure: oral, intravenous, inhaled. Is there any contact with skin or eyes?
- Ensure the scene is safe before approaching. If the casualty is contaminated with chemicals wear disposable gloves, a mask, goggles and use a face shield. In all cases, be prepared to resuscitate.

Treatment

In all cases call emergency help. See Table 3.1 for treatment of poisoning.

Advice about poisoning and overdoses may be obtained from The Poisons Information Centres listed in the British National Formulary (BNF) and the online database TOXBASE.

Musculoskeletal Injuries and Falls

Injuries to muscles, bones, joints and tendons are often due to trauma (e.g., falls, violent blows). Considerable force is usually required to fracture a bone although old or diseased bones (e.g., osteoporosis) may be more brittle and liable to break or crack more easily. Wrenching movements or even violent muscle contractions may cause sprains or dislocations.

Recognition

- Assess the amount of trauma and type of injury. Note external clues, especially if the casualty is unconscious. If the history suggests a fracture then treat as such.
- Ask the casualty about the onset and severity of pain, swelling, bruising and interference with function.
- Look for an unnatural shape or shortening of the limb.
- Check the pulse distal to the site of injury.

Treatment

- Call for help.
- Monitor airway, breathing, circulation and signs of shock.

Table 3.1	Treatment of Poisoning
Ingested poisons	Ensure the casualty does not vomit. For corrosive substances, the casualty should rinse their mouth then take frequent sips of milk or water
Absorbed poisons	Remove contaminated clothing, wash area with cold water for 20 minutes
Inhaled poisons	Help casualty into fresh air
Poison splashed in the eye	Irrigate eye for 10 minutes
Injected poisons	For stings or venom, remove sting if possible

- Steady and support the limb or injured part manually 'in the position found'.
- Prevent casualty eating or drinking.

First Aid and the Elderly

Many older people may have impaired hearing and/or cognitive functions so may need more time to answer questions when carrying out the secondary survey. Casualties with no relatives to corroborate information may pose a particular problem and it may be impossible to get a complete history. Medication, dehydration and confusion may all influence the person's recall of the incident. Some elderly patients are easily confused following a fall, a fit, infection or trauma. Their confusion may be transient but it is important to establish whether it was present before the injury/illness.

The fragility of the skin means that dressings should be bandaged on and adhesive dressings avoided. Pressure sores may develop rapidly.

Dehydration is common in the elderly. This can lead to fainting (vasovagal episodes). The elderly are more easily affected by extremes of heat and cold, i.e., heatstroke and hypothermia.

Accidental poisoning with medication is quite common in persons with cognitive impairment, either by taking too much by mistake or because the body cannot cope with the dose, e.g., digoxin toxicity. Try to establish what medications the person is taking.

There is a high instance of falls, particularly those leading to fractured neck of the femur. Early treatment of fractures, particularly those affecting mobility, is not only essential but life-saving. Many elderly people never fully recover from a fall because their confidence is adversely affected. Emotional support from the first aid point and afterwards could lead to a more positive outcome. An elderly person may have arthritis and therefore pain and reduced mobility prior to any fall, so be aware of this when checking range of limb movement.

Readers interested in furthering their first aid knowledge and gaining a qualification are recommended to attend a training course.

4 Appendix

Medicines and Their Control
TEJAL VAGHELA

Definitions

A medicinal product is:

> *Any substance or combination of substances presented as having properties for treating or preventing disease in human beings; [the first/presentational limb]*
>
> *Any substance or combination of substances which may be used in, or administered to, human beings, either with a view to restoring, correcting or modifying physiological functions by exerting a pharmacological, immunological or metabolic action, or to making a medical diagnosis. [the second/functional limb]*
>
> *(Directive 2001/83/EC)*

Medicinal products may well fall under both limbs of the definition but the European Court of Justice (ECJ) has confirmed that falling under either limb is sufficient to classify a product as a medicinal product.

Medicines Optimization is defined as:

> *A person-centred approach to safe and effective medicines use, to ensure people obtain the best possible outcomes from their medicines.*
>
> (NICE, 2015)

Use of the word 'registrant' throughout this appendix:

Where the word 'registrant' is used this refers to nurses, midwives and specialist community public health nurses who are registered on the Nursing and Midwifery Council Register.

Legislation
Human Medicines Regulations 2012

Humans Medicines Regulations 2012 consolidated most of the legislation regulating the authorization, sale and supply of medicinal products for human use, made under the Medicines Act 1968. The 2012 Regulations govern medicines on the UK market including authorization to market, manufacture, importation, distribution and supply of medicines, and recognition of prescriptions issued in another EU state. The Human Medicines Regulation 2012 classifies medicinal products into the following categories:

1.   Prescription-Only Medicines (POMs)

     A prescription-only medicine (POM) is a medicine that is generally subject to the restriction of requiring a prescription written by an appropriate practitioner: doctor, dentist, supplementary prescriber, nurse independent prescriber, pharmacist independent prescriber, EEA and Swiss doctors and dentists (but not for all Controlled Drugs), EEA and Swiss prescribing pharmacist and prescribing nurse where they exist, community practitioner nurses (for a limited selection of POMs), optometrist independent prescribers (not for Controlled Drugs, or parenteral medicines), podiatrist, physiotherapist and therapeutic radiographer independent prescribers (for certain medicines) before it can be sold or supplied.

2.   Pharmacy-Only Medicines (P)

     A pharmacy medicine is a medicinal product that can be sold from a registered pharmacy premises by a pharmacist or a person acting under the supervision of a pharmacist.

3.   General Sale List Medicines (GSLs)

     General sale medicines (commonly known as GSL medicines) are those that can be sold in registered pharmacies but also in other retail outlets that can 'close so as to exclude the public'.

Exemptions from the general rules are permitted for midwives. These are provided for in the Prescription Only Medicines (Human Use) Order 1997 (SI 1997/1830 the 'POM Order'), the Medicines (Pharmacy and General Sale- Exemption) Order 1980 (SI 1980/1924), the Medicines (Sale or Supply) (Miscellaneous Provisions) Regulations 1980 (SI 1980/1923). Registered midwives may supply and administer, on their own initiative, any of the substances that are specified in the Humans Medicines Regulations 2012 legislation under 'midwives exemptions' provided it is in the course of their professional midwifery practice. They can do this without the need for a prescription, a patient-specific direction from a medical practitioner or patient group direction.

Legislation Applicable to Controlled Drugs

If you are responsible for the storage or administration of controlled drugs (this will also include receipt, key holding and access, record keeping and stock checks), you should be aware of the current legislations applicable to controlled drugs.

The Misuse of Drugs Act 1971 imposes prohibitions on the possession, supply, manufacture, import and export of Controlled Drugs—except where permitted by the 2001 Regulations or under licence from the Secretary of State.

The Misuse of Drugs Regulations 2001 allow for the lawful possession and supply of controlled (illegal) drugs for legitimate purposes.

The Misuse of Drugs (Safe Custody) Regulations 1973 details the storage and safe custody requirements for Controlled Drugs. The enforcement body for Controlled Drug offences is the Home Office, via the police.

The Misuse of Drugs (Supply to Addicts) Regulations 1997 restricts the prescribing of cocaine, diamorphine and dipipanone for the treatment of addiction to doctors licensed by the Home Office (and in Scotland, by the Scottish government).

The Health Act 2006 introduced the concept of an 'accountable officer' and requires health care organizations, and those providing services to health care organizations, to have standard operating procedures in place for using and managing Controlled Drugs. Following the Shipman Inquiry, accountable officers were introduced with responsibility for supervising and managing the use of Controlled Drugs in their organization or setting.

Controlled Drugs (Supervision of Management of use) Regulations 2013 contain measures relating to arrangements underpinning the safe management and use of controlled drugs in England and Scotland.

The Misuse of Drugs Regulations 2001 classifies controlled drugs into five schedules according to the different levels of control attributed to them. Schedule 1 controlled drugs are subject to the highest level of control, whereas Schedule 5 controlled drugs are subject to a much lower level of control.

Schedule 1: Most Schedule 1 drugs have no therapeutic use and a licence is generally required for their production, possession or supply.

Schedule 2: includes opiates (e.g., diamorphine, morphine, methadone, oxycodone, pethidine), major stimulants (e.g., amphetamines), quinalbarbitone and ketamine.

Schedule 3: include minor stimulants and other drugs (such as buprenorphine, temazepam, tramadol, midazolam and phenobarbital) that are less likely to be misused (and less harmful if misused) than those in Schedule 2.

Schedule 4: Part I contains most of the benzodiazepines (such as diazepam), non-benzodiazepine hypnotics (such as zopiclone), and Sativex (a cannabinoid oromucosal mouth spray).

Part II contains most of the anabolic and androgenic steroids, together with clenbuterol (an adrenoceptor stimulant) and growth hormones.

Schedule 5: contains preparations of certain Controlled Drugs (such as codeine, pholcodine and morphine) that are exempt from full control when present in medicinal products of specifically low strengths.

As a registrant, you should be particularly familiar with the regulations concerning Schedule 2 medicines such as morphine, diamorphine and pethidine, and Schedule 3 drugs such as barbiturates.

Queries are often raised in relation to prescriptions for Schedule 2 and 3 medicines (controlled drugs).

Prescriptions for Schedule 2 or 3 controlled drugs must comply with the following requirements:

Name and address of patient
Dose, formulation, strength of the preparation
Total quantity in both words and figures
Prescriber signature, prescriber address and date signed.

In hospitals, requisitioning, receipt, storage and record keeping of controlled drugs are subject to tight control. All hospitals have local their own Controls Drugs Policy, which you should familiarize yourself with.

- Controls drugs must be stored separately in a locked cabinet (which may be within a second outer cabinet) to which access is restricted. The cabinet and room must comply with the technical details of the Safe Custody Regulations. Cabinet must be locked when not in use and the lock must not be common to any other lock in the hospital.
- The nurse in charge of the ward is responsible for the controlled drugs (CD) key and should know its whereabouts at all times. Key holding may be delegated to other suitably trained members of staff but the legal responsibility rests with the nurse in charge.
- Supply from the pharmacy is made to a ward or department only on receipt of a written order signed by a responsible nurse.

- A record is kept of stock held and details of doses given. A special register is used for this and no other purpose, and it is usually the case that each entry is countersigned by two nurses. The records should be regularly checked by the nurse in charge and by a pharmacist, according to Trust policy.

If you have any queries in relation to the misuse of drugs, or if you are aware of illicit substances being in the possession of a patient, you must refer to and act on local policy and/or appropriate Department of Health guidance.

Unlicensed Medicines

An unlicensed medicine is the term used to refer to a medicine that does not have a valid marketing authorization in UK, and is not covered by approval process overseen by Medicines and Healthcare products Regulatory Agency (MHRA). If an unlicensed medicine is administered to a patient, the manufacturer may not have liability for any harm that ensues. The person who prescribes and dispenses or supplies the medicine carries the liability. This may have implications for you in obtaining informed consent. A registrant may administer an unlicensed medicinal product with the patient's informed consent against a patient-specific direction but NOT against a patient group direction.

Off-Label Medicines

Medication which is licensed but used outside its licensed indications (commonly known as 'off-label') may be administered under a patient group direction only where such use is exceptional, justified by best practice, and the status of the product is clearly described.

As a registrant you should be satisfied that you have sufficient information to administer a medicine prescribed 'off-label' safely and whenever possible that there is acceptable published evidence for the use of that product for the intended indication. Liability for prescribing an 'off-label' medicine sits with the prescriber and the dispenser or supplier.

The British National Formulary for children provides useful information for the administration of 'off-label' medication for children. More information on unlicensed and 'off-label' medicines can be found in the NMC publication Standards of Proficiency for Nurse Midwife Prescribers 2006.

Complementary and Alternative Therapies

Complementary and alternative therapies are increasingly used in the treatment of patients. Registrants must have successfully undertaken training and be competent to practise the administration of complementary and alternative therapies. Please refer to The Code: 2015 Professional Standards of Practice and Behaviour for Nurses and

Midwives. You must have considered the appropriateness of the therapy to both the condition of the patient and any coexisting treatments. It is essential that the patient is aware of the therapy and gives informed consent.

Complementary and alternative therapies may interact with other types of medicinal products and laboratory tests. You need to ensure that your employer has accepted vicarious liability for any complementary or alternative therapy you may undertake or that you have indemnity insurance to cover your practice.

It is important to be aware that nurses and midwives remain accountable when practising complementary or alternative therapies.

The Code states: 'You must ensure that the use of complementary or alternative therapies is safe and in the best interests of those in your care'.

Standard 23 of the Standards for Medicines Management states: 'Registrants must have successfully undertaken training and be competent to practise the administration of complementary and alternative therapies'.

Abbreviations Used in Prescriptions

Abbreviations of Latin words are being replaced by English versions, which are considered safer; however, the nurse may still come across the Latin abbreviations given in Table 4.1.

Table 4.1   Abbreviations and prescriptions

Abbreviation	Latin	English
a.c.	ante cibum	before food
ad lib	ad libitum	to the desired amount
b.d. or b.i.d.	bis in die	twice a day
c.	cum	with
o.m.	omni mane	every morning
o.n.	omni nocte	every night
p.c.	post cibum	after food
p.r.n.	pro re nata	whenever necessary
q.d.	quaque die	every day
q.d.s.	quaque die sumendum	four times daily
q.i.d.	quarter in die	four times a day
q.q.h.	quarter quaque hora	every four hours
R	recipe	take
s.o.s.	si opus sit	if necessary
stat	statim	at once
t.d.s.	ter die sumendum	three times a day
t.i.d.	ter in die	three times a day

Guidance
NMC: Standards for Medicine Management (2007)

This document includes standards that cover the process from prescribing, through to dispensing, storage, administration and disposal of medicines. It also incorporates guidance on controlled drugs and provides helpful links to a range of documents on medicines management.

> The administration of medicines is an important aspect of the professional practice of persons whose names are on the Council's register. It is not solely a mechanistic task to be performed in strict compliance with the written prescription of a medical practitioner (can now also be an independent and supplementary prescriber). It requires thought and the exercise of professional judgement…

Many government and other agencies are involved in medicines management, from manufacture, licensing, prescribing and dispensing, to administration. An extensive range of guidance on these issues is provided by the relevant bodies. Sources of information are listed in the references. One of the best sources of advice locally is usually your pharmacist.

Administration of Medicines
Standards for Practice of Administration of Medicines

As a registrant, you are accountable for your actions and omissions. In administering any medication, or assisting or overseeing any self-administration of medication, you must exercise your professional judgement and apply your knowledge and skill in the given situation.

Having initially checked the 'direction to supply or administer' to confirm that a medicinal product is appropriate for your patient you may then administer the medication.

As a registrant, in exercising your professional accountability in the best interests of your patients, you must:

- Be certain of the identity of the patient to whom the medicine is to be administered.
- Check that the patient is not allergic to the medicine before administering it.
- Know the therapeutic uses of the medicine to be administered, its normal dosage, side effects, precautions and contraindications.
- Be aware of the patient's care plan or pathway.
- Check the prescription or the label on medicine dispensed by a pharmacist is clearly written and unambiguous.
- Have considered the dosage, weight where appropriate, method of administration, route and timing of the administration in the context of the condition of the patient and coexisting therapies.

- Check the expiry date of the medicine administered.
- Contact the prescriber or another authorized prescriber without delay where contraindications to the prescribed medicine are discovered, where the patient develops a reaction to the medicine or where assessment of the patient indicates that the medicine is no longer suitable.
- Make a clear, accurate and immediate record of all medicine administered, intentionally withheld or refused by the patient, ensuring that any written entries and the signature are clear and legible; it is also your responsibility to ensure that a record is made when delegating the task of administering medicine.
- Administer or withhold in the context of the patient's condition (e.g., digoxin not usually to be given if pulse below 60) and coexisting therapies (e.g., physiotherapy).
- Where supervising a student nurse or midwife in the administration of medicines, clearly countersign the signature of the student.

Some drug administrations can require complex calculations to ensure that the correct volume or quantity of medication is administered. In these situations, it may be necessary for a second practitioner (a registered professional) to check the calculation in order to minimize the risk of error. The use of calculators independently to determine the volume or quantity of medication should not act as a substitute for arithmetical knowledge and skill.

Registrants must not prepare substances for injection in advance of their immediate use or to administer medication drawn into a syringe or container by another practitioner when not in their presence. An exception to this is an already established infusion which has been instigated by another practitioner following the principles set out above, or medication prepared under the direction of a pharmacist from a central intravenous additive service and clearly labelled for that patient.

In an emergency, where you may be required to prepare substances for injection by a doctor, you should ensure that the person administering the drug has undertaken the appropriate checks as indicated above.

Instruction by telephone to a practitioner to administer a previously unprescribed substance is not acceptable. In exceptional circumstances, where the medication has been previously prescribed and the prescriber is unable to issue a new prescription, but where changes to the dose are considered necessary, the use of information technology (such as fax or email) is the preferred method. This should be followed up by a new prescription confirming the changes within a given time period. The NMC suggests a maximum of 24 hours. In any event, the changes must have been authorized by a registered prescriber before the new dosage is administered.

Text messaging is an increasing possibility in the process of an order to administer a medicine. However, you must ensure there are protocols in place to ensure patient confidentiality and that local policies and procedures are in place to provide robust audit trail and clinical governance, in order to support such practice.

Aids to Support Concordance (Compliance Aids)

Registrants must assess the patient's suitability and understanding of how to use an appropriate compliance aid safely. Before considering the use of compliance aids, you should explore with the patient other possible solutions, for example reminder charts, large print labels, non-child-proof tops. Self-administration from dispensed containers may not always be possible for some patients. If an aid to concordance is considered necessary, careful attention should be given to the assessment of the patient's suitability and understanding of how to use an appropriate aid safely. However, all patients will need to be regularly assessed for continued appropriateness of the aid. Ideally, any concordance aid, such as a monitored dose container or a daily or weekly dosing aid, should be dispensed, labelled and sealed by a pharmacist. The sealed compliance aids are generally referred to as monitored dosage systems.

Where it is not possible to get a concordance aid filled by a pharmacist, you should ensure that you are able to account for its use. The patient has a right to expect that the same standard of skill and care will be applied by you in dispensing into a compliance aid as would be applied if the patient were receiving the medication from a pharmacist. This includes the same standard of labelling and record keeping. Compliance aids, which can be purchased by patients for their own use, are aids that are filled from containers of dispensed medicines. If you choose to repackage dispensed medicines into compliance aids, you should be aware that their use carries a risk of error. You should also be aware the properties of the drug might also change when repackaged and so may not be covered by their product licence. Your employer needs to be aware of this activity and it should be covered by a standard operating procedure (SOP). The NMC would recommend that you confirm the appropriateness of repackaging dispensed medicinal products with the community pharmacist who dispensed the medicines. You also need to consider how the patient will cope with medicines that cannot be included in compliance aids.

Self-Administration of Medicines

The NMC welcomes and supports the self-administration of medicines and the administration of medication by carers wherever it is appropriate. However, the essential safety, security and storage arrangements must be available and, where necessary, agreed procedures must be in place.

For the hospital patient approaching discharge, but who will continue on a prescribed medicines regime on the return home, there are obvious benefits in adjusting to the responsibility of self-administration while still having access to professional support. It is essential, however, that where self-administration is introduced, arrangements are in place for the safe and secure storage of the medication, access to which is limited to the specific patient.

Where self-administration of medicines is taking place, you should ensure that records are maintained appropriate to the environment in which the patient is being cared for.

It is also important that, if you are delegating this responsibility, you ensure that the patient or carer/care assistant is competent to carry out the task. This will require education, training and assessment of the patient or carer/care assistant and further support if necessary. The competence of the person to whom the task has been delegated should be reviewed periodically.

Management of Adverse Events (Errors or Incidents) in the Administration of Medicines

It is important that an open culture exists in order to encourage the immediate reporting of errors or incidents in the administration of medicines.

If you make an error, you must take any action to prevent any potential harm to the patient and report it as soon as possible to the prescriber, your line manager or employer (according to local policy) and document your actions. Midwives should also inform their named Supervisor of Midwives. Registered nurses and midwives who have made an error, and who have been honest and open about it to their senior staff, appear sometimes to have been made the subject of local disciplinary action in a way that might discourage the reporting of incidents and, therefore, be potentially detrimental to patients and the maintenance of standards.

The NMC believes that all errors and incidents require a thorough and careful investigation at a local level, taking full account of the context and circumstances and the position of the practitioner involved. Such incidents require sensitive management and a comprehensive assessment of all the circumstances before a professional and managerial decision is reached on the appropriate way to proceed. If a practising midwife makes or identifies a drug error or incident, she should also inform her supervisor of midwives as soon as possible after the event.

The NMC supports the use of a thorough, open and multidisciplinary approach to investigating adverse events, where improvements to local practice in the administration of medicines can be discussed, identified and disseminated.

When considering allegations of misconduct arising from errors in the administration of medicines, the NMC takes great care to distinguish between those cases where the error was the result of reckless or incompetent practice or was concealed, and those that resulted from other causes, such as serious pressure of work, and where there was immediate, honest disclosure in the patient's interest. The NMC recognizes the prerogative of managers to take local disciplinary action where it is considered to be necessary but urges that they also consider each incident in its particular context and similarly discriminate between the two categories described above.

In the NHS, all errors (patient safety incidents) and near-misses should be reported through local risk management systems.

Reporting Adverse Reactions

As a registrant, if a patient experiences an adverse drug reaction to a medication you must take any action to remedy harm caused by the reaction. You must record this in the patient's notes, notify the prescriber (if you did not prescribe the drug) and notify via the Yellow Card Scheme immediately.

Yellow cards are found in the back of the British National Formulary and online at https://yellowcard.mhra.gov.uk/.

Prescribing Medicines

Detailed guidance on prescribing is contained in the British National Formulary (BNF) and in Medicines, Ethics and Practice: The Professional Guide for Pharmacists. Until 1992, prescribing was essentially restricted to doctors and dentists. Any qualified and registered independent prescriber may prescribe all Prescription Only Medicines for all medical conditions. In addition, Nurse and Pharmacist Independent Prescribers may also prescribe controlled drugs (except diamorphine, cocaine and dipipanone for the treatment of addiction). Independent Prescribers must only prescribe drugs that are within their area of expertise, and level of competence and should only prescribe for children if they have the expertise and competence to do so.

Supplementary prescribers may prescribe in accordance with a clinical management plan in a tripartite arrangement with a doctor or dentist, the patient and the supplementary prescriber.

Prescribing by Nurses, Midwives and Specialist Community Public Health Nurses

The Medicinal Products: Prescription by Nurses Act 1992 and subsequent amendments to the pharmaceutical services regulations allow nurses and midwives, who have recorded their qualification on the NMC register, to become nurse or midwife prescribers. There are two levels of nurse and midwife prescribers.

1. Community Practitioner Nurse Prescribers

   These are registrants who have successfully undertaken a programme of preparation to prescribe from the Nurse Prescribers' Formulary for Community Practitioners. They can prescribe the majority of dressings and appliances and a limited range of Prescription Only Medicines. The Nurse Prescribers' Formulary for Community Practitioners can be found on the British National Formulary website (https://bnf.nice.org.uk).

2. Nurse and Midwife Independent/Supplementary Prescribers

   These are nurses and midwives who are trained to make a diagnosis and prescribe the appropriate treatment (independent prescribing). They may also, in cases where a doctor has made an initial diagnosis, go on to prescribe or review the medication and change the drug, dosage, timing, frequency or route of administration of any mediation as appropriate as part of a clinical management plan (supplementary prescribing).

Nurse or Midwife Independent Prescribers can prescribe Prescription Only Medicines including controlled drugs (except diamorphine, cocaine and dipipanone for the treatment of addiction) and all medication that can be supplied by a pharmacist or purchased over the counter. They must only prescribe drugs that are within their area of expertise and level of competence and should only prescribe for children if they have the expertise and competence to do so.

Nurse, midwife and specialist community public health nurse prescribers must comply with current prescribing legislation and are accountable for their practice.

Prescribing by Other Therapists

Other therapists are now governed by the Health and Care Professions Council. The sixteen health professions include: arts therapists, biomedical scientists, chiropodists/podiatrists, clinical scientists, dietitians, hearing aid dispensers, occupational therapists, operating department practitioners, orthoptists, paramedics, physiotherapists, practitioner psychologists, prosthetists/orthotists, radiographers, social workers in England and speech and language therapists. The Health and Care Professions Council have their own guidance related to medicines and prescribing which permits named professional groups on their register to administer or supply medicines under a patient group direction. However, organizations will have local arrangements and clinical governance structure in place to support the process. Further information can be found on the Health and Care Professions Council website (http://www.hcpc-uk.co.uk/).

Patient Group Directions (PGDs)

A Patient Group Direction (PGD) is a written instruction for the sale, supply and/or administration of medicines to groups of patients who may not be individually identified before presentation for treatment. Guidance on the use of PGDs is contained within NICE Guideline MPG2, 2017.

Patient group directions are drawn up locally by senior doctors or, if appropriate, by dentists, pharmacists and other health professionals. They must be signed by a doctor or dentist and a senior pharmacist, both of whom should have been involved in developing the direction, and must be approved by the appropriate health care organization. The NMC considers it good practice that a lead practitioner from the professional group using the PGD and senior manager, where possible, are also involved and sign off a PGD.

Dispensing

If, under exceptional circumstances, you are required to dispense, there is no legal barrier to this practice. However, this must be in the course of the business of a hospital and in accordance with a doctor's written instructions and in accordance with a registered prescriber's written instructions and covered by a standard operating procedure (SOP). In a dispensing doctor's practice, nurses may supply to patients under a particular doctor's care, when acting under the directions of a doctor from that practice.

Dispensing includes such activities as checking the validity of the prescription, the appropriateness of the medicine for an individual patient, assembly of the product, labelling in accordance with legal requirements, advising in its safe and effective use and providing information leaflets for the patient.

If you, as a registrant, are engaged in dispensing, this represents an extension to your professional practice. The patient has the legal right to expect that the dispensing will be carried out with the same reasonable skill and care that would be expected from a pharmacist.

Information on New and Developing Pharmacy Services and Extended Roles of Pharmacists
Medicines Use Review (MUR)
The MUR service is a free NHS service offered by pharmacies. The Medicines Use Review (MUR) consists of accredited pharmacists undertaking structured adherence-centred reviews with patients on multiple medicines, particularly those receiving medicines for long-term conditions.

New Medicines Service (NMS)
New Medicines Service provides support for people with long-term conditions newly prescribed a medicine to help improve medicines adherence; it is initially focused on particular patient groups and conditions.

Flu Vaccination Service
The service allows community pharmacist in England to provide seasonal influenza (flu) vaccination service for patients in at-risk groups.

Repeat Dispensing Schemes
Under the repeat dispensing service pharmacy teams will: dispense repeat dispensing prescriptions issued by a GP; ensure that each repeat supply is required; and seek to ascertain that there is no reason why the patient should be referred back to their GP

The Supply of Emergency Hormonal Contraception as a Pharmacy Medicine
Pharmacists will supply levonorgestrel emergency hormonal contraception (EHC) when appropriate to clients in line with the requirements of a locally agreed PGD. The PGD will specify the age range of clients that are eligible for the service; it may facilitate supply to young persons under 16 in appropriate circumstances.

Health Care Information and Advice

Pharmacists are encouraged to contribute to the promotion of healthy lifestyles such as advice on alcohol consumption, stop smoking service and weight management service.

By increasing public awareness of health promotion issues and participating in disease prevention strategies pharmacists can work actively towards improving the nation's health.

Diagnostic Testing and Health Screening

Pharmacists working in primary care are well placed to provide diagnostic testing and health screening services to the public. Services include NHS health checks for blood pressure, cholesterol or blood glucose testing, chlamydia screening and pregnancy testing.

Services to Care Homes

Care home residents should receive the right medicines at the right time and in the right way to maximize the benefits of the medication. Pharmacists have the expertise to help achieve this and as part of a multidisciplinary team can be responsible for a whole system of medicines and their use within a care home (RPSGB, 2014).

Needle and Syringe Exchange Schemes

Needle and syringe exchange schemes involve the provision of clean syringes and needles and the collection of contaminated equipment used by substance and drug misusers.

References/Bibliography

British National Formulary 74, 2017–18. Pharmaceutical Press, Basingstoke 2017.
Directive 2001/83/EC of the European Parliament and of the Council of 6 November 2001 on the community code relating to medicinal products for human use. Official journal L–311, 28/11/2004, p. 67–128.
Great Britain, 1972. Medicines Act 1968 (as Amended). HMSO, London.
Great Britain, 1984. Misuse of Drugs Act 1971 (as Amended). HMSO, London.
Great Britain, 2001. Misuse of Drugs Regulations 2001 SI No 3938. HMSO, London.
Medicines & Healthcare product Regulatory Agency (MHRA) 2016: A guide to what is a medicinal product.
National Institute for Health and Clinical Excellence 2014. Needle and syringe programmes public health guideline [PH52].
National Institute for Health and Clinical Excellence (NICE) 2015: Medicines optimisation: the safe and effective use of medicines to enable the best possible outcomes.

National Institute for Health and Clinical Excellence 2016. Controlled drugs: safe use and management NICE guideline [NG46].

National Institute for Health and Clinical Excellence 2017. Patient Group Directions. Medicine practice guideline MPG2. First published 2013 updated on 2017.

Nursing and Midwifery Council, 2006. Standards of Proficiency for Nurse and Midwife Prescribers. NMC, London.

Nursing and Midwifery Council, 2007. Standards for Medicines Management. NMC, London.

Nursing and Midwifery Council, 2015. The Code: Professional Standards of Practice and Behaviour for Nurses and Midwives. NMC, London.

Royal Pharmaceutical Society of Great Britain (RPSGB) 2014: Pharmacist improving care in care homes.

Royal Pharmaceutical Society of Great Britain (RPSGB) 2017: Medicines, Ethics and Practice: The professional guide pharmacists. Edition 41.

Further Information

Adverse reactions to drugs and yellow card scheme: https://yellowcard.mhra.gov.uk/.

British National Formulary: https://bnf.nice.org.uk/.

Department of Health. For information on independent and supplementary prescribing: https://www.gov.uk/government/organisations/department-of-health-and-social-care.

Drug safety update: httpsc://www.gov.uk/drug-safety-update.

Health and Care Professions Council (HCPC): http://www.hcpc-uk.co.uk/.

Medicines and prescribing alerts: https://www.nice.org.uk/news/nice-newsletters-and-alerts/subscribe-to-medicine-and-prescribing-alerts.

Medicines Information/evidence service provided by: https://www.evidence.nhs.uk/.

NHS Choices: https://www.nhs.uk.

National Institute for Health and Clinical Excellence: https://www.nice.org.uk/guidance.

Nursing and Midwifery Council (NMC): https://www.nmc.org.uk/.

Royal Pharmaceutical Society: https://www.rpharms.com/.

Websites accessed 2 March 2018.

Appendix 5

The Legal and Professional Framework of Nursing
JONATHAN GREEN

Accountability

Health care is regulated in a number of ways. The most important of these for nurses are:

- Professional regulation.
- Acts of Parliament.
- Civil law.
- Contracts of employment.
- Ethical standards.

The Nursing and Midwifery Council (NMC) exists to safeguard the health and wellbeing of the public. As the regulatory body for nurses, this is done by maintaining a register of nurses, midwives and nursing associates, setting standards for education and practice and giving guidance and advice to the profession.

The NMC sets the minimum standard of accountability through The Code: Professional standards of practice and behaviour for nurses, midwives and nursing associates. The latest version of The Code was published in December 2018 (and can be found at www.nmc-uk.org and in Appendix 6) to incorporate new responsibilities for the regulation of nursing associates. The Code is regularly reviewed and interprets the boundaries set by Acts of Parliament which set the limits on nursing and midwifery practice and contains the professional standards that registered nurses, midwives and nursing associates must uphold. Those who are registered by the NMC may be the subject of fitness to practice investigations if their conduct falls far below the standards set out in The Code. This may result in restrictions being placed against their ability to practice or their suspension or removal from the register.

Where there is no Act of Parliament, the courts will interpret the law in the civil courts. Examples include the Courts intervening in cases dealing with the right of a patient's family to refuse life-saving treatment, where there are problems regarding patients who appear to lack capacity to make judgements for themselves or cases where no agreement can be reached on what treatment is in a patient's best interests.

The Code will continue to be reviewed periodically by the NMC to ensure that it will reflect the law as well as public and nursing policy.

Contracts of employment set out the rights, responsibilities and expectations of the nurse in the context of his/her employment and may also require that protocols are followed by nursing staff. This is a fourth area of accountability, while a fifth area relates to the ethical scope and practice of nursing, from a professional and a personal perspective.

Law: Criminal Law

The civil and criminal laws of the land bind nurses as citizens and professionals. Criminal law is generally contained in statutes (Acts of Parliament). The violation of criminal law may arise either by an individual performing a prohibited act (e.g., an assault or theft) or omitting to perform a required act (e.g., neglect). A crime is a 'wrong' punishable by the State. Successful prosecution by the Crown will result in a variety of penalties, from monetary fines to imprisonment.

Table 5.1 lists the statutes which relate directly to the clinical and health care environment. They describe clearly what types of behaviour Parliament considers to be unacceptable and unlawful, in response to the perceived demands of society in general.

Table 5.1 Health law statutes	
Statute	**Year**
Offences against the Person Act	1861
Perjury Act	1911
Infant Life (Preservation) Act	1929
Children and Young Persons Act	1933
National Assistance Act	1948
Sexual Offences Act	1956
Suicide Act	1961
Abortion Act	1967

Table 5.1 Health law statutes—cont'd	
Statute	**Year**
Medicines Act	1968
Family Law Reform Act	1969
Misuse of Drugs Act	1971
Congenital Disabilities (Civil Liability) Act	1976
National Health Service Act	1977
Unfair Contract Terms Act	1977
Vaccine Damage Payments Act	1979
Mental Health Act	1983
Medical Act	1983
Public Health (Control of Disease) Act	1984
Data Protection Act[a]	1984
Surrogacy Arrangements Act	1985
Family Law Reform Act	1987
Children Act	1989
NHS and Community Care Act	1990
Human Fertilisation and Embryology Act	1990
Medicinal Products: Prescription by Nurses Act	1992
Data Protection Act	1998
Health Act	1999
Care Standards Act	2000
Health and Social Care Act	2001
National Health Service Reform and Health Care Professions Act	2002
Health and Social Care (Community Health and Standards) Act	2003
The Female Genital Mutilation Act	2003
Human Fertilisation and Embryology (Deceased Fathers) Act	2003
Human Tissue Act	2004
Female Genital Mutilation (Scotland) Act	2005
Mental Capacity Act	2005
Health Act	2006
Human Tissue (Scotland) Act	2006
National Health Service Act	2006
National Health Service (Wales) Act	2006
NHS Redress Act	2006
Mental Health Act	2007
Health and Safety (Offences) Act	2008
Human Fertilisation and Embryology Act	2008
Health Act	2009
Equality Act	2010
Health and Social Care Act	2012
Protection of Freedoms Act	2012
Mental Health (Discrimination) Act	2013
General Data Protection Regulation	2016

[a]Repealed but with savings by the Data Protection Act 1998.
Source: Kennedy & Grubb (1994), updated and Halsbury's Statutes

Civil Law: Professional Negligence

'Negligence' is a tort (or civil wrong), created by the courts, the definition of which has evolved over the years. In contrast to the criminal law, the law of tort regulates the behaviour (in terms of rights and duties) of one individual towards another.

Negligence is centred on the concept of a 'duty of care' or 'responsibility', owed by one individual/organization, to another and the subsequent harm that can be caused to an individual if this duty or responsibility is broken. To establish liability in negligence, three key elements must be present, as follows:

- Did a duty of care exist between the affected parties?
- Was that duty breached by one party to that duty?
- Was the subsequent harm specifically caused by the breach?

A critical part of the test for negligence is to show that harm was caused directly by the negligent (or careless) act or omission of the nurse or health care provider, although it does not have to be the sole or main cause.

If all the elements described above are present, the victim or claimant will be financially compensated. The amount awarded is decided by the Civil Courts (usually the County or High Courts) unless the parties to a claim can reach agreement between themselves.

When a court is making an assessment as to whether a patient has been the subject of negligent treatment, a judge will make an assessment by comparison with two standards:

- The nurse must deliver the standard of care expected from a reasonable competent nurse exercising that professional skill.
- The nurse must act in accordance with practice accepted by a relevant body of responsible and skilled nursing opinion

The legal tests are set out in the Court's decision in Bolam v Friern Hospital Management Committee (1957) and further clarified by the comments of Lord Scarman in Sidaway v Governors of Bethlem Royal Hospital (1985).

If the practitioner has departed from either standard, then negligence can be inferred.

It is essential to recognise here the importance of adherence to The Code and all local policies relating to the clinical environment because both will offer legal protection. The patient will not generally be able to prove professional negligence where the nurse or midwife has followed commonly accepted and up-to-date nursing practice. However, the Courts have also established that a medical professional could be liable for negligence in respect of diagnosis and treatment despite a body of professional opinion sanctioning his conduct where it had not been demonstrated to the judge's satisfaction that the body of opinion relied on was reasonable or responsible. In the vast majority of cases the fact that distinguished experts in the field were of a particular opinion would demonstrate the reasonableness of that opinion. However, in a rare case, if it could be demonstrated that the professional opinion was not capable of withstanding logical analysis, the judge would be entitled to hold that the body of opinion was not reasonable or responsible. See Bolitho (Administratrix of the Estate of Patrick Nigel Bolitho (deceased)) v City and Hackney Health Authority (1997).

Legal Issues Affecting Clinical Practice

An objective of this appendix is to present a concise guide to legal controls on commonly encountered nursing procedures and situations. In doing so, it is essential to bear in mind, firstly, any relevant statutes (see Table 5.1) and, secondly, The Code: Professional standards of practice and behaviour for nurses, midwives and nursing associates (see Appendix 6). Where there is no specific statute to cover a particular area, compliance with professional regulations and protocols from the employer may contribute to a successful defence in the face of any legal claims under civil law, specifically negligence.

Consent

At the heart of the law on consent lies the fundamental principle that every person has a right to control what happens to his or her body. Consent issues generally arise in relation to patients giving consent for physical procedures.

This subject is covered by both criminal law (e.g., Offences against the Person Act 1861) and the judgements of the courts in civil cases (usually in cases involving the civil torts of battery and negligence).

The basic rule is possibly best summed up in the case of Malette v Shulman (1990) where a judge directed 'any intentional non-consensual touching which is harmful or offensive to a person's reasonable sense of dignity, is actionable'. Clearly securing consent makes that interference lawful. To proceed without consent makes the nurse liable for assault (an attempt to apply force to another, such as to put him or her in fear of physical force). The physical force does not have to be substantial and damage does not have to be caused, but intent to carry out the non-consensual contact must be present.

As the major legal defence against assault and battery is consent, the verbal or written agreement of the patient must be sought before any physical treatment can be given. However, the presence of a signed consent form alone is not sufficient. It is a legal requirement that an effective consent must satisfy the following criteria to ensure that it is a true consent (Montgomery, 2003):

- The procedure for which consent is sought must have been explained adequately to the patient. It may be negligent to withhold important information. What must be disclosed is an issue of clinical judgement, but must be sufficient to enable a patient to weigh up the risks and advantages of undergoing the procedure and appreciate any alternative treatments. In the 2015 case of Montgomery v Lanarkshire Health Board, the Supreme Court decided that there was not only a duty to advise of a risk when a patient asked about it but also that the health professional was under a duty to inform the patient of a substantial risk of adverse consequence, even if unasked. The Court stated:

The doctor is therefore under a duty to take reasonable care to ensure that the patient is aware of any material risks involved in any recommended treatment, and of any reasonable alternative or variant treatments. The test of materiality is whether, in the circumstances of the particular case, a reasonable person in the patient's position would be likely to attach significance to the risk, or the doctor is or should reasonably be aware that the particular patient would be likely to attach significance to it.

The assessment of whether a risk is 'material' is therefore fact-sensitive and sensitive also to the characteristics of the patient. Relevant factors here may include the nature of the risk, the effect which its occurrence would have upon the life of the patient, the importance to the patient of the benefits sought to be achieved by the treatment, the alternatives available, and the risks involved in those alternatives.

Essentially, the legal position in relation to consent can be summarized as follows:

- The patient must be able to understand the choices he or she is required to make.
- Consent must then be given freely and voluntarily.
- Consent must not be obtained by duress or deceit.

The Department of Health set out a patient's rights in relation to consent in its Health Circular HC (90)22 A Guide to Consent for Examination or Treatment. The Department has included within its guidance specimen Consent Forms, the use of which are regarded as good practice. A further useful summary is set out in the Reference guide to consent for examination or treatment (second edition), which sets out a comprehensive the legal framework that health professionals need to take account of in obtaining valid consent to examination, treatment or care .

To take account of the nature of medical and nursing practice, three exceptions to the principles above relating to obtaining consent are recognized but practitioners should still proceed with caution.

Firstly, as outlined previously, an informal explanation and verbal agreement between patient and nurse are often sufficient to allow routine clinical care and treatment to be performed, e.g., when obtaining bloods or carrying out routine observations.

Secondly, the principle of 'necessity' will justify treatment of a patient where consent cannot be given, primarily in an emergency situation, perhaps where the patient is unconscious. As such, this exception permits life-saving treatment without a patient's consent (see Re F 1991 (1990)) but should be applied in extreme situations only. The treatment would have to satisfy the 'Bolam' test, being acceptable to a responsible and relevant body of professional opinion and must go no further than is required to safeguard life. Further, the treatment will be unlawful if the patient has clearly communicated his or her objection to such treatment, before becoming 'incompetent'.

Thirdly, and similarly to the above, an 'implied consent' can be relied upon if there is sufficient certainty that the patient would have requested or acceded to the treatment had it been offered in more controlled circumstances. Again, this applies to emergency events where either an initiation of a new treatment or an extension of an existing one is needed. In such events, it is ethically correct to consider that the treatment should be of obvious benefit to the patient, that it would be unreasonable to withhold it, and that no express objection has previously been given.

Children who have reached the age of 16 years are able to consent to treatment in their own right. Children under 16 years of age can still legally give their own consent if they have sufficient intelligence and understanding of what is involved, and the consent is valid. The Guide to Consent for Examination or Treatment referred to above specifies that full notes should be kept of all interactions with the child, attempts made to persuade the child to involve their parents and if there is any doubt that the child does not have sufficient understanding, parental consent should be obtained (save in emergency situations).

Relatives and close friends are frequently involved in care and consultation about patients, although they cannot (save in accordance with the provisions of the Mental Capacity Act 2005) legally give consent on behalf of the patient. This is governed by the legal rule that one adult does not have the authority to give consent for another adult.

Confidentiality

In the course of their duties, nurses handle confidential information about patients. The control of such sensitive details is regulated by statute, specifically the Data Protection Act 1998, and also by The Code.

The Code expressly states that 'you owe a duty of confidentiality to all those who are receiving care. This includes making sure that they are informed about their care and that information about them is shared appropriately.' A nurse should only share information with patients, their families and their carers as far as the law allows, sensitively and in a way they can understand.

Written information can be accessed by an individual to whom the information refers; however, access to it can be restricted if certain exclusions specified in the Act apply. Information entered and stored on a computer is controlled by the Act (not just computer data but also written information).

Nurses are required to prioritise the protection of all confidential information and only disclose it under specific conditions.

Box 5.1 lists the principles concerning the collection and storage of confidential patient data. From May 2018 data protection laws were updated and amended as the

---

BOX 5.1 Principles of holding personal data (Data Protection Act 1998)

1. Data are obtained fairly and lawfully
2. Data are held for one or more lawful purpose only (specified in the Data User's register entry—a legal requirement)
3. Data are used or disclosed only in accordance with the Data User's register entry
4. Data are adequate, relevant and not excessive for the purpose
5. Data are accurate and up to date
6. Data are not kept longer than necessary for a specific purpose
7. Data are made available to data subjects upon request
8. Data are properly protected against loss or disclosure

General Data Protection Regulation and a new Data Protection Act will apply. Both will slightly amend the law although the existing concepts and the principles in the Data Protection Act 1998 remain. However, many things that were considered good practice become a legal requirement. In particular, the new legislation:

- sets a higher standard around obtaining and evidencing informed consent;
- gives greater rights to individuals in relation to data held about them;
- places a greater emphasis on organizations recording and evidencing their compliance with data protection law and designing privacy protection into new or existing business processes.

Breach of confidentiality can lead to three penalties. Firstly, failing to secure confidential information could lead to prosecution under the Data Protection Act 1998.

Secondly, the Nursing and Midwifery Council (NMC) has power to consider whether a charge of professional misconduct applies for breaches of confidentiality or data protection, risking a practitioner's removal from the NMC register. The NMC Code expressly states that a nurse must respect people's right to confidentiality, ensure that people are informed about how and why information is shared by those who will be providing their care and finally, it authorizes disclosure of information if a nurse believes someone may be at risk of harm. The Code makes it clear that a patient's right to confidentiality continues after they have died.

Thirdly, a breach of confidentiality may constitute a breach of contract, leading to disciplinary action and possible dismissal for gross misconduct.

Four clear exceptions to maintaining confidentiality are recognized, as follows:

1. Where the patient consents to disclosure.
2. Where the information is required to continue a patient's care.
3. Where the law (Act of Parliament) requires disclosure, e.g., accidents, firearm incidents, drug-related activities, reporting of notifiable diseases.
4. Where the public interest in disclosure is deemed of greater importance than the public interest in maintaining confidentiality, i.e., where there is a patient safety or public protection reason for doing so e.g., to prevent child abuse.

Nurses should abide strictly by the rules of confidentiality unless one of these exceptions clearly applies. The reason for disclosure should be well documented in a patient's records.

Drug Administration

The responsibility of the nurse for storage and administration of medicines is discussed in Appendix 4.

Safety

Nurses have a comprehensive responsibility for the safety of patients in their care under the NMC Code. Nurses must 'put the interests of people using or needing nursing or midwifery services first' and 'make their care and safety your main concern'. This duty is shared clinically with doctors and with employers; The Code is clear that nurses are expected to 'work with colleagues to preserve the safety of those receiving care.'

Nurses are also legally bound by the civil 'duty of care' principle set out above, which defines in law the responsibility that nurses have to their patients. As stated above, breach of that duty may entitle the injured patient to make a claim for negligence.

Nurses are also subject to the professional duty of candour and the need to be open and honest when things go wrong. In these circumstances the NMC Code requires a nurse to:

- explain fully and promptly what has happened, including the likely effects, and apologise to the person affected and, where appropriate, their advocate, family or carers, and;
- document all these events formally and take further action/escalate if appropriate so they can be dealt with quickly.

Further details on the application of the duty of candour (including case studies) can be found in the NMC's joint statement with the General Medical Council 'Openness and honesty when things go wrong: the professional duty of candour' which was published in 2016.

In the general ward environment, safety is maintained by attention to three main areas. Firstly, by formal identification of the patient and the implementation of a system ensuring correct identification throughout the patient's treatment on the ward, which usually includes the use of non-removable identity bands for patients. The personal details recorded on the bands should be consistent with all documents.

Secondly, the careful compilation of admission, inpatient and discharge charts and care planning documents should ensure that patient safety is not compromised.

Thirdly, the full and conscientious dissemination of information between the patient and all members of the medical multidisciplinary team is essential. This also allows the patient to have an understanding of the plan of care. The NMC Code records specifically that a nurse should:

- maintain effective communication with colleagues
- keep colleagues informed when they are sharing the care of individuals with other healthcare professionals and staff
- work with colleagues to evaluate the quality of their work and that of the team
- work with colleagues to preserve the safety of those receiving care.

The strict application of these safety principles will be enhanced in certain acute and specialist environments. In these areas, identification of the patient and the passing on of accurate and detailed information is critical. Nurses working in extended roles will be accountable for all of their actions in this respect. Nurses should also be aware of their own practical limitations, as encouraged in The Code (The Code expressly states that a nurse must 'work within the limits of [their] competence, exercising [their] professional "duty of candour" and raising concerns immediately whenever [they] come across situations that put patients or public safety at risk'. A nurse should not assume roles or undertake tasks that compromise their clinical ability and the patient's safety.

The responsibility for safety within the physical environment of care and the facilities is allocated to health care management and the health care provider although, under Health and Safety Regulations, all employees must act responsibly in relation to their own health and safety, and that of others (see Section 7, Health and Safety at Work Act 1974).

A nurse must:

- Take care of their own health and safety and that of people who may be affected by what they do (or do not do).
- Cooperate with others on health and safety, and not interfere with or misuse anything provided for your health, safety or welfare.

Within the ward, the relevant management team has specific responsibility for providing adequate basic safety measures, e.g., fire precautions or the control of hazardous substances.

Nurses are instructed in The Code to evaluate the safety of the environment and to take action if this is jeopardised. The Code states that a nurse must raise and, if necessary, escalate any concerns they may have about patient or public safety, or the level of care people are receiving in the workplace or any other healthcare setting in line with NMC guidance and local working practices. These concerns should be recorded in writing if possible. Nursing staff are also required to be professionally aware of other factors affecting safety, particularly quality of care and availability of resources. This applies, for example, to potentially unsafe staffing levels, inappropriate skill mix of staff, or a combination of demanding patients and clinical conditions.

An employee who is in breach of his or her duties under the Health and Safety at Work Act 1974 may be liable to pay a fine on conviction. He or she may also be dismissed from their employment for being in breach of a contractual duty within their employment contract to carry out work with proper care and skill.

Further information on the essential Health and Safety law for nurses as employees or employers can be found at www.hse.gov.uk (accessed 01/01/2018).

Documentation

The range of documentation requiring nursing attention is often voluminous, wide-ranging and detailed. Occasionally, some of it is not directly related to nursing activities. As a result some documents will have a legal significance while others will not. The purpose of documentation is fourfold, as follows:

1. Legal or non-legal record-keeping.
2. Ease of administration.
3. Maintaining standards.
4. Ensuring continuity and safety.

Legal record-keeping is relevant to the nursing environment in several areas, e.g., administration of medicines, recording usage of controlled drugs, and contracts of employment between nurses and employing authorities. Nursing records can ultimately become legal documents, their main function being to evidence the care planned, treatment received and outcomes of a patient's stay. As a comprehensive record of the patient's visit, they form an important defence against allegations of misconduct or negligence. The time within which potential legal actions can be initiated (until a child reaches 21 years or 3 years from the date a victim became aware that he or she had been the victim of potentially negligent treatment) makes the necessity for accurate documentation clear and obvious.

A strong defence of a practitioner's action is much more likely from the basis of clear, precise documentation written at the time of the incident or treatment. The NMC Code requires that a practitioner must complete records at the time or as soon as possible after an event has occurred and it also states that any records must:

- identify any risks or problems that have arisen and the steps taken to deal with them so that colleagues who use the records have all the information they need;
- be completed accurately and without any falsification. A nurse must take immediate and appropriate action if they become aware that someone has not kept to these requirements;
- be clearly written, dated and timed, and should not include unnecessary abbreviations, jargon or speculation;
- be kept securely.

Of equivalent importance to patient records are documents affecting staff, visitors and members of the public that could subsequently acquire a legal significance, e.g., accident reporting forms. Employers are legally required to report accidents, injuries and dangerous incidents to the Health and Safety Executive, and are required to act under the Reporting of Injuries, Diseases and Dangerous Occurrences Regulations 1985 and the Occupiers Liability Act 1957 and 1984.

Decisions Made by Patients

A potentially problematic area for health care providers arises where a patient chooses to make a decision contrary to the professional advice they have received. Having received a full description of proposed treatment, a patient may still exercise their right to refuse to undertake the recommended course of action. The individual patient has an absolute and inviolable right under civil law to decline treatment. Doctors and nurses must ensure that these decisions are recorded (along with details of the action taken or the discussions leading to the patient's decision). The NMC Code declares that all nurses must 'respect, support and document a person's right to accept or refuse care and treatment' but a nurse must be able to demonstrate that they have acted in someone's best interests if they have provided care in an emergency. Only this will prevent a practitioner from leaving themselves wide open to a possible negligence action if there is an adverse outcome as a result of a patient declining treatment.

Secondly, patients may choose to discharge themselves from medical care against the advice from doctors and nurses. Patients cannot be legally detained (unless subject to various sections of the Mental Health Act 1983) and are free to leave at their will. A 'discharge against medical advice' form is valuable as a record of a discussion with a patient and as a place to note that the unplanned and unadvised discharge is the patient's choice. The form should be witnessed by the clinical staff involved, although the patient cannot be legally compelled to sign it.

Patients' Property

Handling of a patient's property requires careful attention from nurses at all stages during a patient's hospitalization—from admission, while an inpatient, during any transfers between clinical areas, and on discharge.

The actions taken to safeguard property are to protect the patient from losing potentially valuable personal property in terms of sentimental as well as financial value. Failure to adequately protect a patient's property during an admission may also lead to a practitioner facing an allegation of theft.

If conscious and capable, the patient will automatically retain control of any property although some facilities for the safekeeping of valuables may be offered by a health care provider. In many cases the patient will be required to sign a disclaimer form, which will absolve the hospital during the patient's stay. If any items are retained for security by the hospital a patient will receive a signed receipt.

If the patient is unable to take responsibility for personal property while unconscious, confused or mentally incapacitated, the nurse will be required to take charge of it. The nurse's legal responsibility in this position assumes that of an 'involuntary bailee' (i.e., technically a person to whom goods are entrusted with no intention of transferring ownership). This demands that the nurse takes care of the property and exercises the same degree of care as the patient would have done had he or she been able.

The well-established procedure of written documentation, double-checking and witnessing with another member of staff, as well as signing in duplicate for property received, is vital to ensure protection against accusations of theft by a patient. Accurate and careful description of all property held is prudent. On discharge all property must be returned to the patient (and on death to authorized receivers). In both cases, this must be in exchange for a signed receipt.

The penalties for inadequate or careless control of a patient's property are individual prosecutions for theft of activation of the health authority's liability for negligence. A nurse may also potentially face dismissal by their employer and be reported to the NMC for professional misconduct.

References

Data Protection Act 1998. Available at: http://www.legislation.gov.uk/ukpga/1998/29/contents (Accessed 01 January 2018).

General Data Protection Regulation 2016. Available at: http://ec.europa.eu/justice/data-protection/reform/files/regulation_oj_en.pdf.

Kennedy, I., Grubb, A., 1994. Medical Law. Butterworth, London.

Montgomery, J., 2003. Health Care Law. Oxford University Press, Oxford.

Re F v West Berkshire HA, 1991. UKHL 1 (17 July 1990).

Further Reading

Brazier, M., 1992. Medicine, Patients and the Law. Penguin, London.

Dyer, C. (Ed.), 1992. Doctors, Patients and the Law. Blackwell, Oxford.

McCall Smith, A., Mason, J.K., 1994. Law and Medical Ethics. Butterworth, London.

Rumbold, G., 1999. Ethics in Nursing Practice, thirrd ed. Baillière Tindall, London.

Tingle, J., Cribb, A. (Eds.), 2002. Nursing Law and Ethics. Blackwell Scientific, Oxford.

Tschudin, V., 1991. Ethics in Nursing. Heinemann, London.

6 Appendix

Professional Standards of Practice and Behaviour for Nurses, Midwives and Nursing Associates

Section 1
Nursing and Midwifery Council (NMC) The Code: Professional Standards of Practice and Behaviour

The Code contains the professional standards that registered nurses, midwives and nursing associates must uphold. Nurses, midwives and nursing associates must act in line with the Code, whether they are providing direct care to individuals, groups or communities or bringing their professional knowledge to bear on nursing and midwifery practice in other roles, such as leadership, education or research. The values and principles set out in the Code can be applied in a range of different practice settings, but they are not negotiable or discretionary.

Our role is to set the standards in the Code, but these are not just our standards. They are the standards that patients and members of the public tell us they expect from health professionals. They are the standards shown every day by those on our register.

When joining our register, and then renewing their registration, nurses, midwives and nursing associates commit to upholding these standards. This commitment to professional standards is fundamental to being part of a profession. We can take action if those on our register fail to uphold the Code. In serious cases, this can include removing them from the register.

The Code sets out common standards of conduct and behaviour for those on our register. This provides a clear, consistent and positive message to patients, service users and colleagues about what they can expect of those who provide nursing and midwifery care.

The professions we regulate have different knowledge and skills, set out in three distinct standards of proficiency. They can work in diverse contexts and have different levels of autonomy and responsibility. However, all of the professions we regulate exercise professional judgement and are accountable for their work.

Nurses, midwives and nursing associates uphold the Code within the limits of their competence. This means, for example, that while a nurse and nursing associate will play different roles in an aspect of care, they will both uphold the standards in the Code within the contribution they make to overall care. The professional commitment to work within one's competence is a key underpinning principle of the Code which, given the significance of its impact on public protection, should be upheld at all times.

In addition, nurses, midwives and nursing associates are expected to work within the limits of their competence, which may extend beyond the standards they demonstrated in order to join the register.

The Code should be useful for everyone who cares about good nursing and midwifery:

- Patients and service users, and those who care for them, can use it to provide feedback to nurses, midwives and nursing associates about the care they receive.
- Those on the register can use it to promote safe and effective practice in their place of work.
- Employer organizations should support their staff in upholding the standards in their professional Code as part of providing the quality and safety expected by service users and regulators.
- Educators can use the Code to help students understand what it means to be a registered professional and how keeping to the Code helps to achieve that.

For the many committed and expert practitioners on our register, this Code should be seen as a way of reinforcing professionalism. Through revalidation, nurses, midwives and nursing associates provide evidence of their continued ability to practise safely and effectively. The Code is central in the revalidation process as a focus for professional reflection. This gives the Code significance in the professional life of those on the register, and raises its status and importance for employers.

The Code contains a series of statements that taken together signify what good practice by nurses, midwives and nursing associates looks like. It puts the interests of patients and service users first, is safe and effective, and promotes trust through professionalism.

Prioritize People

You put the interests of people using or needing nursing or midwifery services first. You make their care and safety your main concern and make sure that their dignity is preserved and their needs are recognised, assessed and responded to. You make sure that those receiving care are treated with respect, that their rights are upheld and that any discriminatory attitudes and behaviours towards those receiving care are challenged.

1. **Treat people as individuals and uphold their dignity**

   To achieve this, you must:

   1.1. treat people with kindness, respect and compassion

   1.2. make sure you deliver the fundamentals of care effectively

   1.3. avoid making assumptions and recognise diversity and individual choice

   1.4. make sure that any treatment, assistance or care for which you are responsible is delivered without undue delay

   1.5. respect and uphold people's human rights.

2. **Listen to people and respond to their preferences and concerns**

   To achieve this, you must:

   2.1. work in partnership with people to make sure you deliver care effectively

   2.2. recognise and respect the contribution that people can make to their own health and wellbeing

   2.3. encourage and empower people to share decisions about their treatment and care

   2.4. respect the level to which people receiving care want to be involved in decisions about their own health, wellbeing and care

   2.5. respect, support and document a person's right to accept or refuse care and treatment

   2.6. recognise when people are anxious or in distress and respond compassionately and politely.

3. **Make sure that people's physical, social and psychological needs are assessed and responded to**

   To achieve this, you must:

   3.1. pay special attention to promoting wellbeing, preventing ill health and meeting the changing health and care needs of people during all life stages

   3.2. recognise and respond compassionately to the needs of those who are in the last few days and hours of life

   3.3. act in partnership with those receiving care, helping them to access relevant health and social care, information and support when they need it

   3.4. act as an advocate for the vulnerable, challenging poor practice and discriminatory attitudes and behaviour relating to their care.

4. **Act in the best interests of people at all times**

   To achieve this, you must:

   4.1. balance the need to act in the best interests of people at all times with the requirement to respect a person's right to accept or refuse treatment

4.2. make sure that you get properly informed consent and document it before carrying out any action

4.3. keep to all relevant laws about mental capacity that apply in the country in which you are practising, and make sure that the rights and best interests of those who lack capacity are still at the centre of the decision-making process

4.4. tell colleagues, your manager and the person receiving care if you have a conscientious objection to a particular procedure and arrange for a suitably qualified colleague to take over responsibility for that person's care.

5. **Respect people's right to privacy and confidentiality**

As a nurse, midwife or nursing associate, you owe a duty of confidentiality to all those who are receiving care. This includes making sure that they are informed about their care and that information about them is shared appropriately.

To achieve this, you must:

5.1. respect a person's right to privacy in all aspects of their care

5.2. make sure that people are informed about how and why information is used and shared by those who will be providing care

5.3. respect that a person's right to privacy and confidentiality continues after they have died

5.4. share necessary information with other health and care professionals and agencies only when the interests of patient safety and public protection override the need for confidentiality

5.5. share with people, their families and their carers, as far as the law allows, the information they want or need to know about their health, care and ongoing treatment sensitively and in a way they can understand.

Practise effectively

You assess need and deliver or advise on treatment, or give help (including preventative or rehabilitative care) without too much delay, to the best of your abilities, on the basis of the best available evidence. You communicate effectively, keeping clear and accurate records and sharing skills, knowledge and experience where appropriate. You reflect and act on any feedback you receive to improve your practice.

6. **Always practise in line with the best available evidence**

To achieve this, you must:

6.1. make sure that any information or advice given is evidence based, including information relating to using any health and care products or services

6.2. maintain the knowledge and skills you need for safe and effective practice.

7. **Communicate clearly**

To achieve this, you must:

7.1. use terms that people in your care, colleagues and the public can understand

7.2. take reasonable steps to meet people's language and communication needs, providing, wherever possible, assistance to those who need help to communicate their own or other people's needs

7.3. use a range of verbal and non-verbal communication methods, and consider cultural sensitivities, to better understand and respond to people's personal and health needs

7.4. check people's understanding from time to time to keep misunderstanding or mistakes to a minimum

7.5. be able to communicate clearly and effectively in English.

8. **Work co-operatively**

To achieve this, you must:

8.1. respect the skills, expertise and contributions of your colleagues, referring matters to them when appropriate

8.2. maintain effective communication with colleagues

8.3. keep colleagues informed when you are sharing the care of individuals with other health and care professionals and staff

8.4. work with colleagues to evaluate the quality of your work and that of the team

8.5. work with colleagues to preserve the safety of those receiving care

8.6. share information to identify and reduce risk

8.7. be supportive of colleagues who are encountering health or performance problems. However, this support must never compromise or be at the expense of patient or public safety.

9. **Share your skills, knowledge and experience for the benefit of people receiving care and your colleagues**

To achieve this, you must:

9.1. provide honest, accurate and constructive feedback to colleagues

9.2. gather and reflect on feedback from a variety of sources, using it to improve your practice and performance

9.3. deal with differences of professional opinion with colleagues by discussion and informed debate, respecting their views and opinions and behaving in a professional way at all times

9.4. support students' and colleagues' learning to help them develop their professional competence and confidence.

10. **Keep clear and accurate records relevant to your practice**

This applies to the records that are relevant to your scope of practice. It includes but is not limited to patient records.

To achieve this, you must:

10.1. complete records at the time or as soon as possible after an event, recording if the notes are written sometime after the event

10.2. identify any risks or problems that have arisen and the steps taken to deal with them, so that colleagues who use the records have all the information they need

10.3. complete all records accurately and without any falsification, taking immediate and appropriate action if you become aware that someone has not kept to these requirements

10.4. attribute any entries you make in any paper or electronic records to yourself, making sure they are clearly written, dated and timed, and do not include unnecessary abbreviations, jargon or speculation

10.5. take all steps to make sure that all records are kept securely

10.6. collect, treat and store all data and research findings appropriately.

11. **Be accountable for your decisions to delegate tasks and duties to other people**

To achieve this, you must:

11.1. only delegate tasks and duties that are within the other person's scope of competence, making sure that they fully understand your instructions

11.2. make sure that everyone you delegate tasks to is adequately supervised and supported so they can provide safe and compassionate care

11.3. confirm that the outcome of any task you have delegated to someone else meets the required standard.

12. **Have in place an indemnity arrangement which provides appropriate cover for any practice you take on as a nurse, midwife or nursing associate in the United Kingdom**

To achieve this, you must:

12.1. make sure that you have an appropriate indemnity arrangement in place relevant to your scope of practice.

Preserve safety

You make sure that patient and public safety is not affected. You work within the limits of your competence, exercising your professional 'duty of candour' and raising concerns immediately whenever you come across situations that put patients or public safety at risk. You take necessary action to deal with any concerns where appropriate.

13. **Recognise and work within the limits of your competence**

To achieve this, you must, as appropriate:

13.1. accurately identify, observe and assess signs of normal or worsening physical and mental health in the person receiving care

13.2. make a timely referral to another practitioner when any action, care or treatment is required

13.3. ask for help from a suitably qualified and experienced professional to carry out any action or procedure that is beyond the limits of your competence

13.4. take account of your own personal safety as well as the safety of people in your care

13.5. complete the necessary training before carrying out a new role.

14. **Be open and candid with all service users about all aspects of care and treatment, including when any mistakes or harm have taken place**

To achieve this, you must:

14.1. act immediately to put right the situation if someone has suffered actual harm for any reason or an incident has happened which had the potential for harm

14.2. explain fully and promptly what has happened, including the likely effects, and apologise to the person affected and, where appropriate, their advocate, family or carers

14.3. document all these events formally and take further action (escalate) if appropriate so they can be dealt with quickly.

15. **Always offer help if an emergency arises in your practice setting or anywhere else**

To achieve this, you must:

15.1. only act in an emergency within the limits of your knowledge and competence

15.2. arrange, wherever possible, for emergency care to be accessed and provided promptly

15.3. take account of your own safety, the safety of others and the availability of other options for providing care.

16. **Act without delay if you believe that there is a risk to patient safety or public protection**

To achieve this, you must:

16.1. raise and, if necessary, escalate any concerns you may have about patient or public safety, or the level of care people are receiving in your workplace or any other health and care setting and use the channels available to you in line with our guidance and your local working practices

16.2. raise your concerns immediately if you are being asked to practise beyond your role, experience and training

16.3. tell someone in authority at the first reasonable opportunity if you experience problems that may prevent you working within the Code or other national standards, taking prompt action to tackle the causes of concern if you can

16.4. acknowledge and act on all concerns raised to you, investigating, escalating or dealing with those concerns where it is appropriate for you to do so

16.5. not obstruct, intimidate, victimise or in any way hinder a colleague, member of staff, person you care for or member of the public who wants to raise a concern

16.6. protect anyone you have management responsibility for from any harm, detriment, victimisation or unwarranted treatment after a concern is raised.

17. **Raise concerns immediately if you believe a person is vulnerable or at risk and needs extra support and protection**

To achieve this, you must:

17.1. take all reasonable steps to protect people who are vulnerable or at risk from harm, neglect or abuse

17.2. share information if you believe someone may be at risk of harm, in line with the laws relating to the disclosure of information

17.3. have knowledge of and keep to the relevant laws and policies about protecting and caring for vulnerable people.

18. **Advise on, prescribe, supply, dispense or administer medicines within the limits of your training and competence, the law, our guidance and other relevant policies, guidance and regulations**

To achieve this, you must:

18.1. prescribe, advise on, or provide medicines or treatment, including repeat prescriptions (only if you are suitably qualified) if you have enough knowledge of that person's health and are satisfied that the medicines or treatment serve that person's health needs

18.2. keep to appropriate guidelines when giving advice on using controlled drugs and recording the prescribing, supply, dispensing or administration of controlled drugs

18.3. make sure that the care or treatment you advise on, prescribe, supply, dispense or administer for each person is compatible with any other care or treatment they are receiving, including (where possible) over-the-counter medicines

18.4. take all steps to keep medicines stored securely

18.5. wherever possible, avoid prescribing for yourself or for anyone with whom you have a close personal relationship.

Prescribing is not within the scope of practice of everyone on our register. Nursing associates don't prescribe, but they may supply, dispense and administer medicines. Nurses and midwives who have successfully completed a further qualification in prescribing and recorded it on our register are the only people on our register that can prescribe.

19. **Be aware of, and reduce as far as possible, any potential for harm associated with your practice**

To achieve this, you must:

19.1. take measures to reduce as far as possible, the likelihood of mistakes, near misses, harm and the effect of harm if it takes place

19.2. take account of current evidence, knowledge and developments in reducing mistakes and the effect of them and the impact of human factors and system failures

19.3. keep to and promote recommended practice in relation to controlling and preventing infection

19.4. take all reasonable personal precautions necessary to avoid any potential health risks to colleagues, people receiving care and the public.

Promote professionalism and trust

You uphold the reputation of your profession at all times. You should display a personal commitment to the standards of practice and behaviour set out in the Code. You should be a model of integrity and leadership for others to aspire to. This should lead to trust and confidence in the profession from patients, people receiving care, other health and care professionals and the public.

20. **Uphold the reputation of your profession at all times**

To achieve this, you must:

20.1. keep to and uphold the standards and values set out in the Code

20.2. act with honesty and integrity at all times, treating people fairly and without discrimination, bullying or harassment

20.3. be aware at all times of how your behaviour can affect and influence the behaviour of other people

20.4. keep to the laws of the country in which you are practising

20.5. treat people in a way that does not take advantage of their vulnerability or cause them upset or distress

20.6. stay objective and have clear professional boundaries at all times with people in your care (including those who have been in your care in the past), their families and carers

20.7. make sure you do not express your personal beliefs (including political, religious or moral beliefs) to people in an inappropriate way

20.8. act as a role model of professional behaviour for students and newly qualified nurses, midwives and nursing associates to aspire to

20.9. maintain the level of health you need to carry out your professional role

20.10. use all forms of spoken, written and digital communication (including social media and networking sites) responsibly, respecting the right to privacy of others at all times.

21. **Uphold your position as a registered nurse, midwife or nursing associate**

To achieve this, you must:

21.1. refuse all but the most trivial gifts, favours or hospitality as accepting them could be interpreted as an attempt to gain preferential treatment

21.2. never ask for or accept loans from anyone in your care or anyone close to them

21.3. act with honesty and integrity in any financial dealings you have with everyone you have a professional relationship with, including people in your care

21.4. make sure that any advertisements, publications or published material you produce or have produced for your professional services are accurate, responsible, ethical, do not mislead or exploit vulnerabilities and accurately reflect your relevant skills, experience and qualifications

21.5. never use your professional status to promote causes that are not related to health

21.6. cooperate with the media only when it is appropriate to do so, and then always protecting the confidentiality and dignity of people receiving treatment or care.

22. Fulfil all registration requirements

To achieve this, you must:

22.1. keep to any reasonable requests so we can oversee the registration process

22.2. keep to our prescribed hours of practice and carry out continuing professional development activities

22.3. keep your knowledge and skills up to date, taking part in appropriate and regular learning and professional development activities that aim to maintain and develop your competence and improve your performance.

23. Cooperate with all investigations and audits

This includes investigations or audits either against you or relating to others, whether individuals or organisations. It also includes cooperating with requests to act as a witness in any hearing that forms part of an investigation, even after you have left the register.

To achieve this, you must:

23.1. cooperate with any audits of training records, registration records or other relevant audits that we may want to carry out to make sure you are still fit to practise

23.2. tell both us and any employers as soon as you can about any caution or charge against you, or if you have received a conditional discharge in relation to, or have been found guilty of, a criminal offence (other than a protected caution or conviction)

23.3. tell any employers you work for if you have had your practice restricted or had any other conditions imposed on you by us or any other relevant body.

23.4. tell us and your employers at the first reasonable opportunity if you are or have been disciplined by any regulatory or licensing organisation, including those who operate outside of the professional health and care environment

23.5. give your NMC Pin when any reasonable request for it is made

24. **Respond to any complaints made against you professionally**

   To achieve this, you must:

   24.1. never allow someone's complaint to affect the care that is provided to them

   24.2. use all complaints as a form of feedback and an opportunity for reflection and learning to improve practice.

25. **Provide leadership to make sure people's wellbeing is protected and to improve their experiences of the health and care system**

   To achieve this, you must:

   25.1. identify priorities, manage time, staff and resources effectively and deal with risk to make sure that the quality of care or service you deliver is maintained and improved, putting the needs of those receiving care or services first

   25.2. support any staff you may be responsible for to follow the Code at all times. They must have the knowledge, skills and competence for safe practice; and understand how to raise any concerns linked to any circumstances where the Code has, or could be, broken.

Throughout their careers, all our registrants will have opportunities to demonstrate leadership qualities, regardless of whether or not they occupy formal leadership positions.

The Code which was published in January 2015 and updated on 10 October 2018 to reflect the regulation of nursing associates is reproduced with the permission of the Nursing and Midwifery Council.

Section 2
Health and Care Professions Council (HCPC) Standards of Conduct, Performance and Ethics
Your Duties as a Registrant
The Standards

1. **Promote and protect the interests of service users and carers**
   Treat service users and carers with respect

   1.1. You must treat service users and carers as individuals, respecting their privacy and dignity.

   1.2. You must work in partnership with service users and carers, involving them, where appropriate, in decisions about the care, treatment or other services to be provided.

   1.3. You must encourage and help service users, where appropriate, to maintain their own health and well-being, and support them so they can make informed decisions.

   Make sure you have consent

   1.4 You must make sure that you have consent from service users or other appropriate authority before you provide care, treatment or other services.

Challenge discrimination

1.5. You must not discriminate against service users, carers or colleagues by allowing your personal views to affect your professional relationships or the care, treatment or other services that you provide.

1.6. You must challenge colleagues if you think that they have discriminated against, or are discriminating against, service users, carers and colleagues.

Maintain appropriate boundaries

1.7. You must keep your relationships with service users and carers professional.

2. **Communicate appropriately and effectively**

Communicate with service users and carers

2.1. You must be polite and considerate.

2.2. You must listen to service users and carers and take account of their needs and wishes.

2.3. You must give service users and carers the information they want or need, in a way they can understand.

2.4. You must make sure that, where possible, arrangements are made to meet service users' and carers' language and communication needs.

Work with colleagues

2.5. You must work in partnership with colleagues, sharing your skills, knowledge and experience where appropriate, for the benefit of service users and carers.

2.6. You must share relevant information, where appropriate, with colleagues involved in the care, treatment or other services provided to a service user.

Social media and networking websites

2.7. You must use all forms of communication appropriately and responsibly, including social media and networking websites.

3. **Work within the limits of your knowledge and skills**

Keep within your scope of practice

3.1. You must keep within your scope of practice by only practising in the areas you have appropriate knowledge, skills and experience for.

3.2. You must refer a service user to another practitioner if the care, treatment or other services they need are beyond your scope of practice.

Maintain and develop your knowledge and skills

3.3. You must keep your knowledge and skills up to date and relevant to your scope of practice through continuing professional development.

3.4. You must keep up to date with and follow the law, our guidance and other requirements relevant to your practice.

3.5. You must ask for feedback and use it to improve your practice.

4. **Delegate appropriately**
   Delegation, oversight and support
   4.1. You must only delegate work to someone who has the knowledge, skills and experience needed to carry it out safely and effectively.
   4.2. You must continue to provide appropriate supervision and support to those you delegate work to.

5. **Respect confidentiality**
   Using information
   5.1. You must treat information about service users as confidential.
   Disclosing information
   5.2. You must only disclose confidential information if:
      - you have permission;
      - the law allows this;
      - it is in the service user's best interests; or
      - it is in the public interest, such as if it is necessary to protect public safety or prevent harm to other people.

6. **Manage risk**
   Identify and minimise risk
   6.1. You must take all reasonable steps to reduce the risk of harm to service users, carers and colleagues as far as possible.
   6.2. You must not do anything, or allow someone else to do anything, which could put the health or safety of a service user, carer or colleague at unacceptable risk.
   Manage your health
   6.3. You must make changes to how you practise, or stop practising, if your physical or mental health may affect your performance or judgement, or put others at risk for any other reason.

7. **Report concerns about safety**
   Report concerns
   7.1. You must report any concerns about the safety or well-being of service users promptly and appropriately.
   7.2. You must support and encourage others to report concerns and not prevent anyone from raising concerns.
   7.3. You must take appropriate action if you have concerns about the safety or well-being of children or vulnerable adults.
   7.4. You must make sure that the safety and well-being of service users always comes before any professional or other loyalties.
   Follow up concerns
   7.5. You must follow up concerns you have reported and, if necessary, escalate them.

7.6. You must acknowledge and act on concerns raised to you, investigating, escalating or dealing with those concerns where it is appropriate for you to do so.

8. Be open when things go wrong

Openness with service users and carers

8.1. You must be open and honest when something has gone wrong with the care, treatment or other services that you provide by:

 – informing service users or, where appropriate, their carers, that something has gone wrong;
 – apologising;
 – taking action to put matters right if possible; and
 – making sure that service users or, where appropriate, their carers, receive a full and prompt explanation of what has happened and any likely effects.

Deal with concerns and complaints

8.2. You must support service users and carers who want to raise concerns about the care, treatment or other services they have received.

8.3. You must give a helpful and honest response to anyone who complains about the care, treatment or other services they have received.

9. Be honest and trustworthy

Personal and professional behaviour

9.1. You must make sure that your conduct justifies the public's trust and confidence in you and your profession.

9.2. You must be honest about your experience, qualifications and skills.

9.3. You must make sure that any promotional activities you are involved in are accurate and are not likely to mislead.

9.4. You must declare issues that might create conflicts of interest and make sure that they do not influence your judgement.

Important information about your conduct and competence

9.5. You must tell us as soon as possible if:

 – you accept a caution from the police or you have been charged with, or found guilty of, a criminal offence;
 – another organisation responsible for regulating a health or social-care profession has taken action or made a finding against you; or
 – you have had any restriction placed on your practice, or been suspended or dismissed by an employer, because of concerns about your conduct or competence.

9.6. You must co-operate with any investigation into your conduct or competence, the conduct or competence of others, or the care, treatment or other services provided to service users.

10. **Keep records of your work**

    Keep accurate records

    10.1. You must keep full, clear, and accurate records for everyone you care for, treat, or provide other services to.

    10.2. You must complete all records promptly and as soon as possible after providing care, treatment or other services.

    Keep records secure

    10.3. You must keep records secure by protecting them from loss, damage or inappropriate access.

Reproduced with the permission of the Health and Care Professions Council published January 2016

Appendix 7

Common Abbreviations

Abbreviation	Meaning
AAA	abdominal aortic aneurysm
AAMI	age associated memory impairment
ABG	arterial blood gases
ABO	three basic blood groups
ACE	angiotensin-converting enzyme
ACL	anterior cruciate ligament
ACO	accountable care organization
ACTH	adrenocorticotrophic hormone
ADH	antidiuretic hormone
ADHD	attention deficit with hyperactivity disorder
ADL	activities of daily living
AED	automated external defibrillator
AF	atrial fibrillation
AFB	acid-fast bacillus
AfC	agenda for change
AHP	allied health professional
AID	artificial insemination with donor sperm
AIDS	acquired immunodeficiency syndrome
AIH	artificial insemination with sperm of husband (partner)
AKD	acute kidney disease
ALL	acute lymphoblastic leukaemia
ALS	advanced life support; amyotrophic lateral sclerosis
am	morning
AMD	age related macular degeneration
AMI	acute myocardial infarction
AML	acute myeloblastic/myeloid leukaemia
ANOVA	analysis of variance

Abbreviation	Meaning
ANS	autonomic nervous system
APEL	accreditation of prior experiential learning
APH	antepartum haemorrhage
APKD	acute polycystic kidney disease
APL	accreditation of prior learning
APTT	activated partial thromboplastin time
ARDS	adult respiratory distress syndrome
ARM	artificial rupture of membranes; age related maculopathy
ASD	atrial septum defect
BCC	basal cell carcinoma
BCG	bacille Calmette-Guerin
BFI	baby friendly initiative
BiPAP	bi-directional positive airway pressure
BLS	basic life support
BMA	British Medical Association
BMD	bone mineral density
BMI	body mass index
BMR	basal metabolic rate
BNF	British National Formulary
BP	blood pressure
BPH	benign prostatic hypertrophy
bpm	beats per minute
BPPV	benign paroxysmal positional vertigo
BSE	bovine spongiform encephalopathy; breast self-examination
BSL	British sign language
Bx	biopsy
./c	with
C	centigrade
CABG	coronary artery bypass graft
CAT	computerized (axial) tomography
CBT	cognitive behaviour therapy
CCF	congestive cardiac failure
CCG	clinical commissioning group
CCU	coronary care unit; critical care unit
CD	controlled drug
CDH	congenital dislocation of the hip
CF	cystic fibrosis
CFS	chronic fatigue syndrome
CHD	coronary heart disease; congenital heart disease
CHF	congestion heart failure
CHO	carbohydrate
CI	cardiac index; cardiac insufficiency; cerebral infarction; confidence interval
CINAHL	cumulative index to nursing and allied health literature

Abbreviation	Meaning
CIP	cost improvement programme
CIS	carcinoma in situ
CJD	Creutzfeldt–Jakob disease
CLL	chronic lymphocytic leukaemia
CML	chronic myeloid leukaemia
CMV	cytomegalovirus
CNS	central nervous system; clinical nurse specialist
c/o	complains of, complaints of
COPD	chronic obstructive pulmonary disease
CPA	care programme approach
CPAP	continuous positive airway pressure
CPD	continuing professional development
CPR	cardiopulmonary resuscitation
CQC	Care Quality Commission
CSF	cerebrospinal fluid
CT	computed tomography
CV	curriculum vitae
CVA	cerebrovascular accident
CVP	central venous pressure
CVS	chorionic villi sampling; cardiovascular system
CXR	chest X-ray
D&C	dilation (dilatation) and curettage
Db	decibel
DEXA	dual energy X-ray absorptiometry
DIC	disseminated intravascular coagulopathy/coagulation
DKA	diabetic ketoacidosis
DMD	Duchenne muscular dystrophy
DNA	deoxyribonucleic acid
DNAR	do not attempt resuscitation
DOA	dead on arrival
DOB	date of birth
DOE	dyspnoea on exertion
DOL	deprivation of liberty
DRG	diagnostic-related groups
DT	delirium tremens
DVT	deep venous thrombosis
EBP	evidence-based practice; epidural blood patch
EBV	Epstein–Barr virus
ECG	electrocardiogram; electrocardiograph
ECHO	echocardiography
ECT	electroconvulsive therapy
ED	erectile dysfunction
EDD	expected date of delivery
EEG	electroencephalogram; electroencephalograph
EIA	exercise induced asthma
EMLA	eutectic mixture of local anaesthetics
ENT	ear, nose and throat

Abbreviation	Meaning
ERPC	evacuation of retained products of conception
ESR	erythrocyte sedimentation rate
ESRD	end-stage renal disease
ET	endotracheal tube
ETT	exercise tolerance test
F	Fahrenheit
FAS	fetal alcohol syndrome
FAST	face arm speech test
FB	foreign body
FBC	full blood count
FEV	forced expiratory volume
FMNF	fetal movement not felt
FOB	faecal occult blood
FSE	fetal scalp electrode
FSH	follicle-stimulating hormone
GAD	generalized anxiety disorder
GCS	Glasgow Coma Scale
GI	gastrointestinal; glycaemic index
GP	general practitioner
GDP	general dental practitioner
GFR	glomerular filtration rate
GIFT	gamete intrafallopian transfer
GMC	General Medical Council
GTT	glucose tolerance test
GU	genitourinary
GUM	genitourinary medicine
GVHD	graft versus host disease
Hb, Hgb	haemoglobin
HbA$_{1c}$	glycosylated haemoglobin
HAI	hospital-acquired infection
Hb	haemoglobin
HCA	health care assistant
HCAI	health care associated infection
HCPC	Health and Care Professions Council
HCT	haematocrit
HDL	high-density lipoprotein
HDU	high dependency unit
HELLP	haemolysis, elevated liver enzymes and low platelets
Hib	*Haemophilus influenzae* type B
HIV	human immunodeficiency (AIDS) virus
HRT	hormone replacement therapy
HSE	Health and Safety Executive
IABP	intra-aortic balloon pump
IAPT	improving access to psychological therapies
IBD	inflammatory bowel disease
IBS	irritable bowel syndrome
ICD	International Classification of Diseases

Abbreviation	Meaning
ICE	in case of emergency; ice, compression, elevation
ICP	intracranial pressure; integrated care pathway
ICU	intensive care unit
IDDM	insulin-dependent diabetes mellitus (no longer—see type 1 diabetes)
Ig	immunoglobulin
IM	intramuscular
IMI	intramuscular injection
INR	international normalized ration
IOFB	intraocular foreign body
IOP	intraocular pressure
IPE	inter-professional education
IPH	intrapartum haemorrhage
IPPB	intermittent positive pressure breathing
IPPV	intermittent positive pressure ventilation
IQ	intelligence quotient
ISC	intermittent self-catheterization
IUCD	intrauterine contraceptive device
IV	intravenous
IVF	in vitro fertilization
IVP	intravenous pyelogram
J	joule
JSNA	joint strategic needs assessment
KPI	key performance indicator
lab	laboratory
LBW	low birth weight
LDL	low-density lipoprotein
LE	lupus erythematosus
LFT	liver function tests
LGBT	lesbian, gay, bisexual, transgender
LH	luteinizing hormone
LMP	last menstrual period
LOC	level of consciousness; loss of consciousness
LP	lumbar puncture
LPA	lasting power of attorney
LSCS	lower segment caesarean section
LSD	lysergic acid diethylamide
LVF	left ventricular failure
MAOI	monoamine oxidase inhibitor
MAST	mandatory and statutory training
MCA	Mental Capacity Act
MDT	multidisciplinary team
ME	myalgic encephalomyelitis
MHRA	Medicines and Healthcare Products Regulatory Authority
MI	myocardial infarction
MND	motor neuron disease

Abbreviation	Meaning
MRI	magnetic resonance imaging
MRSA	methicillin-resistant *Staphylococcus aureus*
MS	multiple sclerosis
MSK	musculoskeletal
MSU	midstream specimen of urine
MUA	manipulation under anaesthetic
MVA	motor vehicle accident
N/A	not applicable, not available
NAD	no abnormalities detected; non-adherent dressing
NAI	non-accidental injury
NBM	nil by mouth
NCT	National Childbirth Trust
NG, ng	nasogastric
NHSE	NHS England
NHSI	NHS Improvement
NICE	National Institute for Health and Care Excellence
NICU	neonatal intensive care unit
NIDDM	non-insulin dependent diabetes mellitus (no longer used—see type 2 diabetes)
NLP	neurolinguistic programming
NMC	Nursing and Midwifery Council
NNT	numbers needed to treat
NOF	neck of femur
NRDS	neonatal respiratory distress syndrome
NREM	non-rapid eye movement (sleep)
NRT	nicotine replacement therapy
NS, N/S	normal saline
NSAID	non-steroidal anti-inflammatory drug
NST	newborn screening test (Guthrie)
NWB	non-weight bearing
OA	osteoarthritis
OCD	obsessive compulsive disorder
ODP	operating department practitioner
ORS	oral rehydration solution
OSCE	objective structured clinical examinations
OT	occupational therapist
OTC	over-the-counter
PA	physician's associate
PALS	paediatric advanced life support; patient advice and liaison service
Pap test	Papanicolaou smear
PBL	problem-based learning
PCA	patient-controlled analgesia
PCI	percutaneous coronary intervention
PCOS	polycystic ovary syndrome
PCV	packed cell volume
PDP	personal development plan

Abbreviation	Meaning
PE	pulmonary embolism
PEFR	peak expiratory flow rate
PEG	percutaneous endoscopic gastrostomy
PET	positron emission tomography
pH	hydrogen ion concentration (alkalinity and acidity in urine and blood analysis)
PICU	paediatric intensive care unit
PID	pelvic inflammatory disease
PKU	phenylketonuria
pm	afternoon, evening
PMH	past medical history
PMS	premenstrual syndrome
POM	prescription-only medicine
PPE	personal protective equipment
PPH	post-partum haemorrhage
PR	per rectum; pulse rate
PRN, prn	as required
PROM	patient reported outcome measure
PSA	prostate specific antigen
PT	physiotherapist; prothrombin
PTSD	post-traumatic stress disorder
PUO	pyrexia of unknown origin
PUVA	psoralen ultraviolet light A
PV	per vagina
QALY	quality adjusted life years
QIPP	quality, innovation, productivity, prevention
RA	rheumatoid arthritis
RAS	reticular activating system
RBC	red blood cell; red blood count
RCT	randomized controlled trial
RDA	recommended daily allowance
RDI	recommended daily intake
REM	rapid eye movement (sleep)
RF	rheumatoid factor
Rh	Rhesus factor
RIP	raised intracranial pressure
RM	registered midwife
RN	registered nurse
RNA	ribonucleic acid
ROM	range of motion
rpm	revolutions per minute; respirations per minute
RSI	repetitive strain injury
RTA	road traffic accident
SAD	seasonal affective disorder
SALT	speech and language therapist
SARS	severe respiratory distress syndrome
s/s, S&S	signs and symptoms

Abbreviation	Meaning
SBAR	situation, background, assessment, recommendations
SC	subcutaneous
SCBU	special care baby unit
SCR	summary care record
SD	standard deviation
SG, sp.gr.	specific gravity
SEN	special educational needs
SFD	small for dates
SGA	small for gestational age
SGOT	serum glutamic oxaloacetic transaminase
SIDS	sudden infant death syndrome
SL	sub-lingual
SLE	systemic lupus erythematosus
SMART	specific, measurable, achievable, realistic, time-bound
SMR	standardized mortality ratio
SOB	shortness of breath
SOBOE	shortness of breath on exertion
SPSS	statistical package for social sciences
SR	sedimentation rate
SROM/PROM	spontaneous or premature rupture of membranes
SSRI	selective serotonin reuptake inhibitors
Staph	*Staphylococcus*
stat	immediately (statim)
STI	sexually transmitted disease/infection
STP	sustainable transformation plans
STM	short-term memory
Strep	*Streptococcus*
SVT	supraventricular tachycardia
T1DM	type 1 diabetes mellitus
T2DM	type 2 diabetes mellitus
TB	tuberculosis; tubercle bacillus
TEDS	thromboembolic deterrents
TENS	transcutaneous electrical nerve stimulation
TIA	transient ischaemic attack
TOP	termination of pregnancy
TPN	total parenteral nutrition
TPR	temperature, pulse and respiration
TSH	thyroid-stimulating hormone
TV	tidal volume
Tx, Rx	treatment
URTI	upper respiratory tract infection
US	ultrasound
UTI	urinary tract infection
VF	ventricular fibrillation
VSD	ventricular septal defect
VS	voluntary sector

Abbreviation	Meaning
VSO	voluntary service overseas
VT	ventricular tachycardia
VTE	venous thromboembolism
VZV	varicella zoster virus
WBC, wbc	white blood cells, white blood count
WCC	white cell count
WHO	World Health Organization
wt	weight
www.	world wide web
X-ray	Röntgen ray

8 Appendix

Common Prefixes, Suffixes and Roots

Prefix/suffix/root	To do with	Examples in the dictionary
a-/an-	lack of	anuria, agranulocyte, asystole, anaemia
ab-	away from	abducent
ad-	towards	adductor
-aemia	of the blood	anaemia, hypoxaemia, uraemia, hypovolaemia
aer-	air, gas	aerobe, aeropathy
angio-	vessel	angiotensin, haemangioma
ante-	before, in front of	anterior
anti-	against	antidiuretic, anticoagulant, antigen, antifungal
arth-	joint	arthritis, arthralgia
bi-	two, twice	biceps, bicellular
-blast	germ, bud	retinoblastoma, osteoblast
brady-	slow	bradycardia
bronch-	bronchus	bronchiole, bronchitis, bronchus
card-	heart	cardiac, myocardium, tachycardia
cephal-	head	cephalography, cephelometry
cerebr-	brain	cerebrovascular
chemo-	chemical	chemoprophylaxis, chemotherapy
chole-	bile	cholecystitis, cholelithiasis
circum-	around	circumduction, circumoral
col-	bowel	colic, colitis
contra-	against	contraindications, contraception
cost-	ribs	costal
cran-	skull	craniostenosis, cranium
cyto-/-cyte	cell	erythrocyte, cytoplasm, cytotoxic
derm-	skin	dermatitis, dermis, dermatology
di-	two	disaccharide, dichromatic, dicrotic

Prefix/suffix/ root	To do with	Examples in the dictionary
dis-	separation	dissociation, distraction
dys-	difficult	dysuria, dyspnoea, dysmenorrhoea, dysplasia
-ema	swelling	oedema, emphysema, lymphoedema
ecto-	outside	ectoderm, ectogenous
endo-	inner	endocrine, endotracheal endothelium
electro-	electrical	electrocardiogram, electronic
enter-	intestine	enterokinase, gastroenteritis
epi-	upon	epithelium, epicardium
erythro-	red	erythrocyte, erythropoietin, erythema
exo-	outside	exophthalmos, extraction
extra-	outside	extracellular, extrapyramidal
ferr-	iron	ferritin
-fferent	carry	afferent, efferent
fore-	in front of, before	forehead, foreskin
gast-	stomach	gastric, gastrin, gastritis, gastrointestinal
-gen-	origin/production	gene, genotype, genetic, antigen, pathogen, allergen
-globin	protein	myoglobin, haemoglobin
gluco-	sugar	glucose, glucocorticoid
haem-	blood	haemostasis, haemorrhage, haemolytic
hemi-	half	hemisphere, hemiplegia
hepat-	liver	hepatic, hepatitis, hepatomegaly
hetero-	different	heterozygous, heterosexual
homo-	the same, steady	homozygous, homologous
-hydr-	water	dehydration, hydrotherapy, hydrocephalus
hist-	tissues	histology
hyster-	uterus	hysterectomy
hyper-	excess/above	hypertension, hypertrophy, hypercapnia
hypo-	below/under	hypoglycaemia, hypotension, hypovolaemia
ileo-	ileum	ileostomy, ileocolitis
intro-	inwards	introitus, introspect
iso-	equal, alike	isometric, isograft
immuno-	immunity	immunodeficiency, immunoglobulin
intra-	within	intracellular, intracranial, intraocular
inter-	between	interstitial,

Prefix/suffix/root	To do with	Examples in the dictionary
-ism	condition	hyperthyroidism, gestaltism, rheumatism
-itis	inflammation	appendicitis, hepatitis, cystitis, gastritis
kerat-	horn, skin, cornea	keratin, keratic
kin-	motion	kinetic
kypho-	rounded	kyphosis
lact-	milk	lactation, lactic, lacteal
lapar-	abdomen	laparoscopy, laparotomy
leuc-/leuko	white, white blood cells	leucocyte, leukaemia
lymph-	lymph tissue	lymphocyte, lymphatic, lymphoedema
lyso-/-lysis	breaking down	lysosome, glycogenolysis, lysozyme
macro-	large	macrocyte, macrophage
mal-	poor, abnormal	malaise, malabsorption
mamm-	breast	mammography
mast-	breast	mastitis, mastalgia
medi-	middle	mediastinum, median
-mega-	large	megaloblast, acromegaly, splenomegaly, hepatomegaly
meso-	middle	mesoderm
meta-	change, between, beyond	metaplasia
micro-	small	microbe, microbiology, micronutrient
mono-	one	monochromatism, monocyte
multi-	many	multicellular, multigravida
myelo-	spinal cord, bone marrow	myelocyte, myeloid
myo-	muscle	myocardium, myohaemoglobin, myopathy, myosin
neo-	new	neoplasm, gluconeogenesis, neonate
nephro-	kidney	nephron, nephrotic, nephroblastoma, nephrosis
neuro-	nerve	neurone, neuralgia, neuropathy
odont-	tooth	odontoma, odontoid
-oid	resembling	myeloid, sigmoid
olig-	small	oliguria
-ology	study of	cardiology, neurology, physiology
-oma	tumour	carcinoma, melanoma, fibroma
onych-	nail	onycholysis, onychomycosis
-ophth-	eye	xerophthalmia, ophthalmology, exophthalmos

Prefix/suffix/ root	To do with	Examples in the dictionary
-ory	referring to	secretory, sensory, auditory, gustatory
os-, osteo-	bone	osteocyte, osteoarthritis, osteoporosis
paed-	child	paediatrician, paediatrics
-path-	disease	pathogenesis, neuropathy
-penia	deficiency of	leukopenia, thrombocytopenia
peri-	around	perinatal, perichondrium
phag(o)-	eating	phagocytosis, phagocyte
phleb-	veins	phlebitis, phlebotomy
phono-	sound	phonology, phonocardiogram
photo-	light	photophobia, photopsia
-plasm	substance	cytoplasm, neoplasm
pneumo-	lung/air	pneumothorax, pneumonia, pneumotaxic
poly-	many	polypharmacy, polyuria, polycythaemia
pre-	before, in front	preterm, presystole
post-	after, behind	postnatal, posthumous
pseudo-	false	pseudocyesis, pseudoangina
psych-	mind	psychology, psychopathic, psychotherapy
re-	back, again	recurrent
rect-	rectum	rectovaginal, rectal
retro-	backward	retrograde, retrobulbar
-rrhagia	excessive flow	menorrhagia
-rrhoea	discharge	dysmenorrhoea, diarrhoea, rhinorrhoea
sarc-	flesh	sarcoma, sarcoid
-scler	hard	arteriosclerosis
sub-	under	subphrenic, subarachnoid, sublingual
semi-	part, half	semicircular, semipermeable
sero-	serum	serological, serotype
supra-	above	suprarenal, supraorbital
tachy-	excessively fast	tachycardia
therm-	heat	thermometer, thermolysis
thrombo-	clot	thrombocyte, thrombosis, thrombin, thrombus
-tox-	poison	toxin, cytotoxic, hepatotoxic
trans-	across	transplant, transmission
tri-	three	trisomy, trimester, triage
ultra-	beyond	ultrasound, ultraviolet
uni-	one	unilateral, uniovular
-uria	urine	anuria, polyuria, haematuria, nocturia

Prefix/suffix/ root	To do with	Examples in the dictionary
uter-	uterus	uterine, uterovesical
vas, vaso-	vessel	vasoconstrictor, vas deferens, vascular
ven-	vein	venous, venepuncture
xer-	dry	xerostomia, xeroderm

Appendix 9

Units of Measurement and Tables of Normal Values

Metric measures, units and SI symbols		
Name	**SI unit**	**Symbol**
Length	metre	m
Mass	kilogram	kg
Amount of substance	mole	mol
Pressure	pascal	Pa
Energy	joule	J

Decimal multiples and submultiples of the units are formed by the use of standard prefixes					
Multiple	**Prefix**	**Symbol**	**Submultiple**	**Prefix**	**Symbol**
10^6	mega	M	10^{-1}	deci	d
10^3	kilo	k	10^{-2}	centi	c
10^2	hecto	h	10^{-3}	milli	m
10^1	deca	da	10^{-6}	micro	μ
			10^{-9}	nano	n
			10^{-12}	pico	p
			10^{-15}	femto	F

Conversion Table for kPa ↔ mmHg (e.g., for capillary pressures)	
1 mmHg	= 0.13 kPa
1 kPa	= 7.5 mmHg
35 mmHg	= 4.66 kPa
25 mmHg	= 3.33 kPa
15 mmHg	= 1.99 kPa
10 mmHg	= 1.33 kPa

Hydrogen Ion Concentration (pH)
Neutral = 7   Acid = 0–7   Alkaline = 7–14

Normal pH of some body fluids

Blood	7.35–7.45
Saliva	5.6–7.9
Gastric juice	1.5–3.5
Bile	6.8–8.05
Urine	5.5–7.0

Some normal plasma levels in adults	
Calcium	2.20–2.60 mmol/l
Chloride	96–106 mmol/l
Cholesterol	<5 mmol/l
Glucose	<7.8 mmol/l
Fasting glucose	4.0–6.0 mmol/l
Potassium	3.5–5.1 mmol/l
Sodium	135–145 mmol/l
Urea	2.1–7.1 mmol/l

Arterial blood gases		
Pao_2	11–13 kPa	(75–100 mmHg)
$Paco_2$	4.7–6.0 kPa	(35–45 mmHg)
Bicarbonate	21–27 mmol/l	
H+ ions	36–44 nmol/l	

Blood pressure	
Normal adult 120/80 mmHg	
<90/60 mmHg	low blood pressure
90/60–120/80 mmHg	ideal blood pressure
>120/80 to <140/90 mmHg	pre-high blood pressure
>140/90 mmHg	high blood pressure

Heart rate	
At rest	60–100/min
Sinus bradycardia	<60/min
Sinus tachycardia	>100/min

Respiration rate	
At rest 12–20/min	
Tidal volume	500 ml

Blood count			
Leukocytes	3.8×10^9/l	to	10.8×10^9/l
Neutrophils	2.0×10^9/l	to	7.5×10^9/l
Eosinophils	0.04×10^9/l	to	0.44×10^9/l
Basophils	0.015×10^9/l	to	0.2×10^9/l
Monocytes	0.2×10^9/l	to	0.9×10^9/l
Lymphocytes	1.3×10^9/l	to	3.5×10^9/l
Erythrocytes			
Female	3.8×10^{12}/l	to	5.8×10^{12}/l
Male	4.5×10^{12}/l	to	6.5×10^{12}/l
Thrombocytes	150×10^9/l	to	400×10^9/l

Coagulation times	
Activated partial thromboplastin time (APTT)	28–37 s
Prothrombin time	12–16 s
International Normalized Ratio (INR)	<1.2
D-dimer	<230 ng/l pulmonary embolism unlikely

Diet	
1 kilocalorie (kcal) = 4.182 kilojoules (kJ)	
1 kilojoule = 0.24 kilocalories	
Energy source	**Energy released**
Carbohydrate	1g = 17 kJ = 4 kcal
Protein	1g = 17 kJ = 4 kcal
Fat	1g = 38 kJ = 9 kcal

Urine	
Specific gravity	1.020–1.035
Volume excreted	1000–1500 ml/day

Glucose is normally absent, but appears in urine when blood glucose levels exceed 9 mmol/l.

Body temperatures	
Normal	36.8°C (98.4°F)
Hypothermia	<35°C (95°F): core temperature

Cerebrospinal Fluid Pressure
Lying on the side 8–15 mmHg

Intraocular Pressure
1.3–2.6 kPa (10–20 mmHg)

Unless otherwise stated, reference ranges apply to adults; values in children may be different.

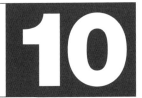
Immunization and Vaccinations

Newborn babies have some temporary immunity to infections as a result of the passive transfer of maternal antibodies to the unborn infant in the last trimester of pregnancy. However, the duration of this protection varies as some antibodies to certain infections are more long-lasting than others.

As an example, a mother's antibodies to measles usually protect her baby against the disease for 6–12 months, but those against whooping cough (pertussis) and Hib (*Haemophilus influenzae* type b) only last a few weeks. This is why the vaccination programme starts at 8 weeks of age (see Table 10.1). Every effort should be made to ensure that all children are vaccinated, even if they are older than the recommended age range; no opportunity to immunize should be missed. **If any course of vaccinations is interrupted, it should be resumed and completed as soon as possible. There is no need to start any course of vaccinations again.**

It is important that premature infants have their vaccinations at the appropriate chronological age, according to the schedule. There is no evidence that premature infants are at increased risk of adverse reactions from vaccines. They are, however, more susceptible to infections because their immune systems are less developed so it is very important they start their vaccination schedule at 8 weeks.

The routine vaccination schedule extends to older children, providing boosters to vaccinations given in the first year as well as vaccinating in older childhood against the human papilloma virus (at 12–13 years) and vaccinating against four strains of the meningococcal bacteria that causes meningitis and septicaemia (at 14 years and to teenagers not previously vaccinated who are going to university for the first time).

Individual considerations always need to be borne in mind, both in terms of possible contraindications and adverse reactions. These concerns can be discussed with the family doctor, the practice nurse or health visitor.

Table 10.1	Childhood immunization programme (UK)	
When to immunize	**What vaccine is given**	**How it is given**
8 weeks	6-in-1 diphtheria, tetanus, pertussis, polio, hepatitis B and *Haemophilus influenzae* type B	One injection
	Pneumococcal meningitis (PCV)	One injection
	Rotavirus	By mouth
	MenB	One injection
12 weeks	6-in-1 (2nd dose) diphtheria, tetanus, pertussis, polio, hepatitis B and *Haemophilus influenzae* type B	One injection
	Rotavirus	By mouth
16 weeks	6-in-1 (3rd dose) diphtheria, tetanus, pertussis, polio, hepatitis B and *Haemophilus influenzae* type B	One injection
	Pneumococcal meningitis (PCV) (2nd dose)	One injection
	MenB (2nd dose)	One injection
1 year	Hib/MenC	One injection
	Measles, mumps, rubella (MMR)	One injection
	Pneumococcal meningitis (PCV) (3rd dose)	One injection
	MenB (3rd dose)	One injection
2–9 years (including children in reception class and school years 1–4)	Children's annual flu vaccine	Nasal spray
Children aged 3 years 4 months	4-in-1 pre-school booster diphtheria, tetanus, pertussis and polio	One injection
	Measles, mumps and rubella (MMR) (2nd dose)	One injection
	Hepatitis B booster (for children immunized in infancy who were born to hepatitis B infected mothers)	
12–13 years old	Human papillomavirus vaccine (HPV)	Two injections given 6 months apart
14 years + young people going away to university or college who may have missed the vaccine	3-in-1 teenage booster diphtheria, tetanus, and polio	One injection
	MenACWY vaccine	One injection

Older people are also at higher risk of contracting certain infections and of getting serious complications if they contract certain infectious diseases. There are vaccinations available to people over 65, including annual flu vaccination and the pneumococcal vaccine. The shingles vaccine is given as a one-off vaccination to people aged 70 years. Carers are also at risk of contracting infections and of not being able to carry out their caring role due to sickness, and are offered the annual flu vaccination. Pregnant women are also offered seasonal flu vaccination.

Other vaccines that are available for at-risk groups, including people with long term or serious conditions and people known to have been exposed to certain diseases. These vaccinations include the BCG vaccine for TB; chicken pox vaccine; flu vaccine; pneumococcal vaccine; and hepatitis B vaccine.

There are also certain vaccinations available on the NHS against common infections for travellers. These include diphtheria, polio and tetanus (combined booster); typhoid, hepatitis A; and cholera. Other travel vaccinations are recommended depending on the destination and are available from private clinics.

When new vaccinations are introduced to the routine schedule there will, in certain instances, be a parallel time-limited 'catch-up' programme to ensure that those who missed the vaccination because they were older than the recommended age when the vaccination was introduced are able to benefit. An example of this is the shingles vaccination.

Vaccination Aftercare and Side Effects
Polio, Diphtheria, Tetanus, Pertussis, Hib and Hepatitis B
The 6-in-1 vaccine is given at 8, 12, and 16 weeks. Some children become irritable and may develop a slight fever, with drowsiness and anorexia, between 6 and 24 hours after vaccination; there may also be erythema, induration and a palpable nodule at the injection site. Children aged 3 years and 4 months are given a further 4-in-1 booster dose of vaccination to protect against polio, diphtheria, tetanus and pertussis. At 14 years they have a further 3-in-1 booster of polio, diphtheria and tetanus vaccination.

Rotavirus
This vaccine is given at 8 and 12 weeks. Some children become irritable and restless, and some may develop mild diarrhoea.

Pneumococcal vaccine
This vaccination is routinely given to babies in three separate doses at 8 and 16 weeks and at 1 year, and to other groups at higher risk of pneumococcal infection, including children and adults with certain long-term conditions, and adults aged 65 years or older. People over 65 years only require a single dose which will provide protection for life. Some children become irritable after vaccination and may develop a slight

fever, erythema, induration and a palpable nodule at the injection site. Adults may also develop mild fever, redness at the site of the injection and a palpable nodule at the injection site.

MenB

Babies are given the MenB vaccine alongside other routine vaccinations at 8 and 16 weeks, and at 1 year. They are likely to develop fever within the first 24 hours after vaccination, erythema, induration and a palpable nodule at the injection site.

Measles, Mumps and Rubella

Given at 1 year, and at 3 years and 4 months. A week to 10 days after the injection, the child may become pyrexial for 1–2 days, and there may also be a rash. Lymphadenopathy in the neck may occur 2–3 weeks after immunization.

MenC

This is given as a single injection with the Hib booster at 1 year. Common side effects include erythema, induration and a palpable nodule at the injection site, fever, irritability, loss of appetite, and sleepiness.

HPV

Offered to girls (and from 2019 to boys) aged 12–13 years with an initial dose and a booster after 6–12 months. Common side effects include erythema, induration and a palpable nodule at the injection site, mild dizziness, nausea and headache.

MenACWY

Offered at 14 years to girls and boys and to young people going away to university for the first time who were not previously vaccinated. Common side effects include erythema, induration and a palpable nodule at the injection site, fever, headache, nausea and fatigue lasting no more than 24 hours.

Influenza

Vaccination is offered every autumn to protect children and people who are at risk of serious illness, e.g., those with long-term conditions or at heightened risk should they catch influenza. It is also advised for carers, pregnant women and everyone over the age of 65, those living in residential and nursing homes, health and social care workers. Repeated annual flu vaccination in October/early November is necessary due to the development of changing strains of the virus. Side effects of the injected flu vaccination for adults include mild fever and aching muscles, plus erythema, induration and a palpable nodule at the injection site. Children's annual flu vaccine is offered to children aged 2–9 years as a nasal spray. Side effects include a runny nose for a few days after vaccination.

Shingles

Shingles vaccine is given as a one-off injection to people aged 70 years. Side effects include redness and discomfort at the injection site, and headache lasting a few days.

References/Websites

NHS Choices. Available at: http://www.nhs.uk/Conditions/vaccinations/

Further details about all immunizations are available at: www.gov.uk/collections/immunisation

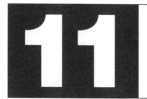

Appendix

Prevention and Control of Infection

Infection control has always been a key component of modern health care but it was in the 1990s that the focus turned to preventing health care-associated infections (HCAI). HCAI are infections that are acquired as a result of health care interventions. Previously, when most complex health care was hospital based, the term 'hospital acquired (or nosocomial) infection' was used but nowadays, as such care frequently occurs in the community, especially the patient's home, the term HCAI is more appropriate.

In England, evidence-based infection prevention guidelines have been published for acute care and primary and community care settings (National Institute for Health and Clinical Excellence (NICE) 2013, 2014, 2016; Pratt et al., 2007: Loveday et al., 2014). NICE standards (2014) for all HCAIs also include antimicrobial stewardship; organizational responsibility; hand decontamination; urinary catheters; vascular access devices; and educating people about infection prevention and control. The 2016 NICE standard which covers preventing and controlling infections in hospitals and other secondary care settings that develop because of treatment or from being in a health care setting additionally include standards on surveillance; collaborative action; responsibilities of hospital staff; planning, design and management of hospital facilities; and admission, discharge and transfer. All three NICE quality standards are reviewed annually. Standard Principles for the prevention of HCAI in hospitals and other acute settings (Table 11.1) (Loveday et al., 2014) are divided into five interventions: hospital environment hygiene; hand hygiene; use of personal protective equipment; safe use and disposal of sharps; and principles of asepsis. As Standard Principles are broad statements of good practice, they need to be incorporated into local protocols to reflect individual circumstances. They must be observed by all health care personnel and should provide a uniform response to infection prevention regardless of setting.

Table 11.1   Standard principles for preventing health care-associated infections 2013.

Standard area number (SP)	Principle	Guideline recommendations according to the strength of underpinning evidence
Hospital environmental hygiene		
SP1	The hospital environment must be visibly clean; free from non-essential items and equipment, dust and dirt; and acceptable to patients, visitors and staff	*Class D/ GPP (Good Practice Points*
SP2	Levels of cleaning should be increased in cases of infection and/ or colonization when a suspected or known pathogen can survive in the environment, and environmental contamination may contribute to the spread of infection	*Class D/ GPP*
SP3	The use of disinfectants should be considered for cases of infection and/or colonization when a suspected or known pathogen can survive in the environment, and environmental contamination may contribute to the spread of infection	*Class D/ GPP*
SP4	Shared pieces of equipment used in the delivery of patient care must be cleaned and decontaminated after each use with products recommended by the manufacturer	*Class D/ GPP*
SP5	All health care workers need to be educated about the importance of maintaining a clean and safe care environment for patients. Every health care worker needs to know their specific responsibilities for cleaning and decontaminating the clinical environment and the equipment used in patient care.	*Class D/ GPP*

Continued

Table 11.1 Standard principles for preventing health care-associated infections 2013.—cont'd

Standard area number (SP)	Principle	Guideline recommendations according to the strength of underpinning evidence
Hand hygiene		
SP6	Hands must be decontaminated: – immediately before each episode of direct patient contact or care, including clean/aseptic procedures – immediately after each episode of direct patient contact or care – immediately after contact with body fluids, mucous membranes and non-intact skin – immediately after other activities of contact with objects and equipment in the immediate patient environment that may result in the hands becoming contaminated – immediately after the removal of gloves.	*Class C*
SP7	Use an alcohol-based hand rub for decontamination of hands before and after direct patient contact and clinical care, except in the following situations when soap and water must be used: – when hands are visibly soiled or potentially contaminated with body fluids – when caring for patients with vomiting or diarrhoeal illness, regardless of whether or not gloves have been worn	*Class A*

Table 11.1   Standard principles for preventing health care-associated infections 2013.—cont'd

Standard area number (SP)	Principle	Guideline recommendations according to the strength of underpinning evidence
SP8	Health care workers should ensure that their hands can be decontaminated effectively by: – removing all wrist and hand jewellery – wearing short-sleeved clothing when delivering patient care – making sure that fingernails are short, clean, and free from false nails and nail polish – covering cuts and abrasions with waterproof dressings.	*Class D/GPP*
SP9	Effective hand washing technique involves three stages: preparation, washing and rinsing, and drying. – Preparation: wet hands under tepid running water before applying the recommended amount of liquid soap or antimicrobial preparation. – Washing: the handwash solution must come into contact with all of the surfaces of the hands. The hands should be rubbed together vigorously for a minimum of 10–15 seconds, paying particular attention to the tips of the fingers, the thumbs and the areas between the fingers. Hands should be rinsed thoroughly. – Drying: use good quality paper towels to dry the hands thoroughly.	*Class D/GPP*

Continued

Table 11.1   Standard principles for preventing health care-associated infections 2013.—cont'd

Standard area number (SP)	Principle	Guideline recommendations according to the strength of underpinning evidence
SP10	When decontaminating hands using alcohol-based hand rub, hands should be free of dirt and organic material, and: – hand rub solution must come into contact with all surfaces of the hand; and – hands should be rubbed together vigorously, paying particular attention to the tips of the fingers, the thumbs and the area between the fingers, until the solution has evaporated and the hands are dry.	Class D/GPP
SP11	Clinical staff should be made aware of the potentially damaging effects of hand decontamination products, and encouraged to use an emollient hand cream regularly to maintain the integrity of the skin. Consult the occupational health team or a general practitioner if a particular liquid soap, antiseptic handwash or alcohol based hand rub causes skin irritation.	Class D/GPP
SP12	Alcohol-based hand rub should be made available at the point of care in all health care facilities	Class C
SP13	Hand hygiene resources and health care worker adherence to hand hygiene guidelines should be audited at regular intervals, and the results should be fed back to health care workers to improve and sustain high levels of compliance.	Class C

Table 11.1 Standard principles for preventing health care-associated infections 2013.—cont'd

Standard area number (SP)	Principle	Guideline recommendations according to the strength of underpinning evidence
SP14	Health care organizations must provide regular training in risk assessment, effective hand hygiene and glove use for all health care workers.	Class D/GPP
SP15	Local programmes of education, social marketing, and audit and feedback should be refreshed regularly and promoted by senior managers and clinicians to maintain focus, engage staff and produce sustainable levels of compliance.	Class C
SP16	Patients and relatives should be provided with information about the need for hand hygiene and how to keep their owns hands clean.	Class D/GPP
SP17	Patients should be offered the opportunity to clean their hands before meals; after using the toilet, commode or bedpan/urinal; and at other times as appropriate. Products available should be tailored to patient needs and may include alcohol-based hand rub, hand wipes and access to handwash basins.	Class D/GPP
Use of personal protective equipment		
SP18	Selection of personal protective equipment must be based on the assessment of the: – risk of transmission of microorganisms to the patient or carer; – risk of contamination of health care practitioners' clothing and skin by patients' blood, body fluids; and – suitability of the equipment for proposed use.	Class D/GPP/H&S

Continued

Table 11.1   Standard principles for preventing health care-associated infections 2013.—cont'd

Standard area number (SP)	Principle	Guideline recommendations according to the strength of underpinning evidence
SP19	Health care workers should be educated and their competence assessed in the: – assessment of risk; – selection and use of personal protective equipment; and – use of standard precautions.	*Class D/GPP/H&S*
SP20	Supplies of personal protective equipment should be made available wherever care is delivered and risk assessment indicates a requirement.	*Class D/GPP/H&S*
SP21	Gloves must be worn for: – invasive procedures; – contact with sterile sites, and non-intact skin or mucous membranes; – all activities that have been assessed as carrying a risk of exposure to blood or body fluids; and – when handling sharps or contaminated devices.	*Class D/GPP/H&S*
SP22	Gloves must be: – worn as single-use items; – put on immediately before an episode of patient contact or treatment; – removed as soon as the episode is completed; – changed between caring for different patients; and – disposed of into the appropriate waste stream in accordance with local policies for waste management.	*Class D/GPP/H&S*

Table 11.1 Standard principles for preventing health care-associated infections 2013.—cont'd

Standard area number (SP)	Principle	Guideline recommendations according to the strength of underpinning evidence
SP23	Hands must be decontaminated immediately after gloves have been removed	*Class D/GPP/H&S*
SP24	A range of CE marked medical and protective gloves that are acceptable to health care personnel and suitable for the task must be available in all clinical areas	*Class D/GPP/H&S*
SP25	Sensitivity to natural rubber latex in patients, carers and health care workers must be documented, and alternatives to natural rubber latex gloves must be available	*Class D/GPP/H&S*
SP26	Disposable plastic aprons must be worn when close contact with the patient, materials or equipment poses a risk that clothing may become contaminated with pathogenic microorganisms, blood or body fluids.	*Class D/GPP/H&S*
SP27	Full-body fluid-repellent gowns must be worn where there is a risk of extensive splashing of blood or body fluids on to the skin or clothing of health care workers.	*Class D/GPP/H&S*
SP28	Plastic aprons/fluid-repellent gowns should be worn as single-use items for one procedure or episode of patient care, and disposed of into the appropriate waste stream in accordance with local policies for waste management. When used, non-disposable protective clothing should be sent for laundering	*Class D/GPP/H&S*
SP29	Fluid repellent surgical face masks and eye protection must be worn where there is a risk of blood or body fluids splashing into the face or eyes.	*Class D/GPP/H&S*

Continued

Table 11.1 Standard principles for preventing health care-associated infections 2013.—cont'd

Standard area number (SP)	Principle	Guideline recommendations according to the strength of underpinning evidence
SP30	Appropriate respiratory protective equipment should be selected according to a risk assessment that takes account of the infective microorganism, the anticipated activity and the duration of exposure.	*Class D/GPP/H&S*
SP31	Respiratory protective equipment must fit the user correctly and they must be trained in how to use and adjust it in accordance with health and safety regulations.	*Class D/GPP/H&S*
SP32	Personal protective equipment should be removed in the following sequence to minimize the risk of cross/self-contamination: – gloves; – apron; – eye protection (when worn); and – mask/respirator (when worn). Hands must be decontaminated following the removal of personal protective equipment.	*Class D/GPP/H&S*
Safe use and disposal of sharps		
SP33	Sharps must not be passed directly from hand to hand, and handling should be kept to a minimum	*Class D/GPP/H&S*
SP34	Needles must not be recapped, bent or disassembled after use	*Class D/GPP/H&S*
SP35	Used sharps must be discarded at the point of use by the person generating the waste.	*Class D/GPP/H&S*

Table 11.1   Standard principles for preventing health care-associated infections 2013.—cont'd

Standard area number (SP)	Principle	Guideline recommendations according to the strength of underpinning evidence
SP36	All sharps containers must: – conform to current national and international standards; – be positioned safely, away from public areas and out of the reach of children, and at a height that enables safe disposal by all members of staff; – be secured to avoid spillage; – be temporarily closed when not in use; – not be filled above the fill line; and – be disposed of when the fill line is reached.	*Class D/GPP/H&S*
SP37	All clinical and non-clinical staff must be educated about the safe use and disposal of sharps and the action to be taken in the event of an injury.	*Class D/GPP/H&S*
SP38	Use safer sharps devices where assessment indicates that they will provide safe systems of working for health care workers.	*Class D/GPP/H&S*
SP39	Organizations should involve end-users in evaluating safer sharps devices to determine their effectiveness, acceptability to practitioners, impact on patient care and cost benefit prior to widespread introduction	*Class D/GPP/H&S*
Asepsis		
SP40	Organizations should provide education to ensure that health care workers are trained and competent in performing the aseptic technique	*Class D/GPP*

Continued

Table 11.1   Standard principles for preventing health care-associated infections 2013.—cont'd

Standard area number (SP)	Principle	Guideline recommendations according to the strength of underpinning evidence
SP41	The aseptic technique should be used for any procedure that breaches the body's natural defences including: – insertion and maintenance of invasive devices; – infusion of sterile fluids and medication; and – care of wounds and surgical incisions.	*Class D/GPP*

In some situations, patients will need to be isolated, in which cases additional precautions are required and Trusts devise their own protocols to manage these occasions. The need for isolation is when there is a risk of microorganisms being transferred from one patient to another, or to protect a vulnerable patient. Isolation is required when a microorganism is spread by air, for example, tuberculosis or measles; when infection can be spread by respiratory droplet, for example, mumps or pertussis; or to prevent spread by contact with the patient or their environment, sometimes known as source isolation. Examples of source isolation include *Clostridium difficile* and influenza. Protective isolation is the term given to situations where a patient is isolated because they are particularly vulnerable to infection.

Understanding infection prevention and control practice requires regular educational updates for all staff. Training in infection prevention and control is part of the UK Core Skills Training Framework developed by Skills for Health, which is the sector skills council for the NHS.

References

Loveday, H.P., Wilson, J.A., Pratt, R.A., et al. 2014 epic 3: National Evidence-Based Guidelines for Preventing Healthcare-Associated Infections in NHS Hospitals in England.

NICE 2013 Surgical site infection Quality standard [QS49].

NICE 2014 Infection prevention and control Quality standard [QS61].

NICE 2016 Healthcare associated infection Quality standard [QS113].

Pratt, R.J., Pellowe, C.M., Wilson, J.A., et al., 2007. Epic2: national evidence-based guidelines for preventing healthcare-associated infections in NHS hospitals in England. J. Hosp. Infect. 65 (Suppl. 1), S1–S69. Available at: http://download .journals.elsevierhealth.com/pdfs/journals/0195-6701/PIIS0195670107600024.pdf, http://www.uwl.ac.uk/academic-schools/nursing-midwifery/research/richard-wells-research-centre (accessed 8 August 2013).

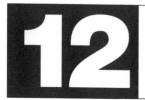

Appendix

Revalidation

Revalidation came into effect from April 2016. From that point on all nurses and midwives wishing to remain on the Nursing and Midwifery Council's (NMC) register must demonstrate that they can practise safely and effectively through the process of revalidation. Revalidation replaces PREP. Nurses and midwives must revalidate every 3 years in order to renew their registration and pay an annual registration fee. Nursing associates in England who were able to join the register from January 2019 will be required to revalidate from 2022.

Revalidation requires nurses, midwives and nursing associates to reflect on the Code: Professional Standards of Practice and Behaviour for Nurses, Midwives and Nursing Associates and complete an on-line application to remain on the NMC register. There are eight components to revalidation.

1. **Practice Hours**

    In order to revalidate nurses, midwives and nursing associates must have practised for a minimum of 450 hours over the previous 3-year period. The minimum number of hours is the same regardless of whether the nurse, midwife or nursing associate works full or part time.

    Nurses who also practise as midwives and vice versa who wish to be registered as both a nurse and a midwife must complete a minimum of 900 practice hours, of which at least 450 hours must be completed in nursing practice and 450 hours in midwifery practice. Nurses and midwives who are also registered as specialist community public health nurses only need a minimum of 450 practice hours.

    The types of activity that count towards practice hours include providing direct patient care as well as managing teams, teaching or running a service as long as those hours draw upon nursing or midwifery skills, knowledge and experience.

Evidence of meeting the required practice hours requires recording dates, the organization where practice took place and the nature of practice on a template.

2. **Continuing professional development hours**

   Revalidation requires nurses, midwives and nursing associates to demonstrate that they have completed a minimum of 35 hours of continuing professional development (CPD) relevant to their scope of practice over the previous 3-year period. At least 20 of those hours must be participatory learning rather than individual self-directed learning. Participatory means that you interact with one or more other professionals but it can be virtual, e.g., a webinar, as well as being in the same physical space. You cannot include statutory and mandatory training unless it is relevant to the scope of practice. For example, you could not include your annual fire training update.

   Evidence of meeting the minimum CPD hours includes keeping accurate records of the method of CPD, e.g., classroom attendance, attending a conference, attending formal clinical supervision sessions, reading journals or a book, taking part in an audit; the topic of the development and how it relates to the scope of practice; the date of the activity and the number of hours of development (including the number of hours which were participatory); how the development relates to the code; and evidence of the activity, e.g., a certificate, notes of the activity, a copy of the journal article that was read.

3. **Practice-related feedback**

   In order to revalidate, each nurse, midwife and nursing associate must gather five pieces of practice-related feedback over the 3-year period prior to revalidation. The five pieces of feedback can come in many different forms such as written or verbal feedback; from patients or colleagues. Feedback can be included if it is about a team that the nurse, midwife or nursing associate works in. Care must be taken to avoid using any patient-identifiable information when recording feedback.

   Evidence of feedback should be recorded, including the source of the feedback; the type of feedback, e.g., written, verbal; and the content of feedback as well as how the feedback influenced the nurse, midwife or nursing associate in their practice.

4. **Written reflective accounts**

   Each nurse, midwife and nursing associate must also produce five written reflective accounts over a 3-year period in order to revalidate. The reflective accounts have to be recorded on an approved NMC form.

Reflective accounts can be about a particular CPD activity; or practice-related feedback; or an event or experience from the nurse, midwife or nursing associate's professional practice. Care must be taken not to include patient-identifiable information in the accounts.

Evidence of the reflective accounts includes a description of the nature of the CPD activity, practice-related feedback, or event or experience from professional practice; what the nurse, midwife or nursing associate learned; how it influenced or changed practice; and how it relates to the code.

5. **Reflective discussion**

The five reflective accounts form the basis of a reflective discussion with another nurse, midwife or nursing associate whose name appears on the NMC register. One reflective discussion can cover all five reflective accounts. The reflective discussion must be face-to-face. Care must be taken to avoid using any patient-identifiable information when having the reflective discussion.

Evidence of the reflective discussion required recording on the approved NMC form the date of the discussion, a brief description of the discussion and details of who it was with, including the contact details and signature of the registrant with whom the reflective discussion took place.

6. **Health and character declaration**

At the time of applying for revalidation each nurse, midwife and nursing associate must make a declaration about their health and character. By making this declaration the nurse, midwife or nursing associate is confirming that their health is good enough for them to be able to practise safely and effectively. Any cautions or convictions need to be declared and any adverse determination about the nurse, midwife or nursing associate's fitness to practise by a professional or regulatory body.

There is no need for the nurse, midwife or nursing associate to collect any evidence for this component of revalidation. The declaration is made at the time of revalidation when the nurse, midwife or nursing associate applies to remain on the register.

7. **Professional indemnity arrangement**

Every nurse, midwife and nursing associate is legally required to have professional indemnity in order to practise. For most nurses, midwives and nursing associates this is provided by the employer, but if this is not the case then the nurse, midwife or nursing associate must make arrangements to ensure professional indemnity is in place.

There is no need for the nurse, midwife or nursing associate to collect any evidence for this component of revalidation. Confirmation that professional indemnity is in place is made at the time of revalidation when the nurse, midwife or nursing associate applies to remain on the register.

8. **Confirmation**

In the final year of the 3-year renewal period each nurse, midwife or nursing associate should meet with a confirmer who will look at all of the components of the revalidation application. If they are satisfied that all the requirements for revalidation are met a confirmation form is completed. This has to be on the NMC approved form which includes the name and contact details of the person undertaking the confirmation and where applicable their professional identification number or equivalent.

The meeting with the confirmer must be face-to-face and at the confirmation meeting the confirmer will look at all of your evidence in order to confirm that you have met all of the requirements of revalidation.

Confirmers do not have to be a registered nurse, midwife or nursing associate. Where possible it should be the line manager of the nurse, midwife or nursing associate.

Making an application is an on-line process. Sixty days before revalidation is due the nurse, midwife or nursing associate receives a registration renewal notification from the NMC. The nurse, midwife or nursing associate sets up an on-line account and must revalidate before the revalidation application date by completing an on-line registration. Information does not have to be submitted or uploaded but information relating to the components must be safely and securely stored by the nurse, midwife or nursing associate. The NMC has the right to request this information through a process called verification.

The nurse, midwife or nursing associate must also pay the registration fee to the NMC. Once the fee has been processed and the revalidation application process has been completed the nurse, midwife or nursing associate will receive confirmation of renewal of registration for a further 3 years.

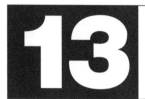

Appendix

Clinical Supervision

Introduction

The supervision of students by qualified nurses is a common event in clinical practice, for example, in mentoring situations. But the ongoing supervision of nurses once qualified is not so obvious, unless participating in a formalized course of study. Prior to qualifying as a nurse, students are entitled to be given the necessary education and support to become registered practitioners. Yet once qualified and accountable, inside the complex world of clinical practice, formalized supervision tends to disappear following induction and a period of preceptorship.

In other health-related disciplines such as counselling, psychotherapy and social work, regular feedback on clinical practice for qualified practitioners is not an unusual feature of practice and is often mandatory. Whilst in nursing is it not mandatory, there is an expectation that clinical supervision will be in place for qualified nurses, nursing associates and other clinicians. The Care Quality Commission (CQC) says that all staff must receive appropriate and on-going periodic supervision in their role. This is to ensure competence is maintained. Therefore all care professionals should have access to clinical or professional supervision as required (CQC, 2015). They state in Regulation 18 that "persons employed by the service provider in the provision of a regulated activity must … receive such appropriate support, training, professional development, supervision and appraisal as is necessary to enable them to carry out the duties they are employed to perform' (CQC, 2015 p.71).

The Nursing and Midwifery Council (NMC) does not stipulate how clinical supervision should be organized but promotes the view that it is best developed at a local level in accordance with local needs and recognises the links between supervision and revalidation. The main principles that underpin any system of clinical supervision are that:

- Clinical supervision should support practice and reflection on practice with a view to maintaining and improving standards of care.
- Clinical supervision involves a practice-focused professional relationship, with the practitioner reflecting on practice guided by a skilled supervisor who is not their line manager.
- Clinical supervision should be developed according to local circumstances and local environments and practice roles. Ground rules should be agreed and a contract entered into so that the supervisor and the supervisee approach clinical supervision knowing what is involved and what each other's roles and responsibilities are.
- All registered practitioners should have access to clinical supervision and each supervisor should supervise a realistic number of practitioners. What may be a realistic number in one environment or field of nursing may differ from another.
- There should be preparation for supervisors and on-going support for them in their role.
- There should be a formal system of recording attendance at clinical supervision which must uphold the principles of good record keeping.
- Evaluation of clinical supervision should be an integral part of a clinical supervision system to assess how it meets the needs of practitioners, influences care and practice standards.

Benefits of Clinical Supervision

There are many benefits to having a structured approach to clinical supervision. Clearly there is a requirement to have systems of clinical supervision in place set out by the regulators, but the real benefits are to the individual supervisee, who is enabled to:

- Have the time to engage in critical self-examination and reflection in practice
- Become more self-aware in clinical practice
- Identify practice issues and approaches to practice-based evidence
- Consider the recipients of practice in terms of their perception of what is happening and their responses to interventions
- Be challenged in a safe environment
- Have opportunity to consider future training and development needs
- Use evidence of participation in clinical supervision for revalidation
- Maintain and promote standards and innovations in practice in the interests of themselves, patients and the service.

Organization of Clinical Supervision

Clinical supervision can be organized in several different ways to meet local needs. There are four modes of clinical supervision that you may experience:

1. **Group**: groups of practitioners meet regularly together with one supervisor. Typically, there will be 10–12 people in the group. The supervisor has responsibility for organizing the meetings. Works well in larger organizations with many staff.

2. **Individual**: one-to-one meetings between a supervisor and supervisee. Works well when staff work in more isolated environments where the work environment makes it difficult for groups to physically meet or in isolated roles.

3. **Peer**: allows sharing and learning from experiences in a non-threatening environment. This works well with groups of staff who might work in very autonomous roles. For example, practice nurses working across a number of general practices might come together as peers and take it in turns to organize supervision sessions; clinical nurse specialists might similarly set up supervision groups and share the organization of sessions.

4. **Network**: for people who work in more isolated or specialist roles but whose roles mean they are part of a wider clinical network that offers supervision.

Contracting for Clinical Supervision

Whether one-to-one, group, peer or network sessions, the participants negotiate and agree a written contract together which identifies ground rules about the supervision process to be undertaken. The sort of issues to consider in agreeing any clinical supervision contract are likely to be:

- The purpose of clinical supervision and knowing what it is not
- Obtaining agreement on how often sessions will occur and be organized
- Protocols for communication
- Managing expectations
- Agreeing an agenda
- Measuring success including feedback
- Structuring the intervention
- Boundaries and ground rules
- Roles and responsibilities
- Confidentiality
- Reporting/recording.

The Structure of Clinical Supervision

The structure of a clinical supervision session will usually be focused around three components which are:

- Normative (managerial/organizational function, with a focus on ongoing monitoring and evaluation, the quality control aspects of clinical practice)

- Formative (learning/educational function, with a focus on the development of knowledge and skills)
- Restorative (supportive function, with a focus on health and well-being and supportive help for professionals working constantly with stress and distress).

These components of clinical supervision were derived from supervision in social work practice. Brigid Proctor's (1986) Interactive Model of Clinical Supervision from youth work and the Supervision Alliance Model (Proctor 2001) provide a 'task framework' of three functions that need to be addressed in supervision. They seem to have stood the test of time in the development of clinical supervision in nursing.

Using Proctor's approach (1986, 2001) enables the supervisor and supervisees to use clinical supervision meetings in ways that best meet their needs. For example, in a group, network or peer clinical supervision meeting, where there are a number of participants, the meeting may take the form of:

- An individual presenting on a predetermined topic
- An individual presenting a personal development topic
- The group discussing issues raised from an audit of practice
- The group discussing a clinical case and how care can be improved.

In individual one-to-one clinical supervision sessions, the supervisee and supervisor can choose to discuss a particular issue, development area, audit or clinical case.

Conclusion

Clinical supervision offers many possibilities for nurses and nursing associates, the organizations they work for and, most importantly, the people that they provide care for. A central aim is about caring for oneself enough to continue to deliver effective care for others, through formalized reflective practice with a clinical supervisor. Accepting the importance of being able to formally stop in practice, and intentionally reflect with others about practice, and putting back that learning for the benefit of others supports the wellbeing of the practitioner and improvements in patient care.

Midwifery Supervision

Following events at University Hospitals Morecambe Bay NHS Foundation Trust (Kirkup, 2015), the King's Fund was commissioned to undertake an independent review into the regulation of midwives. As a result of the King's Fund's report (2015), the Nursing and Midwifery Council accepted the recommendation that statutory midwifery supervision should no longer be part of its legal framework. The change will put the onus of responsibility on the employer to ensure they have processes in place to measure and improve quality. The change will separate midwifery supervision from regulation, and the functions of Local Supervising Authorities and statutory supervision for midwives have been removed.

There is new model of clinical supervision for midwives in England, A-EQUIP—an acronym for advocating and educating for quality improvement was launched in 2017 (NHS England, 2017). In Wales, the Clinical Supervision for Midwives (CSfM) has been introduced. Scotland and Northern Ireland are also testing new models.

References

Care Quality Commission (CQC), 2015. Guidance for Providers on Meeting Regulations. Care Quality Commission, Newcastle upon Tyne.

Kirkup, B., 2015. The Report of the Morecambe Bay Investigation, Preston, Lancashire. The Stationery Office, London.

NHS England, 2017. A-EQUIP a Model of Midwifery Supervision. The Stationery Office, London.

Proctor, B., 1986. Supervision: A co-operative exercise in accountability. In: Marken, M., Payne, M. (Eds.), Enabling and Ensuring – Supervision in Practice. National Youth Bureau, Council for Education and Training in Youth and Community Work, Leicester.

Proctor, B., 2001. Training for the supervision alliance: Attitude, skills and intention. In: Cutcliffe, J.R., Butterworth, T., Proctor, B. (Eds.), Fundamental Themes in Clinical Supervision. Routledge, London, pp. 25–46.

The King's Fund, Baird, B., Murray, R., et al., 2015. Midwifery Regulation in the United Kingdom: Report Commissioned by the Nursing and Midwifery Council. The King's Fund, London.